HOLISTIC VETERINARY MEDICINE

ARE SIMEON THORESEN DVM

For questions on the rights of this book please contact:

Are Thoresen
Leikvollgata 31
N – 3213 Sandefjord
Email: arethore@online.no
Homepage: http://home.online.no/~arethore/

Remark: The author takes no responsibility for the practical use of the methods described in this book.

This book aims to give readers, professional and lay, an understanding of the philosophy, principles and practice of holistic medicine. It is not a "stand alone" textbook of diagnostic and therapeutic veterinary medicine. Unless they work in co-operation with a veterinarian, lay (non-vet) readers should not use the methods to be described. Neither should veterinarians use these methods without a deep and long study of holistic medicine.

Illustrations by Peggy Fleming, Odd Thoresen and Elisabeth Knap.

The book is translated to English from the 3rd Norwegian edition (ISBN 978-82-994172-8-0).

Printed version;   ISBN 978 – 82 – 994172 – 6 – 6
Electronic version;   ISBN 978 – 82 – 994172 – 7 – 3

ISBN-10: 1467991104
EAN-13: 9781467991100

Library of Congress Control Number: 2011961992
CreateSpace Independent Publishing Platform
North Charleston, South Carolina

Norwegian publisher; "Are Thoresen Vererinærservice" (reg. publisher 994172)

HOLISTIC VETERINARY MEDICINE

A HOLISTIC VIEW OF FUNCTIONAL MEDICINE

ARE SIMEON THORESEN DVM

Dedicated to All

Who Seek to Heal

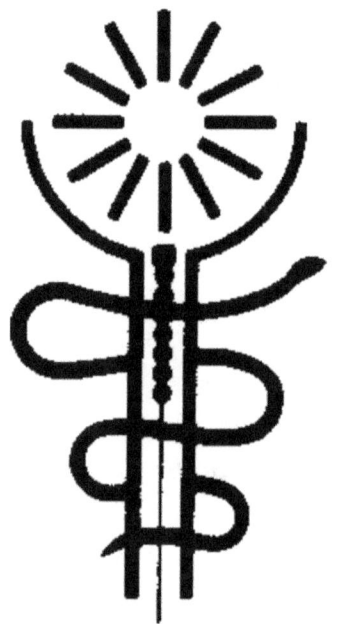

Contents

CHAPTER 1:

Complementary versus Conventional Medicine.   1

This Chapter describes the practical and theoretical differences between complementary and conventional medicine, and how this may make the way for Holistic medicine. Conventional Medicine uses more symptomatic or suppressive therapy than holistic medicine. Holistic medicine is built on the thesis that we must seek and treat the deepest origin, or energetic cause, of the disease. The same deep cause of disease can evoke different Lesion-Symptom Complexes depending on the breed, time of the year and age. To correct the root cause we often must use different methods or different healers. Do not treat an animal without veterinary supervision.

- Holistic Medicine   7

  Describes the principles of Holistic Medicine in detail. Holism states that all of the parts influence the whole and the whole influences all of the parts. This makes the whole greater than the sum of the parts. This Chapter describes holographic photography, the intercommunication of connective tissue and the necessity of knowing the laws of holistic medicine.

- Health and Disease   15

  This chapter describes the basis of health and disease. Bodily function manifests as the integration of 12 Processes, or Fundamental Functions. Health manifests as balance in and between those Processes. Disease manifests as too much or too little of a normal Process at the wrong place or time. The same Process Imbalance may manifest differently in humans than in animals and even differently in different species and individuals of the same species. To live with a Process Imbalance is more harmful to the body than to rebalance the Process by means of the so-called disease symptoms (Lesion-Symptom Complex, or the Syndrome). Each organism almost always has a Weak Structure. Interaction between a Process Imbalance and a Stressor (Pathogenic Factor, the precipitating causal factor) elicits symptoms that usually manifest in the Weak Structure. The body itself evokes the Lesion-Symptom Complex, which is only the manifestation of the Process Imbalance. Therefore, the Lesion-Symptom Complex is the least important defect in the pathogenesis of the disease.

- Bodily Processes   16

  Describes the Fundamental Processes of the body. There are no "Sick Processes". The same Process can manifest differently according to the body's needs to survive.

- Twelve Fundamental Processes of the body   19

  Describes the Twelve Fundamental Processes of the body in general.

- The fundamental laws of the Processes   24

CHAPTER 3:

CHAPTER 4:

CHAPTER 5:

Preface to the English Edition

Are Simeon Thoresen, the author of this book, dedicated it to "**all** *who* **seek** *to heal*". It aims to introduce veterinary, medical and paramedical professionals as well as lay-people to holistic concepts of diagnosis and therapy. Though not intended as a "*vade mecum*" to allow owners to diagnose animal disease without veterinary help, it also aims to help owners to understand and use holistic therapies in their animals in co-operation with their vets. In his introduction, Are cited the prayer for animals by Albert Schweitzer. I will also start this Preface with a prayer that summarises the core of the book:

Qi imbalance causes most disease.
Qi balance causes most good ease -
They who right another's right their own,
Who blight another's blight their own.
Nature is Nature, neither bad nor good.
She is only what she is - sage and fool,
Womb and tomb, savage and kind, warm and cold.
Honor or dishonor her and her might behold.
Spirit, soul, mind and body need each other -
Body from dust, lives in Nature, goes to God;
Besouled it must, nests in twigs
Of body-mind, flies to Sky it must.
Great God! Have pity on Your creatures' moans;
Make us your healers when we will these koans!

The first year of the "third" millennium is an appropriate time for the birth of this book, this love-baby of a caring mind. Like the first Baby of the "first" millennium, it pleads for, and is a beacon to, an integrated, holistic approach to healing of the body-mind-spirit. Today, people and animals need healing more desperately that at any time in history.

This book advocates holistic medicine (Holistic medicine) to treat animal- and human- disorders. It discusses the main differences between alternative medicine (AltMed) and modern conventional (ModMed) medicine. Most practitioners of alternative medicine tend to have a theistic-energetic-immaterial view; most practitioners of modern medicine tend to have an atheistic-mechanistic-materialistic view. Therefore, as Yang needs Yin, or as day needs (cannot support life without) night, there must be mutual interdependence, contrast and tension between those who advocate alternative medicine and those who advocate modern medicine. Both methods are necessary, and have their strengths and weaknesses, but the best method aims to combine the best of both. Holistic medicine embraces both.

Concepts of Holistic medicine involve *all possible component parts,* how they interact and how they fit into the larger plan of Nature. In the end, they are an artistic-intuitive search for aspects of the *transcendent immaterial blueprint* which religious people call God or atheistic physicists see as the infinite interchange of matter and energy. *Holism and holistic concepts of health, disease and medicine contain elements of scientific medicine, art, poetry and mysticism.* Holism has a metaphysical core - the whole is greater than, but depends on, the sum of the individual parts. Each part of the system contains the potential, the image, the dream and the reality, of the whole; each part depends on, serves, and is expendable for, the good of the whole.

ModMed has great value in acute, surgical and immediate life-threatening conditions. It tries to identify the more obvious causal factors in disease and promote healthy living. However, it seldom can identify, or treat the basic causes of disease. In particular, because it relies heavily on symptomatic or suppressive therapy, it has poor success in curing chronic and functional diseases. Also, because it uses potent drugs, vaccines and sera with potent antigens and human- or animal- derived material, and stressful interventions, ModMed has an unacceptably high rate of adverse reactions and iatrogenic disease.

In contrast, Holistic medicine includes ModMed; therefore, it is more powerful than ModMed. Ancient Traditional Chinese Medical (TCM) philosophy said that: "Man stands between Heaven and Earth." This means that: "The organism embodies the characteristics of Heaven (spirit, mind, non-material forces) and Earth (food, physical environment, material forces)". It also means that: "The organism is influenced by spiritual, psychic arid non-earthly forces (cosmic, solar, lunar forces) as well as forces in its immediate environment (nutrition, climate, electromagnetic and geophysical forces).

Holistic medicine as defined her by Are Thoresen, is especially occupied by four main factors in development of disease; (a) *the predisposing factor,* (b) *the initiating factor,* (c) *the weak anatomical structure and* (d) *the syndrome.*

- The **predisposing factor (a)** is an inner unbalance, usually a **deficiency,** in one or more of the 12 main processes (meridians, organs).

- The **stressor** or **initiating factor (b)** is the external or internal *stress,* which trigger the already deficient internal process to collapse.

In addition to these two main factors responsible for the development of disease, it will be important also to be able to consider

- The **weak spot (c)**. This is the "Achilles-heel" of the organism, the *weak anatomical structure* or stressed part where any deficiency most probably will manifest itself.

- In this weak anatomical area the **syndrome (d)** will manifest. The syndrome is the material *manifestation of the disease.* The syndrome is not the disease itself, only the body's own manifestation of the inner deficiency. This manifestation is also very often the body's attempt to help the deficient inner process.

The book discusses animals as sentient beings and criticises the adverse effects that human interaction inflicts on the health and welfare of their animals. It discusses acupuncture theory in detail, the 12 Channel-Organ Systems and their Processes, the Vessels, the Command Points and main Channel Points in humans, horses and dogs.

This is a subversive book. It recognises the strengths of ModMed but challenges its arrogance, its failure to address the basic causes of disease, its heavy reliance on therapies that merely suppress symptoms, and use of surgery when less invasive therapy could be successful. It recognises the innate superiority and wisdom of Holistic medicine but also its failures and weaknesses and its dependence on the ability of the body's adaptive systems to respond. No one system of medicine has, or is likely to have, all the answers to treat or prevent all disease. Although it does not say so explicitly, Holistic medicine implies that one can gain competence in medicine and healing only after long and broad study and experience, and that few people receive the gift of their mastery.

As thunder inevitably involves lightning (discharge of static electricity), Are's ideas will electrify readers whose minds are not insulated by the dull dead drapes of conventional medical thinking. He is the most amazing professional that I have had the privilege to know. He has been my friend and mentor for many years, but that was not always the case. I first heard him talk in 1986 at a European Veterinary Acupuncture Congress in Belgium. Then, I thought that he was crazy because his ideas of medicine and healing were so different from those of mainstream thought, and the success rates that he claimed were so much better than those that I could attain at that time. Later, I realised that my rejection of Are was a "mental knee-jerk" to the severe challenge that his ideas posed to my world-view. I swallowed my egotistical pride and asked if I could visit him to see his methods. Like St. Thomas, I was a doubter. I would not believe unless I could verify his claims for myself. Are agreed to one visit. That was the start of my un-blinding. Since then, I have stayed at his home many times and have talked to his animal-owners and his human patients. They confirmed that his methods are very successful in clinical practice.

In the spring of 2000, Are asked me if I would correct an English draft of this book. Not suspecting the amount of work involved, I agreed. I tore it apart line-by-line and emailed "my corrections", peppered with thousands of queries, to Are. He answered all of these and came to my home in late November to finalise the drafting. So I know this book like I know my hands! I have wrestled with it, mauled it, thrown it away and returned to it time and again. It still amazes me. It has assembled between two covers a wealth of knowledge that I have not seen anywhere before now. I believe that it will be seen as a key influence in the further development of holistic medicine.

Are has been my patient teacher for years; I have learned much from him. However, I suspect that his controversial ideas will scandalise many professionals who do not know him personally. Readers unfamiliar with acupuncture, holistic principles, or natural healing, will find his ideas very difficult initially. After a first reading of the book, if you are tempted to dismiss its ideas as crazy (my first reaction to meeting Are in 1986), I urge you to reconsider. Read it again! And if you do not understand it then, read and re-read it until you do. When you begin to realise and apply his wisdom in your practice, your life and your approach to healing will change; they will differ radically from what they were before.

As I grow older, I am increasingly aware of the meaning behind the myths of Plato's Cave, or the more modern version of the Three Blind Men and the Elephant. Those myths boil down to a debate about subjective versus objective truth. The grace and beauty of science could and should be the study of the natural world in the search for objective truth, and the practical application of that knowledge for the good of all.

Overall, the book inspires wonder and awe, which are the spice of life and the basis of spirituality. It is not "scientific" in the strict sense; indeed it has some ideas that I would reject on my knowledge of science. I must reserve judgement on those few areas but I am content to accept that Are's clinical experiences, described so well in this book, are true. Indeed, for several years I have used his thinking process and some of his acupuncture methods, with better results than I had attained beforehand. I wish Are, his loved ones and this book great success. May its controversial and profound ideas help you (the reader) and others as much as they have helped me.

Phil Rogers MRCVS,
Dublin, Ireland,
Advent, 2000

PROLOGUE

Veterinarians (vets) are trained to diagnose and treat animal diseases; and they are usually the best people to do so. This means that they are the best to find *excessive* symptoms, which are symptoms that express pain, inflammations and degeneration. This book teaches to find *deficient* symptoms, and in this aspect veterinarians are not necessarily the best diagnostics. They may be so, but then they have to educate themselves in a way described in this book. In my opinion, detecting deficient symptoms, lay-people may as good as the veterinarian. This book can be used by the veterinarian as a reference on Complementary Veterinary Medicine, and give useful information on how to treat sick animals; *it is not intended for use as a "Cookbook" on how to treat animals.* Both veterinarians and not-veterinarians must understand this; otherwise they may use it (possibly in vain) only to find a recipe to heal, for example, chronic mastitis in their favourite cow, or lameness in their horse or dog. If they do so, they will miss the whole purpose of the book, which is to give readers basic information on Holistic Veterinary Medicine, based on the detection of deficient processes. The book aims to introduce readers to the concepts of Fundamental Processes from which many holistic therapies have developed, how these methods function and how they can be put to practical use to treat sick animals.

In order to be able to cope with the huge and expanding market of healers, quacks, methods and aids offered today, it is very important to be able to think in a holistic way. *Only by going deeply into the principles of holistic thinking can we give our animals the best treatment and be able to recognise the many charlatans in the area for what they are.*

Only when one has studied and grasped the basic thinking processes of holistic medicine can one use its schemata, recipes or cookbook prescriptions with good conscience. Therefore a list of therapeutic suggestions is included after the chapters on acupuncture (AP) and homeopathy. Every method in this book is discussed in three different ways: first the

- *Theoretical thought processes,* then the

- *Practical thought processes* and finally

- *Therapeutic suggestions,* i.e. recipes and schemata and other necessary details.

For those especially interested, I have included

- *Philosophical and theoretical* approaches in several places. These are printed in italics and marked with an old Celtic sign at the beginning and end.

I hope that English speakers will welcome this updated translation of the second Norwegian edition, and that the book will lead to discussion of a better way to improve animal well being and health world-wide.

"Man has such a predilection for systems and abstract deductions that he is ready to distort the truth. Intentionally, he is ready to deny the evidence of his sense in order to justify his logic".
Fyodor

FYODOR DOSTOYEVSKY

INTRODUCTION

At graduation, each newly qualified veterinarian (vet) swears an oath to act in good conscience and morality and to be a saviour and benefactor of animals. I also swore that oath at my graduation from the Oslo Veterinary School. However, at our graduation ceremony in the scientific bastions of a profit oriented university system, the prayer of Albert Schweitzer was omitted:

> *Hear our humble prayer, O God*
> *For our friends the animals,*
> *Especially for animals who are suffering;*
> *For any who are hunted or lost,*
> *Or deserted or frightened or hungry;*
> *For all that must be put to death.*
> *We entreat for them all thy mercy and pity*
> *And for those who deal with them;*
> *We ask a heart of compassion*
> *And gentle hands and kind words.*
> *Make us, ourselves, to be true friends to animals*
> *And so to share the blessings of the merciful.*

That is a beautiful prayer, but its intent conflicts with capitalistic interests. Capitalism demands that we do not let animals suffer *without a reason*, that we incorporate the *interests of human society* and that we work in the *economic interests of human society*.

The conflict between Schweitzer's prayer and capitalistic ethics arose immediately after my graduation. In spring 1979, I went out into practice to apply the theory that we had learned during 6 years of intensive undergraduate education. In my very first consultation, instead of doing my best to help a cow with a painful condition, I found myself calculating the economic aspects of either treatment or slaughter. I managed to ease the cow's symptoms for a while with antibiotics but I became very aware of my own inadequacy and tried to seek better solutions.

It became clear to me that if we are to find means to really help animals, we must search behind the symptoms, behind the economic calculations and behind the obviously visible. In their enforced service of humans and even in the wild, animals are at high risk and very vulnerable to human wishes and ideas.

In 1978, one year before qualifying as a vet, I began to study homeopathy at Arcanum, Gothenburg (Sweden). Could homeopathy help me to reach my goals and intentions, as in Schweitzer's prayer? Yes! It worked! Cows with longstanding (chronic) mastitis recovered and dogs on cortisone to prevent scratching could be taken off steroids. These results excited me very much and I threw myself more and more into the great area called *complementary medicine.*

I studied Anthroposophical medicine, especially in the study group of Anthroposophical doctors that met regularly in Vidaraasen in Vestfold, Norway.

In 1980 I met Dr. Georg Bentze and studied acupuncture (AP) at his clinic in Oslo. Later, I studied veterinary homeopathy, AP and Holistic Medicine in several countries: Finland, France, Germany, Sweden and USA.

In 1979 I participated in, simultaneously arranging, the first Scandinavian course run by IVAS in veterinary acupuncture, and graduated as a veterinary Acupuncturist.

In 2001 I started on the study of veterinary Osteopathy, excellent taught by Pascal Evrard, and in 2003 I graduated as a veterinary Osteopath.

In my practice, I routinely saw trotters that had various forms of allergies, eczema, metabolic problems and many other disorders. I began to treat them with AP and they improved and won races. It was possible to eliminate quite serious Lesion-Symptom Complexes with methods that I never thought would work when I was studying in university.

After some time I began to use holistic methods more and more. Since 1982, I have given some 150.000 treatment sessions almost exclusively using complementary methods.

As time passed, more and more pet owners asked for lectures and courses on these complementary methods. They asked for literature but I knew of no comprehensive book that I could recommend. The aim of this book is to fill this need. It is an introduction for those who want to treat their animals or patients holistically, or who just want to understand more about the nature of disease in an alternative way of thinking.

In 2002 the existence of this book also gave rise to the founding of the first *"Scandinavian School of Equine Holistic Medicine"*, founded by me and my x-wife, Annica. We are also the main teachers of this school, which is open for all horse-loving and holistic thinking humans.

Originating in this school the *"Association of Scandinavian Holistic Horse Therapists"* was founded in 2003.

Therefore, this book is not only for professional readers (including medical and veterinary readers), but it also will help non-vets to grasp the principles of holistic thinking, and be able to help animals with their vet's co-operation.

I have taken examples from human medicine, to explain the thinking process and as practical examples of how to treat the patient so that readers can understand more easily what I mean. In veterinary education, experimental medicine, research and a great part of the first year in veterinary college it is usual to read books on human medicine. However, it is a grave misunderstanding of the intention of this book to believe that it would be possible to treat humans after reading it.

Pedagogically and structurally this book is divided into four main areas, which partly is divided in chapters. These parts are:

- *Normal* functions of the organism.

- *Pathologic* aspects or symptoms of the organism.

- *Diagnostic* aspects and methods.

- *Therapeutic* methods.

COMMENTARY ON THE 2ND NORWEGIAN EDITION:
I am acutely aware that the ultimate goal of any conscientious work-ing vet or doctor is to find and treat the root causes of the disease. Today, more than was the case some years ago, thorough evaluation of a patient emphasizes the search for the cause of the disease. In their undergraduate years, students also learn this as the ideal approach. However, in routine practice, vets or doctors often fail to identify the root causes. Therefore, to cope with common disorders, they often rely on suppression of the Lesion-Symptom Complexes. That said, in recent years, conventional doctors have advanced very much in their aware-ness of causes of disease that are not taught in university. Originally, this book was intended as **an alternative** *to conventional medicine. Today, however, it aims more to be a* **complementary or holistic text** *to encourage the positive tendencies that are beginning to occur within conventional medicine.*

Are Simeon Thoresen, Sandefjord, 17th of May 2001

COMMENTARY ON THE 3RD NORWEGIAN EDITION:
The third edition has been more thoroughly prepared than the 2nd edition, and has become more holistic. I will mention three main causes for this transformation;

- The first cause is my and Annica's teaching preparations for our school; "Scandinavian School of Holistic Horse Therapy", founded in the autumn 2002. To prepare suf-ficient material for this school we had to go through all our material one more time. All the acupuncture points had to be revised, and in this process several mistakes were corrected.

- Secondly I became more and more aware of the im-portance of "intention", which will be described in the chapters about Homeopathy, Acupuncture and Cranio-Sacral therapy, and explained scientifically as the existence of Mirror Neurons (see Mirror Neurons, page XLIX).

- Thirdly the book was translated to Italian, Spanish, German, Russian and Swedish. All the constructive criticism from the translators was incorporated into the third Norwegian edition, from which this 2nd English edition is translated.

I hope that this second English edition will provide new and important information to the English reading population of the world, both for veterinarians, alternative therapists and animal owners and lovers, who all will contribute to the long and hard road to a more animal friendly veterinary medicine.

Are Simeon Thoresen, Sandefjord, 6th of June 2011

Necessary Definitions And Clarifications

To be able to better understand what I am saying in this book, there are a few concepts that need to be clarified right at the beginning. These are the following:

Yin and Yang: Originally Yin means the dark side of the hill, where the sun doesn't shine. Yang means the bright side of the hill, where the sun is shining. The predictable interaction of Yin-Yang is the most universal law in Asia. It derives from holistic concepts in a cosmological thinking process, or world-view, used to relate all natural phenomena.

In common with modern physics, Yin-Yang Law perceives all things as a balance between reciprocally conflicting powers. This viewpoint is unlike the dualism of later European philosophy, which conceives opposites to be independent. In contrast, Asians view opposites to depend on each other, in a constantly interchanging and dynamic auto-control system with creative and destructive aspects. Anything can be Yang compared to something that is more Yin; anything can be Yin in relation to something that is more Yang. The meaning of this is that all things have something that is beneath and/or above them; that which is underneath is Yin in relation to that which is above.

- **Yin** is more: under, before, inside, cold, dark female, night, hypo, descending, centrifugal, night, diastolic, passive.

- **Yang** is more: above, behind, outside, warm, light, male, day, hyper, ascending, centrifugal, day, systolic, active.

The *Monad*, an ancient Yin-Yang symbol, illustrates the Yin-Yang relationship especially well.

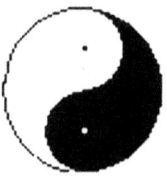

Fig. 1

The dark segment represents Yin, whereas the light represents Yang. The two dynamically oscillate around each other; each needs the other and continuously transforms into the other; they are opposite, mutually complementary and ever changing. Together, they form unity. Everything is relative to something else. Within each main polarity, the small dot of opposite color symbolizes that *there are no absolutes; there is always some Yin in Yang and vice-versa.* The only absolute is the Law of Change; everything must change in time.

Energy (Qi): is a very central concept within most, if not all, alternative or holistic and metaphysical systems throughout the world. With "energy" is meant the very power that makes life possible in its existing image. This energy meet us from the whole creation, from our parents, from the food and water that we eat, from the smells that we smell and from the colours that we see. This energy may work or exist in the body in many ways, and it may usually transform from one function to another, but not always. This energy is dependent on the ability of the different processes to receive this energy. A special form for energy is called *destructive,* or *perverse energy.* This is the only form of energy that cannot be redistributed or used again by the organism.

We have different special forms and for energy:

- **Jing Qi:** this energy comes to us from our parents and from the whole cosmos in the moment of conception and birth. It also may be derived or replenished from the food and air. It is the energy that sustains life and builds up our body, and must not be mixed up with the energy that are used by the meridians, an energy that is used for the control of the Jing Qi. In the West the Jing Qi is often called Etheric energy.

  - **Inherited (Yuan-Qi):** is inherited from our parents.

  - **Acquired (Zong-Qi from the air, Ying-Qi from the food):** this energy is the life-energy that make life living so to say, that make us capable of action. This energy comes from smells, air, colours and food.

- **Etheric energy (resembles Jing Qi / Yuan-Qi)**

  - **Etheric body:** is what we call the structure of the energy that makes our body grow and live. It is this structure (in cooperation with the Astral energy) that makes our body look like it does. This energy streams in the form of lemniscates, see page LVIII.

- **Qi:** is the "ordinary" energy we work with when we do acupuncture. It streams in the meridians (nor in lemniscate movements, but more like spirals), and is used for the regulation of the etheric energy.

  - *Qi in the meridians*

    - **There are several kinds of Qi, one in each meridian:** this sort of energy may perform many kinds of work, after what meridian, organ or process it serves at that special moment. If we stimulate another meridian, then this energy will be drawn to this meridian or process, which it will serve.

- **Destructive energy in specific meridians:** is the only form of energy that may not be used by or transformed to another process or meridian.

° **Qi in a field around the body:** is the part of the meridian Qi, which is transformed from one meridian or function to the next.

- **Wei-Q:** is a form of energy that defends the body against noxious external influences like virus and bacteria. It may be translated to the immune system or the astral energy.

  ° **Wei-Qi in the skin:** is the defensive energy situated in the skin, and may be called the immune system or the astral energy.

  ° **Wei-Qi in the body:** is the defensive energy circulating within the body, also a part of the immune system and the internal parts of the Astral energy or body.

  ° **Wei-Qi in a field around the body:** is the defensive energy circulating around the body, and may be called the astral aura.

- **Astral energy (resemble Wei-Qi):** is the structured energetic body that many see as the aura, and which contain our feelings and soul. The Astral body is the structured totality of the astral energy, and may be found both inside, at the surface and outside the physical body.

- **Shen:** is the energetic part of our spiritual body that resemble our self, what we call ourselves, that make us feel like a self-conscious being.

- **The "I" (resemble the Shen):** is what we think of as ourselves, the eternal living inner core of our spirit.

5   *Elements (phases):* This Law states that all created things can be classified into Five Phases, or Elements. These are fundamental qualities that correspond with common experience of the natural world.

- **Fire**: It warms and is full of emotions and feelings. Excess Fire is destructive and eats up whatever it attacks. We can imagine these forces like those of strong emotions and in craving love.

- **Earth** Controls transformation. It is more purely destructive. It helps to transform each Phase into the next one, for example death and resurrection. Gravity dominates Earth and leads to the detachment of the material lesion from the body.

- **Metal**: Controls the body's gases. Metal/Air Deficiency loses control over the gas Processes. Also Metal dominates or controls pain.

- **Water**: Controls the flowing of all liquids, blood, and lymph and in the excretion of all liquids.

- **Wood**: Controls all growth processes. As a tree grows and produces leaves, Wood is responsible for all tissues and processes that grow in the body, including lumps, nodules and cancers (before they enter the Earth Phase and tend to withdraw from the body).

These five elements interact in a number of ways, mainly by stimulating each other or by controlling each other. This stimulation and control do have a number of aspects, and below I have tried to put up the different ways this control and stimulation may take form.

From the table below we may see that for example the warming forces of the body (fire, temperature) are created by the growth (wood, friction from the creation), commanded by the circulating water (water controls all fire), helped in its work by the gases of the body (metal, gases make the fire grow bigger), ruled by the destructive forces, just as a desire to destroy (earth, the universal destructor) and actually executed by its own "soldiers", the fire itself (fire).

Element	Executes	Rules	Helps	Is Nourished Or Helped By	Is Controlled By
Metal	Metal	Water	Wood	Earth	Fire
Water	Water	Wood	Fire	Metal	Earth
Wood	Wood	Fire	Earth	Water	Metal
Fire	Fire	Earth	Metal	Wood	Water
Earth	Earth	Metal	Water	Fire	Wood

Table 1

The Processes: Life in all its expressions and shades depend on a certain number of processes, which in the old Asian systems are limited to 12 for simplicity, usage and systematic. Throughout recorded history, art, science and religion have reflected on the importance of twelve divisions in all natural phenomena. Twelve is often regarded as a lucky number. It is seen in the months of the year, the hours of the day, the older forms of measurement (dozen), the scale of twelve tones, the twelve star signs, the twelve disciples, the twelve cranial nerves and in a host of other contexts. The ancient Chinese also divided the primary human function into twelve.

Such processes may be excretion, rhythm, building up of tissue (anabolism), destroying or building down of tissue (catabolism) and so on. Such processes may be found in all living creatures, animals as well as plants. In animals these processes do have their own organs to carry out their work, as the kidneys for the excretion, the spleen for the rhythm, the liver for the anabolism and so on, but plants don't have such organs. All the same, they have the processes, and this show that the presence of organs is not necessary for the processes. This we may see in the horse also, as it has the process of the gall bladder although it has no such organ.

The Meridians: The Meridian system is one of several systems that life itself has developed for auto-control and feedback of the processes to balance. The Meridian system is the sum of all the meridians, and this system is controlled by means of an electric/biologic/energetic flow of energy/static current. This energy/static current follows the connective tissue following the veins, arteries and nerves, sometimes also the connective tissue enveloping the muscles. Along the meridians there are specific areas called acupuncture points.

The acupuncture points: are certain areas or points situated along the meridians or also outside the meridians where the activity in the meridians may be stimulated or controlled or regulated. These points are found where the anatomical structure of the veins, arteries or nerves suddenly change, change in direction, making anastomoses or similar "irregularities". They are seldom found where the veins, arteries or nerves are in a continuous direction. They are also found where muscles or bones change their structure, and that is why some of the most effective or important points are found just above or below the joints. See examples of this At page 312 and 322. The energy that flows in the meridians is quite different from the one that sustains the body or life itself (see etheric energy contra meridian energy page XXXIII).

Internal imbalance: is a usual life-long internal weakness in one of the 12 processes. For example an animal may have a weak (deficient) liver, which give this particular animal different problems throughout his entire life.

- *Excess:* means that there is too much energy in an area, process, meridian or organ. This will lead to symptoms as painful muscles, painful points and painful movement. Such excess is usually better if the animal is working, as the excessive energy then is used and diminished. It is most important to know that when we find excess, we may usually find a causative, underlying and primary deficiency. In my opinion, this underlying deficiency is usually the real cause of the excess, and just treating the excess is to me symptomatic treatment. Unfortunately, many of my veterinary colleges tend to just diagnose areas of excess, and leave the underlying deficiency undiscovered and untreated. With this book I hope to shed light on the importance of finding and treating the deficiency.

- *Deficiency:* means that there is too little energy in an area, process, meridian or organ. This will lead to symptoms, but it is difficult to recognise these symptoms, as a deficiency seldom shows up as painful conditions. Such a deficiency usually will lead to secondary excess, which is more easily diagnosed.

- *Destructiveness:* is when the energy is neither in excess nor in deficiency, but in a form that in itself is pathological. This form of energy may be mistaken for a form of extreme excess.

Stressor (external and internal): is a factor that influences the body, either it be the weather, food, emotions or any other stress that stresses and thereby weakens the body (further).

Weak spot: is an anatomic part of the body that has a weak construction, and is where stress and disease usually manifest. It may be the back (dachunds), the sinuses, the shoulder muscles (humans), the udder (cows) or the joints (horses).

Anatomical expressions to be known: It is important at this stage of learning to get to know certain anatomical expressions to be able to understand simple locations of muscles, acupuncture points and so on.

- Proximal: above (the elbow is proximal to the hand)

- Distal: under (the hoof is distal to the elbow)

- Lateral: more to the side of (the nipple is lateral to the sternum)

- Medial: more to the middle (the front teeth is medial to the molars)

- Caudal: more to the tail (the ears are caudal to the nose)

- Cranial: more to the front (the navel is cranial to the penis)

- Dorsal: more to the back (dorsum = back)

- Ventral: more to the stomach (ventrum = stomach)

- Rostral: more to the nose (rostrum = nose)

- Palmar: on the side of the palm (palma = palm)

- Plantar: on the side of the sole (planta = sole of the foot)

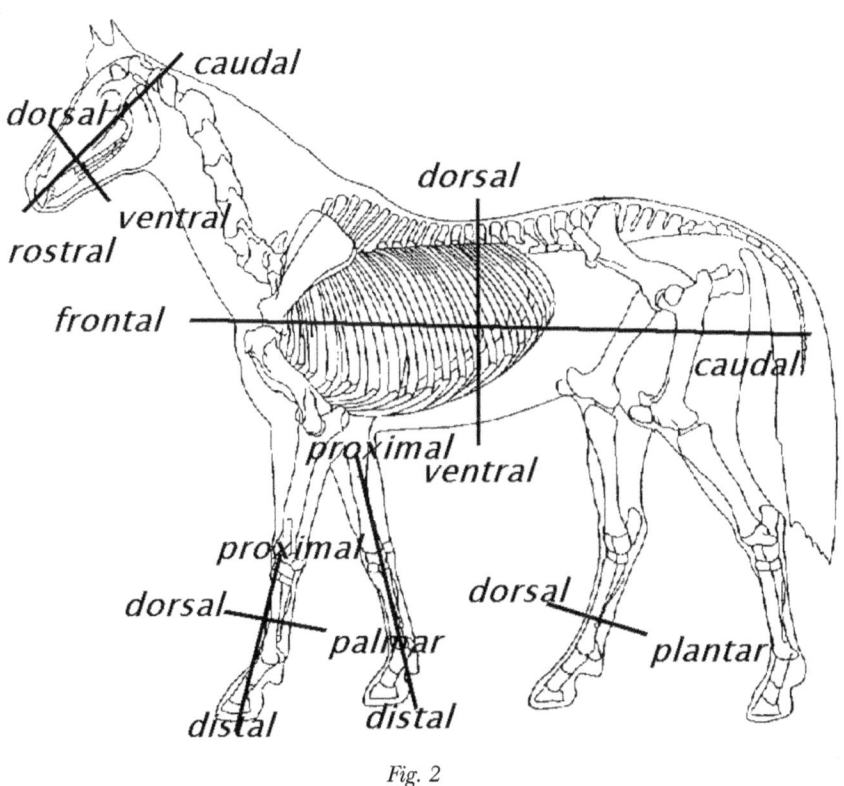

Fig. 2

SELF-HEALING, A NECESSITY FOR THE SURVIVAL OF LIFE

When reading this book, it is important to understand that all we do to our patients the animals or our fellow men to obtain healing concerning alternative medicine, actually all kind of medicine, is build on our ability to stimulate the self healing of the body.

In itself, per se, the alternative methods or tools, like the acupuncture needle or homeopathic remedy, have no effect. Their only effect is that they may stimulate self-healing. Therefore, if the self-healing is disrupted or compromised by radiation, chemotherapy, β-blockers or cortisone, there will be no effect from most alternative methods. Also, in double blinded trials, where most of the effects from the body itself are taken away, the effect will be minimal.

But it is the self healing we will try to stimulate.

Control over our self and our processes are the foundation for a good life.

Disease is loss of control.

`Self-healing* does happen, - at least sometimes, when we, for some reason have been able to reclaim the control over our body and its processes.

And even if it is rare, it is no less a possibility – to all of us.

- If we can only find out how it can be regained, which button we have to push..

The Catholic Church classifies such self-healing as a *miracle*, when no doctor or medicine is used.

In a medical dictionary as Zetkin/Schaldach the term self-healing is not even mentioned.

It is not found in a common dictionary either.

On Google I found 6.990.000 hits on "Self-healing", especially, if not solely, within alternative medicine.

Within ordinary medicine such incidents as self healing are considered as non explicable incidents, as incidental healing, as self lying or self deceit or illusion or as the patient's wish of getting better. Self-healing is in a way not considered "real", and very few scientists investigate the processes that lie behind this kind of treatment. And if self-healing appear in any scientific investigation, the patient is excluded from the investigation.

But, if self-healing really exists, then the *possibility* of these phenomena must be present in the body, not only for those few that experience this blessing, but also for all of us.

The truth is of course that self-healing occurs all the time, in each and every one of us. All the time our body is fighting inflammation, bacteria, fungus and virus, even prions. All the time cancer cells are killed.

We are in complete control all of the time, or at least most of the time.

It is only when this continuous control or constantly self-healing fails, halts, stops or goes wrong that disease occurs. And if then our body, our selves or that we by means of any other factor, manage to put the self-healing into work again, we call this for a miracle, for self-healing, for placebo.

Because of this I have been interested in finding and mapping out these self-healing processes through my entire professional life, and then to find ways to restart them in diseased animals and people, in patients; make the patient able to regain the control in his own body.

From this knowledge, gathered during a long professional life, I have observed quite many factors or methods that are able to restart the missing self-healing; psychic factors, meditation, artistic activity, medical plants, acupuncture, zone-therapy, music or osteopathy. Therefore it is possible that there are numerous ways or doors to re-establishing the self-healing.

Within school medicine self-healing is often labeled as "Placebo".

Placebo is, when a patient, from unknown factors, often as simple as belief, really has been cured from a disease.

Our bodies own self-healing mechanisms, which may be restarted by acupuncture or psychic factors, are often exactly the same processes that are stimulated by traditional therapies. It is shown that the placebo effect leads to changes in the brain identical to those leading to a "real" healing, like "real" medicines or therapies may. How this is possible is still under discussion.

This subject is discussed and documented by Dr. Ario Conti, a Swiss scientist, in his description and introduction of neuro-immunomoduling. In this science it has been shown that the human mind and psyche has direct and real connections to the nervous system, the hormonal system and the immune system; that is of great importance to most diseases.

This is why different therapists do have very different results, and if we remove the personal and human influence (placebo) in double-blinded investigations, we remove the possibility here described and lessen the outcome of a successful therapy.

The foundation for self-healing: a functioning body without too much medication, β-blockers, chemotherapy, radiation or stress.

All real healing is self-healing.

It is only our own body, our own self-healing systems, which can provide a total and lasting healing.

A wound cannot heal or grow if not the body itself lets it grow.

A hair cannot grow unless the body lets it grow.

Many years ago I was on a horse-riding holiday at *"Dovre"*, a Norwegian mountainous area. There I met a medical professor, and started a conversation about self-healing. He said, "Self-healing is the only true healing". Several years later when I was writing an article about self-healing, I confronted him with this opinion. Then he denied ever having said something like that.

A presupposition that a sick person can regain the control over his body by the help of re-establishing the self-healing is that at least one of the command lines leading to the self-healing in the body is intact, and that the self-healing processes are not destroyed, in short; that the mechanisms function.

Several things may destroy or damage the mechanisms, especially in sick people;

- The medication one get may hinder the self healing, as;

    ○ Cortisone

    ○ Chemotherapy

    ○ β-blockers

- Radiation therapy minimizes or temporarily destroys many of the restoring processes of the body, for example the immune system. In such case it might be difficult to stimulate the immune system.

- Difficult psychological situations, for example work related.

- Chronic stress and psychological strain as divorce, death, loss of friends, animal companions and such like.

The regulatory mechanisms of the self-healing

The self-healing systems have several levels

GENES

Several genetic components regulate the growth and death mechanisms of the cells, and by such cancer.

What turns these genes on or off is then the same regulatory processes that serve self-healing.

THE ELECTRIC SYSTEM

Bjørn E. W. Nordenstrøm, M.D. has found and described BCEC, "Biologically Closed Electric Circuits". He has shown that a static electrical field regulates the whole organism. He has shown that this field is able to create entirely new anatomical structures as fibrous membranes, organ capsules and different kinds of tubes or channels. This electromagnetic field is created by the ionic migration in the blood channels, the lymphatic channels and in the interstitial channels.

When the blood vessels divide, they often do so in an angle of ~90⁰. The vessels also often make a loop. These structures function as transformer coils for both the ionic current and the electromagnetic field. This field regulates the multiple functions of the body, including the self-healing processes.

THE NERVOUS SYSTEM

This system involves all the bodily processes, and by stimulating this with needles most of the processes may be regulated.

THE MERIDIAN SYSTEM

This system is fundamental within Chinese traditional medicine, and is considered a potent regulatory mechanism for the entire body. This system is probably a combination of the nervous system, the blood system, the peptide system and the electric system all together.

THE BLOOD CIRCULATION SYSTEM

The abundance of blood in the different anatomical structures regulates the activity of these structures. Without blood no activity. So, if the blood supply to an area diminishes, disease will result. If the blood supply is restored, health is regained. In this way the blood supply is an important part of the self-healing capacity of the body.

PEPTIDES, AN IMPORTANT CONTROLLING AND SIGNALING SYSTEM

Proteins are some of the fundamental molecules of life (proteios = primary). Lately, science has become aware of that segments of these proteins also are very important, may be even more so. These segments are called *peptides*. These peptides exist everywhere in the body, and are a part of a number of sophisticated processes and functions, varying from toxins to antibiotics and signaling substances. The peptides have been considered to be produced at need, but the investigations that I have done show that just cutting them off from already existing proteins, like for example hemoglobin, creates the peptides. In this way great amounts of peptides may be produced in the matter of seconds, always at need.

THE MULTIPLICITY OF THE SELF-HEALING

It is important to understand that the self-healing mechanism is very complicated, with several levels of function, several processes to work on, several ways of restarting and several ways of action. It may thus be activated in several ways, depending upon which organ process is diseased, what the cause of the disease is and the susceptibility of the patient.

What may reactivate the self-healing?

It is important to know that self-healing is a specific process, varying with the different diseases. This means that the stimulation of the self-healing demand a specific stimulus, varying with the disease and the location of the symptom.

ACUPUNCTURE
Within acupuncture there is two ways to re-establish the healing process;

1. Stimulate the organ process that is failing
2. Stimulate the area where the symptom is situated

OSTEOPATHY
All the tissues in the body are in intercommunication. This means that stimulating the areas that are diseased or under-stimulated may trigger a healing process where it is needed.

IMAGINATION
As Dr. Ario Conti has shown the brain is connected to all the processes in the body, and also that imaginations of special events may trigger the self-healing processes related to the specific diseases.

VITAMINS AND MINERALS
Lack of specific minerals and vitamins may shut down fundamental processes. To supply the body with the lacking substance may re-establish the failing healing process

PSYCHOLOGICAL FACTORS
As shown by Dr. Ario Conti, our psychic state of mind may influence the self-healing processes.

PLANTS
As several plants are known to stimulate certain organ systems, they will also be able to stimulate the self-healing processes connected to these specific organ systems.

The soldiers of self-healing; the peptides

Bioactive peptides are amino acid chains consisting of 2-40 amino acids. Their task is, among others, to be part of a signaling or communication system inside and outside the cells. These bioactive peptides have a flexible structure, and they can attach to specific areas on bigger molecules like proteins, RNA or DNA. This attachment is reversible or not, and may have a sedating or stimulating action.

Professor Rocca in Turin performed the following experiment:

A rabbit was acupunctured at a point that induced reduced pain sensitivity in the jaw area, nowhere else. Blood from this rabbit was then transferred to another rabbit, and this other rabbit then also developed decreased pain sensitivity in the jaw area.

This effect was due to the transference of the peptides from the one to the other rabbit, and which were produced because of the acupuncture.

Self-healing; the future of medicine

A science, based on understanding and insight in the body's own healing mechanisms, developed through ages, with specific remembrance and a multitude of possibilities for re-establishing the function and re-starting of the processes, related to plants, points, meditation and music ....

Yes, it sounds like a bird's song.

About Mirror Neurons

My whole practice and thinking in medicine is based on the following two axioms;

- It is always a deficiency that is the cause of the disease, and secondary excesses are the cause of the so-called symptoms.

- It is an intimate and real connection between all living creatures.

To understand this connection between all living creatures, it will be helpful to know about "Mirror neurons".

MIRRORING BRAIN ACTIVITY IN ACTION AND OBSERVATION
In "New Scientist" the following was to be read; "A child watches her mother pick up a toy. The child smiles: Mum wants to play. A husband watches his wife pluck car keys from a table. He shivers: she really is leaving this time. A nurse watches a needle being jabbed into an elderly patient. She flinches: it must have hurt.

How do these people know what the other person is thinking? How do they judge intentions and feelings, or assign goals or beliefs to the other? It sounds simple, but the child could just as easily have decided that Mum was leaving or the husband that his wife wanted to play. Yet they didn't. They knew.

"Reading" the minds of others is something we take for granted. Yet philosophers, psychologists and neuroscientists alike have been baffled by our ability to anticipate other people's behavior and empathize with their feelings. At the University of Parma scientists have identified an entirely new class of neurons. These neurons are active when their owners perform a certain task, and in this respect are wholly unremarkable. But, more interestingly, the same neurons fire when their owner watches someone else perform that same task. Yes, even when somebody else just is *thinking* of performing this task. The team has dubbed the novel nerve cells "mirror" neurons, because they seem to be firing in sympathy, reflecting or perhaps simulating the actions of others.

Many neuroscientists are starting to think that in higher primates, including humans, these neurons play a pivotal role in understanding the intentions of others. Mirror neurons may be one important part of the mosaic that explains our social abilities. So they presented monkeys with things like raisins, slices of apple, paper clips, cubes and spheres. It wasn't long before they noticed something odd. As the monkey watched the experimenter's hand pick up the object and bring it close, a group of these neurons leaped into action. But when the monkey looked at the same object lying on the tray, nothing happened. When it picked up the object, the same neurons fired again. Clearly their job wasn't just to recognize a particular object. Most importantly, the very same action that made a neuron fire when a monkey performed it would almost always make that neuron fire if the monkey saw the experimenter doing the same thing. It soon became clear that the motor system in the brain is not limited to controlling movements. In some way it is also reading the actions of others.

Mind reading, or theory of mind, is an ability that all healthy humans possess. We are particularly good at representing the specific mental states of others. These can be basic, such as seeing someone crying and understanding that they are sad, or realizing that when someone is yelling and gesticulating wildly at you they may be angry and might even mean to harm you.

But we intuitively understand more complex mental states too. When a mother loses a baby, other parents get lumps in their throats. When you hear that a colleague has been cheating on their spouse, you share the hurt and shame.

A dominant theory, championed mainly by philosophers like Goldman, is known as simulation theory. It's based on the idea that people understand what is going through the minds of others by mentally mimicking what the other is thinking, feeling or doing—in essence, putting themselves in the other's shoes. The discovery of mirror neurons backs up this theory nicely.

Luciano Fadiga, now at the University of Ferrara in Italy, was the first to find some evidence that humans may have a system analogous to that found in monkey brains, when he measured the excitability of particular muscles in the hand. He found that when the volunteers were watching grasping actions, the very muscles that would be needed to copy that movement seemed primed to act—as if they were preparing to make the same movement themselves. "The interesting thing was that the pattern of activated muscles changed according to the observed actions," says Fadiga.

This is preliminary evidence of a far-reaching neural mechanism. Could this explain how we are able to "feel" what others feel? Could it underpin the sensations behind empathy?

Mirror neurons and the way they facilitate imitative learning help to explain why we only developed things like tool use, art and mathematics about 40,000 years ago, despite the fact that our brains had reached their full size some 150,000 years earlier. These cultural inventions, he contends, probably popped up accidentally, but they were disseminated quickly because of our amazing, imitative, learning brains—made possible by a more sophisticated version of the monkey mirror neuron system."

HOW CAN THIS BE OF IMPORTANCE FOR A THERAPIST?
The knowledge that all creatures influence each other, especially through their thinking, willing, feeling and intention, is very important to a therapist.

Let me create an example in your mind; a horse has blocked vertebra, a locked and aching back. A therapist wants to unlock this vertebra. He is thinking and imaging this vertebra to loosen up. This thought, imagination, will and intention leads to a stimulation and activation of those neurons in his own brain connected to this task. This activation of his own neurons will in turn lead to an activation of the same neurons in the horse's brain. This will in turn lead to a loosening of the locked vertebrae. The horse itself thus performs the healing.

To be able to intend such a task, some details are important;

1. We have to know anatomy, so that it is possible to imagine what we want to perform
2. We have to place the image in our lower stomach

The contact between all living creatures, which is felt in all ancient cultures, is now then scientifically shown, to a certain extent, in the existence of the "Mirror neurons". Men in primitive cultures felt or saw that all living creatures were connected to each other through a network of energy that included the whole cosmos.

Skiing in the forest on the 4th of February 2006, I suddenly, and for the first time, saw this network, this matrix of living energy. It was like black, shining snakes that flowed or moved between all living entities, from tree to tree, from animal to animal, from human to human. It also flowed between species; from trees to humans, from animals to trees. This matrix merged the whole of nature with its presence. The matrix included all living things, even the farms that I passed, especially those having animals. I saw how these energy power lines streamed from the forest, embracing the houses where cows were living, where pigs were living, and also the houses where people were living. However where animals were present, the matrix was stronger than where humans were living.

The network was stronger between trees of the same kind, between animals of the same kind.

This observation made me understand that the whole creation was inter-tangled in wholeness, and if anything in this wholeness is changed or made to disappear, the whole will suffer.

After this experience I have written a whole book on my experience with this phenomenon, and all the observations I have made. In this book it would be too much to go into all the specificities of this matrix, except the one I will describe, which has some importance to our friends, the animals.

At several occasions I have observed fishermen or hunters, when killing their prey. Usually fishermen or hunters are not aware of the described matrix, they don't even feel it. But, in the moment of killing, it seems that the whole matrix opens up for them, and they feel connected to the wholeness of creation. For a few minutes they are one with everything, and will have an intense communication with cosmos. This might be one explanation that hunters and fishermen so often justify their actions with nature experiences. While people that have this feeling or connection all the time do not have to kill to experience the wholeness of creation.

This will explain why sacrifical offering was an important part of the old connection to God. In the blood of the lamb, the closeness of God was felt.

But it is better to have this feeling all the time, and not killing.

THE ETHERIC
ENERGY-CIRCULATION
OF THE BODY
(THE ETHERIC-BODY)

When reading this book, it is important all the time to bear in mind the energy that creates and sustains the life and development of the body, called Jing-Qi or the etheric energy. This form of energy moves in **lemniscates.** This is 8-formed movement. Such a circulation may be observed in all nature, in all beings that contain life. Try to observe an old pine-tree, see how the lemniscates are physically seen in the growth of the stem. Look at the movements of the water running out of the bathing tub. See the form of the horns of the animals and the spin of the atoms.

Everywhere we may see the form of life, the lemniscate movement.

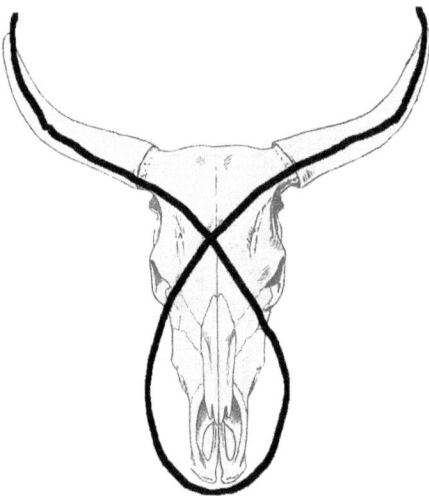

Fig. 3; We may see the lemniscate form in the horns of animals, especially in the Gazelle.

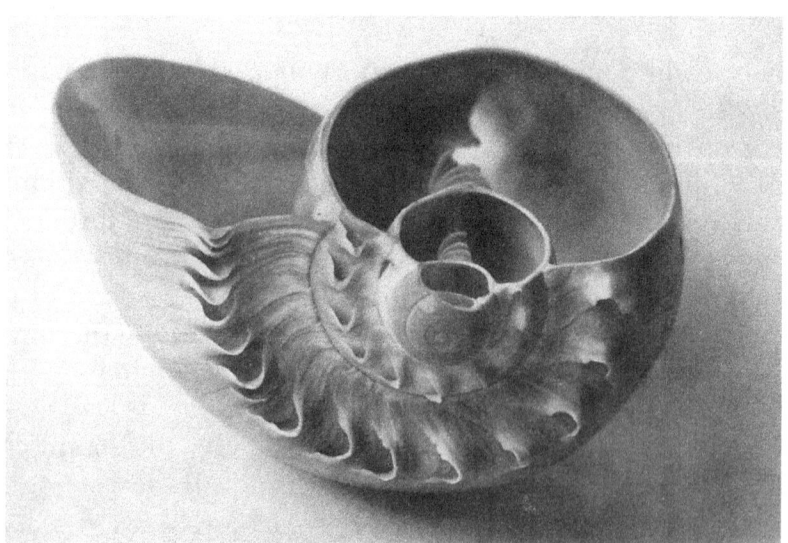

Fig. 4; the lemniscate is obvious in the snails shell

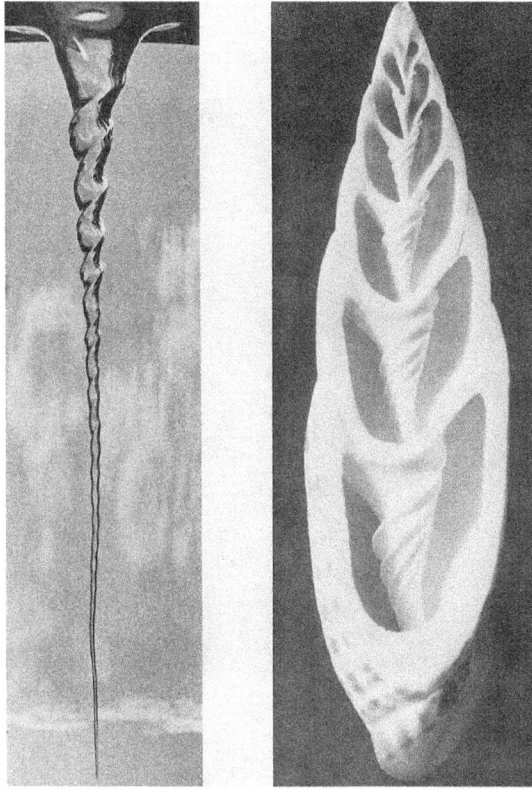

Fig. 5; We may see the lemniscate movement in the movement of the water.

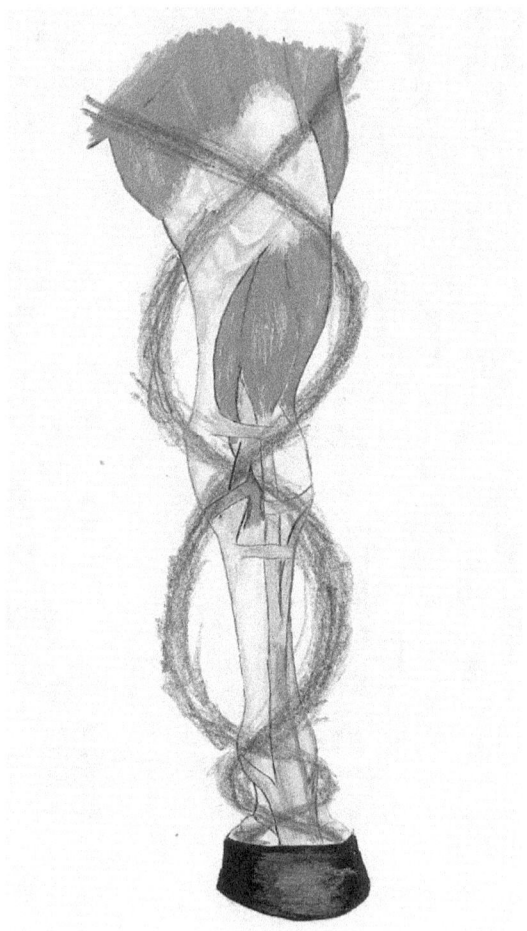

Fig. 6; In the joints of all mammals the etheric energy-movements cross, and just here the energy does not belong to any particular element. Under and above the energy has a certain elemental colour, but just over the joints the command-point have no elemental connection, and form the source-points.

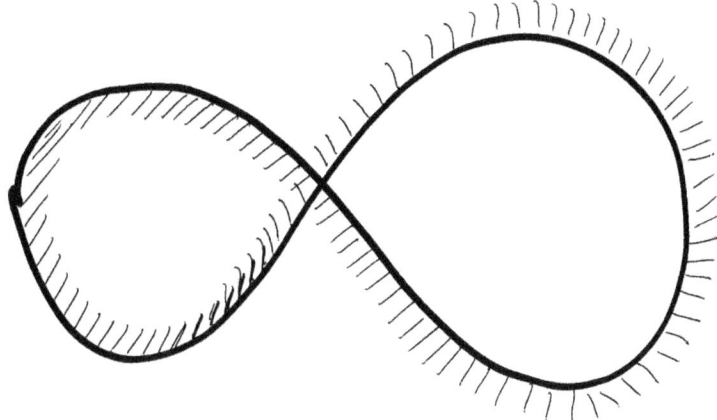

Fig. 7; demonstration of how the energy change from below to above the joint. See how the inside becomes the outside after the crossing, and in the same way the energy also becomes "twisted" or changed to the opposite!

Chapter 1

HOLISTIC VERSUS CONVENTIONAL MEDICINE

H olistic medicine tries to understand and find the root causes, the Imbalanced Inner Functions (Processes) that lie behind (beneath) the disease; the energetic deficiency that cause the Lesion-Symptom Complexes to appear and recur, even though the Lesion-Symptom Complexes may differ from time to time in the same patient. Because the holistic practitioner tries to find and stimulate the deficient organic process, he has few if any symptom suppressing remedies or methods available. In this way, holistic medicine can not cope with conventional medicine in dealing with the symptoms, but it tries to change or remove the root causes of disease, or helps the organism to adapt to "the disease", or to live in better harmony with it.

Conventional medicine also tries to understand the causes that precipitate the Lesion-Symptom Complexes. However, it

1

knows little about biorhythms, Qi circulation, Processes and several other fundamental biological mechanisms. The conventional doctor only knows the appearance of the numeral symptoms, which the patients ask him to remove, and to his availability he only has symptom-suppressing medicines that the pharmaceutical industry support him with.

Conventional medicine has many effective remedies that easily suppress or mask the Lesion-Symptom Complexes. The pharmaceutical industry is also interested in how Lesion-Symptom Complexes work and how they can be reduced. For example, instead of tackling the primary energetic causes of mental disease, infectious disease or hormonal imbalance, conventional medicine and allopathic pharmacology use mood-altering drugs, anti-microbial drugs and hormone replacement therapy to "correct" the Lesion-Symptom Complexes. In summary, rather than addressing the root energetic causes, allopathic therapy is symptom-suppressive.

Failure to address the root causes and the energetics of disease has important consequences for doctors and their patients. Patients who are not educated in the natural progression and cure of disease often demand that their doctors provide rapid suppression of the symptoms. In turn, doctors ignorant of other ways, prescribe such medicines. Dr. Marvin Cain, veterinarian, an American colleague, says that allopathic practitioners forget that the best and most permanent way to stop the alarm bells´ from ringing is to shoot the bell ringer and not the bell. Even better, solve the conflict that necessitated the ringing of the alarm bells in the first place.

The expectation of a "pill for every ill" is widespread in today's frenetic western societies. For those uneducated in the realities of disease and the ways to adapt to it, "time (lost) is money (lost)". Many people want the "quick fix"; they are not prepared to take the time needed to heal themselves or their animals. They do not realise that symptom suppression merely drives disease "underground", to recur later in another form.

Example:

- Because no lesions could be found, a patient with back pain took painkillers and muscle relaxants that suppressed the symptoms. However, as he was not satisfied with this treatment, he went to a complementary therapist. The therapist diagnosed an excess with pain in the bladder-meridian, and drained this excess with acupuncture. The patient got better for some weeks, but then the pain came slowly back again. The poor patient then went to a holistic therapist who diagnosed an excess in the KI Qi as the root cause of the back pain and prescribed a homeopathic remedy and an herbal tea to sedate the kidney process. This took away the pain for a longer time, but eventually the symptoms reappeared. The patient's disorder improved but he was not completely cured. Finally, he went to an orthodox doctor, who diagnosed that the man had kidney problems originating from tonsillitis. The throat infection had a negative toxic influence on KI, which referred pain to the back. The doctor prescribed an antibiotic, which cured the tonsillitis, the disorder in KI and bladder, and the backache. Afterwards I can resonate or think that the tonsillitis could also have been treated in a holistic way with herbs, or acupuncture of the TH-meridian (as a deficient TH-process may lead to a kidney problem, usually an excess). However, this was a real example from my own experience, and this example show that the most important is to find the real underlying cause, and not just treat the symptoms.

This example shows us three very important things:

a. It is not the most obvious underlying cause that is necessarily the real cause. There may be several layers of underlying causes, and few of us are really capable of finding the ultimate cause, which the doctor really did. Often we must be satisfied with acknowledging the cause that made the disease disappear for a considerable time, like the complementary and the holistic therapists did.

3

b. Holistic medicine is not always about giving a "natural remedy" instead of conventional medicine; it is essentially about to find the deepest cause of the symptoms and treat this, whether it is a usual antibiotic remedy or a homeopathic one. The real alternative to conventional medicine is the search for the ultimate cause. Conventional medicines or pharmaceuticals do not necessarily conflict with holistic medicine. Indeed, in some cases, they are not only valuable, but also absolutely essential.

c. Natural medicine (medication) is not to be considered just as an alternative for conventional medicine (medication): *We should not necessarily substitute natural medicine for conventional medicine.* Indeed, in many cases, conventional medicine or surgery is the best clinical option for our patients on the basis of conventional diagnosis. However, *holistic thinking processes and concepts of health and disease* help us to search for the deeper cause of disease. *This is where holistic medicine has its real alternatives to conventional concepts.* This thinking must of course be based on a considerable amount of knowledge about the interaction between the causes and the symptoms, the biorhythms, and the interactions between the organism and the surroundings. Ideology without knowledge becomes fanaticism, and knowledge without Ideology becomes cynicism.

I emphasise that the **diagnosis**, finding the original or deepest cause of the disease, which in practise means to find the starting deficient process or trauma, is the most important work of holistic medicine. This is the main or essential difference between holistic and conventional medicine, or rather causative and symptomatic medicine. Alternative medicine may also be used symptomatically if the therapist is only searching for secondary symptoms like excesses and pain. A real causative or holistic medicine will search for the underlying deficiency or initialising trauma and treat this.

Conventional medicine also aims to diagnose accurately, but it overlooks many important causal factors and usually prescribes treatments that are symptom suppressive. By this I mean that, without doing anything about the cause, it tries to remove the Lesion-Symptom Complexes by using medication. It is so easy to see the Lesion-Symptom Complexes (both in conventional and in alternative medicine) while the real cause is often more difficult to see (as it is usually related to painless deficiency syndromes).

Like conventional medicine, complementary medicine also can be used to suppress Lesion-Symptom Complexes if the therapist fails to find the original (root) cause of the disease. As Lesion-Symptom Complexes often manifest in different places, *it requires a deep level of knowledge to see their interactions or connections. Unfortunately, much of this knowledge is **not taught** in university.*

For example:

Symptoms that may arise from a poor blood circulation (the deficient process) are very variable. Symptoms differ according to the time of the year, the age and the species or breed of the patient. Poor blood circulation manifests differently with species and age:

Species and age	Poor blood circulation manifests as
Children	Otitis media
Young girls	Acne
Older women, menopausal women	"Heat" Syndromes (internal Heat after menstruation); hot flushes (vasomotor disorders)
Puppies	Red skin infections around the nose
Young dogs	Furunculosis, skin infections of the paws
Trotters	Fetlock, or navicular disorders, especially on the right forelimb
Cows	Mastitis

Table 2

Holistic practitioners try to diagnose the deepest (usually energetic) cause of the disease, the deficient process. They regard the Syndromes (Lesion-Symptom Complexes of body, mind and spirit) only as clues to indicate the deeper underlying energetic deficiency. Throughout this book, this diagnostic method or procedure is called the *Holistic Method.*

The Holistic Method

Holism tries to describe how the separate parts influence each other and how all the different parts and Processes affect the wholeness of the organism, and the relationship of the organism to its environment. Holistic medicine looks for relationships between *all* Lesion-Symptom Complexes, Processes and causes *within the complex of the disease and of the internal and external environment.* Holistic thinking processes demand deep knowledge in several areas, including areas not directly connected with medical disciplines. Holistic practitioners must also know how the weather, music, colours, time of the day, and many other factors, influence the physiology and rhythms of the organism.

THE VETERINARIAN'S ROLE

Before they call a holistic or complementary therapist who is not a veterinarian, owners or handlers first should call a veterinarian to examine a sick animal and diagnose its disease by conventional methods. Depending on the country and the university, veterinarians spend 4-8 years in full-time undergraduate study. During that time, they study anatomy, animal behaviour, animal management and husbandry, biochemistry, conventional diagnostics, embryology, medicine, nutrition, pathology, pharmacology, physiology and surgery, etc. Legally, diagnosis of animal disease is a veterinary responsibility. *Veterinarians who are properly trained in holistic methods are better to diagnose and treat the root than both ordinary veterinarians and lay people trained in holistic veterinary medicine.*

Holistic (Complementary) methods combine well with conventional veterinary medicine. The use of effective holistic or complementary therapy, on its own or together with conventional medicine, can only be done properly by a person properly educated in both systems.

One should note that the system of linear thinking (cause-reaction-cause-reaction) that is taught at the scientific faculties often interferes with good holistic diagnosis and therapy.

It is important that animal owners recognise the strengths and weaknesses of the veterinarian, chiropractor, osteopath, herbalist, neural therapist, acupuncturist or homeopath (in one or in several people) and that these methods complete or complement one another. The word "complementary", or "holistic" is more correct than the word "alternative". "Alternative" implies *instead of,* whereas "complementary", or "holistic" embraces *the best of conventional therapy plus the best of unconventional therapy.* The combination of both medical approaches is the basis of a powerful holistic approach to veterinary medicine. The ideal situation would be that the same vet could apply both therapies, conventional as well as complementary. This is likely not to happen in the near or distant future, as these systems are so different and require such different thinking that they are most likely not to meat, even though veterinary students and colleges today are far more positive towards holistic medicine than they were a few years ago.

HOLISTIC MEDICINE

Holistic medicine has a unique philosophy that is most satisfying professionally, intellectually and spiritually. Its philosophy crosses many boundaries: physics and metaphysics, form and function, material and energy, microcosm and macrocosm, science and art, experience and intuition.

Holistic medicine is founded on a certain view of life. In this view, nothing happens in the universe (macrocosm) without an impact on the smallest subatomic particle (the microcosm) and *vice-versa.* Every thought and action has its effects. All parts of the ecosystem (the cosmos and the local environment) and of the body (soma, psyche and spirit) depend on each other and interact. Most importantly, the whole is more than the sum of the individual parts.

Holistic medicine aims to diagnose and correct (where possible) the primary cause of the disease, whether it is traumatic, dietary or energetic. *It aims to heal the whole individual, not just the elbow pain, muscle spasm, diarrhoea, ovarian dysfunction or insomnia.* The sum of all the symptoms points to the deep cause, also the **interaction** between the symptoms and the environment. All parts influence each other and the whole influences every single part.

Holistic Diagnosis investigates and depends on relationships between seemingly independent phenomena. It depends on the observation of possible:

- Relationships between separate phenomena, more than the study of the single factors

- The Process Imbalances, which are the root energetic causes, of different Syndromes.

The imbalanced process may be divided into

     º   The deficient process, which is primary

     º   The excessive process, which is secondary

As holistic practitioners, if we find that a patient's eczema varies in the same way as a chronic cough and the diarrhoea that often bothers him/her, insofar as all symptoms are aggravated after drinking cold drinks or water, we can conclude that the total Lesion-Symptom Complex has the same root cause. We will see later how LU and LI (the Yin-Yang organs in the Metal Phase), connect with each other and that HT control both. Therefore an effective treatment of HT *helps the eczema and the diarrhoea.*

Also, if the eczema is at the upper part of the body and the symptoms are burning, the cough is from the upper respiratory tract and is painful and the diarrhoea also is burning, we may deduce that this triple Lesion-Symptom Complex is linked within the same Fundamental Process. They are just manifesting in different microcosms, but all are depending on the deficient heart.

As mentioned before, an important factor within a holistic system is that the macrocosm manifests or mirrors itself in several different microcosms. The next chapter, which discusses holographic photography, illustrates this. Microcosms that mirror the whole organism are found in the ear (Ear-AP), eye (iris diagnosis), nose (nose-AP), palm of the hand (hand analysis), back (Back-Shu Points), coronary band of horses (Ting-Points) and several other places.

In recent years, such microcosmic systems have been called "ECIWO Systems" (**E**mbryo **C**ontaining **I**nformation of the **W**hole **O**rganism). ECIWO biology is a theory where such Microsystems are used to explain biological mechanisms and also therapeutic and diagnostic properties in such diverse body parts as those mentioned.

*Recent western science contains traces of holistic philosophy. For example, the field theory of physics accepts that the whole influences the parts and that every single part influences the whole and not only the next part of the chain. We see that the single part works as part of a process, and influences the whole organism. This is a different concept to one that sees one factor influencing the next in a chain of linked processes. We can see the same in the relationship between **photons**. A photon is a light particle, a minimum packet of light energy that travels at light speed. Two photons that come from the same energy source are always connected. Even if they travel many light years from each other, anything that influences one immediately influences the other. These photons are a part of a holistic system, where everything that influences one part also influences the other parts and as a result change the whole. Therefore, the whole is more than the sum of the individual parts. These aspects of modern physics support ancient holistic medical theories. **Yin-Yang** theory states that all phenomena have their counterpart within themselves and that the balance between the counterparts changes all the time. Western science recognized this concept around 1930. In quantum mechanics there is no stability in the same meaning as in classical physics. Every "stable" mechanical* *system vibrates around its balancing point, and is also dependent on the mind of the person that watches the phenomenon (Heisenberg's uncertainty principle).*

*The concept of **Yin-Yang** in traditional Chinese Medicine (TCM) differs from the more modern concept of dualism. One should not confuse these two concepts. Modern dualism sees the counterparts in every phenomenon but does not see the relationship to the whole. Holistic principles abound in oriental philosophy, especially in TCM. TCM sees every little part as a mirror of the bigger whole: the microcosm reflects the macrocosm. This view is also relative and changeable; every big organization can be viewed as a macrocosm compared to a smaller organization. In TCM, man stands between (mirrors) heaven and earth. Man is the microcosm in relation to the heavens and man is the macrocosm in relation to the microcosm (atom). The same applies to animals. The **Bible** expresses the same view when it says that Man is created in the image of God and that Man mirrors God. Other philosophers add that God needs Man to realise His love of Creation and to be His Hands and Helper in the evolution of Creation.*

Holographic Photography and ECIWO Biology

Most of us have seen a *hologram, or holographic picture.* This is a 3-dimensional image, where we can "see into" the image (it must not be mistaken for the new computer-generated fractal images where we really must make an effort to find out what the motive is in the image). A picture like that astonishes us and yet it is just a piece of paper, like any other picture.

A special technique is needed to make a holographic photo. A laser beam is used to light the object. A prism, that splits the light in two laser beams, captures this laser light. These two beams are sent to a photographic emulsion where the interference between the two light patterns creates a photographic pattern that looks 3-dimensional. This far it is technically understandable and interesting for photographers. It also is interesting for us as medical professionals because it can serve as a model to explain Holistic Medicine.

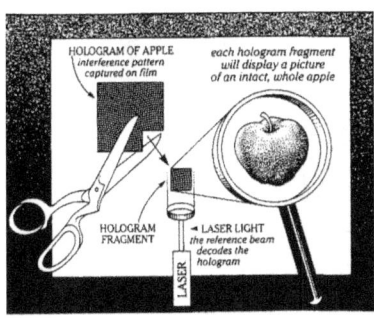

Fig. 8; Illustration of a holographic picture.

For example, let us consider a holographic picture of *an apple.* From this picture, let us cut off a corner, where we see no apple. If we then put laser light on this corner, we can see the whole apple as a complete picture. No matter what part of the picture we remove and no matter how tiny the removed part is, all parts of the picture contain the image of the complete apple. These removed pieces also show another very interesting phenomenon. In the empty space that the pieces had occupied, using laser light one can make the picture reappear, as a sort of mirage, or illusion, as one may experience in the desert, or at the sea. One has the impression of seeing the oasis, but the oasis is not where one sees it.

This example shows that the whole manifests in the smallest parts. If the body functions in this way, it is no wonder that the whole body can be found in the ear, the palm of the hand, etc.

Ying Qing Zhang, a Chinese professor, put these systems into a new and very interesting context. In 1981 Zhang published a "new law of nature", namely the

- *"bio-holographic law"*

Zhang had noted that many pathological bodily Processes manifested as tender points along metacarpal bone 2. This was a similar observation to that of the ingenious French doctor, Paul Nogier. In 1954 (see page 137 & 146), Nogier found that pathological bodily Processes manifested as tender points in the human ear.

In one sense, Zhang's discovery of a biological micro system was not really new. *What was new, however, was that this is a universal phenomenon that is valid for all areas of the body.* He stated that his metacarpal 2 system and the Nogier's ear system are just a part of a universal system, which he called ECIWO biology.

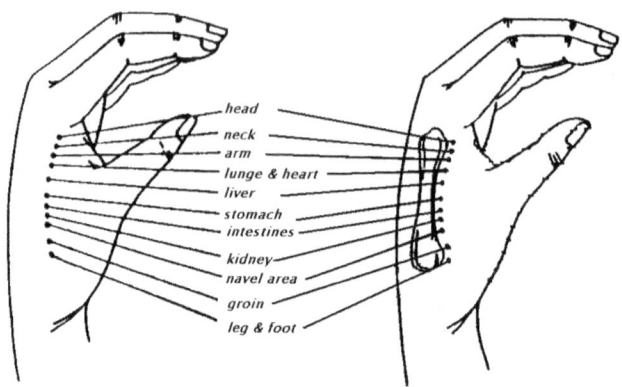

Fig. 9; Diagram where the different reflex-points are found along the 2nd. metacarpal bone.

ECIWO is an acronym that means **E**mbryo **C**ontaining **I**nformation of the **W**hole **O**rganism. It indicates that all cells and parts of the body contain information of the whole body. Zhang further said that all these systems communicate with each other and with the whole organism. Because of this, all microsystems (ECIWO Systems) may be used in therapy and in diagnosis.

There are different levels of ECIWO-systems. The lowest, or primary level is the DNA-molecule as such. This molecule contains information on the whole organism, and can give rise to all the cells in the organism. The next level is the cell, then the organ, the organ system and then the whole organism as such. We see this most clearly within botany. We may place a part of a leave in water, and a whole new plant may arise from this. The same will happen if we put the whole leaf in water, or the branch. All these levels are able to create a new plant.

Another important issue that characterize an ECIWO-system, which is of great importance to a therapist, is that all the ECIWO-systems are interconnected and by such *self-maintaining and self-repairing*. The DNA-molecule has enzyme-systems to detect and repair all possible damage. Such self-repairing and self-maintaining systems are also present in all higher ECIWO-systems. As self-repairing systems they are of great value, if not of crucial importance, to the self-healing systems. It is possible that these systems *are* the self-healing systems.

These are the systems that are activated by the so-called *"placebo-effect"*, or by the help of *"mirror-neurons"*. All the systems we use to heal the body is nothing but different kinds of or levels of self healing ECIWO-systems.

Professor Zhang postulated further that all the ECIWO-systems are interconnected, and that is why they may be used as a healing device. Interference in one system will automatically restore all the other systems as well, and by such the entire body.

How this interconnection and intercommunication happen is unclear, and the theories here are multiple. What is certain is that the connective tissue is central.

We do not know the mechanisms that underlie this communication. However, Soviet research showed that bodily cells communicate by a signal system that does not depend on nerves. This system uses bioluminescence or chemiluminescence, a form of electromagnetic signal in the light range, and this light can transmit through connective tissue. If this proves to be correct, it will explain to a large extent the existence of the Channels described in TCM, the existence of the different microcosms and the importance of the connective tissue in different therapies.

Dr. Björn Nordenström, who has given evidence for an additional circulatory system, which he call "closed electric circuits", has showed the same. This circulatory system uses the connective tissue as the transportation way, and low static currents as the circulating information. This system is of vital importance in balancing the processes of the body, and is possible the same as the meridians. The meridians may thus be found along the vessels and nerves in the connective tissue that surrounds all nerves, vessels and muscles.

The laws governing the actions of the universe have been verified over the centuries by the use of scientific modalities such as physics, thermodynamics and chemistry. We have come to understand and respect the laws of physics and chemistry. We learned in our chemistry classes about the behaviour of fluids in varying environmental conditions. The biological sciences have to a large extent explained the method by which our bodies digest, assimilate, metabolise, detoxify and excrete what we ingest. These are the physical laws inherent in nature, the laws we innately follow as physical beings living in a physical universe. However, we are also energetic beings living in an energetic universe. And as specific laws bind the physical universe, a separate and distinct set of laws binds the energetic aspects of life also. These are the principles one must comprehend before truly understanding and practising holistic medicine.

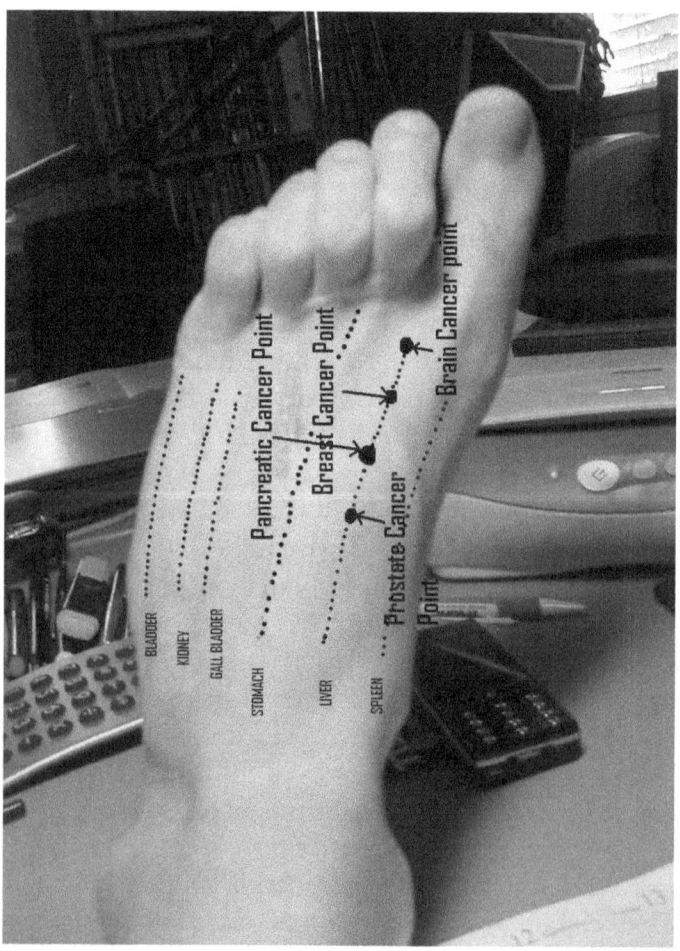

Fig. 10; Different ECIWO-systems along each of the metatarsal bones.

Health and Disease

One can view health and disease in several ways and the nature of these approaches has changed through time. Ancient cultures view health as a complex state consisting of a sound mind in a sound body (mens sana in corpore sano), as in ancient Rome. Whether this just applied to the upper classes I don't know, but this view varied with the wealth of the society. When the daily struggle to survive changes into a search for spiritual values, then we demand more from life than just physical function. In medieval Europe, most people considered health to be the absence of physical complaints. Modern definitions of health are more complex than such definitions. They stress not only the absence of physical, mental and spiritual symptoms of disease but also that we need to experience positive elements like the possibility to fulfil oneself, to be in balance, to have joy and success, etc. This agrees very well with holistic ideas of health and disease in complementary medicine, which defines health as an absolute balance of physical, mental and spiritual energies. Conversely, disease is defined as any physical, mental, spiritual or energetic imbalance, even if it is preclinical at the time, i.e. the imbalance (as detected by Pulse or other diagnostic methods) does not necessarily manifest as symptoms of disease at that time.

How is a healthy balance achieved?

All life-regulating Processes must balance Internally and Externally in a very fine harmony. Anabolism balances catabolism; building up balances breaking down; sleep balances wakefulness; excretion balances absorption and uptake; joy balances sorrow and good balances evil. To be able to help a sick organism we must get as much knowledge of the special properties of the Processes as possible; at least we must know them and recognise them and know the typical Lesion-Symptom Complexes which can manifest if the Processes become imbalanced.

BODILY PROCESSES

Vital Inner Functions (Processes) are necessary to maintain health and life, and lie behind all expressions of life. To survive and thrive in an ever-changing environment, all plant and animal life forms have developed adaptive internal Processes to sustain life, and complex systems to regulate these Processes in always changing feedback systems. Even if all the details were known (and that is not the case), no human brain could hope to store or recall all the complex details of these processes and their controlling systems. In keeping with the Theory of the "Survival of the Fittest", these processes have adapted by passage through countless generations of the myriad of life forms (species). Thus, they manifest as great differences between the different species.

These Processes balance each other in a complex system based upon stimulation and sedation, feedback and feedforward. An excessive disturbance of this balance activates different homeostatic or self-balancing systems and mechanisms, such as the earlier described ECIWO-systems and the acupuncture system. If the Processes remain unbalanced (usually deficient), that is if the different ECIWO-systems of different levels cannot restore equilibrium, then the body must activate compensation to help the deficient Process, *which cause symptoms of disease to arise.* Such compensation (symptoms) will, if it is allowed to persist over a longer period of time, lead to irreversible and chronic changes in the organism (chronic disease symptoms).

However, the innumerable individual processes can be reduced to 12 essential/adaptive Fundamental Processes. In all living creatures like fish, birds, plants or insects, waste excretion occurs in very different ways. However, the differing methods of waste excretion are still manifestations of the same Fundamental Process, which in mammals is called the Kidney Process. Trained clinicians can use their knowledge of these Fundamental Processes in their daily diagnostic and therapeutic work. The vital Processes are expressed in the different organs. When Imbalance of these vital Processes occurs and last for some time without the controlling mechanisms being able to restore the balance, we become ill or weakened, until, eventually, disease can manifest as Lesion-Symptom Complexes.

THERE ARE NO SICK PROCESSES

It is easy to consider bodily actions (compensatory processes) that allow disease to manifest as "*bad Processes*", and the processes that lead to health as "*healthy Processes*". However, we must not consider the vital Processes as healthy or bad *per se*, in the same way as we cannot say that a rifle is good or bad. As a Marxist said during the 1970s "A tractor can be either communistic or capitalistic".

It is very important to understand that life does not develop sick Processes. Instead we must understand that the Lesion-Symptom Complexes of disease appear when the normal Processes become **imbalanced (usually deficient),** and when this unbalance is not rebalanced by the natural balancing systems, of which acupuncture (AP) is but one.

Below are five examples of Processes essential for life and what happens when these become Process Imbalances, i.e. become a Qi Deficiency or a Qi Excess.

	Process	Normal function	Excess of normal Function	Deficiency of normal function
1	**KI-Water Process**	Urine excretion	Incontinence (leaking)	Urine retention
2	**KI-Water Process**	Ca, P and Mg deposition in and resorption from bone	Calcification, spondylosis	Brittle bones, osteomalacia
3	**LI-Metal and GB-Wood Processes**	Excretion of waste via LI (feces) and GB (bile to SI)	Diarrhea	Headaches, congestion
4	**LU-Metal Process**	Gaseous exchange	Dizziness	Dyspnea, fear of suffocation
5	**TH-Fire and SP-Earth Processes**	Hormone production in the glands	Nymphomania, pseudo pregnancy	Amenorrhea, no menses

Table 3

17

This way of thinking becomes clearer if we make a list of Process Imbalances. For example, Process Imbalances include:

- **Weak states** (Qi depletion, deficiency, weakness, hypoactivity);

- *Excess states* (Qi repletion, excess, fullness, hyperactivity);

- **Qi Stagnation - Obstruction;**

- Or when **Qi, Blood or Body Fluids** appear at the

  ° **Wrong place** (for example, oedema of the limbs), or

  ° **Wrong time** (premature ejaculation, premature birth or aging, etc.).

All normally balanced Processes exist to maintain life. However, heavily stressed Inner Functions (Process Imbalances) allow Lesion-Symptom Complexes of disease to manifest in the Weak Structure. Disease is no more than too much or too little of the normal Processes occurring in the wrong place, or at the wrong time. This is what we mean by imbalance or disease.

MANIFESTATION OF NORMAL AND IMBALANCED PROCESSES
CAN DIFFER

It is very important to note that the same Process can manifest differently in different species, both in its normal state, in its deficient state and in its excessive state (as for example love, hate and anger expresses itself differently in different people, different cultures, different species and at different times). Expression of normal Processes can differ in the same species, or between different times in the same animal. We must learn all the existing Processes and how these different Processes manifest themselves in humans and in different species of animals. Similarly, the Lesion-Symptom Complexes of the same disease (i.e. the manifestation of the same Process Imbalance) can vary widely between and within species.

To treat the under-function

In 1980 I had an experience that changed my medical thinking forever. I visited the office and clinic of the very famous and skilled doctor and acupuncturist Dr. Georg Bentze, who by the way became my teacher and benefactor after that visit. He presented me for a patient suffering from torticollis; the head was constantly bent to the right in an angle of about 50⁰. "This condition", Bentze said "is due to a diaphragmatic hernia". I looked at him surprised. He then directed a green light beam towards the patient's diaphragm, and after a few seconds the torticollis vanished. He then directed a red light beam towards the same area, and after some seconds the torticollis reappeared. Later the patient was operated for his hernia, and the condition and the torticollis were solved.

Dr. Bentze's thinking was in short to treat the process, the organ, the muscle or the tissue that show the less activity, the under-function, the deficiency (in this case the diaphragm). Such a deficiency will create a compensatory over-function, an excess (in this case the muscles of the neck), possibly as an attempt to compensate in ways that I do not understand presently, and this excess is usually the symptoms that people see, feel, suffer, and which the doctors usually try to eliminate.

An example of this under-function from the world of trotters. All horse people interested in trotters know of the lame trotter, injected several times in his front right knee (carpus). The problem reappears several times, but the under functioning joint is actually the right Ilio-sacral joint. After treating this joint, the horse will work better with his right hind leg, and the strain and over work on the right front will be relieved, and the symptomatic problem will not reappear.

The 12 Fundamental Processes of the body in its normal (physiological) aspect:

Twelve Fundamental Processes (Inner Functions) interact in the body to maintain homeostasis and health. Each of the 12 Processes relates to one of the 12 Channel Organ Systems

(Process) and their TCM Processes; they relate directly with the 6 Yin and 6 Yang Organs and their Processes in paired Yin-Yang Couples within specific Phases as follows:

	Yin-organs	Phase	Yang-organs	
1	LU-Lung	Metal	LI-Large Intestine	2
4	SP-Spleen	Earth	ST-Stomach	3
5	HT-Heart	Fire	SI-Small Intestine	6
8	KI-Kidney	Water	BL-Bladder	7
9	PC-Pericardium	Fire	TH-Triple heater	10
12	LV-Liver	Wood	GB Gall Bladder	11

Table 4

So as not to confuse the reader or resign a possible veterinary or medical reader, it is important to underline that the processes here described are not synonymous to the organs we call by the same name in western medical terms, even though the names are not by chance either. First of all, we must understand that the processes described here are present in every living creature, man, animals and plants. To realize that the processes are also present in plants will make us understand the difference between our organs and the processes. In the plants the processes are not "condensed" or "materialized" to organs yet, as they are in mammals.

- For example the kidney process is present in all cells in all living creatures; all cells are excreting waste, via the skin, the cell wall, the urine, the saliva and numerous other channels.

- Likewise the heart process is present everywhere nutrients are brought to the working cell, is be via the blood, the sap or different kinds of fluid.

I will also shortly discuss why we have chosen to work with 12 processes. To be able to function or be active in the material world, we have to categorize the different things of the world. To do so, we have to choose a system that may be used for our intentions, for our goals.

We have to choose which system we want to work in.

- We can reduce all the bodily processes to a minimum, for example two. The anabolic processes and the catabolic (building up and breaking down). Every symptom may be characterized according to this system; if tissue is broken down or if it is built up.

- We can divide all the processes to three categories, as in Anthroposophical medicine (See page 605).

- We can divide the processes in four, after the four European element; fire, water, air and earth.

- We can divide the processes of the organism in five, as they do in Asia; fire, earth, metal, water and tree.

- We may decide the processes in twelve, after the 12 fundamental processes used in Asia.

- We can even, after some Tibetan sources, divide the processes in fifty-four.

We must, in order to work effectively in the world, actually *choose* the way we divide the phenomenon of the creation. In medicine several practitioners have experienced that a 12-partitition is the best way, and the most profitable way.

1. **LU-Lung** and exchange of bodily gases is a Yin Process, sharing its functions with LI, the connected Yang-Process. LU controls gaseous exchange, the intake of oxygen (O_2) and excretion of carbon dioxide (CO_2) and other waste gases. LU is also the boundary or interface between the internal and external environments, the inner and outer worlds. LU connects us with the material outer world. LU develops from embryonic ectoderm, the skin, which shares interface function between the Internal and External. Thus, LU and skin are closely related. Love and reliance of and to the surroundings are the psychic aspect of the LU Process (love for the world). LU also governs pain, as pain is a means to be aware of the world.

2. **LI-Large Intestine** is the Yang or psychic aspect of LU, with which it shares its functions. LI Process is both to keep and excrete the more condensed food particles and the more condensed matter that the body can't use. It is very important to differentiate between the excretion of KI (KI dominates the rectum) and the retaining/excreting Process of LI. LI symptoms may manifest everywhere in the body. In the horse the LI is also responsible for metabolism of water. The psychic aspect of LI (Metal) is to be inflexible, stubborn or single minded.

3. **ST-Stomach** Process is the Yang aspect of the SP Process. ST Process is to "store and ripen" the food. Different organs handle that Process in the different species of animals. In humans, at this time of our evolution, the stomach has that function. The large intestine (the cecum) and rumen mainly handle this function in horses and cows, respectively. The psychic aspect of this Process is the joy for life (which is the deeper aspect of philosophy).

4. **SP-Spleen** and digestive tract rhythm is a Yin Process, the Yin-aspect of the ST-process, and is responsible for the maintenance of all the bodily rhythms and habits. This is, as we surely know, most important for the digestive apparatus, which is most dependent on regularity. The psychological aspect of the Spleen is thinking, philosophy and inner peace (as well as the rhythms of the mental life).

5. **HT-Heart** is a Yin-process, linked to the SI-process that is the Yang-process in the HT/SI-pair. HT relates to too much or too little blood circulation, especially arterial circulation. The blood circulation in every corner of the body is dependent of a good and strong HT Process. The psychological aspect of HT is love, joy and friendship to other creatures.

6. **SI-Small Intestine** is the Yang Process of HT, and it has by this to do with the psychic abilities of love and joy. But SI Process also has its own Yin-process, namely in the digestive function to control the absorption of food.

7. **BL-Bladder** is the Yang-process of the KI/BL pair. The BL-process is mainly of a psychic character (astral or yang), especially related to the bravery of the Kidney. It may be said that generally all Yang processes are the psychic aspect of their Yin counterpart or companion Processes. *It is important to note that all Processes have psychological symptoms to some degree but when psychological symptoms in general are marked, it is likely that BL is involved.* Of course BL Process (the bladder process) also relates to the physical urinary bladder and its work in collecting and excreting urine.
The psychological aspect of the Bladder is bravery, the same as for the Kidneys.

8. **KI-Kidney** has an excreting Function. KI controls not only urine excretion but also the excretions and the Yin orifices (anus, vagina and urethral opening) including perspiration (sweat). It also controls uro-genital function and dominates the rectum, the excretion orifice of the LI. KI also relates to the bones (bones are deposited minerals). KI influences especially certain body regions, especially the stifles, lower back, forehead, throat and ears. It also governs essential parts of the reproduction. The psychological aspect of the Kidneys is bravery.

9. **PC-Pericardium** is the Yin-partner of the PC/TH-pair. It is also called the Heart Constrictor or Circulation Sex, is responsible mainly for the control or regulation of blood circulation. The whole function of the Heart-process is dependent on the PC-process, but mainly the blood flow to the middle part of the body, especially the sexual organs. The psychological aspect of the PC is sexual joy, or to be "horny".

10. **TH-Triple Heater** Process is the Yang Process of the PC/TH-pair, and is important for hormonal balance. It is also, like PC Process, important to the circulation of blood, especially in the mucosal membranes. It relates also to the hypophysis, adrenal glands and gonads (i.e. to hormone balance and reproduction), and is thus important to hormonal balance and libido (sex-drive, etc). The psychological aspect of this process is "incarnation", to be present in the flesh.

11. **GB-Gallbladder** Process is the Yang Process of the LV/GB-pair. The main role of this astral Wood Process is to overcome or subdue the Earth Processes within the body, or those that are to be included in the body. This means in clear language to digest the food we ingest, the digestion of all the impulses we get through the senses like sight, sounds and smells. The psychic aspect of GB is aggression (resistance against External Stressors, the external world in general) and self-consciousness.

12. **LV-Liver** is the Yin-process in the LV/GB-pair. The LV-process expresses itself in the physical body in the venous blood circulation, and by this it controls muscles in general. Especially the muscles around the hips and neck depend on the LV Process. The immune system is also one of the more important functions governed by LV Process. The psychological or psychic aspect of the LV is will.

The Laws of the fundamental processes:

The fundamental processes relate to each other through a refined and ingenious feedback system. If this system is not enough to keep up the sound balance of the body, then external help is required like the stimulation of skin-areas, herbs and other external influences. But this will be dealt with under the chapter on therapy.

Here we will first deal with the internal and physiological ways that the processes keep their balance, and which laws they obey.

The fundamental processes obey the following laws:

- **The Five Phase Law**

- **The Yin-Yang Law**

- **The flow of energy (Chinese Qi Clock (biorhythm)**

- **The Husband-Wife Law**

These four laws are the most important ones dealing with the normal physiology of the processes.

The two following laws are mostly active concerning the pathology of the processes, and they are dealt with in more detail under the chapter of therapy, acupuncture.

- **The Deficiency law**

- **The law of the mirrors**

1. FIVE PHASE LAW

This Law states that all created things (Processes) can be classified into Five Phases, or Elements. These are fundamental qualities that correspond with common experience of the natural world. The Phases interact or influence each other directly in two ways, the Sheng Cycle and the Ko Cycle. These Cycles either support (Sheng) or control (Ko) each other. Some practitioners call the Ko Cycle the Control Cycle. The Sheng and Ko Cycles are explained further in the section on diagnostic methods (see page 99). Thus, there are two cycles:

- The Sheng Cycle supports or nourishes its Sheng Son Phase

- The Ko Cycle dominates or controls its Ko Son Phase (see page 28)

The main characteristics of the Five Phases are:

Fire	Earth	Metal/Air	Water	Wood
It warms and is full of emotions and feelings. Fire Excess is destructive and eats up whatever it attacks (the Weak Structure). We can imagine these forces like those of strong emotions and in craving love.	Controls transformation. It is more purely destructive. It helps to transform each Phase into the next one, for example death and resurrection. Gravity dominates Earth and leads to the detachment of the material lesion from the body.	Controls the body's gases. Metal/Air Deficiency loses control over the gas Processes. Also Metal dominates or controls pain.	Controls the flowing of all liquids, blood, and lymph and the excretion of all liquids.	Controls all growth processes. As a tree grows and produces leaves, Wood is responsible for all tissues and processes that grow in the body, including lumps, nodules and cancers (before they enter the Earth Phase and tend to withdraw from the body).

Table 5

In another version, Earth is viewed as a transitional Phase, placed in the centre, between all the other Phases. The force of Earth can be either destructive or transformational, helping to change one Phase into the next. Although the Five Phases originated in ancient Chinese philosophy, especially that of TCM, they are identical to the European tradition as taught, for example, by Rudolf Steiner.

Classification of the created universe into different Phases is a very old idea and we see such classifications in most cultures. In European tradition, existence usually is classified into Four Elements, although some ancient philosophies used five (Apollonius from Tyana). The Asians usually divided all creation into five categories and named them after Fire, Earth, Metal/Air, Wood and Water. By this we mean that all things, in their own forms, follow the Laws, which in turn follow that Phase to which each created thing relates.

Classical physics, in which all things can be divided into three aggregate states, has parallels to this. The states are solid, liquid and gas. Each Phase can come under one of these three states and each state follows its own Laws. Liquids flow, solids retain their form and gases adapt themselves to the shape of their environment.

We can classify and characterize precise Laws for the various Phases. Phenomena that belong to the Fire Phase all act similarly, as do all phenomena that belong to the Water Phase. If we combine phenomena from Fire and Water, they neutralize each other. Therefore, it is practical to categorize all things and Processes by Phases; thereby we can predict their effects more easily. In this way TCM evolved its concepts of physiopathology. TCM categorized all the phenomena in nature and in the body by the Phase(s) to which they belonged. They could then predict what the reaction of the organ would be to specific medicines or treatment that was categorized by the same Phase system. Thus, treatment of HT (Fire Phase) with a plant like Equisetum Arvense (Water Phase), would subdue the activity of HT.

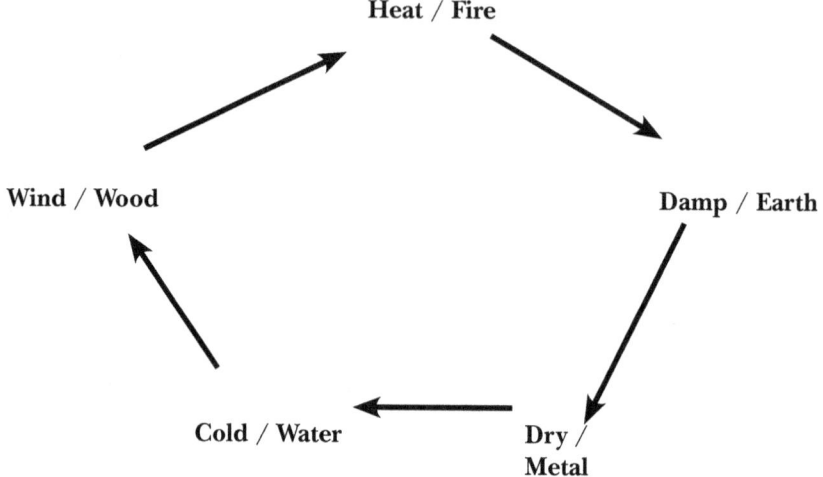

Table 6; Diagram of the Sheng-cycle

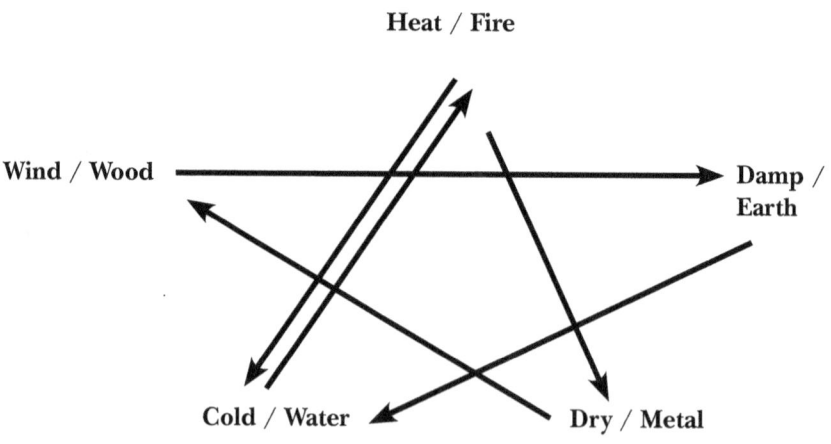

Table 7; Diagram of the Ko-cycle

FURTHER COMMENTS ON THE FIVE PHASES (ELEMENTS):

Since its origins, several thousand years ago, two paradigms dominated the philosophy of TCM: (1) Yin-Yang Theory and (2) Five Phase Theory. Chinese culture incorporated the latter not only into medical theory and practice, but also in all other facets of life including food, architecture, art, politics and war. Thus, Five Phase Theory is central to Chinese philosophy, classical TCM and Acupuncture. The Five Phases have a sequence: Fire, Earth, Metal, Water, and Wood. In some paradigms, Earth is viewed as a central transferring Phase between all other Phases. Since Metal = Air in European tradition, we get this order: Fire, Metal/Air, Water and Wood, with Earth between each Phase. The sequence of the Phases is identical to traditional European viewpoints, which we find in the fundamental theory of the Rosicrucians, Paracelsus and by Rudolf Steiner.

In medicine, one must understand the Five Phase Theory in order to understand the relations of the Back Shu Points to the Phases. The Five Phases represent a cybernetic, auto-controlling cycle with two main parts, the Sheng Cycle and the Ko Cycle.

Each of the Five Elements/Phases relates to both a Yin and Yang organ Channel pair, as follows:

	Fire	Earth	Metal	Water	Wood
Yang Organ	SI and TH	ST	LI	BL	GB
Yin Organ	HT and PC	SP	LU	KI	LV

Table 8

2. YIN-YANG LAW

The predictable interaction of Yin-Yang is the most universal law in Asia. It derives from holistic concepts in a cosmological thinking process, or world-view, used to relate all natural phenomena.

In common with modern physics, Yin-Yang Law perceives all things as a balance between reciprocally conflicting powers. This viewpoint is unlike the dualism of later European philosophy, which conceives opposites to be independent. In contrast, Asians view opposites to depend on each other, in a constantly interchanging and dynamic auto-control system with creative and destructive aspects. Extreme Yang creates Yin and extreme

Yin creates Yang, just as each season follows the next, turning from the heights of its power to the depths of its weakness. Day proceeds night and crying creates the following laughter.

Anything can be Yang compared to something that is more Yin; anything can be Yin in relation to something that is more Yang. The meaning of this is that all things have something that is beneath and/or above them; that which is underneath is Yin in relation to that which is above. The shoulders are Yin in relation to the head, but are Yang in relation to the chest. The chest is Yin in relation to the shoulders, but is Yang in relation to the abdomen. Yin and Yang are terms used to describe states of relativity between different things or functions. They can be viewed as material and energetic polarities, where Yang is positive or active (+), and Yin is negative or passive (-).

Relative to the *thing* to which it is being compared:

YIN IS	LESS	UNDER	BEFORE	INSIDE	COLD	DARK (UN-FEELING)	FE-MALE	DARK	ETC
Yang is	More	Above	Behind	Outside	Warm	Light (feeling)	Male	Bright	Etc

Table 9

Relative to the *function* to which it is being compared:

YIN IS	HYPO	DESCEND	CENTRI-PETAL	NIGHT-ACTIVE	DIASTOLIC	ATONIC	PASSIVE	ETC
Yang is	Hyper	Ascend	Centrifugal	Day-active	Systolic	Spastic	Active	Etc

Table 10

The Monad, an ancient Yin-Yang symbol, illustrates the Yin-Yang relationship especially well.

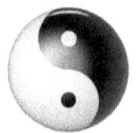

Fig. 11; The Monad, or Yin-Yang symbol.

The dark segment represents Yin, whereas the light represents Yang. The two dynamically oscillate around each other; each needs the other and continuously transforms into the other; they are opposite, mutually complementary and ever changing. Together, they form unity. Everything is relative to something else. Within each main polarity, the small dot of opposite color symbolizes that *there are no absolutes; there is always some Yin in Yang and vice-versa.* The only absolute is the Law of Change; everything must change in time.

3. BIORHYTHMS, THE CHINESE QI CLOCK OR CIRCADIAN CLOCK

As life in its totality and as in our mental processes, the activity of the fundamental processes varies during the day, the week, the month, the year and the life.

The most usual and observed changes are during the day. The table below indicates at which time the different processes are most active, or when the bodys demands of that particular process are at their highest.

The relationship between the processes and the changing demands throughout the week, month, year and life easier to see in a table. The moments, states or times indicated are when the most work is demanded or expected from the process.

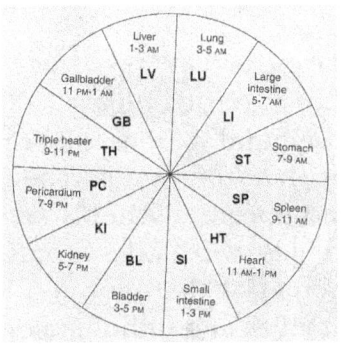

Fig. 12, the biorhytms

31

	Week-day	Season	Part of life	Mental state	Activity
Lung	?	Late summer	Late life	Tolerance	Breeding
Large Intestine	?	Late summer	Late life	Tolerance	Excreting
Stomach	Saturday	Autumn	60-70´s	Holism	Keeping
Spleen	Saturday	Autumn	60-70´s	Holism	Making Rhythms
Heart	Sunday	Summer	Grown up Loving	Joy	Regulating
Small Intestine	Wednesday	Summer	Grown up	Joy	Food absorption
Bladder	Friday	Winter	Dying	Courage	Gathering
Kidney	Friday	Winter	Dying	Courage	Excreting
Pericardium	Monday & Sunday	Summer	Grown up	Sexual desire	Leading
Triple Heather	Sunday & Monday	Summer	Grown up	Feeling present	Blood microcirculation
Gall Bladder	Tuesday	Spring	Young	Will to dominate	Traveling
Liver	Thursday	Spring	Young	Will to do something	Doing

Table 11

4. THE HUSBAND-WIFE LAW

The interpretation of ancient Chinese calligraphy is that harmony within organisms and seasons is best preserved when the husband is stronger than the wife is. The Chinese had noted that the most harmonious households had a strong husband and a somewhat weaker wife. Likewise, if summer becomes stronger (more energetic) than autumn, this creates imbalance and illness in nature and in human or animal bodies.

The Husband-Wife Law states that the man should be stronger than his woman, otherwise there may be conflict in the house. Therefore, the male processes should be stronger than the female. *The husband/wife pairs are* NOT the same as the coupled processes within the Phases (the Yin-Yang Phase Mates).

Husbands	Wives
HT	LU
LV	SP
KI	PC
SI	LI
GB	ST
BL	TH

Table 12, The relationships between Husbands and Wives:

5. THE DEFICIENCY LAW

This law states that we always shall treat or stimulate the weakest process. Whenever there is an excess (painful condition, mainly in the Yang Channels), there must be a deficiency (not painful condition, mainly in the Yin Channels).

The inferior acupuncturist treats the excess, but the superior acupuncturist treats the deficiency.

The Nei Ching states that: "The inferior doctor treats the thousands of symptoms (local, symptomatic treatment), the good doctor treats the underlying excess (excessive Channel), but the superior doctor treats the underlying deficiency (usually the Ko-father of the symptom-carrying meridian).

6. THE MIRROR LAW

The Law of Mirror applies to all life. It applies to the reoccurrence of symptoms after treatment, to life-parts (the seventh 7-year period mirrors the first 7-year period and so on), to Karma, to time, to symptoms in the body (right arm mirrors left arm), to treatment (right leg points cure left leg pain) and so on.

That earlier symptoms reappear after treatment in opposite order, can be explained in connection with this law, which states that the energetic body or the etheric body's "mirror-relation" to the physical body.

According to occult tradition the etheric body and the physical body are exact mirror images of each other, as the two loops in a lemniscates (see figure 7).

In this way pain in the right arm may be treated with points in the left arm or in the left leg. In the same way we may consider symptoms placed in time. The etheric time moves from present to past, while the physical time moves from present to the future. As we treat a symptom in the present, this will resonate with the past and the future. Philosophically this may explain "deja vu", cycles in appearance of phenomena and karma.

How disease emerges

We must learn to observe the animals: In everyday life, different species and different animals within a species have different abilities to meet heavy work, irregular or poor nutrition and the many and varied stresses. The more specialized an animal or an organ is, the less it can cope with new or ongoing stressors involved in everyday wear and tear. This is due to differences in breeding (genetics), natural environments, special needs for feed, special areas of use and varying stresses.

In holistic thinking, **a Process Imbalance (usually deficiency) is the root cause of disease**; an imbalance in one of the 12 Fundamental Processes of the body allows disease to manifest. For example, consider the high yielding dairy cows. Such cows have extremely "stressed" udders. For them, the udder is often the Weak anatomical Structure and mastitis is one of their most prominent disorders. Conventional veterinary medicine usually treats mastitis with antibiotics or other remedies to reduce infection, in addition to other udder supporting treatments. Treatment is aimed at the mastitis producing pathogens. In contrast, holistic medicine has a very different approach. It regards a Process Imbalance as essential to allow the Stressor to manifest as Lesion-Symptom Complexes in the Weak Structure. In this example, the Process Imbalance allows the mastitis to manifest. It might have been a Process Imbalance (deficient) in KI, due to too many calvings, allowing a Stressor, such as severe Cold, or Wind to weaken it even more. It might have been a Process Imbalance in LV Process, due to chronic malnutrition and in which LV was weakened further by a sudden change in feed.

When deciding on which treatment to institute, conventional medicine ignores the underlying and/or initiating cause:

- The *underlying* (predisposing) *cause* is the *Process Imbalance* that allows the stressor to precipitate mastitis.

- The *initiating* (precipitating) *cause* may be an *External or Internal Stressor* that overcomes the capacity of one or more of the Processes to adapt, i.e. it imbalances one or more Processes over its limit.

  a. *External Stressors* include the *Six Evil Qi Factors* of TCM (Heat / Summer Heat, Damp, Dryness, Cold and Wind), change of feed, food spoilage, or trauma. It also includes other environmental stressors, as recognized in western medicine, such as heavy infectious or parasitic challenge, allergens, toxicity, serious defects of management or husbandry, geopathic effects, or adverse effects of lunar, solar or other cosmic stimuli, etc.

  b. *Internal Stressors* include emotional imbalance, particularly serious Excess or Deficiency of excitement, obsession, grief, fear and anger, or their related emotions.

- The *weak structure* of the body is where the symptom may emerge or express itself.

It takes a great challenge (External or Internal Stressor) to precipitate serious illness if the body has perfect inner equilibrium, i.e. if all Processes are balanced. Unfortunately, few individuals are perfectly balanced. That is why there is so much international interest in training programs that help people to become physically and mentally "fit". Such programs include physical fitness and exercise training, the martial arts, Tai qi, meditation and stress-control programs (yoga, Qigong, etc) and state-sponsored schemes to encourage healthy living. The latter schemes include legislation on pollution and sanitation, safety-at-work, personal- and food- hygiene, nutritional health, antismoking campaigns, control of alcohol and drugs, etc. In spite of all these efforts, many people do not take steps to develop a full physical and mental balance.

*A Process **Imbalance** seriously weakens the adaptive capacity of the body to withstand **Internal** or **External Stressors;** both act as stressors. If a cow also has a **Weak Structure**, then this combination allows disease to manifest (mastitis, if the udder is the Weak Structure), even if the Stressor is relatively minor.*

Recent research in high-yielding cows shows that fertility (conception rates, days from calving to conception, etc) decreases as milk yield increases. In nature, to feed her suckling calf, a cow needs to produce only 400-600 kg milk per lactation. She can do this with minimal intake of feed dry matter and minimal metabolic stress on the gastrointestinal tract, LV, SP and KI. Today however, because of genetic manipulation and selection for high milk yield, many dairy herds produce an average 7000-9000+ kg of milk per lactation. This puts enormous metabolic stress on all the systems of the cow. Apart from mastitis and lameness, sub fertility is a huge problem in such herds, which often have conception rates to a given service of <40 %, as compared with 60-70 % in lower yielding herds. Such cows have "prioritized" milk yield over pregnancy. In TCM, pregnancy / reproduction falls under the control of KI (Water Phase) and LV (Wood Phase).

In those cows, KI and LV can be the Deficient Processes, and KI and LV Deficiency can be the foundations of mastitis or reproductive problems.

1. PROCESS IMBALANCES

We, humans, are proud of our unique individuality. Even if we may seem to be as alike as peas in a pod, or drops of water, even if we have the same Weak Anatomical Structures springing from the same kind of work, no two of us are the same. We all have our genetic differences, our specialties, our strengths and weaknesses, our joys and sorrows, our fears and loneliness. And it is subtle differences in these that make one individual unique from another. We are each unique beings, and so too are animals. The more I work with animals, the more I am astonished at how different and individual they are. Two trotters that may perform the same kind of work, have the same training and eat the same food, and yet may have totally different weak Processes that are unique to them. One may have a weak BL-process, and get easily scared and one may have a weak spleen and thus get digestion problems after change of feed.

On initial assessment, it is *very important to distinguish between* the **Weak Structure** *and the* **Process Imbalance** *of the same animal.*

- The Weak Structure is a physical weakness because of a special anatomical structure, or because of special use.

- The Process Imbalances (dysfunctions of Internal Jing-Qi balance) may be due to Deficiency (Weak Jing-Qi) or to Excess (Full Jing-Qi).

It is also very important to have in mind that *different* Process Imbalances may elicit *similar* Lesion-Symptom Complexes because the Weak Structure is like "an accident waiting to happen". As water or electricity find the lines of least resistance, differing Process Imbalances may manifest in the Weak Structures of the animal.

It is equally important to distinguish between the *Internal Stressor* (destructive emotions) and the *Imbalanced Process*. The latter usually is a lifelong weak Internal Process, while the Internal Stressor usually is the combination of day-to-day mental stressors that are an inevitable part of living. All Internal Stressors more or less weaken the Imbalanced Process. However, if the Internal Stressor correlates with the Imbalanced Process, it has much more adverse effects than if it did not correlate. This is explained in more depth at page 151 & 155.

It is very important to understand that all animals or people have their own individual Process Imbalances. Under attack by an acute or prolonged Stressor, the Process Imbalances are the main determinants that elicit Lesion-Symptom Complexes at their individual Weak Structures.

In trotters, which normally have great stress on their joints, especially on the right carpus, any strain or stress combined with a Weakest Process can elicit pain in this joint. Many owners ask me to treat horses with such carpal disorders. Instead of treating the joint, I search for the Weakest Process. In some cases it may be a KI Deficiency due to giving birth (and exaggerated by cold weather or prolonged Wind), a SP Deficiency due to many changes of the feed (and worsened by irregular feeding) or a LU Deficiency present at birth (and worsened due to dust inhalation). Having determined the Weakest Process, I treat that as the root cause. If I have managed to identify the Stressor, I will of course try to eliminate that also (keep the animal away from cold wind, irregular feeding or dust). Having done all this it is usually not necessary to treat the painful joint, but we may of course treat the painful joint as well.

This holistic concept is very important. It *means that two horses with the same symptom (right carpal pain) are treated very differently, depending on which Process Imbalance is the underlying energetic cause.* Conversely, if we correctly diagnose and treat the Process Imbalance, the carpal disorder disappears sooner (usually much sooner) than usual and the disorder usually does not recur for a long time. Other complaints as headache, bad skin and dandruff will also disappear if we treat the deficient process.

In contrast, if one treats the Lesion-Symptom Complexes only, for example using "Cookbook Points" for carpal pain, or conventional symptom-suppressive analgesic/anti-inflammatory drugs, the clinical results may be as good, but the disorder recurs sooner. Additional complaints will not disappear together with the main ailment if the treatment is just symptomatic.

2. THE STRESSOR

A Stressor is necessary for Lesion-Symptom Complexes to manifest in the Weak Structure. Stressors, whether physical, psychic or spiritual, include all influences that stress and weaken the body. We often are aware of this Stressor. For example, we often see that the "cause" of a disorder is that we eat too much for supper, that the racetrack was harder or much wetter than usual, or that the animals had undergone much more stress, or a totally different routine than usual. But the Stressor is not the real cause of the disease; it is not even the most important factor, unless it is *extremely* strong. The same applies for the Weak Structure, unless it is *very* weak. Also, it is very difficult for a mild Stressor to manifest as disease in a body that is well balanced (i.e. has no Process Imbalance).

A strong Stressor may precipitate Process Imbalances
It is important to consider all the factors in diagnostic evaluation, and to decide if the Stressor may have been strong enough to create a deficient process by itself.

- A horse exposed to cold weather (say -20^0 C), or that stands in (or drinks!!) too much cold water, may develop a deficient KI.

- A horse submitted to frequent changes of feed may develop a deficient SP (digestive disorder or weak iliopsoas muscle)

If a Stressor is strong enough to trigger disease, one should try to eliminate the future Stressors of the same kind. This is really good *preventive medicine.* The main aim is to create a strong and well-balanced animal, an animal that can withstand ever-changing conditions and everyday wear and tear, without reacting to these influences by manifesting disease.

In TCM, the best therapy is one that builds up or balances Qi, (if there is a Process Imbalance), or removes the Stressor, Qi Obstruction, Phlegm, etc. All symptomatic therapy is inferior.

If a **Stressor overcomes the Wei Qi** (Antipathogenic Qi of the organism), it leaves its "fingerprint" (its peculiar set of signs) behind. A deep knowledge of the Five Phases is especially useful to help us categorize the Stressor. Once we recognize it, we can deduce the origin of the initiating factor (Stressor). Classification of the Lesion-Symptom Complex is based on the specialty or peculiarity of the Lesion-Symptom Complex. The symptoms may be dry, painful, hot or damp (edematous). TCM designated or symbolized this after the Phase to which the symptom belongs (also see page 28, 155 & 238). This is very important. Such observations can indicate

- Which element the Stressor belongs to

- Which element the deficient process belongs to

- Which remedy or acupuncture-point to use

- How deep the disease is rooted in the body (6 divisions, see page 219)

3. THE WEAK (ANATOMICAL) STRUCTURE

All humans and animals are mortal creatures. Each creature has its "Achilles' Heel", its Weak Structures or points where disease, strain or stress develop, or manifest more easily. Stress manifests in different ways in different people. Some develop angina or heart infarction. Others develop one or more of the following Lesion-Symptom Complexes: acid reflux, gastro-du-odenal ulcers, muscle spasm, asthma, constipation, colitis, uro-genital or reproductive disorders, arthritis, arthrosis (restricted joint movement), headaches, etc. Some develop the psychic or mental equivalents of these physical symptoms: insomnia, ex-citability or mania, obsession, apathy or mental fixation, claus-trophobia, tension, impotence, aggression, or fear etc.

Every stress, disease or imbalance appears at the Weak Structure. Therefore we reach the wrong conclusion if we think that LU symptoms must originate in the lungs, KI symp-toms in the kidneys, HT symptoms in the heart etc. If an ani-mal has a predominant Weak Structure, for example the udder of the high yielding cows, all Process Imbalances will manifest primarily as mastitis. If an animal has no Weak Structures, then disease cannot appear easily. In that case, the Lesion-Symptom Complex usually relates to the specificity of the Stressor or the Process Imbalance. Bur usually disease can manifest only if the Stressor is strong enough, or if the Process becomes imbalanced enough relative to the weakness of the weak structure. If we know the Weak Structure of the animal, we should **usually look elsewhere to find the real origin (Process Imbalance, the Predisposing Cause) and precipitating cause (Stressor)** that induced the disease to manifest in the Weak Structure.

For example:

- Dogs have very different individual constitutions. Some are big and heavy and have great stress on the joints, especially the elbow and the hip. Such dogs often develop elbow arthrosis and hip dysplasia. (HD). Small "sausage dogs", like dachshunds, suffer less stress on the joints but their backs are vulnerable because of their length and C shape; this is also the case in pigs. Small dogs kept as pets (lapdogs) get too little exercise and too much food; these dogs usually suffer stress on their digestive and metabolic system, circulation and heart. Such dogs usually react to Process Imbalances and Stressors by developing circulatory disorders, heart disorders and epilepsy. Generally the dogs assume their owners' disorders, because the dog usually shares the owners' lifestyle.

- Cows in intensive dairy herds are under extreme stress from selective breeding and management to produce higher and higher milk yield. This weakens the udder, which often is the main Weak Structure in high-yielding cows. Combined with very little exercise, most of our cows are balancing on the brink of mastitis and diarrhoea. For most of the year, most cows in Scandinavia are kept in a barn; this makes their legs grow weak. Very little extra stress inevitably precipitates disease, such as laminitis, mastitis, etc. A change of relief-milker for one weekend may be a sufficient stressor to precipitate an increase in somatic cell count in the milk, followed by mastitis some days later.

- **Horses** have very different lives. Riding horses are usually less stressed than trotters and the disorders of riding horses usually vary more than those of trotters. Trotters suffer from repetitive stress every day. They are forced to trot in an abnormal way and at a speed that should be a canter or gallop. They are forced to do this day after day in the same trails, races or tracks. This is grossly abnormal for horses. These stressors induce extreme wear and tear on the joints, and manifest then especially in the fetlocks and the carpus (the Weak Structure). The slightest change in feed, care, surroundings or training (the Stressor) can then precipitate joint disorders if a Process Imbalance is present. In all types of riding horses like dressage-, jumping- or event-horses the weak structure is usually the same, namely the joints. In the development of the disease, the Stressor varies as well as the Internal Process. Usually the rider/handler is the main Stressor of these horses. Personal communication from a German physiotherapist has shown me that all horses that are ridden over a period of two years "take over" the problems (symptoms) of their rider. They develop malfunction in the same structures or joints where the rider has problems.

We must learn to assess and integrate all the presented data and clinical findings holistically, in such a way that we are able to see and recognize the real disorders and to distinguish between the External and the Internal causes (Process Imbalances, imbalanced emotions). This must be done in a way that enables us to deduce these factors back to environmental-, feed-dependent-, breed-dependent-, psychological-, acquired-, or inherited- Process Imbalances.

In most cases of disease, *all three factors (Process Imbalance, Stressor and Weak Structure) must interact.* This interaction allows disease to manifest, and the most important *root cause of disease is the Process Imbalance.*

The relationship and dependence between the Weak Structure, the Stressor and the Process Imbalance in the development of Lesion-Symptom Complexes may vary from disease to disease. It is very important to evaluate all these three factors when we are to evaluate every patient.

CONCLUSION:
In our diagnostic work we must be able to differentiate three causal complexes and in every individual case be able to interpret the different parts of each of these three complexes.

- *An inherited or congenital individual Weak Structure* (cystic fibrosis, cerebral palsy, strabismus, etc.), or a *stress-induced Weak Structure*, **due to overuse, stress or bad environment (for example the udder, liver, gastrointestinal tract and hindlimbs of high yielding cows, or the right fetlock or carpus in trotters).**

- *Process Imbalance* **(LU Deficiency, SI Deficiency, etc.).**

- *Acute and varying Stressors*, **for example change of feed, Cold and Wind, or psychological shock.**

The Lesion-Symptom Complex as an auto-therapy

Why does a particular Lesion-Symptom Complex develop and what is its purpose? I will show below that the *body itself chooses the Lesion-Symptom Complex*. This choice is crucially important. It allows the organism to survive with a Process Imbalance (Deficiency, Excess or Obstruction of a normal Process), to adapt to the Stressors and to cope or live with its Weak Structures. In order to understand more easily that the body itself chooses the Lesion-Symptom Complex, we will take a closer look at some examples.

Examples of symptoms that "help" the body:
- *Excretion of urine* is a key function of the kidney (KI). If the kidney fail in doing its tasks, the subject first tries to adjust this by different feedback mechanisms such as thirst, changed salt intake, etc., the body try to re-establish the normal blood values. If it fails to do so, urea and other urinary toxins (metabolites) that KI should have excreted, instead overflow throughout the organism. It is most important that the body

can eliminate these because death is inevitable if it continues. Then s/he seeks self- or AP stimulation of different systems, such as ECIWO-systems (including acupuncture). Then s/he may seek medicinal plants, such as Chamomile and Equisetum. If these attempts are not sufficient, the body seeks to recruit help from other cell-systems to help KI function. Other organs and tissues of the body have great capacity to adjust to different functions; they are multipotent (see the effectiveness of ECIWO Systems on page 12, 148 & 498). Therefore, the excretory function normally controlled by KI may occur in other body sites also. The symptoms emerging at these sites are usually due to excess (the local KI-process is elevated). If we then just diagnose according to excess (painful areas, smelly areas, wet areas), we will be able to relieve the symptoms, but then we miss the real cause of the disease, namely the deficient kidney. It is then of the utmost importance not only to treat the symptoms with medication, herbs or acupuncture, but that we address the underlying deficiency.

    º   If abnormal excretion occurs in the joints, it can induce arthralgia and arthritis, and can damage the joint. The body "recruits" pain to minimize joint damage; pain reminds the subject to spare the joint while this excretion continues.

    º   If abnormal excretion occurs in the skin it may lead to a bad body odor or pruritus.

    º   If abnormal excretion occurs in the mouth (via the saliva), it can lead to gingival and mucosal ulcers, stomatitis and halitosis.

• *The daily activities and functions of LV* are very broad and different. They have many aspects, including the very important sugar-, fat- and protein metabolism and detoxification. In mild LV Deficiency, LV function usually remains normal. However, if nutrition changes markedly, the workload on LV function becomes more stressful, the toxin-load to be neutralized increases, etc. These Stressors put extra strain on LV and render it unable to maintain its functions effectively. Then, having tried to recruit help from the feedback mechanisms and stimulation methods, including ECIWO-stimulation and ingestion of Dandelion, LV must recruit help from other tissues because it cannot handle the metabolism of sugar or toxins (among other things) on its own. Several other tissues must then take over to help LV. The different compounds that should have been metabolized in LV are transported to the other tissues or organs in a partly metabolized state. These "incompletely detoxified" substances then overflow throughout the organism and can lead to

- ° Pain, migraine, rheumatism or headaches (according to the Weak Structures).

- ° We may also see fluctuating levels of blood sugar, dirty skin, disorder of concentration and general symptoms of minor poisoning.

- ° For example, we may see a depressed dog instead of one that previously was happy and approached us with eagerness, wagging his tail. Now it is reluctant to approach, gives an impression of scruffiness, has eczema and dandruff and shows clearly that it is depressed.

- If some Stressor or Process Imbalance weakens the *blood circulation*, the organism compensates by weakening the circulation in places where a strong circulation is not absolutely necessary. For example, we often feel sleepy after a heavy meal and we know that we should not swim at that time. This is because blood diverts to the gastrointestinal tract, leaving relatively less blood for the muscles and brain; at that time we are not as strong as we think we are.

- *A weakened immune system* must be seen in relation to its related Processes; especially LV and SP. Immune function is sacrificed first in LV and SP Deficiency, in order to strengthen more important functions (digestion and metabolism) and to spare more important tissues, such as muscle and nerve tissue. The same occurs in stress, acute or chronic. In stress, the immune system is suppressed (sacrificed) for the benefit of fight or flight mechanisms. The Lesion-Symptom Complex that then arises is a good example of what was discussed before, i.e. that the Weak Structure tells us very little of the **cause** of the disease. The predisposing **root cause is the Deficient Process (Imbalance)**, in this case LV or SP, both of which strongly influence the immune system. A weak immune system may manifest differently in different species or different individuals according to their relative weak structures, for example as:

   ° Pharyngitis

   ° Pneumonia

   ° Allergy

   ° Chronic infections in *humans*

   ° Infection in the paws (furunculosis), demodectic mange or otitis externa in *dogs*

   ° back pain in *horses.*

- *The same principle applies in calcification,* for example in dogs with spondylosis (calcification of the spine) or hip dysplasia. These dogs have great pain but AP treatment can give rapid pain relief, long before the calcification disappears. This suggests that the calcification itself is not the cause of the pain but that the body calcifies special joints to prevent movements that are painful. Thus, *calcification is the body's way to prevent painful movements.* It is a sort of auto-therapy or self-help.

It is important to understand that **the Weak Structure,** *in which the Lesion-Symptom Complex manifests initially,* **is seldom the site of the Primary Process Imbalance.** The Primary Process Imbalance or Weakest Process (the Qi imbalance, the root cause of the symptoms) usually lies elsewhere, often far away from the Weak Structure. For example, in the initial stages of oliguria, when KI excretes too little urine, it is difficult to see this initially in the physical kidneys (or in standard kidney tests); often the primary cause does not lie in KI. Instead we see it in places where KI Deficiency is compensated, especially at the Weak Structures of that particular body.

The best therapy is to correct the Process Imbalance (tonify the Deficient Process, and by this, automatically sedate the Excess Process) wherever that may be. The Process Imbalance can lie in any of the organs or Phases. Correction of the Primary Process Imbalance restores balance to KI. This eliminates the Lesion-Symptom Complex, i.e. the symptoms disappear and/or the tissues at the Weak Structure normalize, thus the lesions disappear. In summary, by correcting the Process Imbalance, effective energetic treatment removes the need for the Lesion-Symptom Complex, so that the manifestations, warning signs that represented the disease, disappear.

Practical Examples:
- In rheumatism and painful joints due to KI-excess and HT-deficiency, we might stimulate HT-function to sedate the KI. If this succeeds, it removes the need to excrete urinary metabolites in the joints.

- In rheumatism due to LV-deficiency, we might stimulate LV-GB function and biliary formation and excretion. If this succeeds, it removes the need to excrete uric acid in the joints.

- In a chocolate- or alcohol- induced migraine due to LV-deficiency and SP-excess, we might stimulate LV. This activates LV-Wood to bring control to SP-Earth, thereby regulating sugar or alcohol metabolism more effectively.

Holistic medicine aims to treat disease by correcting its root energetic cause. It is a profound "root and branch" therapy, a therapy that treats the real origin of the disease. The essential thinking process of holistic medicine is to differentiate the Lesion-Symptom Complex from its primary energetic cause, the deficient Process Imbalance. *It regards the Lesion-Symptom Complex only as the manifestation of disease and not the disease per se.* One may apply such principles to all sorts of diseases and symptoms. *Experts seldom treat disease where the Lesion-Symptom Complex appears.* Unless the Weak Structure and/or symptoms are very severe or threaten life, experts seldom treat the Weak Structure directly, or the symptoms *per se.* To do so in routine cases would be inferior, disease-suppressing therapy. *Instead, they try to help the body to rebalance the Process Imbalance.*

CONCLUSION:
Disease as a form of auto-therapy

To recapitulate on this section, we may regard disease as an auto-therapy. The organ or tissue that really should have done the actual Process, has for some reason, failed in its duty. This can lead to serious complications, if other tissues or organs do not help to fulfill the task. Of course the symptom itself can lead to certain disorders, for example bad body smell, calcification etc. but from the viewpoint of the body, this is far better than the "original disease". We must view the Lesion-Symptom Complex that our patient manifests as the best way for the body to solve the disorder at that moment. If we try to suppress this Lesion-Symptom Complex without addressing the real cause (the Process Imbalance or primary internal Qi imbalance), we just aggravate the disease or drive it "underground" to manifest elsewhere. We force the body to choose another, usually worse, solution than the one with which we were confronted initially.

Ethical concepts of chronic pain

We may often wonder why many humans or animals manifest chronic muscular spasm and pain for years. Why can the body not eliminate chronic symptoms in the same way as it can heal wounds or bone fractures? One may argue that healing of bone fractures is essential for survival. It is the same with serious wounds, even with more serious organic dysfunction, which can compensate over time by producing different symptoms. But it is NOT essential for survival to heal chronic pain and muscular spasm that originate in psychological tension or in reflex areas of Process Imbalances. Such tensions usually are the result of an inappropriate lifestyle, physically or psychologically. If we fail to change our way of life, the disorders continue, or change to other Lesion-Symptom Complexes. This change often follows the Ko-Cycle. For example, symptoms that originally manifested as HT problems may change to LU problems (coughing at night). Lesion-Symptom Complexes are only warning signals to remind us constantly that we need to change our lifestyle, or correct our faults and our wrongdoing. Without such warning signals, we would probably change nothing. In this way some chronic pain functions as the physical expression of our inner voice, our conscience.

Relationships between humans and animals

By now, readers should have some understanding of the importance of holistic relationships in the internal environment of the soma, psyche and spirit. We also must learn to evaluate holistic relationships in the external environment, i.e. the immediate and more distant surroundings. These also influence health and Qi status. We must learn to see the whole farm, the whole stable, the whole barn with its animals, humans, houses and surroundings as one unit, one large, interactive organism. We must consider this organism as a holistic system, a system where all of the individual parts influence and depend on each other and where the totality is more than the sum of all the parts.

Humans have an obvious and profound influence on animals in their care. The human leader of the system, be it the farmer, keeper or stable girl, is the most important part in this system. Humans influence this totality, not only by the fact that they decide the overall management and husbandry (what to do, what and when to feed, when to vaccinate and train, the type of housing and shelter, etc). However, humans also influence animals in more subtle ways that we will discuss in more detail later (See page 617).

Domesticated animals react to our behavior, voice, temperament, movements and our whole being. But we also influence animals in more subtle ways. A sequence in a Walt Disney film showed different owners with their respective pets. Owners and their pets may be so alike in appearance and habits that the likeness calls for laughter. We might say that special owners tend to choose pets "in their own likeness" but the similarity goes far beyond this. In my experience, most species of animals regard their owners or handlers as so totally sovereign and dominating that the energetic structure of the animal tends to change to mirror that of the owner in temperament and behavior. An animal in very close contact with a human can develop a whole inner Qi balance that mimics that of the human. On several occasions, I have been able to decide the best treatment for the animal only by observing the owner.

The same may be seen in couples that have been married for a long time; they often grow more and more alike. Rudolf Steiner says that married couples develop similar "etheric bodies" as they have been together for a long time. When one dies, it takes three years to break down this "intermingled" etheric structure. That is why, in old traditions, a widow or widower should remain unmarried for three years.

VARIATION OF THE IMBALANCE

Those who do not understand the many causes of disease recognized in holistic medicine may find it difficult to accept that animals often adopt the Process Imbalances (especially Qi Weaknesses) of their human "group leader".

Here is an example from human medicine. TH Channel relates strongly with the endocrine system, blood circulation and metabolism. However, depending on the sex and age of the human, TH Deficiency manifests its imbalance very differently:

Sex and age of human	Usual Lesion-Symptom Complex of TH Deficiency
Children	Otitis media
Young women	Contact allergy, Menstrual pain
Young men	Contact allergy, acne vulgaris, mumps
Menopausal women	Internal Heat (vasomotor disorders, hot flushes) and obesity

Table 13

All these symptoms and lesions manifest differently but have their origin in TH Deficiency. All are due to the same imbalance and stimulation of the same acupoint can treat all these cases. To tonify TH Qi, one could use the classical Mother Point (Wood - TH03), or the Source Point (TH04), or really almost any point on TH Channel.

When Lesion-Symptom Complexes vary so much in humans, they clearly can vary even more in animals. Huge variation in and between the many different species of animals relates to different uses and adaptations for each species, each of which has its own specialized Weak Structure. For example, TH Channel Deficiency manifests as:

Animal	Usual Lesion-Symptom Complex of TH Deficiency
Puppies	Infection around the mouth
Older dogs	Dry eczema, outer ear infection (otitis externa), furunculosis
Horses	Hoof-crack, weak fetlocks and tenderness in the back, especially between the 17th rib and L3
Mares	Changes of behavior (nymphomania) and disorders of estrus (heat)
Cows	Mastitis, as described earlier

Table 14

However, careful study shows that human owners or handlers often transfer their own Process Imbalance to their animals. The animals may then develop Lesion-Symptom Complexes related to their owners' Imbalances. This often occurs in psychiatry and in parent-child relationships. Often, the disorders of a child are nothing but the disorders of the parents, though in a very transformed fashion. The same applies concerning human animal relationships, especially in the energetic or etheric areas.

Animals as sentient beings

Animals probably have highly developed feelings (as developed, or even more highly developed or containing different feelings than humans), and this is an extremely important part of animal behavior and disease. The owner and the veterinarian often overlook or at least underestimate the sentient ability of animals. These feelings are the reason for the above-described relationship between humans and animals. There is also evidence that some animals, especially dogs and cats, dream. Usually we admit that animals have feelings like fear and aggression but many researchers believe that animals have the whole range of feelings, just like humans do, maybe even more. These include feelings like sorrow, joy, depression, elation, grief, compassion, melancholy, longing etc. They may even have feelings that we do not understand or cannot imagine, since we may not have the full range of animal feelings.

I have often observed how the emotions of the keeper or stable-girl have influenced the animals through the whole day. Many farmers report that the frequency of mastitis increases when they have weekend-help in the barn. It can be very stressful for cows to be milked by an unknown and insensitive person. The stress reaction can precipitate immunosuppression, which can allow mastitis to arise.

I have noted that a change of staff or riders often is associated with decreased performance in thoroughbred horses. This is especially marked when the former staff or riders had a close and good relationship with the horses and maybe even worked overtime to make life easier for the horses. I have noted a long-lasting decrease in racing ability, and more infections and injuries, when staff that is much tougher or heavy handed replace good staff.

I will, to demonstrate the advanced sensitivity of the animals, cite the following

Two examples from my practice;

- A Norwegian horse was to be sold in Germany. At home it showed no lameness and was a very stable and friendly horse. But as soon as it arrived in Germany it became lame, got bruises, wounds and other serious problems. It was not sold. Accidentally, I was in the area and had the opportunity to treat the horse. In investigating the animal with the help of Pulse Diagnosis, I found the energy in the HT meridian to be almost zero. The horse showed severe signs of sorrow, knowing it was to be sold. I treated the HT meridian, and the horse changed radically, and all the problems vanished like dew to the sun. As the owner realized this connection, she immediately took the horse home again to Norway.

- Another horse was to be sold, and it had been free of problems for a long time, but as it was examined in Oslo it showed severe lameness in several legs. It was sent back to Sandefjord, where I live, and I found a severe Qi deficiency in the HT meridian (via Pulse Diagnosis), which led to a decreased blood circulation in the front legs. The horse had mourned being sold, and developed what we by humans call a bruised and broken heart. The horse was treated, and all the problems disappeared quickly.

I have also noticed that noise from fans, bad smell from manure, humidity due to bad ventilation, irregular feeding and careless husbandry, highly influence meat or milk quality,

In the more relaxed and easygoing days, the old farmers in the West of Ireland had a saying "Look after your animals and they will look after you". Compassion towards animals involves treating animals as individuals, treating them with respect, dignity, patience, gentleness and kindness. It also involves close physical contact (massaging, scratching and rubbing the animals), talking and singing to them, and *playing with them.* Today, these aspects of animal care are not taken as seriously as they should be. The reasons for this are multiple. One reason is that modern labor is scarce and expensive. One worker must handle many more animals today than was the case in the past. Therefore, animal handlers do not have the time to get to know the individual natures, likes and dislikes of their animals. Even if they do know, they cannot, or will not, take the time to cater for individual needs or preferences in their animals.

Another important factor is that quantity rather than quality is the measure of animal productivity today. This is not so obvious in pork meat (even though many studies show the relationship between stress and meat quality) as in the objectively recorded race times in horses. Race times certainly decrease in stressed animals.

Chapter 2

DIAGNOSTIC METHODS

Diagnosis is the recognition of the nature, location and extent of disease, especially of the factors that are involved in, or cause, its expression. Thus, if we want to understand why an animal is diseased, for example why it suffers from recurrent infections in the paws or itchy eczema, we must know what we seek and where to look for it. As discussed in several places in this book, *the root cause of disease is due to imbalance of the vital energetic Processes* (the Process Imbalance, or Imbalanced Inner Function). External or Internal Stressors can precipitate the Process Imbalance, and many different Process Imbalances can manifest as Lesion-Symptom Complexes in the Weak Structures.

The cause of the disease usually manifests in the way that the Lesion-Symptom Complex presents itself. But, to recognize the cause, we must recognize the external and internal clues. In order to do this, we must know the clues (what it is that we seek), where to look, or which door to open. People in many civilizations and cultures were aware of this through the ages. For example:

- The Bible say: "Seek and ye shall find; knock and it shall be opened unto ye".

- Medieval mystics said that the seeker that knew the sought would find it and see it even if it was hidden in the spiritual worlds. True clairvoyance requires that one must know what one seeks.

- Goethe's phrase "eine offenbare Geheimnis" = "an obvious secret" or as he also said: all hidden phenomena manifest in the revealed, expressed the same idea.

This applies also for diagnosis of human and animal diseases. The Lesion-Symptom Complexes reveal both the Stressor that made it appear and the Process Imbalances; we only must know what to look for. A correct diagnosis is 90 % of the work; for those with a good training in holistic therapy, the rest is plain sailing.

Correct diagnosis of the Deficient Process Imbalance is essential for effective treatment

Correct diagnosis of the Stressor is essential for correct etiology and effective prophylactic work

For effective therapy, it is of the utmost importance to find the Primary Deficient Process and to stimulate it. In KI-deficiency, we may consult

- A herbal dictionary (or see below) to find a KI-stimulating herb, or

- An AP textbook (or see below) to find KI-stimulating points or zones

- KI-stimulating diets or remedies.

But if our diagnosis (i.e. our identification of the Primary Deficient Process) is wrong, all the remedies or points in the world will be of little help. We must expect poor results if we fail to help the deficient Process, or just treat symptomatically, or just focus our treatment on the Weak Structure.

Of course it can be helpful to **combine causal and symptomatic treatment**, i.e. to treat the cause of the disease (the deficient Process) and the secondary excessive process (with pain and tensions) and the Lesion-Symptom Complex (Weak Structure and/

or the manifestations of the disease). Sometimes, especially in serious or life-threatening conditions, it is necessary to combine these approaches. Therefore, some ways to treat the most common symptoms are listed below after each method of therapy.

Chronic diarrhea improves with a "contracting" remedy like "Cortex Querqus", or a chronic BL infection improves with the herb "Uva Ursi". But we can expect only temporary symptomatic relief from any other therapy if we fail to identify and correct the deficient Process, the real underlying cause of the disease that called forth the Lesion-Symptom Complex.

A very strong Stressor may precipitate a Lesion-Symptom Complex **without** a pre-existing Process Imbalance, or may cause a Process Imbalance directly. If we sit outside in the cold all night in the Norwegian winter, we will probably catch pneumonia, even if we have an excellent Qi balance. An extreme Stressor can precipitate many diseases. Then we may treat this disease with symptomatic remedies, or just give western symptomatic treatment like antibiotics. Sometimes, such diseases auto-cure and remain cured without direct intervention by a therapist. For example, the body's Wei Qi, or homeostatic mechanisms can dispel some diseases without any direct treatment.

We must look for deeper causes of the disorder when a Lesion-Symptom Complex recurs over and over, or becomes chronic, or is induced by just a moderate Stressor. In such cases we need good methods to be able to find this cause, the pre-existing Process Imbalance.

Homeopathic case taking (repertorizing) may suggest an effective remedy without suggesting a diagnosis from the viewpoint of western pathology or TCM diagnosis. In other words, in homeopathy the correct remedy (the perfect match for the symptoms and Modifying Factors) is considered the correct diagnosis. We talk about a Silica case, a Sulphur case etc. However, this approach makes it impossible to be able to recognize the deeper and causal origin of the disease. If we want to prevent further disease, it is of utmost importance that we recognize the primary Qi imbalance, or primary cause of the disease. Depending on the cause, we may need to prescribe a change of diet, change of sleeping place, change of work etc.

2 main types of symptoms

It is, as I have said several times, very important to differentiate between to main types of symptoms, which is:

1. *Symptoms that come from a deficiency*
2. *Symptoms that comes from an excess*

What we *don't learn to see* are symptoms that come from a deficiency.
What we *don't learn to see* are symptoms that are numb.
What we *don't learn to see* are symptoms that are cold and painless.

What we usually learn to se is symptoms that come from an excess.
What we usually learn to se is symptoms that are painful.
What we usually learn to se is symptoms that are warm and tender.

Symptoms that originate from an excess are usually acute, traumatic and painful. They have Yang-character, and they usually show up within a Yang-process or along a Yang-meridian. Such symptoms are primary in all primary traumas, but in all chronic diseases they are usually secondary.

Symptoms that originate in or from a deficiency are usually chronic. They have Yin-characteristics, and usually they show up within a Yin process. Such symptoms are primary in all chronic diseases.

If we are able to find this type of symptoms, we will be able to find the primary deficiency in most cases.

If not, we may from the more easily observe excessive Yang-symptoms deduce where the primary energetic deficiency is from the table at page 61.

*Of course, it is no problem/hindrance to treat **both** the deficient cause of the disease, **and** the excessive symptom, even at the same time. I will though add here a very important observation; if we treat the deficient cause correctly, the excess energy in the symptoms will, in a matter of seconds, flow directly to the deficient process. Then it is usually not necessary to treat the excessive symptom, if we treat the deficiency correctly. But, if we don't treat the deficiency correctly, it might take some time until the excesses and pain is resolved, and then it might be correct to also treat the excess according to symptomatic treatment.*

Therefore I have, after each chapter, added a list of symptomatic treatment according to symptoms and diagnoses.

*Chronic diarrhea will always be better if we add a constricting remedy like the bark of the oak, finely powdered of course. A chronic infection of the urinary tract will always be better if we give the patient bearberry (Arctostaphylos Uva Ursi). **But if we don't find the cause of the disease, and treat the energetic deficiency, all therapy will be temporary.***

Within homeopathic diagnosing, (repertorizing), we may find the right remedy (causal treatment) without having to make a "correct" diagnosis, as the correct diagnosis within homeopathy is the name of the correct remedy, (a silica-case, a sulphur-case).

*But going this way will not make us able to **realize** the true weakness of the animal or patient, the true weak process. This is important in my opinion, as we then will not be able to prevent further disease in different ways as changing the diet, the work, the sleeping place, the clothing and so on.*

4 levels of making a diagnosis

Following this there are in my opinion 4 main levels or levels to make a correct diagnosis:

- Observation of the symptoms and lesions
    - ° Of the deficient processes
    - ° Of the excessive processes
- Observation of the reflex and sensitive zones
    - ° Of the deficient processes
    - ° Of the excessive processes
- Observation of the Modifications
    - ° Of the deficient processes
    - ° Of the excessive processes
- Direct observation
    - ° Of the deficient processes
    - ° Of the excessive processes

1. Noting the symptoms and lesions (see page 98)

A	In what order did they appear	Important for diagnosis by the 12 Processes
B	How the symptoms appear	Important for which Command Point (Element/Phase) to use, or which remedy to choose
C	Where they appear	Important for a Channel diagnosis. Important to find the correct microcosm (ECIWO)

Table 15

We also ought to differentiate between:

- The Process Imbalance.

- The Stressors that precipitate the disease.

- The Weak Structure of the animal.

It is very important to remember that the symptoms usually are expressions of the excessive reflections of the underlying deficient process. Usually the obvious and painful symptoms are related to the following Yang-process in the Ko-cycle (see page 28).

2. Noting the reflex and sensitive zones (see page 103)

Noting the reflex zones and the sensitivity in the acupoints (especially the Back-Shu and Front-Mu Points) may give important information to the diagnosis. This relates especially to Zone Therapy, AP, auriculomedicine and Ear-AP.

The reflex zones, especially the Shu-points, are situated on Yang Channels, and thus show areas of excess. As the origin of most diseases are deficient Processes, we then have to consider which process is in deficiency, and then stimulate this special Process. The deficient process is usually the Ko-father.

Symptom-carrying meridian	Deficient cause of the symptoms
Gall Bladder	Lung
Liver	Lung
Heart	Kidney
Small Intestine	Kidney
Pericardium	Kidney
Triple Heather	Kidney
Spleen	Liver
Stomach	Liver
Lung	Heart
Large Intestine	Heart
Kidney	Spleen or Heart
Bladder	Spleen or Heart

**Table 16; shows the probable deficient origin
in excessive Yang-conditions.**

3. Noting the Modifications (see page 151)

Noting the Modifications means how and when the Lesion-Symptom Complex varies. This may tell a lot about which

- Stressors and which
- Deficient Process

Are the cause of the symptoms.

The Modifications, by the individuality of their appearance, then often show the real cause of the problem, the deficient Process. These observations are of special importance in AP and homeopathy.

4. Direct observation (see page 163)

Direct observation of the Stressors (precipitating factors) and Process Imbalances may also be of great importance. By direct observation, we mean sensing the energy imbalance directly through our subjective, emotional, or intuitive skills.

Note for professional therapists: In this book, I stress the need for unconventional methods of diagnosis. These methods are essential to determine the primary energetic imbalance – the Imbalanced Process. However, veterinarians must NOT use these methods INSTEAD of conventional diagnostic methods; they should use them IN ADDITION TO conventional methods. Veterinarians who overlook a Western diagnosis (such as a definite endocrine or neoplastic condition because they have neglected to use standard diagnostic tests do themselves, their profession and their patients a great disservice. They also leave themselves open to a charge of professional negligence, which may be upheld in court).

It is most important that we exercise our subjective skills in observing the cause of disease directly, as discussed above. This elevates our sensitivity and develops our extrasensory skills. In this way we have great opportunities to develop as diagnosticians and clinicians. There are many methods for direct observation, such as Pulse Diagnosis, Iris Diagnosis and methods where the therapist can feel or "see" things that are hidden or difficult for others to see. Unfortunately, such methods are open to fraudulent exploitation and all types of charlatanism. However, extrasensory diagnostic methods are of such importance and interest that I will describe one of the better-known methods, namely the Pulse Diagnosis. This is a method that I use with good success (see page 164). On page 180 I will describe several other ways to develop a higher level of diagnostic sensitivity.

It is of course no problem in both treating the deficient cause of the symptoms, the excessive meridian, the painful area and the symptoms themselves. Sometimes it will even be beneficial to combine therapy of all these levels.

*Chronic diarrhoea will be better with pulverized oak, and a chronic cystitis will be better with tee made from Uva Ursi. **But without the treatment of the deficient cause, all therapy will only be symptomatic.***

Within homeopathic diagnosis, repertorizing, we may arrive at the right remedy without having to make a correct diagnosis, as the remedy IS the correct diagnosis in homeopathy.

*But along this way it is impossible to **really understand** the weak process of the patient. This is of the utmost importance if we shall be able to prevent further problems by change in diet, air, sleeping-place, and work or by any other means.*

Before we will go into depth with the description of the 4 methods described above, it is important that we learn to recognize the 12 processes in their pathological aspect.

Thus we will start with the description of this.

The pathology of the 12 Fundamental Processes

TCM theory and its methods of classifying natural phenomena are of great clinical value in my practice of veterinary medicine and human healing.

If, as in allopathic medicine, we focus on local symptoms, we must consider hundreds of possibilities in clinical diagnosis. However, if we use holistic fundamental principles and focus on finding the Process Imbalance, we reduce to a minimum the number of variable disease factors to be considered.

Now we must choose the thinking process, within which we want to work. We may reduce the Processes of the body to a minimum, for example two, the anabolic or building Processes and the catabolic or lytic Processes. We could then categorize all diseases into one of these two Processes or categories and then give a general remedy to stimulate one Process in Deficiency states (e.g. Sulphur to increase anabolism) and the other Process in Excess states (e.g. salt to increase catabolism). Alternatively, we may consider 4 Processes, after the Four Elements of ancient Greco-European medical philosophy. In that philosophy, too much or too little of Fire, Earth, Water or Air was the triggering factors for disease.

We may in fact divide the Bodily Processes in 1, 2, 3, 4, 5, 7, 9 or 12. There are even systems that operate with 54 variable Processes. We must find and use classifications that fit best with our thinking processes and knowledge. Above all, those classifications must help us to find the best methods to diagnose and treat holistically. For thousands of years, TCM has classified 12 Fundamental (main) Processes in the organism. It used those 12 Processes diagnostically and therapeutically. Each of these Processes relates to a multitude of different phenomena, including the zodiac signs, different plants, states of mind, days in the week, muscles and also, as we shall see later, specific Channel-Organ Systems. Ancient oriental knowledge, especially TCM theory, has been especially helpful in my clinical practice with humans and animals. The following part describes how the Processes of the 12 Process work in the organism in relation to pathology, in deficiency and in excess as well as in destructive energy.

TCM classifies bodily Processes into those that mainly involve **Substance** (Material, Yin) and those that mainly involve **Process** (Immaterial or Energetic, Yang). There can be no Yin without Yang, no substance without function. There can be no function without substance, no Yang without Yin.

THE 12 MAIN PROCESSES ARE:

YIN PROCESS		PHASE		YANG PROCESS
Lung	LU	Metal	LI	Large Intestine
Spleen	SP	Earth	ST	Stomach
Heart	HT	Fire	SI	Small Intestine
Kidney	KI	Water	BL	Bladder
Pericardium	PC	Fire	TH	Tripel Heather
Liver	LV	Wood	GB	Gall Bladder

Table 17

These processes may be classified as:

    ° **6 Yin Substantial**

    ° **6 Yang Functional**

- **Yin Substantial Processes** are more materially based (bound to the body); they give more visible Lesion-Symptom Complexes, such as infections, exudations, excretions, etc. They are the most important Processes, in non-human animals. They are the most organ bound, dynamic and energy giving. They are more important in veterinary medicine (i.e. in animals) than the Yang Functional Processes. This contrasts with human medicine, where the Yang Processes are more important than in animals.

- **Yang Functional Processes** are more immaterial; they govern the material functions and give more non-physical symptoms like anger, pain, etc. They govern, or direct biological processes; they regulate and divide. Without government or regulation from the Yang Processes, the Yin Processes would overflow the organism totally. Therefore the Yang Processes are more linked or bound to the psyche and they are conscious or subconscious controlling processes. Such processes are thus much more important in the humans.

All the Processes may be found in the following three variants:

- In excess (usually in Yang-processes with painful symptoms, usually secondary to deficient Yin-processes).

- In deficiency (usually in Yin-processes with failing functions as the main symptoms, also usually with the compensating Yang-functions in excess).

- As destructive energy (may be present in both Yin- and in Yang-processes).

NOTE: *It is important to remember that painful symptoms or conditions usually point to a deeper deficiency. If you decide to diagnose by the help of painful areas, SHU-points or muscles, please remember to make sure if not:*

- *The Yin-Ko-father is in deficiency. If so, this deficiency must be treated if a lasting amelioration shall be obtained.*

- *The paired process is in excess.*

- *The symptoms derive from destructive energy (perverse energy). Such energy must be deleted and not recycled in the energetic system of the body.*

It is very important to remember that symptoms originating from a deficiency in a Yin-process may give quite similar symptoms as from the same process in excess.

1. LU-Lung Processes and gas exchange

LU is the Yin Process (Mate of LI) in the Metal Phase. The main Process of the LU is to connect us to the surrounding world, put us in contact with the world. Physiologically it also dominates Qi, controls respiration, dominates dispersing and descending, dominates skin and hair, and regulates the water passages. The LU Process dominates not only the lung organ, but also the anatomical structures belonging to the "lower airway" (pulmonary blood vessels and capillaries, alveoli, bronchioles, bronchi) and the "upper airway" (trachea, larynx, tonsils, the connections to the inner ear, the nose and nasal sinuses).

In both TCM and western medicine, one of the functions of LU is to direct respiration (gaseous exchange) and purify the Blood (expel Toxic Air, or carbon dioxide). LU Yang Process (inhalation) takes in the Vital Air (oxygen, O_2); LU Yin Process (exhalation) expels the Toxic Air (CO_2). This vital relationship between LU, HT and Blood occurs via gaseous exchange.

The Process also helps to control blood pH; respiratory acidosis can arise in lung failure, or severe pneumonia. Gaseous exchange depends on balanced Process between HT, LU and Blood. But TCM also attributes to LU the action of developing a Vital Qi from this exchange, similar to the intake of caloric energy via the gastrointestinal tract.

A *deficiency* in the lung-process may express itself as:

- Eczema, especially dry

- Exhaustion, especially after running or races

- Asthma, dust allergy

- Chronic infections of the respiratory tract

- Dandruff and dry scaling of the skin

- Lameness in the front-feet, especially in horses

- Elbow-arthrosis, especially in dogs

- Tension between the right wing of the Atlas and the Occiput

- PRA in dogs (Progressive Retinal Atrophy)

- Lung bleeding

- Claustrophobia

- General tendency to painful conditions

An *excess* of the lung-process may express itself as:

- Pressure in the chest

- Great endurance

A *destructive energy* may give the following symptoms:

- Fear

- Deep infections of the skin

LU and LI play a critical role in the health and function of the skin and hair. LU Excess may thicken the hair of the head (KI controls the head hair) and body. Other symptoms of LU Excess may include a full pulse, heat in the upper body and a difficult and sonorous respiration. In contrast, LU Deficiency may produce short and thin hair. Other symptoms of LU Deficiency may include an Empty pulse and dyspnoea with a weak respiration.

The patho-psychological aspect of the lung in deficiency is claustrophobia, fear of the outer world, in which the lungs purpose is to introduce the entity. In excess there are no special psychological symptoms that I have observed.

All people (patients) can help themselves by doing the following exercise for 10 minutes twice a day; press the right nostril down during inspiration, and press the left nostril down during expiration through the nose (shut the mouth).

A deficient LU Process often tends to create excessive states in the GB Process.

2. LI-Large Intestine Processes

LI is the Yang Process of the Metal Phase. The main Processes of LI are to receive the waste material sent down from SI, absorb its fluid content, and form the remainder into feces to be excreted. Pathological changes of LI lead to dysfunction in this transportation Process, resulting in loose stools or constipation. As in the case of most organs, LI also has a role unknown to western medicine. TCM is unique in recognizing painful conditions that appear along the course of the Channels. Painful areas along LI Channel correspond to the shoulder and arms (se page 263). Pain in these areas often indicates an excessive pathological state of LI, usually with the origin in a deficient HT or PC. Parasitism and inflammatory bowel disease are examples of such disease states. Remember that also KI may be either in excess or deficiency like-wise the LI, as the KI often dominate the last part of LI, the Rectum.

LI is a main depository of Qi; its functioning is crucial to an ample supply of Qi to the body. A very old energetic procedure is to stand with the anus facing the rising sun. It is said to give energy to the entire body.

An excessive state of the LI Process is often combined with a deficiency of any of the Yin Fire processes, which are HT and PC.

A *deficiency* in the large intestine-process may express itself as:

- Diarrhea or constipation

- Elevated hematocrit by the horse (thick blood, see commentary on this page)

- Furunculosis around the nose in dogs, puppy-furunculosis

- Stiff shoulder muscles, especially subclavius muscle

- Lameness in the front feet

- Eczema

- Chronic infections of the respiratory tract

- Dandruff and dry scaling of the skin

An *excess* of the large intestine-process may express itself as:

- Pressure in the lower stomach

- Strong and lasting diarrhea

- Pain around the shoulder and lower neck

- Headache

A *destructive energy* may give the following symptoms:

- Bloody diarrhea

- Deep infections of the skin of the face

Commentary on the diagnosis "thick blood", a Scandinavian myth.

Overtraining or *"unexplainable lowering of the stamina syndrome" may be defined as; long standing (even after 2 weeks of rest) unexplainable (without a serious disease) lowered stamina, which appear in horses that have been trained quite hard without periods of rest. The diagnosis often includes behavioral problems.*

Main cause; *too much training,too little rest. Another factor is stress; too many competitions and transportations, muscular pain and tensions, mental stress and inadequate feeding. This may strongly add to the development of "overtraining". Over time overtraining will lead to changes in the nervous system and change the behavior of the horse. Neither in humans nor in horses have any standard changes or factors in the blood been found.*

During the last 40 years veterinarians in Sweden and Norway have thought or believed that the main causative factor in overtraining is production of too many red blood cells. This is actually a paradox, as science very well knows that there is a link between blood volume, the number of red blood cells and the aerobic capacity in both humans as in horses. Further it has never been shown that athletes have produced too much red blood cells due to overtraining. The production of red blood cells is a fine tuned process governed by the hormone erythropoietin (EPO). This hormone is controlled through a negative feedback system, and in scientific investigations it is shown that strong training or overtraining never has led to elevated concentration of EPO in the horse. In several long term studies of horses in hard training it is clearly shown that too many red blood cells do not lead to decreased stamina in horses that are "over trained"!

Diagnoses; *there is no help in blood tests or muscle biopsies. The diagnosis is based upon the fact that over trained horses show decreased stamina over several weeks although training is reduced. Horses that are better after two weeks get the diagnosis "over-extending", which of course may be an early stage of "overtraining".*

3. ST-Stomach Processes

ST is the Yang Process in the Earth Phase. The main Process of ST is to receive, contain and decompose food. Food enters the mouth, passes through the esophagus, and is received by ST where it is decomposed and transmitted down to SI. In this way it provides the organism with the Qi needed to provide nutrient energy. This Qi provides more than the total digestible energy measured by western medicine, but also the specific Qi of each Process. After ST completes its digestive Process, the purified Qi derived from the digestive tract is sent to SP by the help of TH.

A Process Imbalance in ST can manifest in several combinations of symptoms, depending on whether the Process Imbalance is ST Excess or ST Deficiency. ST Excess manifests as pain, hyperacidity, heartburn or fullness; ST Deficiency manifests with opposite symptoms – hypoacidity, poor digestion and loss of appetite.

A *deficiency* in the stomach-process may express itself as:

- Eczema on the stomach

- General lack of energy

- Loss of appetite

- Poor digestion and hypoacidity

- Depression and melancholy

- Lameness of the back feet due to shortening of the stride

An *excess* of the stomach-process may express itself as:

- Pain in the stomach due to hyperacidity

- Angina, pain in the heart region

- Pain in the quadriceps muscle

- Manic behavior

- Brest-cancer in both women and dogs

A *destructive energy* may give the following symptoms:

- Aggression

- Bleeding stomach ulcer

- Cancer of the breast

An important function of the stomach process is to receive a significant part of cosmic Qi. Ancient Chinese texts rarely refer to this form of energy. In order to understand this aspect of Qi one must refer to texts from India or from Rudolf Steiner. For an organism to properly digest and assimilate food they need to possess an ample amount of Gu Qi (Qi derived from digestion) as well as a supply of cosmic Qi. This type of Qi is derived from the universe and enters the body via conduits at the apex of the skull (at GV20, Baihui, Hundred Meetings). Some authors theorize that the presence of horns in cloven-hoofed animals (usually ruminants) actually act as receivers of such Qi allowing effective digestion and assimilation of fibrous foods that monogastric animals find relatively indigestible. Personal experience, and reports from farmers, supports these theories, as cows often suffer from digestive disorders after dehorning. (Needles and moxa at ST36 and SP03 or SP06 can treat patients suffering from cosmic Qi Deficiency).

The Earth Phase, of which ST is the Yang part, relates to the emotion of worry or obsession, which stress may precipitate. Treating ST is important in the treatment protocol for patients suffering from excessive worry and the wish to die, including gastric and duodenal ulcers. ST Deficiency is one cause of vertigo and treatment of ST often helps patients with vertigo.

Excess in the ST Process often have its origin in a deficient SP- or LV Process.

4. SP-Spleen Pancreas Processes and the rhythms of digestion

SP is the Yin Process (Mate of ST) in the Earth Phase. The main Processes of SP are to maintain the different rhythms of the organism. An important symptom of SP Deficiency is that the different symptoms are related to rhythms in a certain way. Either they appear in a certain frequency, or they are connected to the disappearance of rhythms. It is then interesting to note that after splenectomy (removal of the spleen), the patient has to eat in a much more rhythmical manner to avoid further complications.

Further the SP controls transportation and transformation, controls Blood, dominates the muscles and limbs, opens into the mouth and manifests on the lips. SP Processes include pancreatic Processes. Diabetes, a disease manifestation of the pancreas, can be a result of either a Process Imbalance in SP or LV. LV may be involved due to its role in glycogen metabolism, and also as the husband of the Spleen.

A *deficiency* in the spleen-process may express itself as:

- Eczema

- Exhaustion

- Asthma

- Chronic infections of the respiratory tract

- Dandruff and dry scaling of the skin

- Decreased function of iliopsoas muscle

- Recurrent Mediterranean fever

- Stomach ulcer

  - In humans we often find a deficiency in the spleen and an excess in the stomach

  - In dogs we often find a kidney in deficiency and a stomach in excess

  - In the horse we often find a lung in deficiency and a stomach in excess

An *excess* of the spleen-process may express itself as:

- Kidney-problems due to the controlling action of SP to the KI

- Cramps in the stomach

- Colic

A *destructive energy* may give the following symptoms:

- Painful colic

- Bloody stools or vomit

Digestion: Although digestion is a Yang function, SP, a Yin organ, plays an important role in this Process. This can be justified by the fact that Yin produces Yang. SP Process Imbalance often manifests at the root of the tongue, another example of how SP relates closely with digestion. The Neijing says: *"when SP is full, solid and fluid, food is digested; skin and flesh (connective tissues) are oily. If the spleen is empty, the body becomes thin, the extremities are not lifted and the navel stands out. It is hard to live, easy to die. The mouth is bluish black".* The Neijing further states, *"As long as you can rely on SP functioning well, you can eat and drink as much as you like. But excessive fatigue or exertion can hurt SP Qi. When SP and ST Qi are injured, food can no longer be assimilated and the mouth does not sense tastes any more. The extremities become weak; the epigastrium is full; there is expectoration and diarrhea and the intestines are filled up".*

Blood and immunity: A main function of SP is to control blood and to keep it in the vessels. This refers to both blood that surges through the vessels and the blood that makes up one's Yin Qi. This is why SP is called the "House of Blood". SP function also involves the reticuloendothelial system. This system covers all the connective tissue in the body and consequently controls the function of the immune system. (As we shall see later on, Xue Hai (Sea of Blood, SP10) is an important acupoint for blood disorders and allergies).

Digestion of thoughts and ideas: SP controls reflective thought or intention (Yi); it "digests and regurgitates" ideas and is involved with the cognitive aspects of thinking and intelligence. An Imbalanced SP (or KI) Process can lead to obsession, worry (interminable "looping" of thought without the possibility of constructive action) and inability to decide.

Growth: The Neijing also says that SP influences growth directly. Although SP depends on sugar, large amounts harm SP Qi; the same applies to LV, the Husband of SP. SP and LV-meridians (See page 426) run close together on the lower extremity as they both follow the Vena saphena (the great saphenous vein), and pain caused by these two Channels has similar locations (apart from the branch that LV Channel sends to the genitals which follow the superficial external pudendal artery and vein). One must use other diagnostic methods to differentiate which meridian causes such pain.

Depression is the pathopsychological aspect of SP.

I have cured many patients with SP-Deficiency just by asking them to concentrate on rhythms, live and eat rhythmically, listen to rhythmical music etc. This approach usually works well. The color of the excretions may indicate a SP Process Imbalance, as they usually are yellow. The yellow color may also be used to tonify SP. A middle-aged woman, an acknowledged painter in south Norway, was especially famous for her yellow pictures. I treated her for a digestive problem, and after I had corrected the imbalance in her SP Qi, her complaints disappeared. After some months she returned in anger and despair. She told me that after I had corrected her SP Qi, she was unable to paint her yellow pictures any more. Her art had been a self-curing attempt, and when she was well, she did not need this activity any more. Much of what we do **instinctively** is aimed at restoring our balance. Finally, ingestion of beef or rye may be used to tonify SP.

A deficiency in the SP Process will often lead to excessive and painful conditions in the BL Process.

The spleen, the kidneys, the liver and the lungs may dominate the skin. Deficiency in the different processes may give the following changes in the skin;

- *Spleen deficiency*; the hairy coat gets a dirty, not shiny impression

- *Kidney deficiency*; dandruff, losing hairs, thin hairy coat

- *Liver deficiency*; fatty impression

- *Lung deficiency*; dry impression

5. HT-Heart Processes and arterial blood circulation

HT is the most dominant Yin Process of the entire Fire Phase. HT is the solid organ, Yin, and SI is its coupled hollow organ, Yang. The main Process of HT is to dominate the Blood and vessels.

HT manifests on the face, houses the mind, and opens into the tongue. Both HT and PC regulate the circulatory aspects of physiology. While HT is involved in the physical movement (including the mechanical pumping) of blood, PC covers all other aspects of circulation.

*Here I must add a consideration on what really makes the blood flow. The human heart has an effect of 1,7 watt, and this is of course way too little to drive or push a large amount of blood cells and fluid (5 litres) through an enormous network of tiny vessels, often as small as one single red blood cell. If we then consider the fact, usually unknown to most, that in so called bypass-operations (the heart is eliminated from the circulation) then the blood flow is **faster and larger** than if/when the heart was connected to the entire circulation. That death occurs when the heart for some reason stops, is of course due to the fact that the valves in the heart stop the blood if the heart is not beating. If we make an obstruction to a water pipe, the water will stop even if the water pipe is not the driving force.*

This indicates that there are other forces that make the blood flow in the veins, and that the heart is only there to regulate the flow. If this force is connected to the vessels themselves, the electric field or the blood itself will not be discussed here, but it is this totality of flow we will have in mind when we talk about the process of the heart.

HT and PC control the spirit and social intelligence (EQ) of humans. HT represents the same function in ruling and coordinating within the organism as the emperor does in the state. HT is considered the most important organ in TCM, acting as the supreme controller of the entire organism. Due to its important role, one may observe within acupuncture that all the other Channel systems protect HT against pernicious influences.

HT also houses the *Spirit (in Chinese it is called the Shen)*. This is considered the consciousness (and vitality) of an entity.

HT has a direct action on body temperature. Its fullness causes hyperthermia, with a feeling of excessive Heat (Heat and Excess). Its emptiness causes hypothermia, with a feeling of Cold (Cold and Deficiency).

The symptoms can also be quite serious as a consequence of deformation of the heart itself or its valves (the heart as an organ, not as a process), and not functioning, as it should. All types of heart problems as deformation of the valves, "hole in the heart" (patent foramen ovale, Foramen ovale persistens) and other valvular defects are all symptoms on a deficient heart. Decreased stamina, heavy breathing and general depression may also be symptoms of a deficient heart. Also in the patients where there are specific and anatomical problems, as valvular degenerations, I have, believe it or not, often had excellent results. I have seen (heard) heart murmurs completely disappear after just one treatment with acupuncture.

A typical symptom in horses with a heart deficiency is that they perform a good race, but in the last part of the race they fall back and get tired. The horse don't breed, there is no lameness, but the acceleration just disappears.

Often such problems have started with;

- Extreme strain (hard races)

- Congenital heart failure (in dogs)

- Psychological reasons (they are sold, separated from their mother, lost a friend)

Extreme strain may lead to what we in old times called a "broken heart".

Congenital heart failure is of course always a cause we have to consider, but the third cause is quite new for most people (psychological reasons). Quite often, when the horse is sold, or separated from its friends by death, divorce and other causes, the horse will suffer sorrow, and this sorrow will weaken the heart. The same as in humans after a breakup in a relationship; "his heart was broken", "the heart was close to being broken", "she broke his heart" and so on. Likewise, a chronic lack of love leads to a heart deficiency, as in women with a loveless marriage. In humans often women suffer from this condition, but in horses this is more common in stallions, who suffer extremely by being separated from the mares.

The process of the heart is circulating love.

A *deficiency* in the heart-process may express itself as:

- Coldness in the limbs
- Exhaustion after hard work or races by horses
- Reduced endurance
- Asthma, due to poor blood-circulation in the lungs
- Pain in the joints, chronic deformation of joints
- Sorrow, depression and lack of joy
- Heart-dysfunction
- Changes in the blood-values
- Anemia

An *excess* of the heart-process may express itself as:

- Pressure in the chest

A *destructive energy* may give the following symptoms:

- Strong pain all over the body

The symptoms may also be more severe, due to the fact that the heart itself (the organ) may not function, as it should. Heavy breathing, low stamina and a general depression can be symptoms to consider in HT Qi Deficiency. Such symptoms may develop after extreme hard work, or they may even have been congenital. Less important symptoms may have just an energy deficiency as the cause, often due to chronic lack of love. The Process of HT is warmth, circulating warmth as in love. The color of the symptoms be it wounds, infected mucosal membranes, urine or joint fluid is red, and all lesions bleed easily.

The pathopsychological symptom of HT is loneliness, the opposite of love.

The two extremes of the Process (Yin & Yang).

As regards HT Process, it may show its pathology as two opposites, either as a decreased or an accelerated blood circulation. In the horse we usually see the pathological version of a decreased circulation, and in dogs we usually see the version with an accelerated circulation. The same principle applies to all Processes – they may manifest pathology by a decreased or increased activity of their basic functions.

6. SI-Small Intestine Processes and digestion

SI is the Yang Coupled Process of HT in the Fire Phase. The main Processes of SI are to receive and digest. SI receives and further digests the food from ST, separates the clear from the turbid, and absorbs Essential Substances (Essence), and some water from the food, transmitting the residue of the food to LI, and that of the water to BL. Since SI includes the Process of separating the clear from the turbid, dysfunction may not only influence digestion, but also give rise to an abnormal bowel movement and disturbance of urination. Anatomically, the functional aspects of SI include the jejunum, ileum and the duodenum.

A *deficiency* in the small intestine-process may express itself as:

- Chronic diarrhea
- Reduction of weight

An *excess* of the small intestine-process may express itself as:

- Pain in the area of the Scapula

A *destructive energy* may give the following symptoms:

- Severe colic and pain in the stomach
- Bleeding from the intestines

In TCM, as Neijing states, it "presides over the division of food into solids and liquids. It sends the liquids to KI and the solids to LI. It separates the pure from the impure", i.e. the pure Qi is sent to SP and then into the Qi Flow system. The impure part goes to BL and LI (colon). The latter milieu is further separated in order to send even more pure Qi to SP. The final by-product is then excreted. Decreased absorption of food is a pathological sign of SI Qi Deficiency; malnutrition and diarrhea may follow. Like HT Process, SI Process dominates the flow of fluid, especially the blood.

Just like HT Process, loneliness and lack of joy and love is the pathopsychological symptom of a Deficient SI Process.

Painful symptoms connected to the SI Process usually have their origin in a deficient KI Process.

7. BL-Urinary Bladder Processes

BL is the Yang Process of KI in the Water Phase. The main Process of BL is the temporary storage of urine, which is discharged through Qi activity when a sufficient quantity has been accumulated. KI Qi helps this Process of the BL. Physiologically, the bladder organ stores, transports and excretes urine. Disease of BL leads to symptoms such as anuria, urgency of micturition and dysuria; failure of BL to control urine may lead to frequency of micturition, incontinence of urine and enuresis.

In TCM, BL also has an important psychological role. In cases of BL Excess, the mental symptoms may include bitterness and internal unrest. Physically this patient may have difficulty in bending forward and straightening up again. The pulse feels full. In contrast, BL Deficiency (Weak BL Qi) manifests as a weak pulse, incontinence, intestinal pain irradiating towards the loins, difficulty in bending and straightening; tight and contracted leg muscles and reduced hearing.

A lack of energy in the Bladder (as well as in the Kidney), often give the patient a feeling of being cold, or freezing.

A *deficiency* in the bladder-process may express itself as:

- Urine-leaking

- Head ache

- Nocturia

- Urinary infections

- Fear and fright

- Aggression in dogs

- Cold feet

An *excess* of the bladder-process may express itself as:

- Pain in the back, Ichias, Lumbago

A *destructive energy* may give the following symptoms:

- Strong and wild fear

Psychologically BL deficiency often manifest as lack of bravery, which is fear. Lack of bravery may also manifest as a tendency to be uncertain, problems in taking decisions or just a feeling of terror. In practice this lack of bravery may show up as generic unpleasant and overwhelming feelings. We may then say that general symptoms accompanied by strong and overwhelming feelings may belong to the Process of the Bladder.

In the description of the pathological Bladder we may very well picture the little frightened Bichon Frise. Everything is dangerous, and if the situation becomes a little too dangerous it urinates in the owner's lap. We may ourselves experience the connection between coldness, fear and the Bladder. If we go out in the cold, or if we feel a sudden fright, both conditions may cause us to "pee in our pants".

In conditions with a painful BL-meridian, we must usually seek the origin or underlying cause in a deficient Spleen or Heart Process.

8. KI-Kidney Process and the function of urinary excretion

KI is the Yin Process (mate of the BL-Process in the Water Phase). KI is the solid organ, Yin, and BL is its coupled hollow organ, Yang. The main Processes of KI are to store Essence, dominate reproduction and development, dominate Water metabolism and the reception of Qi, and produce marrow to fill up the Brain, dominate bone and manufacture Blood. Kidney manifests in the hair, opens into the ear and it dominates the Lower Orifices (anus, urethra, vulva). KI is considered the most Yin of all the Yin organs, although some consider the Heart as the most Yin organ. Therefore KI plays a critical role in the regulation of fluid substances (as the Heart also does). As fluids are considered Yin in nature, KI controls the regulation of urine. On this point, TCM and western medicine agree.

Besides this obvious western medical function of controlling urination, KI has several other functions not considered by conventional medical science.

KI is the root of Jing-Qi, the vital energy that sustains life. Jing-Qi has two main sources, prenatal and postnatal. Prenatal Jing-Qi (Yuan-Qi) is congenital, inherited from the parents; *Yuan Qi is the most essential energy for life;* without it the fetus would not have been born. Postnatal Jing-Qi is acquired after birth (Zong-Qi).

KI is intricately involved in the development and maintenance of bones, as well as bone marrow.

KI is also closely linked with the quality of head hair; KI Deficiency may result in premature greying and baldness.

As mentioned in Chapter 1, psychologically *KI dominates bravery.* This quality of a healthy KI Qi empowers one with a strong sense of willpower as well as the aspect of intellect having to do with "cleverness"; KI controls also other more cognitive aspects of intelligence. Therefore, KI Deficiency may manifest with symptoms such as indecision.

The KI-Process also regulates the function of the gonads (ovary, testis) and adrenal glands. This KI function involves its Yang quality (not the same as the BL-process, more like the Qi of the Triple Heather, TH), and is often referred to as *KI Yang.* KI Yang dominates sexual physiology and rheumatic disease is one pathological process that stems from a malfunction in this subsystem.

A *deficiency* in the kidney-process may express itself as:

- Fear

- Infections of the skin, furunculosis

- Coldness and edema, especially of the back legs

- Color-less urine, also without smell

- Polyuria and polydipsia

- Chronic infections of the urinary tract

- Eczema, dandruff and dry scaling of the skin
- Lameness, sciatic pain, pain in the joints
- Epilepsy
- Furunculosis in the dog
- Migraine
- Sleep problems, fearful dreams
- Diarrhea
- Aggression
- Rheumatism of the joints

An *excess* of the kidney-process may express itself as:

- Thirst
- Little and dark urine
- Too much sexuality
- Difficulty to sleep

A *destructive energy* may give the following symptoms:

- Deep and strong fear
- Destructive infections of the skin
- Mental disturbances

Body structures tend to help the kidneys, especially the skin. Here ill smelling sweat will appear. Also waste will be excreted into the joints to help the kidneys, and rheumatic symptoms will appear. This starts in the knees, but will spread to the entire body after some time.

The areas in the body, which are specially influenced by the kidneys are the knees, the back (lumbar part) and the forehead (all the parts that are hurt by cold, just as the kidneys themselves).

The kidneys do also have another function that is important to be aware of. In addition to the downward directed and excreting function, they also have an upward directed "fire-process", which is connected to sexuality. A weakness here shows up as a decreased libido, decreased blood circulation in the upper body, tiredness and often tinnitus. It is this function that connects the kidneys to the hormonal process, Triple Heather.

The pathopsychological symptom of the Kidney is fear, the lack of bravery.

In a Kidney Deficiency the excess or painful symptoms usually appear in connection to one of the fire meridians or processes. The usual symptoms may be several painful areas or spots in the shoulder area.

9. PC-Pericardium Processes and blood circulation

PC is another Yin Process of the Fire Element (Phase), and it is coupled to the TH Process in the Fire Phase. PC is the Yin partner, and TH is the Yang partner. The main Process of PC (also called the Heart Protector or the Heart Constrictor (HC)) is to defend the emperor (HT) from injury. When Pathogenic Qi invades HT, PC is always the first to be attacked, and invasion of PC by Pathogenic Qi will often affect the normal Process of HT. For example, Pathogenic Heat describes invasion of the interior by Pathogenic Heat, which precipitates symptoms of mental derangement such as coma and delirium, although the clinical manifestations are the same as those of HT. For this reason, the PC Process is not generally regarded to have an expression or representative among the physical organs, but the process is obviously closely related to HT. According to the Neijing this organ system "has a name but no form", which means that the PC Process does not express itself in an organ, just as the GB Process don't expresses itself in an organ in the horse; it is without any organ.

In northern Europe this process is seldom the sole cause in problems with the flexor tendons, and we should look for Liver involvement also. But, in warmer areas like Florida, a PC-deficiency may be the sole cause. In such areas there are much PC-deficiency, up to 30% of all patients.

Neijing also states that PC is the *"Mother of Blood"*. In the context of the Neijing, the word "blood" implies more its circulatory function than its actual physical quality. PC is also called the Heart Constrictor, or the Circulation Sex Channel, due to its function in regulating local blood flow to the sexual organs. Other sexual functions of this "organ system" include assisting the development of spermatozoa and facilitating ovulation. Symptoms that are accompanied by sexual diversities or abnormalities or changes usually have their origin in an Imbalanced PC Process.

A *deficiency* in the pericardium-process may express itself as:

- Arrhythmic heart-beating

- Decreased blood-flow to the sexual organs

- Unbalanced hormonal status

- Decreased blood-flow in the flexor tendons at the front legs

- Frigidity and impotency

An *excess* of the pericardium-process may express itself as:

- Pressure in the chest

- Hyper sexuality

- Red face

A *destructive energy* may give the following symptoms:

- Hyper sexuality

Symptoms of PC imbalance are direct result of an imbalance in the above-mentioned functions. In PC Deficiency, the patient exhibits fatigue, weakness in the extremities, dizziness, ear pain and a reduced libido. If Cold (External Stressor) causes Deficiency in PC Channel, the genital apparatus becomes weak and the extremities show profound weakness. In contrast, the Stressor of excessive Heat may cause PC Deficiency to manifest as melancholy and dysuria. In PC Excess, Lesion-Symptom Complexes like pressure and pain may arise in the thorax and abdomen, and also cause pain or discomfort along the sides of the body.

The pathopsychological aspect of the PC is frigidity or impotence.

A deficient PC Process often shows symptoms of excess and pain in the BL- or the ST Processes. Painful areas will then be the back or the ventral parts of the animal (where the BL- and/or ST Channels transverse).

10. TH-Triple Heater ("Sanjiao") Processes and hormonal balance

The Chinese name for TH is "Sanjiao" (Three Jiao, Heaters or Burning Spaces). *TH is one of the two Yang Processes (linked to PC) in the Fire Phase.*

The Processes of PC and TH do not manifest in physical organs in the same way as the other 10 Processes. TH Process is very complex, and it is wide ranging in its scope and effect on the body. The Classic on Medical Disorders says "TH [controls] the passage of water and food". The book Plain Questions says "TH is the irrigation official who builds waterways".

The main Processes of TH are to be present (to be present in this connection means that the controlling mind, the self-consciousness is present in all parts of the body, that the connection between the nervous system and the blood is functioning), and to control the digestion, absorption, distribution and excretion of food and water. All of those functions are performed by the joint efforts of various organs, including TH.

A *deficiency* in the TH-process may express itself as:

- Eczema and dry skin

- Unable to be present in conversations

- Otitis interna and externa

- Asthma and infections of the upper respiratory tract

- Unbalanced hormonal excretion

- Hypothyroidism

- Dandruff and dry scaling of the skin

- Tinnitus

- Sinusitis

An *excess* of the TH-process may express itself as:

- Pain at the Scapular area

A *destructive energy* may give the following symptoms:

- Sleeplessness

- Easy breakable bones

The universal importance of TH Channel for the whole organism is shown nicely in a passage (often cited by Georg Bentze, my benefactor): "Ah! To contemplate the wonderful usefulness of TH is to know that the Zang (Solid Organs, Yin) and Fu (Hollow Organs, Yang) are united as well as different from each other. Divided, they are twelve; united, they form the Three Heaters". The word Heater (or Burner) implies central Qi - "Yuan-Qi, the Source Qi, or Original Energy". The Classic on Medical Disorders says, "TH is the ambassador of Yuan-Qi. It circulates the Three Qi and distributes them to the other organs and functions". Some texts refer to TH as the Father of Qi as well as the Father of Yang. In this context TH directs the function of the body involved in heat production (the intake of food, its assimilation and conversion into Qi and heat, and the elimination of waste food and heat). TH Process is also involved in directing the reproductive processes.

In summary, the main TCM Processes of TH are to govern various forms of Qi, and serve as the passage for the flow of Yuan-Qi and Body Fluid. Yuan-Qi has its root in KI but requires TH as its pathway for distribution in order to stimulate and promote the Processes of the other processes and tissues of the whole body.

TH (Fire) normally controls LU (Metal) via the Ko Cycle. In TH Deficiency, control of Metal is lost and the Metal Process may show imbalance. Thus, a weak TH Process may manifest in Lesion-Symptom Complexes that include LU chilliness, congestion and swelling in the mid section of the body. Other symptoms of severe TH imbalance (Deficiency or Excess) include tinnitus, urinary dysfunction, weakness of the extremities and a feeling of exasperation.

The Stressor of Heat Invasion of TH manifests as fullness in the thorax, thirst and swelling of the pharynx.

TH has three parts, called the Three Heaters (or Burners, or Burning Spaces). Each Heater dominates specific Organs and has a specific sphere of influence.

	Upper Heater	Middle Heater	Lower Heater
Location	Thorax	Upper abdomen	Lower abdomen
Sphere of influence	Respiration and circulation	Digestion and extraction	Elimination and reproduction

Table 18

Lesion-Symptom Complexes of a Process Imbalance in each of the Three Heaters are unique. For example:

- Upper Heater Deficiency may induce dull thinking, due to deprivation of energy to the brain. Other symptoms may include tinnitus, a despondent expression and darkening of the eyes. In contrast,

- Middle Heater Deficiency can manifest as irregular stool formation and intestinal damage.

- A Process Imbalance (deficiency) in the Lower Heater may manifest as paresis and arrhythmia.

A painful condition related to the TH Process, usually have its origin in a deficient KI Process.

11. GB-Gallbladder Processes

GB is the Yang Process (Coupled Mate of LV) in the Wood Phase. In western medicine, the physiological GB function is quite rudimentary; that of storing and excreting bile. In both Oslo and Dublin Vet Schools, students learned about biliary function as follows: "The bile of the liver saponifies fat; it helps to absorb and emulsify it; it saves putrefaction and purges a bit and stercobilogen colors the feces".

The role of GB in Chinese physiology is much more complex. The main Process of GB is to combat the external impulses that threaten to extinguish our personal and individual being. Its role is also to store bile and continuously excrete it to the intestines to aid digestion.

The strength of the pulse of GB can reveal the presence of biliary calculi. Often the pulse seems seriously in excess. This is somewhat of a false finding, as the Qi Full is a direct result of these calculi. One can often stimulate the expulsion of bile stones by tonifying the GB Process, but care must be taken if the calculi are especially large, as such a removal could cause trauma to the bile duct.

A *deficiency* in the GB-process may express itself as:

- Bad digestion

- Apathy, anemia (too little iron in the blood)

- Underdeveloped muscles

- Trotting problems, especially in the bends

    ° Into the curves means a deficiency in the right GB

    ° Out of the bends means a deficiency in the left GB

- Colic around midnight

An *excess* of the GB-process may express itself as:

- Pain along the side, especially around the hip-joint

- Pain in the stomach, colic at night

A *destructive energy* may give the following symptoms:

- Biliary calculi

Like the LV-Process, GB-Process dominates the joints and tendons of the entire body. Although horses have no physical gallbladder, they have all the functions and aspects of GB.

The pathopsychological aspect of the GB Process is inability to cope with the external impulses, which then lead to aggression. This is clearly seen in discussions; when we don't cope with the arguments of our opponent, then we get angry.

Painful conditions or symptoms related to the GB Process may often have their origin in a deficient LU Process.

12. LV-Liver Processes and venous blood circulation

Although many LV functions resemble those recognized by western medicine, TCM recognizes many unique differences. The main functions of LV Process are to maintain the immune system, store Blood, nourish muscle, maintain the free flow of Qi and control tendon and sinew.

LV-Process manifests in the nails and opens into the eye.

The immune system is one of the first functions to suffer in LV Deficiency. This system depends mainly on LV (and SP). The symptoms of immune deficiency may be multiple. Usually we find a tendency to infections, especially chronic, long-lasting infections.

LV Process primarily regulates metabolism. Inefficient or incomplete LV metabolism can allow many un-metabolized or un-detoxified compounds from the digesta (or metabolites, such as ketones, from the liver itself) to escape into the circulation. This can cause migraine (Horton's disease or Cluster headache), hepatic encephalopathy and other general states of intoxication. This gives the skin and hair a certain dirty appearance. (However, loss of *Shen* indicates SP Deficiency). This is very obvious in liver-deficient calves fed with fats other than real milk-fat. As a deficient liver is unable to cope with the fatty acids derived from these new fats, they are excreted directly over the skin, and such calves are called "fat-calves" in Norway. In normal calves with healthy liver function, fats usually are not absorbed or excreted intact, as calves with a functioning liver can handle reasonable amounts of vegetable fats. LV symptoms often involve the color green; the skin may be green, the eyes may be green and the pus or excretions from all orifices may be more or less green if the symptoms originate in LV Deficiency. The symptoms also tend to wander around in the body. Rheumatism that wanders is usually due to LV Process Imbalance; rheumatism of fixed location usually is due to KI Process Imbalance.

A *deficiency* in the liver-process may express itself as:

- Allergy
- Hip-joint problems, HD (hip dysplasia)
- Migraine and headaches (Cluster headache, Horton disease)
- Digestive problems, poor digestion
    - Hyperglycemia
    - Hypoglycemia
- Eczema and skin dermatitis
- Allergic asthma
- Breast cancer
- Anemia
- Azoturia, Monday morning disease, Easter disease
- Hyperactivity
- Stiffness in the neck
- Groin pain (football players)

An *excess* of the liver-process may express itself as:

- Beginning allergy
- Anger

A *destructive energy* may give the following symptoms:

- Strong anger

- **Blood and Qi (vitality and energy):** TCM and western practitioners both recognize the function of LV in haematopoiesis, storage of vitamins including B_{12}, and in glycogen and protein metabolism, neutralization or detoxification of absorbed toxins. Severe stress on LV (as in patients undergoing cytotoxic chemotherapy for cancer, or severe hepatitis) is very debilitating; it greatly reduces Qi. Human sufferers report great depletion of energy they feel "as weak as a kitten".

- **Sleep patterns:** TCM also included sleep habits under its domain of LV influence. Exposure to the harmful effects of Cold on LV results in the inability to sleep. In contrast, the patient may sleep too much if LV is exposed to excessive Heat. Excessive sleeping is also a sign of great depletion of Qi, as occurs in the terminal stages of disease or old age. Patients with an insufficient liver activity often report waking up at 0300 in the night without any obvious reason.

- **Tendons and muscles:** In TCM, although SP dominates the muscles, LV provides their nourishment. Therefore, anything that damages LV function, also wreaks havoc on the muscular system. Pernicious factors, which can attack LV, include Wind and a sour (acidic) environment. Often, Internal Wind in LV can create muscle spasms or muscular pain that often moves around in the body. The muscles that primarily are weakened are the hip-muscles and the neck-muscles. Therefore, liver deficiency is the primary cause of the development of hip dysplasia in dogs and neck stiffness in humans and dogs.

- **Nails/hooves:** The LV-process also plays an important role in the health of the nails. The Neijing states that "the liver flourishes in the nails". Therefore tonifying LV helps the nails. It is also interesting to note that stimulation of the LV Process can also cure nail biting.

- *Eye and sight:* TCM texts state that LV has an important action on the eye. A chronic LV Deficiency may weaken sight and may lead to atrophy of the optic nerve. Though LV is the classical Channel related to eye disorders, in my opinion all 12 Processes (especially LU, GB, BL, ST, TH and LI) influence the eye, as well as all the other sense organs. To treat progressive retinal atrophy in dogs, I have found all of those Processes involved, although at different times.

- *Genitalia:* The LV Process is important for the male genitalia. We will later see that the acupuncture meridian of the liver (LV Channel) passes exactly through the genital area.

- *Immune system:* The immune system is one of the first functions to suffer when the liver is suffering. This is seen very often in children's allergies. The main cause of this in children is their excessive eating of sweets. I often cure allergies in children just by ordering a complete absence of sweets between 3 am and 3 pm (between 0300 and 1500). Also the need to eat sugar or chocolate is a symptom in liver- or LV Deficiency. This shows that the body does not always know what the best thing to do would be.

The hip area, the hip joint, the gluteus medius muscle, the pelvis, the back, the jaw, the neck and the head are areas that are especially influenced by the liver process. Calcifications, stiffness, pain or decreased movement are symptoms that these areas may show. This makes the liver process especially important concerning the hip area, the hip muscles and by this the whole speed in the horse as well as all kind of problems like azoturia and elevated muscle transaminases. Within the muscles cells the liver process governs the sugar metabolism, the building up of glycogen and the breaking down of the same. If the concentration of glycogen, the result of a deficient liver process, gets too large, the muscle cells will be destroyed, and azoturia occurs. A deficient liver process will also decrease the blood circulation in the pelvic area, and this will also aggravate a tying up condition.

Here, at this point, I would like to tell an interesting aspect of the story of how I realized the importance of the liver in the horse, and also that many horses do have problems with this process.

I had just started to practice the pulse diagnosis, and had found that about 60% of all horses had liver deficiency. They also got much better after I treated the liver, so I was convinced that I was right.

All veterinarians have to report all their diagnosis every month, as I did. I then reported 234 horses with a liver deficiency during the year 1983. This result was reported to the European veterinary statistic, situated in Brussels. The Norwegian veterinary authorities then immediately got a worried question from Brussels "what is wrong up in Norway"? What has happened with your horses? Each year there are about 12 horses in the whole Europe that have a liver problem, and now you have 234 horses just in Norway.

The veterinary department in Oslo found out quite quickly that the "sinner" was I. I received a worried call from the department, asking me what the problem was. I told then that according to my diagnosis 60% of the horses had a liver problem, resulting in problems with the hip area.

The man from Oslo asked me if I could make another diagnosis, but I said that it was difficult to lie.

He then asked me if I could stop reporting at all, to which I agreed. All my colleagues have to report every month, and they sit and sweat over the papers for hours, at least before the computer programs were available, while I just take a nap.

The most interesting part though, is that some 20 years later, a more sensitive test for liver problems in the horse was introduced, it is called GLDH. This test showed that about 60% of all horses have liver problems..

The gluteus medius muscle is especially under the control and influence of the liver process, and within this muscle we may find fibers that governs and balance the whole dynamics of the pelvic area, via the Ilio-Sacral-joint. This joint may be characterized as a sort of gyroscope for the whole pelvic area. Therefore the liver process is of crucial importance for the movement and speed of the horse.

As the liver has to do with the glycogen metabolism of the muscles, problems in this process will lead to chronic stiff and acidified muscles, and this will lead to muscular rheumatism and headache, tension headache.

A special variation of this kind of headache is called "Horton's´ migraine". I have treated this type of migraine only through stimulating and regulating the liver process, and the results have been very good. Out of 19 Horton patients (2010), 16 have been more or less cured, the first patient have now been without pain for > 20 years. The healing percentage is 84%.

The liver process is central also in the development of hip dysplasia, mainly through its relevance for the hip area and the gluteus medius muscle. The treatment works as well in humans. The effect both in dogs and in humans is > 90% disappearance of the symptoms, and restoring the quality of life in most patients. Norwegian TV has also made a program about this method.

A summary of factors that harm the liver process;

- Too much sugar, especially between 0300 and 1500.

- Food additives.

- Antioxidants used in food. It is a paradox that veterinarians themselves sell this kind of food.

- Fungus in the food.

- Pelleted food.

- Too much protein in the food.

The **pathopsychological** aspect of the liver is lack of will power, which is indecision.

A deficient LV Process usually shows symptoms of excess and pain in the ST Process, especially the ventral parts of the animal and Quadriceps muscle.

RELATIONSHIPS BETWEEN THE PROCESSES AND THE CHANNELS

It is usual to think or observe relationships between Structure and Process. If we see a spade, we can at once deduce from the form of the spade, that it may be used for digging (the Process). Such a view also dominates concerning the internal organs. Anatomists have studied organic structure macroscopically and microscopically. From this they have deduced the main functions of each organ. Such studies are important but they may limit our medical thinking. Take for example KI, the most important organ for excretion of urine. But, as stated earlier, all mammalian cells, especially mucosal cells, can excrete urinary metabolites to a greater or lesser extent. In other words, all body cells can assist KI Process of urine excretion, especially when KI is stressed to the point that it cannot perform its Processes alone.

If we want to understand the functions of the organism, we must be able to separate the Processes from the Organs and from the structures. Most of the Vital Processes occur all over the body and not only in their classical organs. This is why we should consider that different tissues might substitute or compensate the Processes of the main Organ. This is why Lesion-Symptom Complexes may appear far away from the main organ or far from the true origin of the disease itself.

*This way to view the Lesion-Symptom Complex is also important concerning the part of therapy. Most acupoints, remedies, herbs and other effective therapies not only work or act on the organ they are "meant for", but primarily they work or stimulate the Process itself. **The Process is the primary function.** If we give a treatment meant for HT and KI, then this therapy also works on the blood circulation and the urine excretion in general. These Processes may be stimulated all over the body, even if they are stimulated most of all in the main related Organ.*

This is the real reason why we usually get initial aggravation of the symptoms when we start therapy. The specific Process that the acupoint or the remedy stimulates is especially active at the site of the symptom; stimulation of this Process first manifests at the Weak Structure. The symptoms disappear first after this initial aggravation, when the therapy has "reached" and stimulated the main organ. Thus, this organ may take over for the symptoms and compensation no longer is necessary.

RELATIONSHIPS BETWEEN THE PROCESSES AND THE BRAIN (THINKING AND CONSCIOUSNESS)

Historically the Chinese did not consider the brain as a separate organ but rather as an extension of (or substance secreted from) the kidney. The brain was not even considered as the main area of the thinking, but only as an instrument to make this thinking conscious; to make the whole body conscious of the processes at work. The act of thinking was done within the processes, and the existence of the brain is only to make the thoughts and decisions conscious. In a way, we observe our own thinking with the brain. The brain thus functions as a mirror, the mirror of consciousness; the body itself thinks, and just experiences its thoughts in this mirror. This is what we mean when we say that some people "think" with their testicles, or "speak" from their liver etc. It is very interesting that, just before this book went into printing for the first time (2nd. March 2001), a most astonishing report was discovered by the scientific world. German and American scientists have now discovered that there are more brain-cells in the intestinal area than there is in the spinal cord. It seems that thoughts and decisions are made here before they are made conscious in the central nervous system. This observation is just in line with the old knowledge cited above.

The brain is often linked to the moon, and is compared with this in mythology. The moon reflects or mirrors the light of the sun in the same way as the brain reflects the feelings and the consciousness of the heart and other organs.

4 Methods to find the deficiency

1. Observation of the symptoms, page 98
2. Observation of the reflex zones, page 103
3. Observation of the modifications, page 151
4. Direct observation, page 163

1. Noting the symptoms and lesions (The Lesion-Symptom Complex)

a) The succession of the Lesion-Symptom Complex

According to the Law of the Five Phases, the order (succession) of appearance and disappearance of Lesion-Symptom Complexes does not arise by chance. Usually the succession follows the Ko-Cycle, sometimes the Sheng-cycle (page 28). Therefore, to be able to start therapy at its root, it is important to decide in which Process the problem started, i.e. which was the primary deficient Imbalanced Process, and which was the secondary excessive Process. In traumatic origin, the excessive Process may be the primary one.

Classification of the Lesion-Symptom Complex related to the 12 Processes and their succession, according to the Ko-cycle or the Sheng-cycle:

The Sheng (nourishing, or Mother-Son) Cycle is an anabolic, generative or creative cycle. Each Mother Phase creates, nurtures, stimulates or strengthens its Son (succeeding) Phase. Each Son Phase needs or receives its Qi from its Mother (preceding) Phase. The Sheng Cycle creates (>>) the succeeding Phase in a clockwise circle, where:

Fire >> Earth >> Metal >> Water >> Wood >> Fire

Fire is the Mother of Earth and the Qi of Fire is nourished by the Qi of Wood (Fire is the Son of Wood), etc.

As an aid to remember the Sheng Sequence, make a mental picture of the Phase relationships as follows: Fire burns to, or creates, ash (Earth). Earth produces ore (Metal). Metal when melted produces liquid (Water), or mist condenses on Metal to produce Water. Water is necessary for (produces) vegetation (Wood). Wood burns to make Fire, completing the auto-generating cycle. In the Sheng Cycle, the circular sequence discussed above, each preceding Phase (the Mother) nurtures, strengthens or engenders the subsequent one (the Son).

The KO (Controlling Father) Cycle *is a controlling cycle. It is also known as the Restraining Cycle. Each Ko Father Phase controls its Son Phase in the Ko Cycle. Each Ko Son Phase is obedient to or has its Qi controlled by its Father Phase in the Ko Cycle. The Ko Father Phase controls (X) the Ko Son Phase in a clockwise pentagram, where:*

Fire XX Metal XX Wood XX Earth XX Water XX Fire

In the Ko Cycle, Fire Qi is the Ko Father of (controls) Metal Qi and Fire Qi is the Ko Son of (is controlled by) Water Qi.

As an aid to remember the Ko Sequence, make a mental picture of the Phase relationships as follows: Fire melts Metal. Metal controls (the axe cuts) Wood. Wood controls Earth (lack of vegetation allows soil erosion). Earth (sandbanks, dykes, earth dams) controls Water. Water controls (extinguishes) Fire, completing the auto-controlling cycle.

b) How the symptoms appear

In order to be able to do this, we must decide to which Phase (Element) the symptom(s) belong. *The important diagnostic tool here is the Phase not the Process.* This may be the same Phase as the Imbalanced Process that was the origin of the disease, but it also may be a different Phase. For example, the disease may start in the KI Process (Water Phase), but the symptoms may be characterized by pain (the Metal Phase). When we must decide how the symptoms appear, we must determine to which Phase the symptom belongs. This will tell us which Phase point we should use on the Channel in question.

To answer this question, we must look in more depth on how one can recognise the *Phases* in pathology (we will deal with how the *Processes* are recognised in pathology below).

- *Heat* relates to the *Fire Phase and* "attacks" the Fire Process (HT, PC, SI and / or TH (hormonal balance)). It increases body temperature. The skin is red, the blood circulation increases, the sweat is hot and the patient wants to drink cold water.

- **Damp** relates to the **Earth** *Phase* and "attacks" the Earth Process (SP and ST). It leads to stagnation of the body fluids, edema and tumors (excess of body tissue, cancer). The external material parts of the Lesion-Symptom Complex tend to detach from the rest of the body, i.e. the lesions disassociate. For example, warts fall off, blood seeps out, viscera descend (prolapse), etc.

- **Dryness** relates to **Metal** and "attacks" the Metal / Air Process (LU and LI). It weakens the mucous membranes and the airways by its drying action. The Lesion-Symptom Complex manifests as dandruff, scaly skin, pain and stiffness.

- **Cold** relates mainly to the **Water/Air** *Phase* and "attacks" the Water Process (KI and BL). It weakens the body so that body temperature and blood circulation decreases. The subject has a cold sweat, trembles, does not want to drink, has dark urine and mucosal membranes and cold sensations.

- **Wind** relates mainly to the **Wood** *Phase* and "attacks" the Wood Process (LV and GB). It precipitates Lesion-Symptom Complexes that tend to move around in the organism and also that the pain and the discomfort vary considerably.

c) Where the Lesion-Symptom Complex manifests

- **In relation to the acupuncture-meridians (Channels):** If we note the location of the Lesion-Symptom Complex, we may diagnose with great certainty the Channel that carries the excessive reactions to the deficient process (see diagram on page 61). This diagnosis requires knowledge of the superficial and deep pathways of the different Channels. (We will discuss this later).

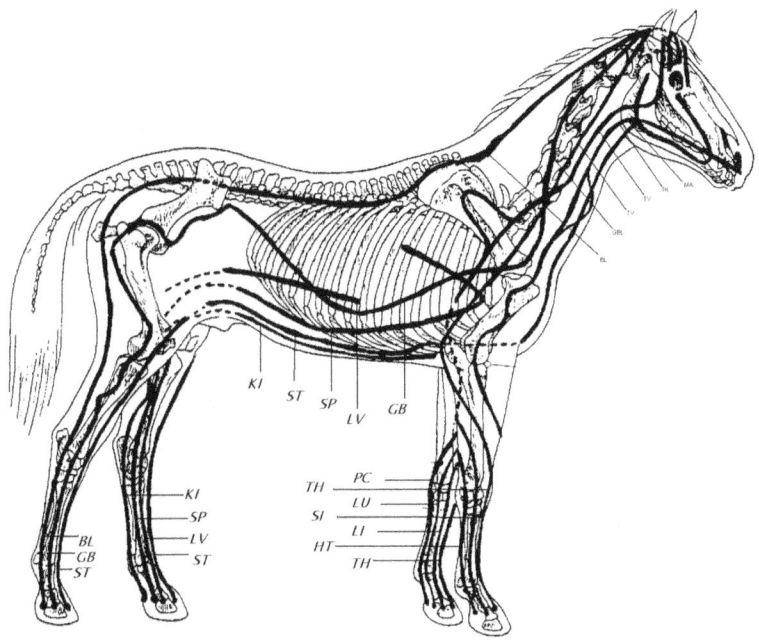

Fig. 13; Illustration of the meridians in the horse.

ii) In relation to different microcosms: Often several Lesion-Symptom Complexes, such as pain, eczema or other skin changes, may manifest within several different microcosms at the same time and develop in parallel with the disease process (the Process Imbalance). This really is holistic thinking. Knowledge of these different microcosms may give information on the cause of the disease. This way of thinking is today developed within the so-called ECIWO biology, which really is more like Zone Therapy rather than AP. ECIWO theory states that many different micro-cosmos or micro-systems mirror every part of the body. It also states that any pathological changes in one or more organs or parts manifest or reflect themselves at many different places of the body. A neck trauma may then manifest at all the different "neck zones" of the different microcosms of the body, which means all distal parts of the limbs, fingers etc.

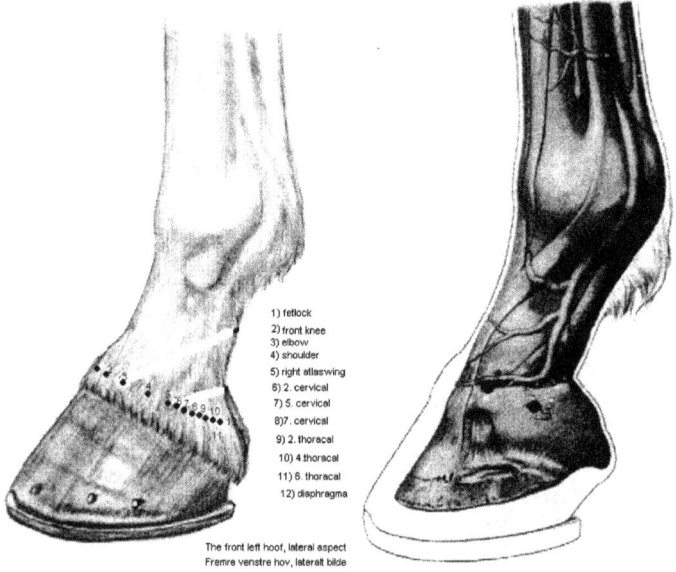

1) fetlock
2) front knee
3) elbow
4) shoulder
5) right atlaswing
6) 2. cervical
7) 5. cervical
8)7. cervical
9) 2. thoracal
10) 4 thoracal
11) 6. thoracal
12) diaphragma

The front left hoof, lateral aspect
Framre venstre hov, lateralt bilde

Fig. 14; Illustrations of one of the microcosmos in the horse, in this case the coronary band.

Then we have to find out if the process is in excess or in deficiency.

- Excess

- Deficiency

To do so we should observe how the symptoms vary with work and relaxation.

- If the symptoms get better after work, or worse after relaxation, they are in excess

- If the symptoms get worse after work, or better after relaxation, they are in deficiency

2. The Reflex Zones: Diagnostic Acupuncture and ECIWO biology

Over aeons of time, the body has developed reflex-zones for almost every process, organ and structure. This enables the body to cure and stimulate the parts that need treatment. The ways the body has chosen to stimulate these points (before there were doctors or acupuncturists) are:

- Electric stimulation through environmental charges; reducing the electric resistance in the point does this.

- Direct stimulation by getting the patient to scratch the area. Have you considered the deeper meaning of the urge to scratch? Almost all living creatures scratch themselves, some even vigorously. Some scratch each other, and some only themselves. There is a reason for all bodily needs: Thirst is the signal to seek water, for example in dehydration; hunger is the signal to seek food, etc. Thus, the urge to scratch has its cause; it is a system to autoregulate or autostimulate the Processes that are underactive (Deficient) at that time. If we watch where birds, animals or humans press, scratch, massage, preen or stimulate themselves by other means, we may be able to make a diagnosis even before we have investigated the patient.

- Change the point in some way by means of circulation, pigmentation or other means to urge stimulation by community members or by oneself.

From a holistic viewpoint, the whole body is mirrored in every single part; for example, in the ear, the nose, the tongue and the eye. It is also possible to say that the processes are mirrored in the whole body as such, and by this look at the whole acupuncture system as a great ECIWO-system.

It is possible to find Reflex Zones in the acupuncture system as well as in those microcosmic wholes; the so-called ECIWO Systems of a lesser degree. This gives us the opportunity to diagnose and treat with different methods and in different places of the body (microcosms). For example we have Ear-AP, Foot Zone Therapy, Tongue Diagnosis, Iris Diagnosis, Scalp-AP, Nose-AP, diagnosis by analysing the palm of the hand, etc.

THE MOST IMPORTANT REFLEX SYSTEMS IN ANIMALS

Our knowledge of holographic photography suggests that these reflex microsystems have value, but it is also clear that no single person can master all of these different microcosms. However, in my opinion, six of these systems are most applicable in veterinary medicine. These are as follows:

- **The General AP System**
- **The command-point system**
- **The Back Reflex Zones** (Back Shu Points)
- **The Equine Coronary Band System**
    - ° **The Ting-point system**
    - ° **The Coronary Band ECIWO System**
- **The Ear Zone System**
- **All 12 metatarsal and metacarpal ECIWO systems**

The General Acupuncture System

A System for Treatment and Diagnosis

All of the acupuncture-points may also be used as a tool for diagnosis, much in the same way as described for the Shu-points, the Ting-points and the Ear-points.

All acupuncture-points change in regards to several aspects, if they need treatment. If we are able to detect these changes we may also diagnose changes in the processes. The changes in the points tell us if the process relating to the point is in excess or in deficiency.

Changes relating to:

- In deficiency:
    - ° Less tenderness
    - ° Decreased blood-flow
    - ° Sunken appearance of the skin
    - ° Decreased electrical resistance
    - ° Hairs are more stiff and loosen more easily
    - ° Skin temperature is decreased

- In excess:
    - ° More tenderness (pain)
    - ° Elevated blood-flow
    - ° Swollen skin
    - ° Decreased electrical resistance in the skin
    - ° Skin temperature is elevated

The Command-point Acupuncture System

A System for Treatment and Diagnosis

1. **THE COMMAND POINTS**
- *Jing-well or the Ting-points;* is the very point where the Qi either enters or leaves the meridian. Here Qi also changes from Yin to Yang or from Yang to Yin. All the Ting-points belong to the *wood*-element.

- *Ying-spring points;* is where the Qi flows quietly to the superficial part of the skin. Ying means "source." All Ying-points belong to the Fire-element.

- *Shu-stream points;* is where the energy (Qi) of the meridian flourishes. Shu means to transport. They belong to the *earth*-element.

- *Jing-river points;* is where the Qi flows or streams through. Jing means to pass. They are connected to the *metal*-element.

- *He-sea points;* where the energy dives deeper into the body. He means to join. These points belong to the water element.

- *Yuan-source points;* are points that belong to the command-points as it commands the meridian and does not act only as a local point. It has no connection to the elements, and stimulation of a source-point stimulates the whole meridian in a non specific manner.

The changes to look for and detect in diagnosis are the same as described under the general acupuncture system, see last page.

Command Point	Key energetic functions
Fire Point	Commands, or influence the Fire Aspects of the Processes represented by that Channel
Earth Point	Commands, or influence the Earth Aspects of the Processes represented by that Channel
Metal Point	Commands, or influence the Metal Aspects of the processes represented by that Channel
Water Point	Commands, or influence the Water Aspects of the Processes represented by that Channel
Wood Point	Commands, or influence the Wood Aspects of the Processes represented by that Channel
Horary (Own Phase) Point	Is the name of the elemental point that correlates with the element of the meridian itself. It is used like the other elemental points.

Table 19

Back Shu Points

The Back Shu Points are also called the Association Points. They lie in symmetrical pairs along the inner path of BL Channel lateral to the vertebral spines, from vertebra T1 to S4. The points are situated in:

- Humans 1.5 cun lateral to the midline

- Dogs 2 cun lateral to the midline

- Horses 3 cun lateral to the midline

The reason why the points are situated at different distances from the midline is because the M. longissimus dorsi is of a different size in the animals mentioned.

An Imbalance in the Channel-Organ-Process Systems and the related Shu Point(s) manifest(s) as localized changes in several parameters such as:

- Tenderness of the point.

    º Hypertenderness.

    º Hypotenderness.

- Blood flow locally in the point.

- Hair quality.

- Colour of the skin.

- Electrical resistance (Ohm).

- Also other qualities.

Elevated tenderness (sensitivity) must not be mistaken for a common backache.

It is important to remember that painful points along the BL Channel usually are signs of excess. When diagnosing these, we must always think of the possibility that these excessive projections are the results of more underlying states of deficiency. Always then look for a deficiency in the foregoing process in the Ko Cycle.

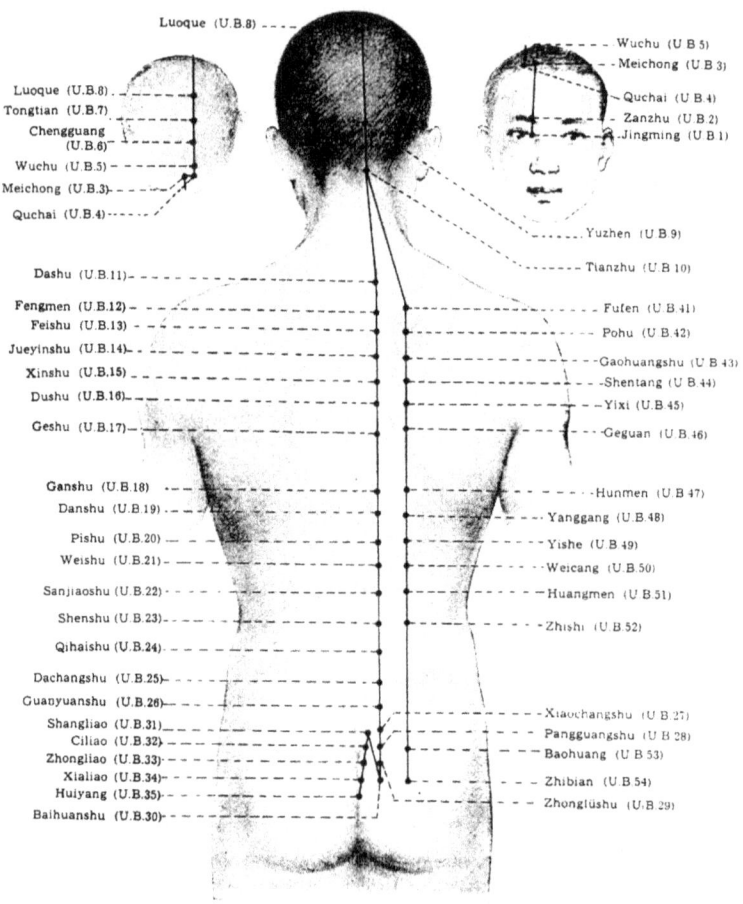

Fig 15; Illustration of the Shu-points at the man

Summary of the relations between the Paravertebral (inner path of BL Channel) Back Shu Points and their related organs or functions and vertebral locations in humans

Shu Point	Related function	Vertebrae
-	Blood pressure	C7-T1
BL11	Dashu Great Shuttle (Bones)	T1-T2
BL12	Fengmen Wind Gate (Wind)	T2-T3
BL13	Feishu LU Shu	T3-T4
BL14	Jueyinshu PC Shu	T4-T5

BL15	Xinshu HT Shu	T5-T6
BL16	Dushu GV Shu (spine)	T6-T7
BL17	Geshu Diaphragm Shu (also respiration and haemorrhage)	T7-T8
-	-	T8-T9
BL18	Ganshu LV Shu	T9-T10
BL19	Danshu GB Shu	T10-T11
BL20	Pishu SP Shu	T11-T12
BL21	Weishu ST Shu	T12-L1
BL22	Sanjiaoshu TH Shu (Endocrine)	L1-L2
BL23	Shenshu KI Shu	L2-L3
BL24	Qihaishu Qi Sea Shu	L3-L4
BL25	Dachangshu LI Shu	L4-L5
BL26	Guanyuanshu Gate Origin Shu (Uterus)	L5-S1
BL27	Xiaochangshu SI Shu	S1-S2
BL28	Pangguangshu BL Shu	S2-S3
BL29	Zhonglushu Central Backbone Shu	S3-S4
BL30	Baihuanshu White Circle (Anus)	S4-S5

Table 20

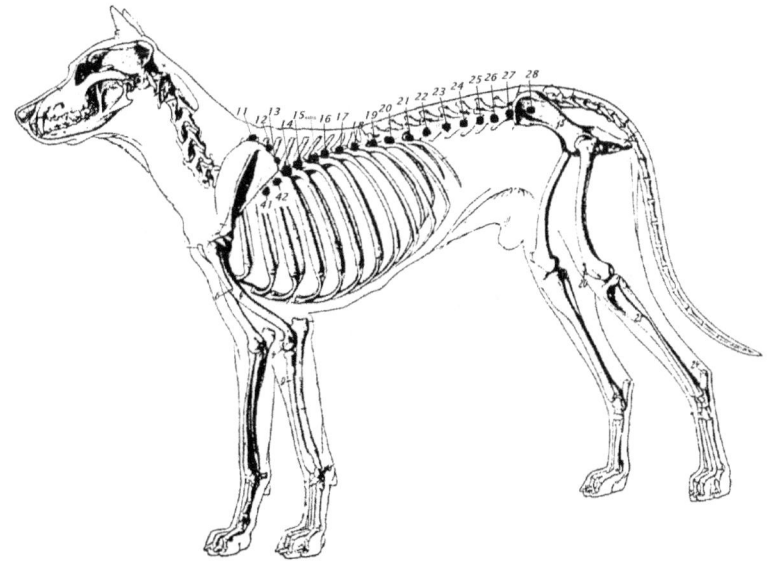

Fig 16; Illustration of the Shu-points at the dog.

Summary of the relations between the Paravertebral (inner path of BL Channel) Back Shu Points and their related organs or functions and vertebral locations in dogs

Shu Point	Related function	Vertebrae
-	Blood pressure	C7-T1
BL11	Bones	T1-T2
BL12	Wind	T2-T3
BL13	LU	T3-T4
BL14	PC	T4-T5
BL15	HAT	T5-T6
BL16	GV and spine	T6-T7
BL17	Ge-Diaphragm; also respiration and haemorrhage	T7-T8
-	-	T8-T9
-	-	T9-T10
BL18	LV	T10-T11
BL19	GB	T11-T12
BL20	SP	T12-T13
BL21	ST	T13-L1
BL22	TH hormones	L1-L2
BL23	KI	L2-L3
BL24	Qihai-Sea of Energy	L3-L4
BL25	LI	L4-L5
BL26	Guanyuan-Gate Origin (Uterus)	L5-L6
BL27	SI	L6-L7
BL28	BL	L7-S1
BL29	Zhonglu-Midback (lowback)	
BL30	Baihuan-White Circle (Anus)	

Table 21

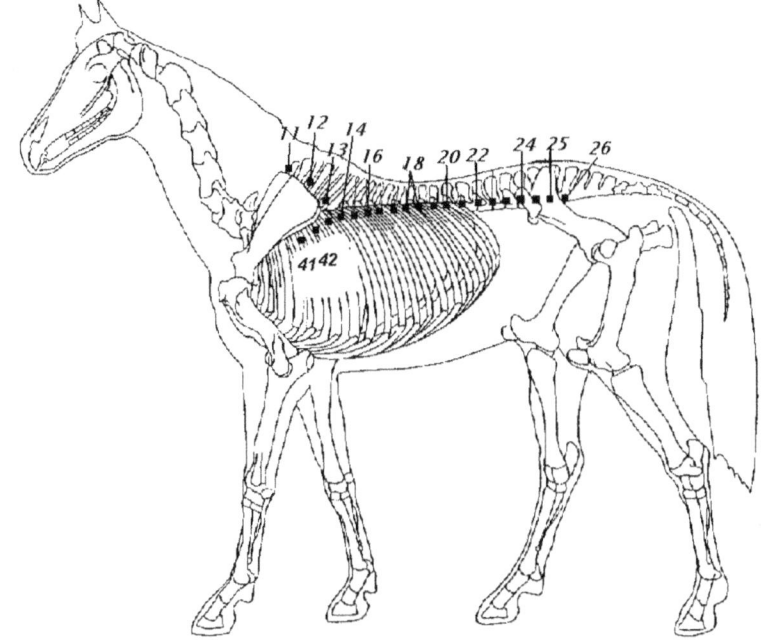

Fig. 17; Illustration of the Shu-points at the horse.

Summary of the relations between the Paravertebral (inner path of BL Channel) Back Shu Points and their related organs or functions and vertebral locations in horses

Shu Point	Related function	Vertebrae
-	Blood pressure	C7-T1
BL11	Bone	T1-T2
BL12	Wind	T2-T3
-	-	T3-T4
BL13&42	LU	T4-T5
		T5-T6
BL14&43	PC	T6-T7
-	-	T7-T8
BL15&44	HT	T8-T9
BL16	GV and spine	T9-T10
-	-	T10-T11

BL17	Ge-Diaphragm; also respiration and haemorrhage	T11-T12
-	-	T12-T13
BL18	LV	T13-T14
-	-	T14-T15
BL19	GB	T15-T16
-	-	T16-T17
BL20	SP	T17-T18
BL21	ST	T18-L1
BL22	TH hormones	L1-L2
BL23	KI	L2-L3
BL24	Qihai-Sea of Energy	L3-L4
BL25	LI	L4-L5
BL26	Guanyuan-Gate Origin (Uterus)	L5-L6
BL27	SI	S1
BL28	BL	S2
BL29	Zhonglu-Midback (lowback)	S3
BL30	Baihuan-White Circle (Anus); also tarsus	S4

Table 22

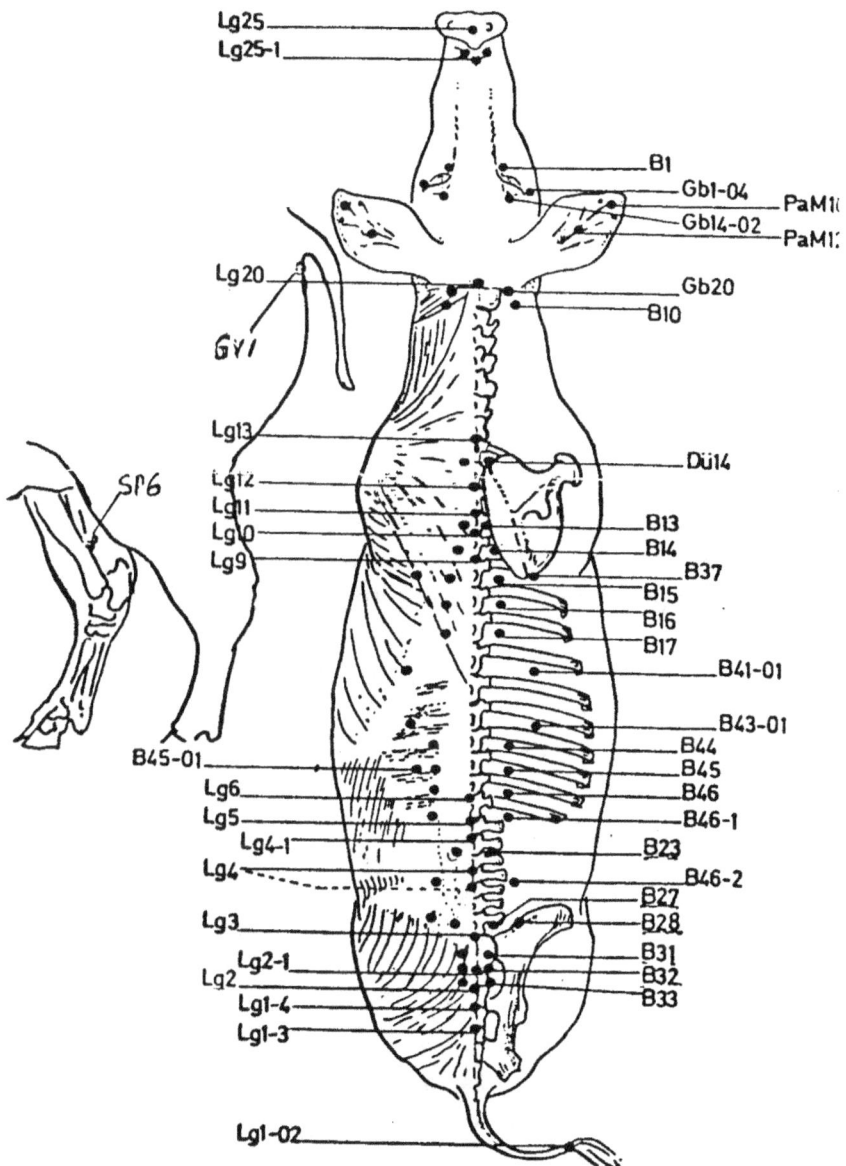

Fig. 18; Illustration of the Shu-points at the pig (Dr. Vet. Oswald Kothbauer)

Point tenderness, per se, can be a very subjective parameter. It depends on how hard one presses each point and on the basic sensitivity of the subject. Therefore, one should develop a consistent, evenly applied pressure-palpation technique.

In practice, I have myself watched many skilled and famous acupuncturists "fooling themselves" (consciously or subconsciously, preferably the last) in their examination by pressure-palpation before and after AP therapy; they apply less pressure after their therapy than before. This gives the impression to observers that point sensitivity is lost after the therapy, when, in fact, it may have changed little, or not at all. Therefore, in addition to pressure-palpation, other techniques to measure pain reactivity should be used more often and new techniques (such as objective pressure-manometers) should be developed for use in animals.

An unskilled practitioner uses point reactivity only (point sensitivity, or pain reaction from the animal) to indicate which Process(es) is/are imbalanced. This is a mistake; it is very often misleading and causes the practitioner to misinterpret the diagnostic significance of the reactive points. Diagnostic interpretation improves markedly when one includes the structure, colour, temperature or attitude and many other physical clues to the health of the tissues, etc. in the assessment. To a great extent, reactions to pain (and to palpation of pain points) depend on the fitness, stamina, tolerance and temperament of the animal and how hard the therapist presses the points. In this way the expectations of the therapist or other factors may bias the results greatly. It is much better to try to assess (and select the relevant) Back Shu Points more objectively than when based solely on their reactivity to uneven, unskilled palpation.

Therefore, for example, Ting Point Diagnosis in horses is much more accurate than the usual method of Shu-Point palpation. In time, the therapist becomes more experienced and sensitive. Then, the qualities of the skin (whether Hot, Cold, Dry, Damp (oedematous)) and its electrical resistance become much more informative than simple assessment (even if objective) of the basic reactivity (tenderness) of the Back Shu Points. Also, to diagnose the root cause of the disorder (the Primary Process Imbalance) one should try to ascertain *the nature and cause of the tenderness* at the Back Shu Points.

Should one remove all point reactivity at each session? This is a controversial topic in AP therapy, and its answer depends on which philosophy one follows. There is a very important difference in philosophy in *how fast* the healing response should be. Some therapists want to see an *immediate* response, i.e. that the indications of pain should be gone immediately at the end of each session. However, even allowing that this might be possible (and it is possible in some cases), in my opinion, it usually takes some 3-10 days for the body to adjust to the new balance. Also, all pain cases have an underlying Deficiency as the real cause. If one drains the Channels in Excess (Excess = pain), one *usually* gets an immediate result, but it does not last as long as when one treats the underlying Deficiency correctly. Underlying Deficiency seldom causes pain in itself, but frequently causes an Excess elsewhere. With correct Command Point treatment of the Deficient Channel, one can *sometimes* see an immediate effect that *lasts*. One *need* not see the immediate effect, and yet one can get excellent results some days later. Treating Deficiency can be a preventative method because it can be done before pain would otherwise manifest. However, recognition of Deficiency in pain-free animals demands very good diagnostic skills, such as the Pulses, skin drag, etc. Therefore, one must decide whether one wants a "fast but transient" or a "slower but more long-lasting" clinical result.

To be able to decide which point is the primary, we must know the relationships between the points relating to the Processes/Channels and the Elements/Phases.

The most important law regulating the interrelation of the Back Shu Points is the Law of the Five Phases (see page 28).

Three examples:

- *In horses,* a reactive BL18 in

    ° *Excess* indicates pain or sprain of the muscles of the hip area (Weak Structure, related to a Process Imbalance in LV). This leads to pain, muscle spasm and/or lameness in the gluteal area. Then the horse puts weight on the forelegs to relieve the hip pain and pain manifests in the joints in the foreleg, especially the right carpus or fetlock (Weak Structures). Furthermore, we may expect urticarial reaction on the belly (LV controls ST Channel).

o   *Deficiency* indicates degeneration of the muscles of the gluteal area with decreased muscular activity of Musculus gluteus medius. This will also lead to more work for the front legs and joint-problems here may result.

- *In dogs* a reactive BL18 in

    o   *Deficiency* indicates an underactive liver process. This leads to eczema, allergy or weakness in the hip muscles (also a weak structure in heavy dogs), with development of hip dysplasia later. We may also expect mammary cancer (if LV is weak it will not be able to control ST, and an uncontrolled ST is the first step towards a mammary cancer) and different psychic changes, such as aggression.

    o   *Excess* indicates an excessive process in the liver process. This may lead to aggression, colic or other symptoms due to over-activity in the hyperchondriac region.

- *In cats* a reactive BL18 in

    o   *Deficiency* usually indicates digestion problems.

    o   *Excess* usually indicates psychic changes, such as aggression because of an excessive liver process.

Equine Ting (Jing-Well) Points:

A Special Diagnostic and Therapeutic System

The coronary band in horses is an extremely important area. Here we have;

- The foundation of the hoof growth.

- The most important acupuncture points for all the processes.

- The most important ECIWO-system for the joints.

- The most important self regulatory system for self healing.

Ting (Jing-Well) Points are the most distal acupoints of the 12 Meridians (Channels). In horses, 10 of them are situated in the coronary band and 2 in the bulb of the heels on each hoof.

Ting points may serve as Diagnostic Points in all species, but only in the horse can they be used diagnostically without any form of refined measurement, apparatus or the like; one may observe physically whether or not the point is in deficiency (or in excess). *This is a very special characteristic of the equine Ting points.* This may be done in four ways:

- By inspection and palpation of the skin at the point.

- By inspection of the way the hoof-wall is growing beneath each point.

- By measuring how fast the hoof wall is growing beneath each point.

- By observing where the hoof wall receives the most pressure. That is where it is the most worn down.

In this way, the Ting Points may be used diagnostically in much the same way as the Back Shu Points, only that in the Ting Points it is much more easy to find deficiencies, while in the Shu-Points it is more easy to find excesses (if we only use pain-palpation as our diagnostic parameter, and not the finer detection of deficiency described on page 107).

We may observe that the blood supply to the coronary band is very extensive and abundant, and knowing that the most important acupuncture-points are situated just over arterial and venal anastomoses, we may assume that the points situated in the coronary band are very important. Also, such abundance of vascularisation gives a lot of room for changes in the consistence of the skin over the points.

1. Ting Point Diagnosis on the Basis of Local Changes in the Skin

The method simply investigates the equine coronary band in all four feet, looking for areas of change in the texture of the skin over/in the Ting-points. When examining Ting Points on one limb, do not ask for the opposite limb to be lifted up. This would increase the pressure in the foot being investigated so that it's deficient Ting Points would more or less disappear. However, it is permissible to have one of the hind limbs lifted while investigating a foreleg and *vice-versa*.

To perform Ting Point investigation, one gently palpates all around the coronary band, circa 1.5 cm above the hoof, especially in the area where the Ting-points are expected to be found.

Forelimb Channel Ting Point	Degrees lateral from 0°	Hindlimb Channel Ting Point
TH	0°	ST
SI	55°	GB
HT	115°	BL
PC	180°	KI
LU	245°	SP
LI	305°	LV

Table 23

One uses one finger in a gliding search with a pressure of circa 200 gram (see picture page 130). One seeks to locate one or more Ting Points with changed skin texture, which then indicates a Process Imbalance (a Channel imbalance, i.e. an Excess or a Deficiency state in the corresponding Channel).

The findings may be classified in two groups:

- Points in *deficiency* (which indicates that the energy in the meridian also is deficient, which also indicates that the correlating process is in deficiency). Such points are covered with a skin that feels:

    ° Thinner.

    ° Colder.

    ° Stiffer.

    ° More in-sunken.

    ° The hair is stiffer.

- Points in *excess* (which indicate that the correlating meridian also is in excess, which again indicate that the correlating process also is in excess). Such points are covered with a skin that feels:

    ° Thicker.

    ° Warmer.

    ° More spongy.

    ° The hair is softer.

The locations of these reactive points indicate which Channel / Organ / process are imbalanced (see picture page 122).

The changes are demonstrated in the micro-slices I have made from different Ting-points that are in different stages of pathology (see next page).

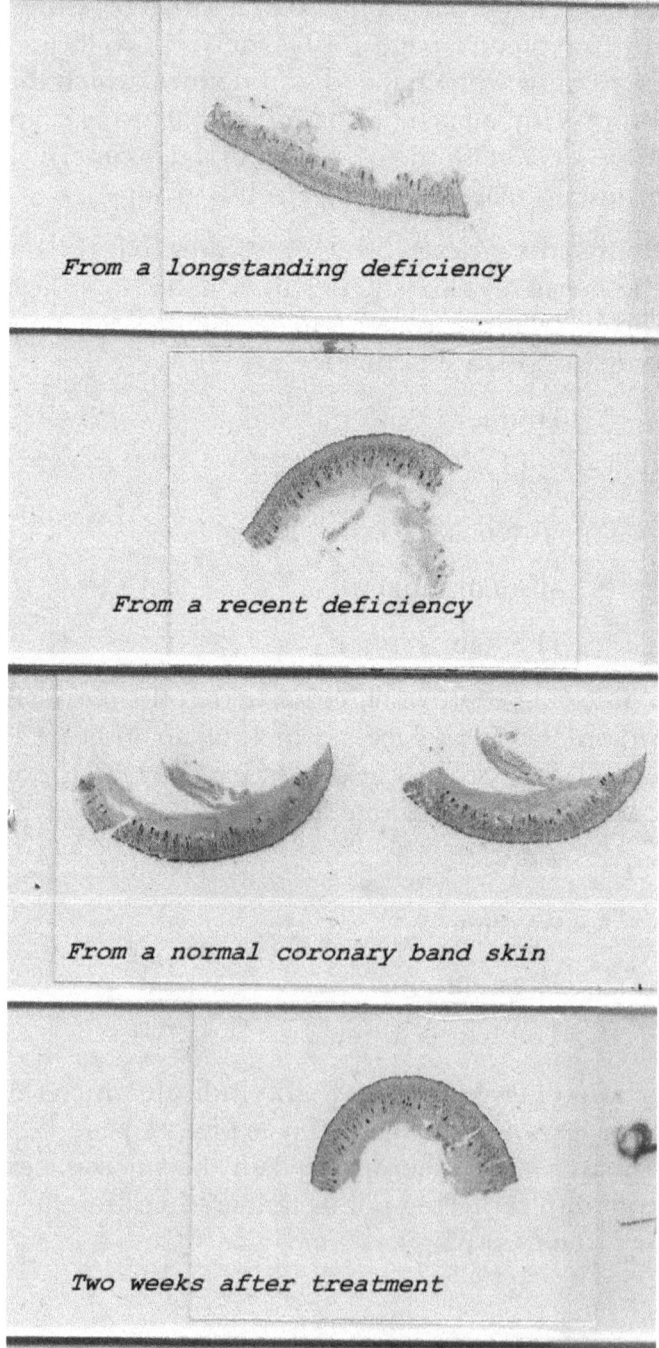

Fig. 19; the skin at the Ting-points at different faces

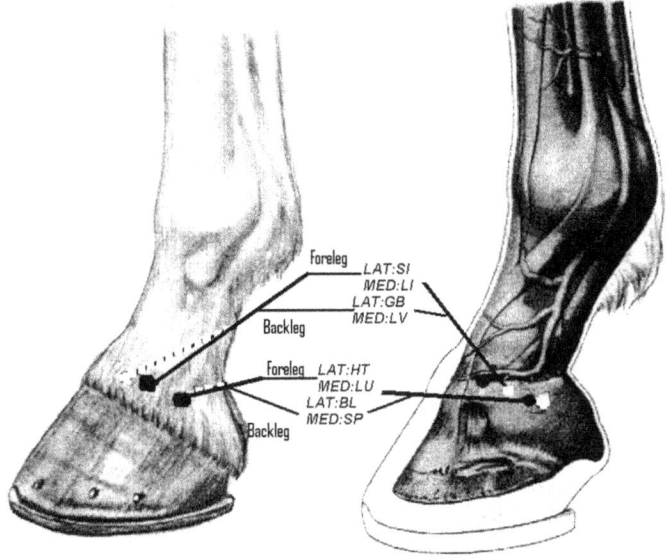

Fig. 20; Illustration of the lateral and medial Ting-points on both the front and the hind-leg in the horse.

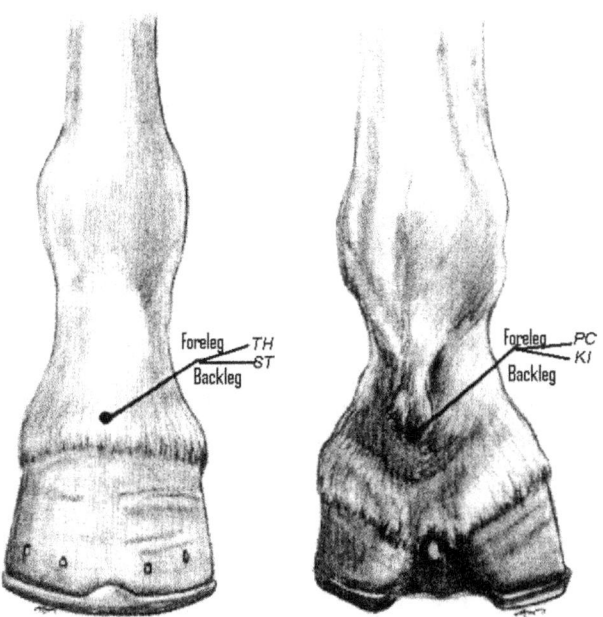

Fig. 21; Illustration of the cranial and the caudal Ting-points on both front and hind-leg in the horse.

Diagram showing the placement of the TING-points

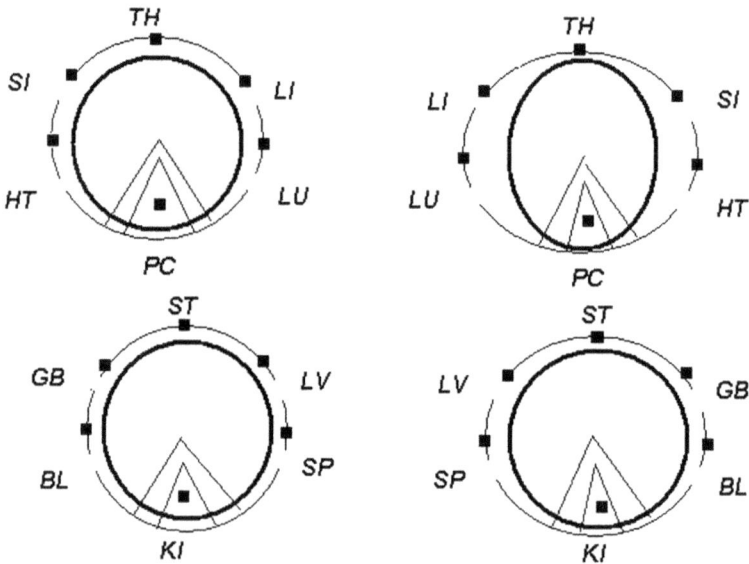

Fig. 22; diagram showing the placement of the Ting-points

At this point, I find it appropriate to make some comments on how the Ting-points in the horse were discovered. This is done to avoid unnecessary discussions about who did what in years to come.

As I learned human acupuncture from my initiating benefactor, **Dr. Georg Bentze MD (1979)**, I mainly used command points and especially the Ting-points. Therefore, I was very interested in finding out where these Ting-points were situated in the dog and the horse. At that time, within the acupuncture society, this was unknown, at least in the horse. Georg Bentze stated quite certainly that, **"All meridians must go to the earth. The Ting-points of the horse have to be found at the coronary band."**

This was my first step towards the Ting-point system, which was a step based on philosophy. I then thought that the sequences of the points were similar to humans, namely counted after the numbers in the illustrations above. From laterally: front leg: SI-HT-TH-PC-LI-LU (zones 1-6), and back leg: BL-KI-GB-ST-LV-SP (zones 7-12). I also had quite good results with them in horses from 1979 on.

The next step was my meeting with **Dr. Dominique Giniaux (1983)**. This step was based on observation. Dominique had observed that the growth of the *hoof changed according to the syndrome of the horse (as described above), and he corrected my sequence of the Ting-points to the following: front leg: HT-SI-TH-LI-LU-PC (zones 1-6), and back leg: BL-GB-ST-LV-SP-KI (zones 7-12). This proved to be correct (I think).*

The third step towards the Ting-point system was made scientifically by **Dr. Emiel van den Bosch (1984)**. *He had measured the electrical resistance in different points around the coronary band, and he confirmed the opinion of Dr. Giniaux.*

The fourth step in the development of the Ting-point method was my own finding of the diagnostic part of this method, which is the pathological sponginess or dry pitting of the Ting-points. This step was based on observation.

The fifth, and presently the last step, was my finding of the ECIWO-system of the coronary band. This finding was, of course, based on earlier findings by, among others, Dr. Nogier, which had led me to the knowledge of the presence of ECIWO-systems in general.

Two of the Ting Points, those of KI and PC, are difficult to investigate in the way described. These Points are between the heel bulbs of the hind- and fore- limbs, respectively. The structure of the tissue here is such that it is difficult to feel the change, although it is there and may be felt by an experienced practitioner. Novices must diagnose a Process Imbalance in KI and PC Channels by other means. However, these two points have good therapeutic value when their use is indicated.

2. Ting-point Diagnosis on the Basis of the Growth of the Hoof

Changes in a Ting point (deficiency or excess of the blood circulation in the skin covering the point) coincide with equal changes in blood circulation in that specific area of the coronary band that give growth to the hoof wall, and will also lead to changes in the growth of the hooves;

- **Decreased** blood circulation leads to decreased growth of the hoof wall right under the area.

- **Elevated** blood circulation leads to faster and more growth of the hoof wall right under the area.

To determine which Channel lacks Qi and which Channel has abundance of Qi, we may note the changed hoof growth. This may be done merely by looking at the hoof wall itself.

Reduced blood circulation in the coronary band will result in reduced growth of the hoof wall in the same segment as the reduced blood circulation. We must then observe;

1. Where the hoof wall is lowest
2. Where the ferrier cuts less

Or directly measure the growth of the hoof wall directly below the Ting-points.

To measure the growth every third day will give a very good measure on the energy in all the processes or meridians.

This system developed by the horse, has also a system for self therapy incorporated. To decide which meridian the horse itself "chooses" to stimulate, we only have to decide where on the hoof there has been put most pressure, where the hoof wall or horse shoe is most worn away.

3. Where there has been most wear and tear at the shoes.

The decreased hoof growth in one area will lead to a change in the weight-bearing system of the horse, which will lead to an elevated pressure at other areas of the hooves.

So, we must then also observe where there will be more wear and tear than usual than other areas of the hooves. This is to decide how the horse itself tries to treat itself through the self-adjusting system that the hooves, Ting-points and hoof-growth make up.

In this system, we may then be able to consider *why* the Channels start or end at the precise points where they do. For example, if LU Channel is Deficient, the hoof wall will grow slower at the medial side of the front foot. This puts greater pressure on the lateral side, where the HT and the SI Channels are situated. Then the Ting-points of HT, HC (partly) and SI are stimulated (and lead to more wear and tear here). These points are all related to the Fire Element, which is the Ko-Father of the Metal Element (LU); as a result, it corrects LU. In other cases the horse itself puts on extra weight on the Ko-father of the deficient meridian, so that also this area will be exposed to more wear and tear. The horse may also put on extra weight on the already lowered deficient area, so that this part will show additional lowering of the hoof wall. I guess that the horse puts on extra weight out of a feeling of what is nessesary, or by a certain feeling of need (like ourselves when we put on extra weight on a tooth suffering from gingivitis).

To summarise: if this system is to be used in its full content and possibility, we must map out exactly where there is:

1. Decreased growth, by measuring the growth of the hoof-wall.
2. Increased pressure on the hoof-wall by observing where the shoes or sole is thinner, or having marks from pressure.

Then we may see **if** the relationship between the Ting-points and the Channels is an automatic treatment procedure *per se*, based on the location of the Channels. This system of self-regulation is supposed to work in the wild horse. In shoeing the horse we destroy this possibility.

Then it makes sense of what I learned at veterinary school; *"If a horse is lame, then take off the shoes and it will heal itself."*

In practice, this will mean that decreased growth in the:

- Cranial aspect of the front hoof(s) may be corrected by increased pressure, either by growth (the hoof wall will be higher) or pressure (the hoof wall will be lower) at the caudal or lateral aspect of the hind hoof(s) (according to the Ko-cycle), or at the medial aspect of the hind hoof(s) (according to the Shen-cycle).

- Lateral aspect of the front hoof may be corrected by stimulation at the caudal (the heels) or lateral aspect of the hind hoof(s) (according to the Ko-cycle) or at the medial aspect of the hind hoof(s) (according to the Shen-cycle).

- Medial aspect of the front hoof may be corrected by stimulation at the lateral aspect of the front hoof(s) (according to the Ko-cycle), or at the medial aspect of the hind hoof(s) (according to the Shen-cycle).

- Caudal (the heels) aspect of the front hoof may be corrected by stimulation at the caudal aspect of the hind hoof(s) (according to the Ko-cycle) or at the medial aspect of the hind hoof(s) (according to the Shen-cycle).

- Cranial aspect of the hind hoof may be corrected by stimulation at the medial aspect of the hind hoof(s) or at the frog (according to the Ko-cycle) or at the lateral aspect of the front hoof(s) (according to the Shen-cycle).

- Caudo-lateral aspect of the hind hoof may be corrected by stimulation at the cranio-medial aspect of the hind hoof(s) or at the cranial aspect of the front hoof(s) (according to the Ko-cycle) or at the medial aspect of the front hoof(s) (according to the Shen-cycle).

- Cranio-lateral aspect of the hind hoof may be corrected by stimulation at the medial aspect of the front hoof(s) (according to the Ko-cycle) or at the caudal (the heels) aspect of the hind hoof(s) (according to the Shen-cycle).

- Cranio-medial aspect of the hind hoof may be corrected by stimulation at the medial aspect of the front hoof(s) (according to the Ko-cycle) or at the caudal (the heels) aspect of the hind hoof(s) (according to the Shen-cycle).

- Caudo-medial aspect of the hind hoof may be corrected by stimulation at the cranio-medial aspect of the hind hoof(s) (according to the Ko-cycle) or at the lateral aspect of the front hoof(s) (according to the Shen-cycle).

- Caudal aspect of the hind hoof (the heels) may be corrected by stimulation at the caudal, cranial or lateral aspect of the front hoof, (according to the Ko-cycle) or at the medial aspect of the front hoof(s) (according to the Shen-cycle).

If humans have evolved from quadrupeds, then such a consideration will explain why the Channels have evolved just where they actually are, and why they are still where they are also in the humans.

Cranial means straight forward towards the head.

Lateral means on the outside, away from the midline.

Medial means on the inside.

Caudal means towards the tail.

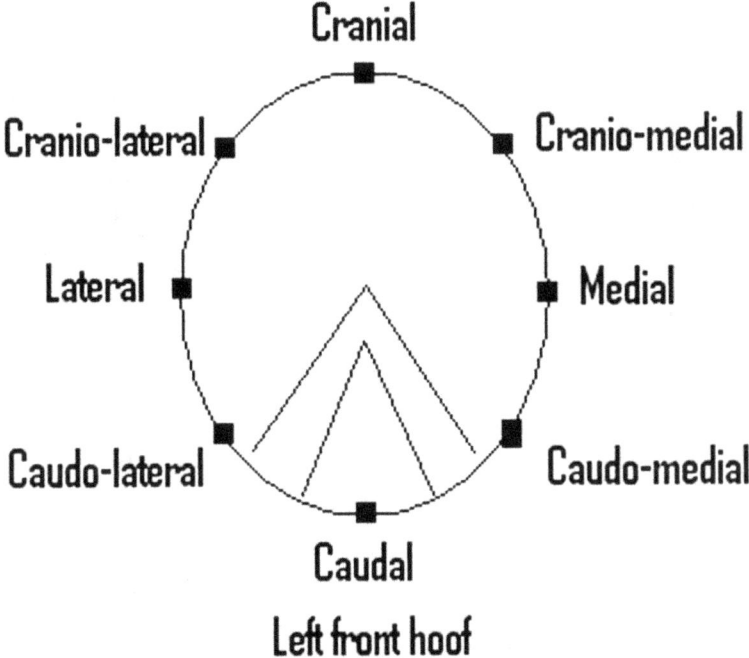

Fig. 23; showing the directions of the hoof

SOMETHING ABOUT THE TING-POINTS IN THE COW.

In the coronary band in the cow's cloven-hoofs we also find the same Ting-points as in all other species. As my bovine practice is minimal, I do not have the same experience as with the horses´ hooves; although, I have managed to localise some of the Ting-points in the cow, and I have also made some observations concerning their function.

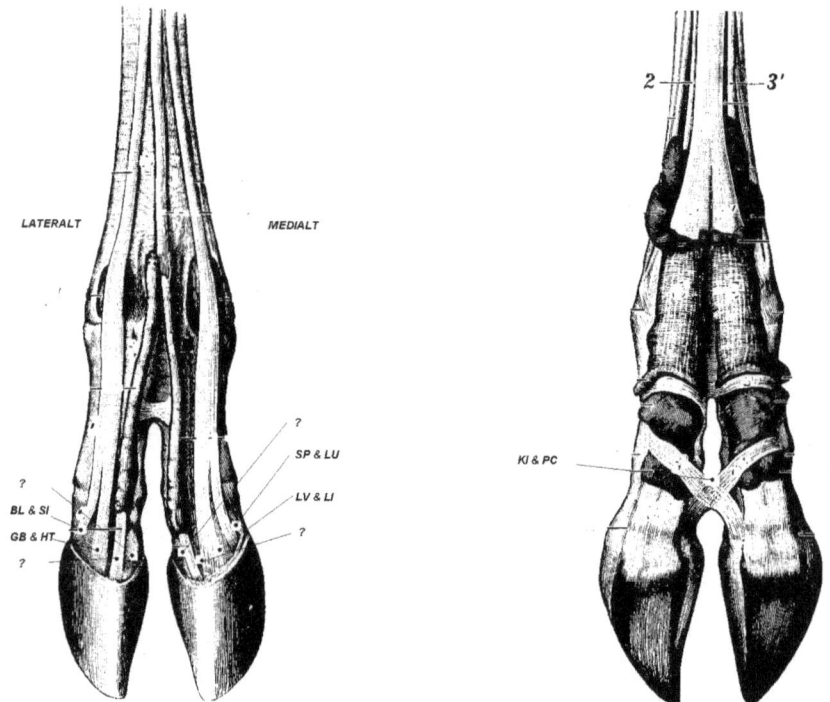

Fig. 24; Illustration of the Ting-points in the cow.

The most important observation is that the growth of the cows hoof stagnates at the medial side of the back hoof after calving.

This correlates with the liver-depression most cows (if not all) go through after giving birth to her calf. The birth and the too high amount of milk are two very strong stresses for the liver, and these result in a marked decrease in the growth of the hoof below the liver Ting-point.

THE EQUINE CORONARY BAND AS AN ECIWO SYSTEM:
Further Studies on the Equine Coronary Band

In 1989 I published an article in the "American Journal of Acupuncture" on the Ting Points after using them and studying their effect for 7 years. Since then I have diagnosed thousands of horses with this method. In 1998 I suddenly had a most interesting experience. A horse I was to diagnose was extremely aggressive. To protect myself, I stood behind a wall when I tried to find the Ting-points. I stretched out my hand, but was unable to hold the thumb correctly as it must be held when searching for the Ting-points. I instead held my thumb as showed in the picture below, namely horizontally. As shown in this picture, I instead came to hold the hand with my thumb´s end vertically.

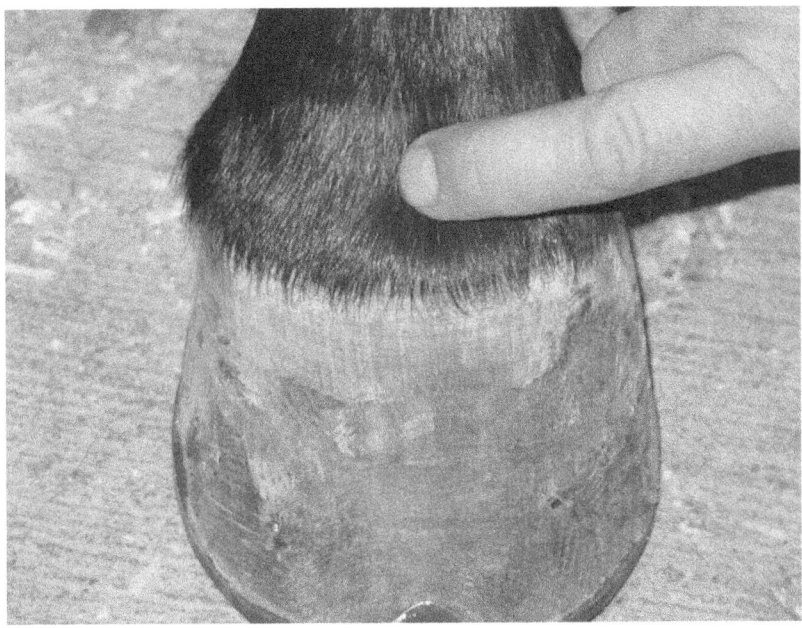

Fig. 25; Picture of how to hold the fingers when investigating the coronary band in search for ECIWO-points.

And suddenly it was like a new world opened to my mind. I suddenly found a whole new set of points. These points were elliptical, and the diameter was smaller than the diameter of my thumb held horizontally. Therefore, I had not discovered them before. Now, while holding my thumb vertically, the thumb was able to slip into one of these points. I found later that the coronary band has many of these elliptical points; many more points than the expected 12 Ting Points of the main Processes.

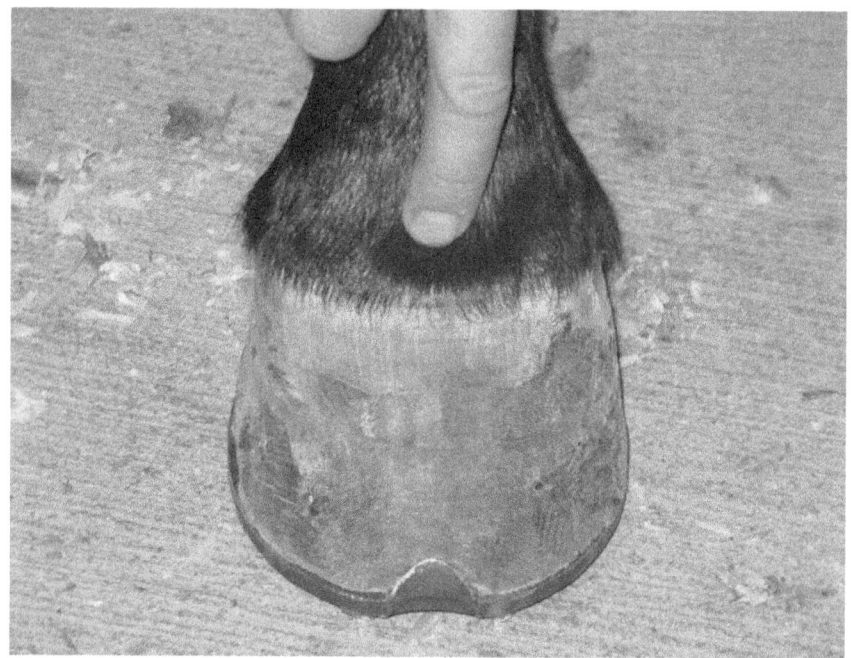

Fig. 26; Picture of how to hold the fingers when investigating the coronary band in search for Ting-points.

Today, I know that the equine coronary band is an ECIWO System (**E**=Embryo, **C**=Containing, **I**=Information, **W**=Whole, **O**=Organism). It may be used as a new diagnostic and therapeutic microsystem. Once grasped, the method is easy to learn, easy to perform and requires very little time.

*ECIWO biology is a newly **re**-discovered and simple method that has proven to be very effective both in medicine and in agriculture. The efficacy of the system is well documented through documents gathered from thousands of cases and several large clinical studies.*

ECIWO biology also has great theoretical interest. It introduces a more detailed understanding of the relationship between the whole and its parts in biology. It also gives a new approach to explain the capacity for self-repair and spontaneous healing that characterizes living beings.

There are many microsystems of AP. Ear-AP is one of the best known, rediscovered c 1953 by Nogier. We also have AP microsystems of the Scalp, Forehead, Nose, Face, Eye, Hand, Foot, etc. These are just part of a much greater law, namely that all parts of the body can serve as a microcosm. This theory has been called the theory of ECIWO biology and this phenomenon may be seen in all living organisms, in plants, animals and man.

As all cells of an organism have developed from one cell, the fertilised ovum or cuttings (in the case of some plants), each single cell contains information about the whole organism. It also has an embryonic potential. This means it can turn into an embryo or a foetus that can grow into a new organism. It has the potential to form a new organism; what we call "total potential". For example, under certain conditions even highly differentiated cells can change into unspecialised cells with more embryonic-type properties, which potentially may differentiate into cells of another type. The science fiction of cloning dinosaurs, as in the film "Jurassic Park" may soon be a reality. Already, several mammalian species have been cloned successfully from non-germinal cells, i.e. cells from tissues not normally recognised as directly related to the ovary or testicle.

The novelty of ECIWO biology is that it is a general phenomenon, found not only at a cellular level but also at higher levels of biological organisation. The following sections will show that ECIWO organisation may be found at the equine coronary band also.

LOCATION OF THE EQUINE CORONARY BAND POINTS

For orientation purposes, the Zero Point (0°) is at the anterior midpoint of the coronary band above each hoof. Moving laterally and horizontally in a circle from the Zero Point, we count 360° around the coronary band until we arrive at the Zero Point again, in the same way as the Ting-points are localised at page 122.

Thus, we move laterally along the coronary band from the Zero Point (0°) at the anterior to about 135°, where the coronary band goes around the bend to the lateral hoof-bulb. There we meet an empty space for about 80° until we meet the medial coronary band at about 210° above the medial hoof-bulb. From there, one moves anterolaterally along the coronary band to the front to meet the Zero Point and complete the circle of 360°.

To assist in precise location of points in the coronary band, each point is characterised as follows:

Fore- or hind foot.
Left or right foot.
Number of degrees (°) lateral from Zero Point (0°).

To illustrate this, go to page 118 and the well known equine Ting Points.

Points on the coronary bands of the left and right forelimbs are mirror images of each other, each representing the side they are on. So also are those of the coronary bands of the left and right hindlimb. The points are located in degrees laterally in opposite directions on the left and the right hoof, i.e. anticlockwise from 0° on the left and clockwise from 0° on the right.

ECIWO EQUINE CORONARY BAND POINTS

The degrees from the Zero Point (0°) to the ECIWO point and its related body parts and structures reflected on the coronary bands of the fore- and hind- feet are:

Forelimb	Degrees lateral from 0°	Hindlimb
Fore fetlock	0^0	Hind fetlock
Carpus, foreknee	15^0	Tarsus, hock
Elbow	35^0	Stifle
Shoulder	55^0	Hip
Atlas	60^0	Sacral area, L6
C2	65^0	L5
C3	70^0	L4
C4	75^0	L3
C5	80^0	L2
C6	85^0	L1
C7	90^0	T18
T1	95^0	T16

T2	100^0	T15
T3	105^0	T14
T4	110^0	T13
T5	115^0	T12
T6	120^0	T11
T7	125^0	T10 – T9
T8	130^0	T8
Diaphragm*,**	135^0	Diaphragm*,**
Diaphragm*,**	225^0	Diaphragm*,**

*   It is possible that there are also several other points in the gap between the bulbs of the heels (between 135^0 and 220^0) but I have not been able to map these out yet.

**   It seems that all 8 cartilages represent the diaphragm (probably different parts of it).

Table 24

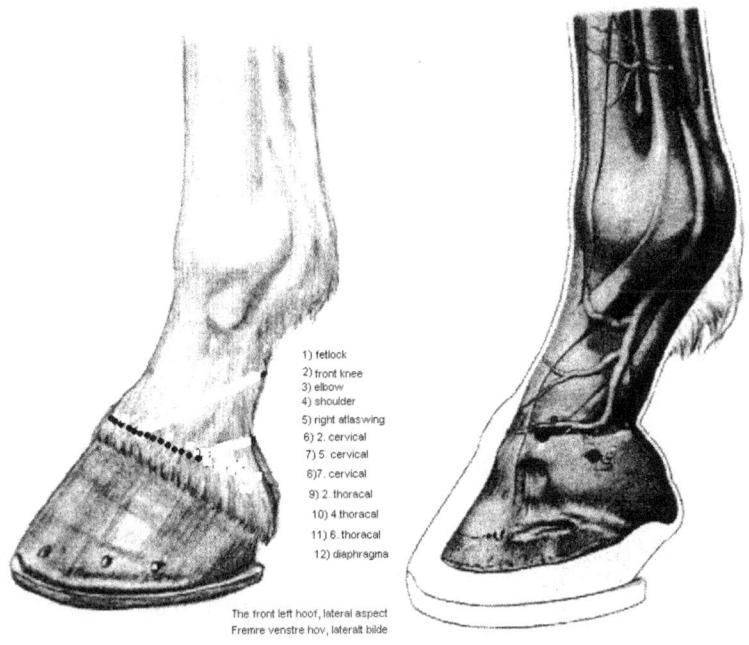

1) fetlock
2) front knee
3) elbow
4) shoulder
5) right atlas wing
6) 2. cervical
7) 5. cervical
8) 7. cervical
9) 2. thoracal
10) 4 thoracal
11) 6. thoracal
12) diaphragma

The front left hoof, lateral aspect
Fremre venstre hov, lateralt bilde

Fig. 27; Illustration of the ECIWO-points at the coronary band at the lateral side of the fore leg of the horse.

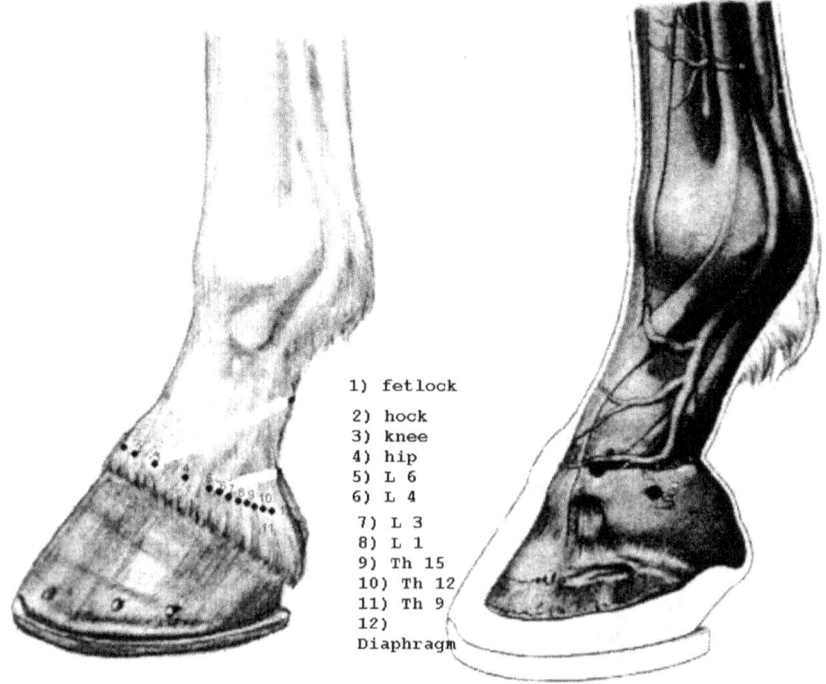

1) fetlock
2) hock
3) knee
4) hip
5) L 6
6) L 4
7) L 3
8) L 1
9) Th 15
10) Th 12
11) Th 9
12) Diaphragm

Fig. 28; Illustration of the ECIWO-points at the coronary band at the lateral side of the hind leg of the horse.

THE EAR ZONES (THE EAR ECIWO-SYSTEM)

The ear is a very interesting microcosm. It has been used for diagnostic (and therapeutic, see page 497) purposes since ancient times. There are reports of this both from Egyptian and Arabic sources.

DIAGNOSTIC EAR POINTS

The ear-points are very interesting because "reactive ear-points" are:

- Absent in perfect health (balance) or when there is nothing wrong with the organs or anatomical structures to which they relate.

- Unstable in their location. They can "wander" several millimetres during treatment, especially between several sessions, and this indicates both prognosis and therapeutic effect of the treatment.

The fact that the ear-points are present or can be found only when there is something wrong or pathological makes the ear a very useful diagnostic tool.

Reactive ear-points are found by many different methods. All aim to find points with changes sensitive to probe pressure, heat, electricity or other physical stimuli.

- In deficient states, the reactive ear-points can be:
  - Pale.
  - Cold.
  - Show lack of sensibility to:
    - Pressure.
    - Heat.
    - Cold.
- In excessive states, the reactive ear-points can be:
  - Painful.
  - Red.
  - Show elevated sensitivity to:
    - Pressure.
    - Heat.
    - Cold.
    - Electricity.

The easiest way to find reactive points is to search with a sensitive acupoint detector and a good ear chart. However, the method of Nogier is the most advanced way to find reactive points. Between these two extremes are several other methods.

The *diagnostic parts* of these two extremes will be discussed in this section.

TOPOGRAPHIC EAR-AP:

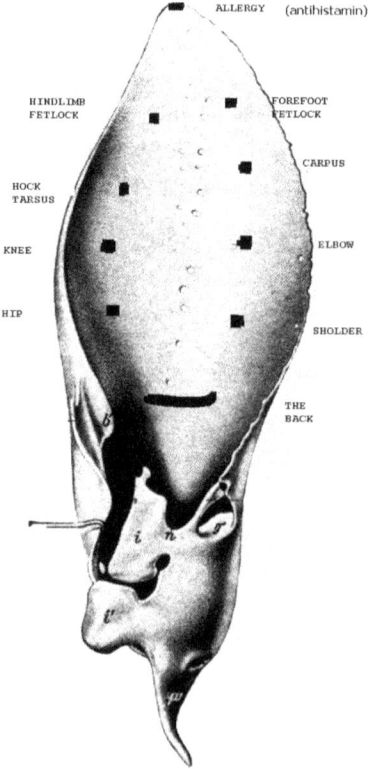

Fig. 29; A very simple ear-point chart, but in animals it is highly usable.

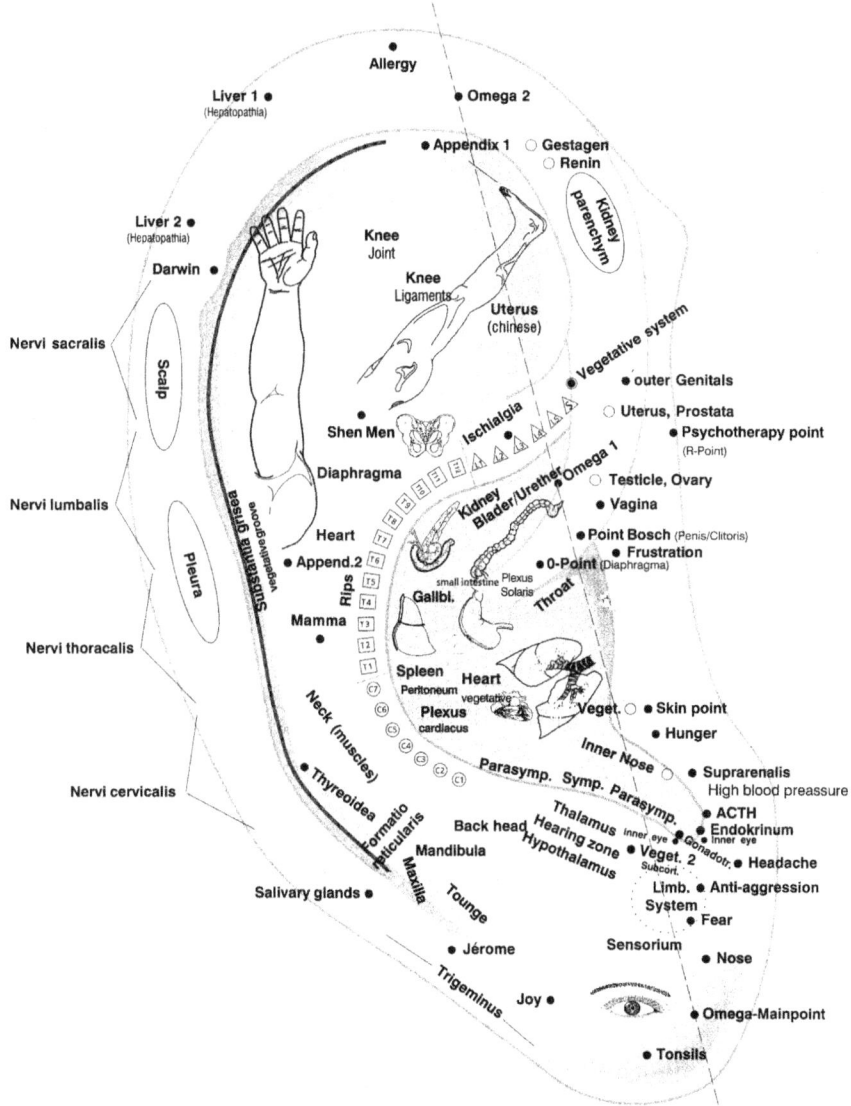

Fig. 30; A much more advanced ear-point chart developed in humans.

AURICULOMEDICINE:

Simple forms of Ear-AP were known for several thousand years. From India and China, Ear-AP spread to Egypt and North Africa. In the early 1900s, there were many French people, including soldiers in the Foreign Legion, in the French colonies in North Africa. Some of these people asked the local healers to treat their common disorders, such as back pain.

The French doctor, Paul Nogiér, began to develop Ear-point therapy in 1952. He had noticed that some soldiers who had served in North Africa had burn marks in certain areas or their ears. On inquiry, he was told that the local medicine men had applied heat to these points to treat lumbago, sciatic and other back disorders. Nogiér began to investigate whether there were reflex points for the whole body in the ear. He stimulated distant areas of the body in volunteers by using clips or forceps and he observed the skin of the ears for any visible changes. When he noticed a reflex change in the ear, he marked the exact reactive point or zone. In this way, he meticulously mapped the main reflex zones on the ear for the main body parts and organs. He developed this later into ear-point therapy and auriculomedicine.

THE EAR AS AN INVERTED EMBRYO

After a long period of study, Nogiér had a revolutionary idea that would solve many questions and develop the Ear-point therapy further. He imagined the ear as an image of an embryo turned upside down. This opened up to the complete picture of the body's reflex points in the ear. China, the homeland of AP, welcomed this discovery with enthusiasm. Auriculomedicine, however, was not developed until many years later, when Nogiér discovered RAC (**R**eflex **A**uriculo **C**ardiac), or more correctly VAS (**V**ascular **A**uricular **S**ignal).

*In my practise I have discovered that the VAS really is a DVR (**D**ermal **V**ascular **R**esponse) because all areas of the skin give a reaction in the entire vascular system. Really it might even be called a TEVR (**T**otal **E**nvironment **V**ascular **R**esponse) as the total influence of the environment including the skin, atmosphere and cosmos reflect its influence in the vascular system.*

He discovered also how different colours and frequencies influence the skin so that the detection of certain points got easier.

Ear-point diagnosis, the name for Nogiér's method before he discovered the VAS and the sensitivity of the skin to different colours, is a reflex-point diagnosis. This form of diagnosis is simple and symptomatic.

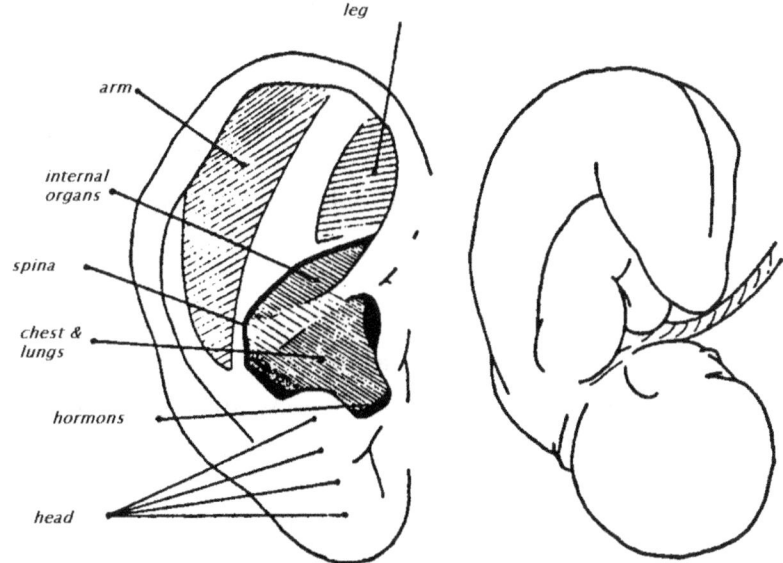

Fig. 31; The ear as an inverted foetus.

Modern auriculomedicine differs radically from Ear-AP. Auriculomedicine is based mainly on the principles of conventional medicine, while Ear-AP is based on the teaching of reflexes, something like Foot Zone Therapy.

After his discovery of the VAS, Nogiér discovered that different and specific colours made the body react more specifically and clearly on the different stimuli of the skin. If the body was influenced by these colours, it was much easier to get a response through the RAC, so easily that the skin of the ear (and also the rest of the body) only had to be stimulated with a light beam to give a detectable response.

In this way, the *Auriculomedicine* was born.

This method is a form of diagnosis (and therapy) that is more complicated, more comprehensive and much more informative as to the energetic causes. It is based on the principles of conventional medicine, but we often see that the discoveries correspond to the Laws of AP and that the TCM pulses normalise after successful treatment.

The equipment needed for a complete Auriculomedicine examination is:

- A pair of sensitive hands.

- 7 Colour filters + one filter with all the 7 colours.

- A thin ray of light (penlight, lamp, or laser).

- A diagnostic hammer with a black and white head.

ACR / VAS

The pulse reaction, called the ACR or VAS by Nogiér, is an essential part of a thorough examination in auriculomedicine (as in "controlled AP" as well). This pulse response is a reflex from the skin to the heart or arterial blood circulation. Stimulation of the skin over a reactive area or a point or Weak Structure activates an autonomic reaction or recognition that induces a special VAS Pulse reaction.

The VAS-reaction may be found anywhere at an artery, but is most usually found at:

- Arteria radialis (radial artery) right under the radial Processus styloideus (the styloid process) between the second and third classical Chinese Pulse-Positions (for GB-LV and BL-KI, respectively)

- Arteria carotis externus in front of the ear.

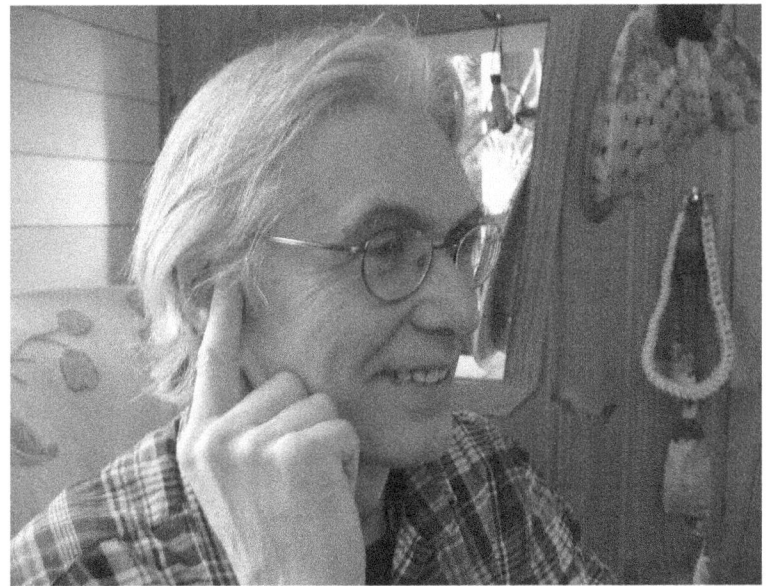

Fig. 32; Picture of how to hold the hand while investigating the VAS at Arteria carotis externus.

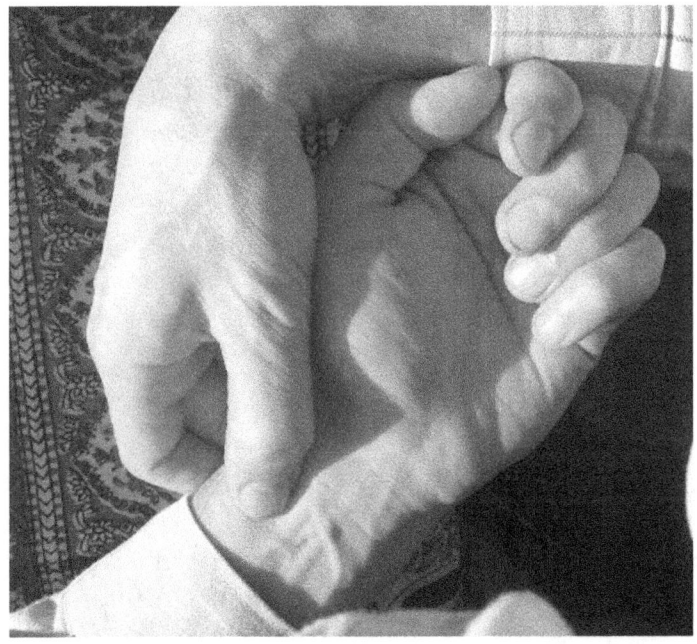

Fig. 33; Picture of how to hold the hand while investigating the VAS at Arteria radialis.

VAS manifests as an altered quality in the pulse. VAS Pulse-changes can not be proven objectively, since pulse quality is a subjective parameter.

It usually takes some time before the VAS occurs. The number of pulse beats:

- Before it occurs, is called the "*VAS latency time*", usually 1-20 beats.

- Before the reaction go away again [the duration of the VAS (i.e. the time until the Pulse normalises again) is called the "*VAS reaction time*" (range 1-10 beats)].

These times have diagnostic value. Young and strong (Qi Excess) individuals have a short latency time (2-4 beats) and a long reaction time (8-10 beats). Old and weak individuals (Qi Deficiency) have a long latency time (8-12 beats) and a short reaction time (2-4 beats). If the reaction time is long (especially with a short latency time) the prognosis is good.

Stimulation of effective acupoints usually gives a reaction in VAS.

The 12 Chinese Pulses mirror the Qi Status of their related Process. Thereby, they also indicate the presence and nature of a Process Imbalance (Deficiency or Excess) in one or more Channels. In contrast, the VAS reflects the location of the injury anatomically.

Chinese- or VAS- Pulse quality is a subjective phenomenon. It has not been possible to prove objective changes in these Pulses, nor to correlate such changes with objective pathology. Therefore, diagnosis based on these Pulses may be regarded as a form of diagnostic dowsing or divining for Energetic Imbalances, see page 164.

THE COLOUR FILTERS

Colour filters are used to locate reactive ear points more easily. A colour filter gives a message to the body to release certain information or select information. It reinforces the response from the ear so that we can better find the points. A filter placed:

- On the head reduces the amplitude of the signals or response from the body.

- On the body elevates the amplitude of the signals or response from the body.

The filters are colour-filters made from Kodak Wratten colour filters, and are as follows:

Filter A	2,28 Hz	Nervous system	Kodak Wratten 22	Yellow
Filter B	4.56 Hz	Metabolism	Kodak Wratten 25	Red
Filter C	9,125 Hz	Movements	Kodak Wratten 4	Yellow
Filter D	18,25 Hz	Internal organs	Kodak Wratten 23A	Dark pink
Filter E	36,50 Hz	Spine	Kodak Wratten 44	Petrol blue
Filter F	73 Hz	Emotions	Kodak Wratten 98	Dark blue
Filter G	146 Hz	Personality	Kodak Wratten 30	Margent pink

Table 25

The filters correspond to and reinforce the response from 7 important areas or functions or organ-systems of the body. The filter numbers relate to Kodak Wratten colour filters. The 7 main colour filters may be purchased in any photo store, but today they are only made a few places and may be more difficult to find. The filters may then be bought from "Sedatelec" (see internet). Each filter is cut to size so that it fits into a slide frame. This frame is placed wherever one wishes on the patient's body. We only need to ensure that light shines through the filter onto the body. The program-filter contains the colours of all the 7 colours.

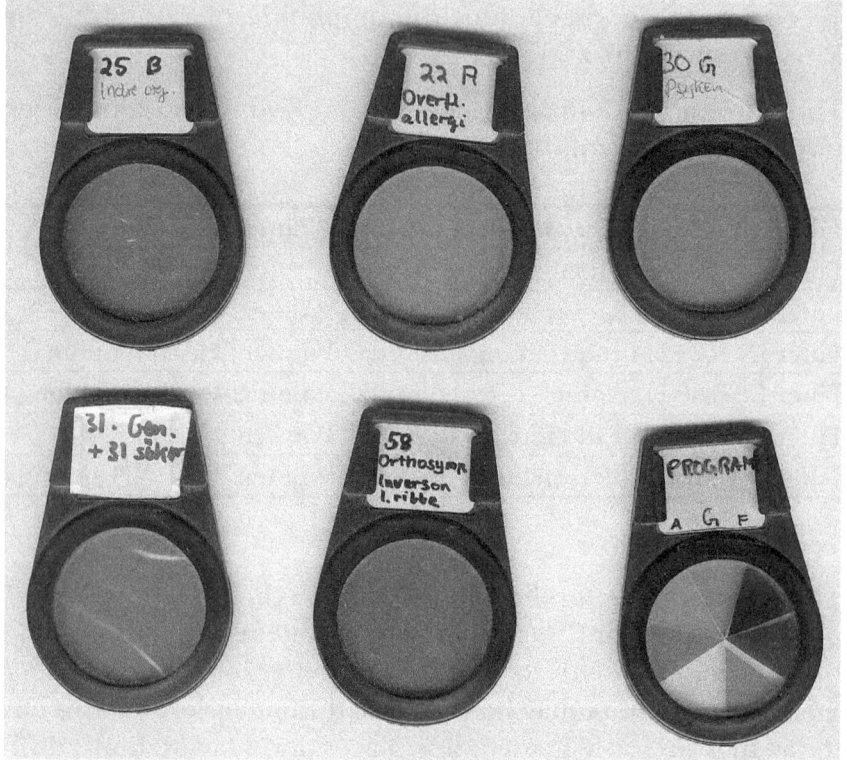

Fig. 34; Examples of filters that I use in my daily practise.

Detailed Description of the Methodology

1. **Finding the dominant side:** The first step is to decide the laterality of the patient. We mainly want to treat and diagnose on the dominant side. The dominant side is usually where we get the most clear RAC (a clear RAC is when the pulse suddenly gets weak after some sort of stimulus) after touching the ear with the program filter.

2. **Finding the correct filter to use:**

   A. We may then place the program-filter on the head on the dominant side and send a strong light-beam through each and every colour of the filter. When we arrive at the correct filter, the VAS is at it most clear response.

B. We may take the Chinese pulses and "holding" the weakest pulse, we may place each filter on the head of the patient. The correct filter will re-establish the energetic balance of the pulses (explained in greater detail on page 179).

3. *Finding the correct ear-point to use:* After finding the correct filter to use, we place this filter on the body of the patient. Then we go over the entire ear with the light-beam and the correct point will result in a clear and strong VAS. If we want to use body-acupuncture, we may also in a similar way test all the usual acupuncture points, as described by several authors as "Controlled acupuncture".

Bill Wagner, an American veterinarian who works with these colours, places the colour-filter in a dias-frame, as a slide in a projector, and exposes the whole animal to the projected colour. In this way, he does not need to worry whether the slide is in place or has fallen down. When these colour slides are used, the skin of the ear (and the body) becomes more reactive to the VAS Pulse method. Usually we must stimulate the skin quite strongly (with a needle) to get a VAS reaction. But, in using the colour filters, it is sufficient to expose the skin to a thin light-beam from a Heine-lamp in order to elicit a VAS reaction.

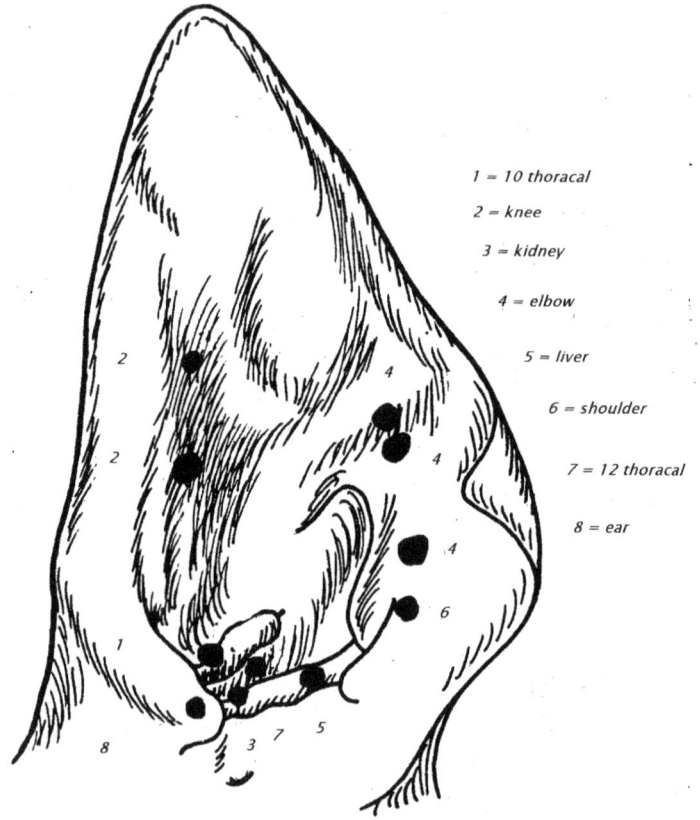

1 = 10 thoracal

2 = knee

3 = kidney

4 = elbow

5 = liver

6 = shoulder

7 = 12 thoracal

8 = ear

Fig. 35; Some results from my own auriculomedical investigation on the dog-ear.

Use of the Nogier Colour-Filters in the Chinese Pulse Diagnosis
As the filters of Nogiér may be used to strengthen or weaken
the responses from the body, they may also be used in Chinese
pulse diagnosis to further evaluate the origin of the different
deficiencies found in the pulse.

Filter A	Nervous system	Yellow-orange
Filter B	Metabolism	Red
Filter C	Muscles and legs	Yellow
Filter D	Internal organs	Dark pink
Filter E	Spine	Petrol blue
Filter F	Feelings	Dark blue
Filter G	Personality	Margenta pink

Table 26

146

- If we place the filter that "represents" the area that is the cause of the deficient process on the head, it will lead to a weakened response from the body; that is a deficiency that will be harder to detect (the pulse will be stronger and more balanced at that particular position).

- If we place the filter that "represents" the area that is the cause of the deficient process on the body it will lead to a stronger response from the body; that is a deficiency that will be easier to detect (the pulse will be weaker and more unbalanced at that particular position).

If we, for example, have a horse with a deficient kidney process, we may try to place the filters on the head, one after each other, and then observe which filter restores the pulse on the kidney position; that is, to weaken the response of the weak process.

An example:

- My own horse, Balder, had a weak kidney process. When I placed the G-filter on his head, the pulse felt quite normal again (the filter took away the weak pulse). Then I may conclude that his personality is the underlying cause of his weakened kidney. He is a nervous horse and that weakens his kidneys due to his personality.

THE 12 METACARPAL AND METATARSAL ECIWO SYSTEMS

In the year 2001 I made a very interesting observation. I found out that there is a separate ECIWO-system related to every single process located along the metacarpal and metatarsal bones.

In man, these ECIWO-systems at the hand are situated as shown in the photograph on the next page. For the foot see figure 10, page 14.

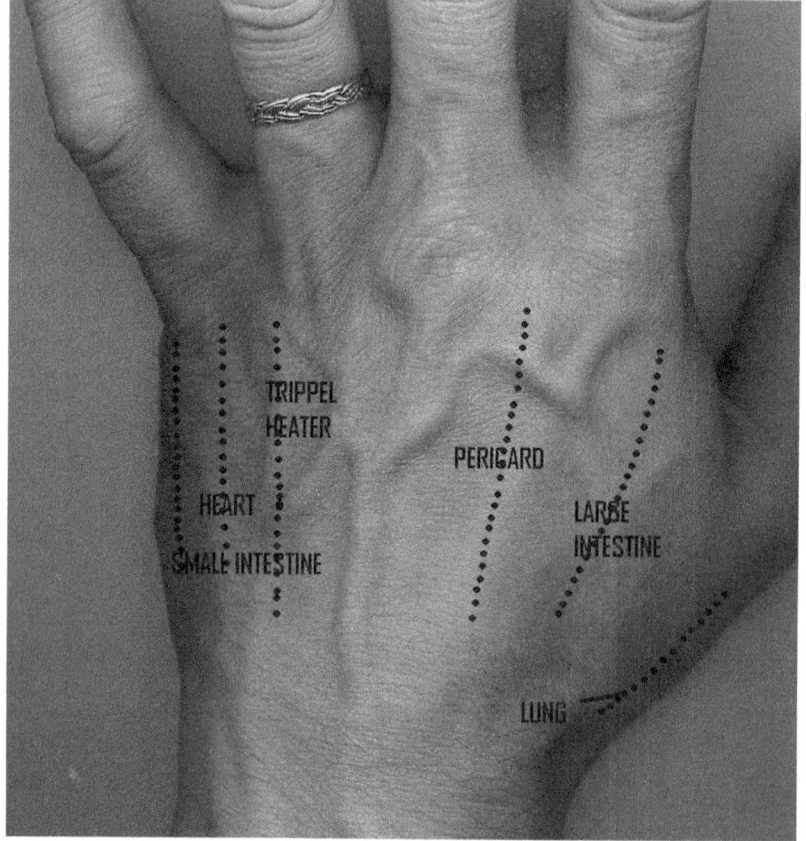

Fig. 36; The ECIWO-systems at the human hand

In the horse, there are equal systems along each of the meridians where they pass the canon bone. There are 6 ECIWO-
systems along each one of the metacarpal and metatarsal bones.
On the pictures on the next page I have illustrated 3 of these
systems, those situated on the medial side of the front leg.

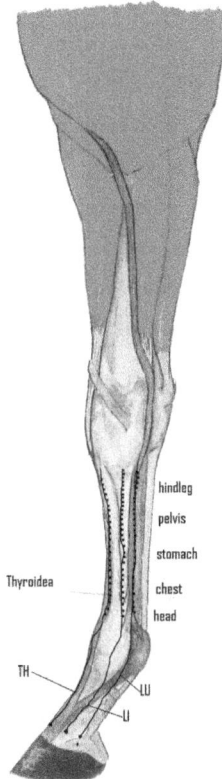

Fig. 37; The ECIWO-systems in the horse (medial front leg)

These ECIWO-points may be used in the following way;

- ***For diagnoses:***

1. First you decide which meridian is deficient.

2. Then you feel along the ECIWO-system with your finger.

3. Where you find a point that is deficient or excessive, you have located about where on the body the symptom from the deficient meridian is (where on the body the symptom is situated)

- ***For therapy:***

1. You put a needle in the point that you have found through the diagnosis.

2. You locate where on the body the most prominent symptom is situated.

3. Then you put a needle in that point.

An example:

A woman has breast cancer. The deficient process is the liver. The breast is situated about one third distal along the medial side of the first metatarsal bone (see figure 10, pag 14).

Sacrum as an Effective ECIWO-System

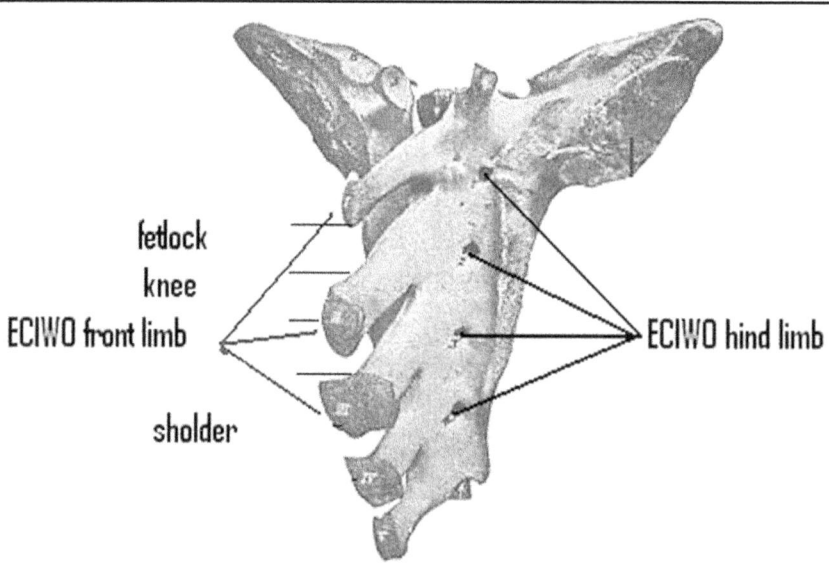

fetlock
knee
ECIWO front limb

ECIWO hind limb

sholder

Fig. 38; The ECIWO-systems at the Sacrtum

Os sacrum is one of the most important bones in the entire body due to its close connection to the Ilio-sacral joint and Musculus gluteus medius.

It is also an ECIWO-system, as are all other bones also, but some are more important that others.

Within the sacral ECIWO-system there are points especially important to the lumbar area and the hip. They are situated on the right side of the bone, with the most distal parts of the hind leg situated most cranial, and the most proximal areas of the hind leg situated most cranial on the sacral bone.

The way to diagnose the problem is to tap through both sides of the bone and where you hear a distinct muffling of the sound that is where the projection of the problem is situated (and there you should treat).

3. MODIFYING FACTORS

These are factors that alter the manifestation of disease or influence disease in any way, by improvement, aggravation or other change. If we can find the Modifying Factors, we can find with good precision the ultimate cause of the disease.

External factors influence the processes and either weaken them or strengthen them. If such weakness or strength is the cause of the symptoms, then the modifying factors will also change the symptoms.

As the symptoms themselves also are part of the process in question, then the external or internal factors will also be able to influence the symptoms more directly. The different bodily Processes, microsystems (ECIWO Systems) and organs continuously exchange communication with equivalent Processes in the external world. If such External Processes (outside of the organs and the body) influence us, the corresponding Process in the body responds by improvement, aggravation or change in some way.

- *Strong Cold weakens Water, while moderate Cold strengthens (KI-BL).* We know this very well if we have had cystitis or nephritis. If Cold causes Modification of any symptom (for example if a dry eczema is aggravated when exposed to cold weather) we may deduce that its energetic root cause (Process Imbalance) is a deficient Process in KI.

  ° If strong cold make:

    ▪ The symptoms better, then the symptoms come from an excess of the kidney

- - The symptoms worse, then the symptoms come from a deficiency of the kidney

  o If moderate cold make:

  - - The symptoms better, then the symptoms come from a deficiency of the kidney

    - The symptoms worse, then the symptoms come from an excess of the kidney

- *Strong Heat weakens Fire, while moderate Heat strengthens (HT-SI and PC-TH).* If strong Heat aggravates a migraine, we may deduce that its Process Imbalance lies in an imbalance of one or more of the Fire Phase Channels (HT, SI, PC or TH) or in LV Channel, which controls venous blood circulation. This applies also if a migraine is aggravated on Sundays (sun = Fire) or in red light (red = Fire) or on ingestion of hot spices or by Heat of any kind. All of these "modifiers" suggest a Process Imbalance in Fire.

  o If strong heat makes:

  - - The symptoms better, then the symptoms come from an excess.

    - The symptoms worse, then the symptoms come from a deficiency.

  o If moderate heat makes:

  - - The symptoms better, then the symptoms come from a deficiency.

    - The symptoms worse, then the symptoms come from an excess.

- *Strong Wind weakens Wood, while moderate Wind strengthens (LV-GB).* If symptoms vary with Wind and unstable weather, this is a strong indication of an LV imbalance as the cause of the symptoms. If symptoms also vary with the intake or ingestion of sugar, chocolate or especially margarine, this also suggests an imbalance in LV Process. LV is the main organ governing the metabolism of sugar and fat.

- If strong wind makes:
  - The symptoms better, then the symptoms come from an excess.
  - The symptoms worse, then the symptoms come from a deficiency.
- If moderate wind makes:
  - The symptoms better, then the symptoms come from a deficiency.
  - The symptoms worse, then the symptoms come from an excess.

- *Strong Damp weakens Earth, while moderate damp strengthens* (SP-ST). If strong Damp or humidity aggravates a gastrointestinal problem we may deduce that its Process Imbalance lies in an imbalance of one of the Earth Phase Channels (SP-ST). This applies also if the problem aggravates with worry or on ingestion of too much sweet or citrus food, etc. (sweet, yellow, worry = Earth). All of these "modifiers" suggest a Process Imbalance in Earth.
  - If strong damp makes:
    - The symptoms better, then the symptoms come from an excess.
    - The symptoms worse, then the symptoms come from a deficiency.
  - If moderate damp makes:
    - The symptoms better, then the symptoms come from a deficiency.
    - The symptoms worse, then the symptoms come from an excess.

- *Strong Dryness weakens Metal, while moderate Dryness strengthens* (LU-LI). If strong Dryness aggravates a respiratory or abdominal problem, we may deduce that its Process Imbalance lays in an imbalance of one the Metal Phase Channels (LU-LI). This applies also if the problem is aggravated with grief or bereavement or on ingestion of too much spicy food, etc. (spicy, grief = Metal). All of these "modifiers" suggest a Process Imbalance in Metal.

  ° If strong dryness makes:

    - The symptoms better, then the symptoms come from an excess.

    - The symptoms worse, then the symptoms come from a deficiency.

  ° If moderate dryness makes:

    - The symptoms better, then the symptoms come from a deficiency.

    - The symptoms worse, then the symptoms come from an excess.

And this thinking also goes for all the other things that modify the symptoms showed in the table on the next page.

By feedback from human patients and especially when we examine our own Lesion-Symptom Complexes, it may be easy to document how different Stressors influence the Lesion-Symptom Complexes (the manifestations of disease). For example, careful questioning or self-examination can elicit very important information on what aggravates or improves the symptoms, say a cough, rhinitis, headache, stomach ulcer, eczema, conjunctivitis, etc. We should determine how these Lesion-Symptom Complexes vary with different Stressors, food intake or different states of mind, etc.

The relationships between the Phases, Process and Stressors are easier to see in a table:

	Fire	Earth	Metal	Water	Wood
Season	Summer	Late summer	Autumn	Winter	Spring
Growth and development	Growth	Transforma-Tion	Harvesting	Storing	Germina-Tion
Climate (good and bad)	Heat	Damp	Dryness	Cold	Wind
Direction	South	Centre	West	North	East
Yin Organ	HT, PC	SP	LU	KI	LV
Yang Organ	SI, TH	ST	LI	BL	GB
Colour	Red	Yellow	White	Blue black	Green
Emotion	Joy	Worry	Grief	Fear	Anger
Sound	Laugh	Sing	Sob	Groan	Shout
Orifice controlled	Tongue	Mouth	Nose	Ears, anus, vagina, urethra	Eyes
Sense organ controlled	Speech	Taste	Smell	Hearing	Sight, vision
Body fluid	Sweat	Phlegm	Mucus	Urine	Tears
Manifests in	Face	Lips	Skin	Hair (head)	Nails
Nourishes	Vessels	Fatty tissue	Skin	Bones	Tendons
Stores	Psychic Qi	Ideas	Vital Qi	Will	Spiritual
Flavour	Bitter	Sweet	Spicy	Salty	Sour, like vinegar

Table 27

IMPORTANT!

If the external factor strengthens the internal process, then all excessive symptoms will be aggravated.

If the external factor weakens the internal process, then all excessive symptoms will be ameliorated.

If the external factor strengthens the internal process, then all deficient symptoms will be ameliorated.

If the external factor weakens the internal process, then all deficient symptoms will be aggravated.

However, it may be difficult to observe these types of changes in animals. It requires very careful observation to be able to see such variation but it is important to be aware of this possibility of diagnosing because it is important to see the total picture. It also makes our job as veterinary clinicians so much more interesting.

TIME OF DAY (SEE ALSO PAGE 31)

It is important to note the time of day at which the disease or symptoms arises or change markedly (begin, aggravate, improve or in any way change significantly). These changes relate to the body's diurnal rhythms (see page 31). In TCM, it is often said that Qi flows through the 12 Main Channels in a definite diurnal sequence. I personally would rather express it by saying that each of the Twelve Fundamental Processes has a certain time or period when the body needs maximal effect from that Process. At this time, the Process must work maximally. Therefore, if a Process is weakened, the symptoms tend to manifest only at this time as the symptoms are designed by the body only to help the deficient process; just as when we require maximal work from an already exhausted worker then we will really observe how tired he is.

The activity of the process is minimally 12 hours away from its maximal time. These Biorhythms have diagnostic and therapeutic significance. The Qi Clock relationships are:

Hour	02	04	06	08	10	12
Channel	LV-	LU-	LI+	ST+	SP-	HT-
	X	X	X	X	X	X
Channel	SI+	BL+	KI-	PC-	TH+	GB+
Hour	14	16	18	20	22	24

Table 28

In the table above, "-" signifies Yin, "+" signifies Yang and "X" signifies Qi Clock Opponents. Note that the Opponents are always of opposite polarities (- / +). For example HT (Yin) is the Qi Clock Opponent of GB (Yang), at 12 noon and 12 midnight, respectively.

Elem.	met		jord		ild		van		ild		tre
Yin-prosess	LU¹		SP⁴	>>	HT⁵		KI⁸	>>	PC⁹		LV¹²
	‖		‖		‖		‖		‖		‖
Yang- prosess	LI²	>>	ST³		SI⁶	>>	BL⁷		TH¹⁰	>>	GB¹¹
Lem	arm		ben		arm		ben		arm		ben

Table 29; Detailed description of how the energy flows in the body.

TWO EXAMPLES:

- A headache that increases in intensity up until noon and then eases after noon may indicate imbalance (deficiency) in HT Process as its cause. As HT governs circulation, the imbalance may change blood circulation to the head, triggering the headache. As the work for or the demands on HT Qi should be maximal around noon, the need for compensation (the cause of the symptoms) also is maximal at this time. Such symptoms also may be due to a GB Excess Process, as GB is the Qi Clock Opponent of HT.

- Waking up every night at 0100-0300h without any obvious cause (no desire to drink water or urinate) may indicate LV Deficiency (Weakest Process in LV). Those symptoms may arise because the demands on LV are high at this time. Waking at that time may occur also when SI Process is Excess; SI is the Qi Clock Opponent of LV.

It may be difficult to see diurnal variation in Lesion-Symptom Complexes in animals. This is because we usually do not observe the animals as closely throughout the whole day as way we may observe ourselves. However, in some cases, one may observe such variations of the symptoms. Such information from an observant owner often helps the vet to diagnose the deficient Process, especially in itchy dogs that scratch more during specific times of the day.

The table above summarises the Qi Clock biorhythms and shows the time of maximum stress for each Process. It also is important to be aware that each organ also has its time when its Qi is minimal; exactly 12 hours out of phase with the time of its maximal Qi. The time of lowest GB Qi is the same as the Qi peak time of HT and this must be considered. In the first example above, HT Deficiency or GB Excess may provoke the migraine.

The table following here is a more detailed table concerning the time of day that the symptoms vary. If the table on page 31 is difficult to apply to animals, then this one must be almost impossible.

But, as I have had great use of it in my human practise, I will bring it to your attention.

If for example the symptoms change in some direction between 0400 and 0430, then the stomach is the origin of the problems.

This table may be used in preference to the 2-hour cycle. This one is the most reliable.

LUNG	0300-0330	0900-0930	1500-1530	2100-2130
LARGE I.	0330-0400	0930-1000	1530-1600	2130-2200
STOMACH	0400-0430	1000-1030	1600-1630	2200-2230
SPLEEN	0430-0500	1030-1100	1630-1700	2230-2300
HEART	0500-0530	1100-1130	1700-1730	2300-2330
SMALL I.	0530-0600	1130-1200	1730-1800	2330-2400
BLADDER	0600-0630	1200-1230	1800-1830	2400-0030
KIDNEY	0630-0700	1230-1300	1830-1900	0030-0100
PERICARD	0700-0730	1300-1330	1900-1930	0100-0130
TRIPPEL H.	0730-0800	1330-1400	1930-2000	0130-0200
GALL B.	0800-0830	1400-1430	2000-2030	0200-0230
LIVER	0830-0900	1430-1500	2030-2100	0230-0300

Table 30

SEASONAL INFLUENCES ON THE MANIFESTATION OF DISEASE (LESION-SYMPTOM COMPLEXES)

In Five Phase Theory, each season influences a different Phase and all of its Correspondences:

Phase	Fire	Earth	Metal	Water	Wood
Season	Summer	Late Summer	Autumn	Winter	Spring
Process	HT-SI-PC-TH	SP-ST	LU-LI	KI-BL	LV-GB
External Stressor	Heat	Damp	Dryness	Cold	Wind

Table 31

If the energy of the seasons becomes too strong or too weak, this influences the misbalanced process and acts as Stressors that influence the organism and modify the Lesion-Symptom Complex. By depleting Qi in the body, extreme weather conditions or seasonal expressions, *per se,* can precipitate disease. This thinking applies to all the seasons and their Phase Correspondences, including their related Channels and Processes.

- *Spring (Wood / Wind)* influences LV-GB. Typical cattle diseases in Spring include muscular dystrophy (in selenium-vitamin E deficiency), muscular spasms in hypomagnesaemic tetany, and ketosis. Process Imbalances in LV-GB are more common in spring and in weather with a lot of Wind. Wind "moves the leaves and branches" and Wood/Wind diseases typically have Lesion-Symptom Complexes that move from place to place unpredictably. The Wood Phase, to a great extent, relates to the nutrition of tendons and muscles and to that which grows and germinates, including tumours. If the Lesion-Symptom Complex changes with Wind, we may deduce that the cause probably lies in one of the Wood Processes.

  ° Moderate spring will stimulate the wood-element.

  ° A too strong spring will weaken the wood-element.

159

- *Summer (Fire / Heat)* influences HT, SI, PC and TH. Typical human diseases of Summer include heart attack, circulatory disorders, heatstroke and gastroenteritis due to food poisoning. Typical cattle disorders include hormonal disorders (infertility, repeat-breeders, nymphomania, anoestrus, pseudopregnancy and early foetal loss), etc. Occasionally, unusual summer-like weather may appear in the autumn or in the spring; such weather can weaken the Fire Process. Also, in the case history, if the Lesion-Symptom Complex changes with warmth or Heat, we may deduce that the cause probably lies in one of the Fire Processes.

  - ° Moderate summer will stimulate the wood-element.

  - ° A too strong summer will weaken the wood-element.

- *Late Summer (Earth / Damp)* influences SP-ST. Typical animal diseases of Late Summer are of digestive origin, like diarrhoea. If the Lesion-Symptom Complex changes with Damp or is most marked in late summer we may deduce that the cause probably lies in one of the Earth Processes, etc.

  - ° Moderate late summer will stimulate the wood-element.

  - ° A too strong late summer will weaken the wood-element.

- *Autumn (Metal-Air / Dryness)* influences LU-LI. Typical cattle diseases of Autumn include coughing, hoose (lungworm), fog-fever, viral pneumonia in weaned suckler calves, parasitic gastroenteritis, chronic diarrhoea in molybdenum-induced copper deficiency. If the Lesion-Symptom Complex changes with Dryness or is most marked in autumn, we may deduce that the cause probably lies in one of the Metal Processes, etc.

  - ° Moderate autumn will stimulate the wood-element.

° A too strong autumn will weaken the wood-element.

- **Winter (Water / Cold)** influences KI-BL. Typical cattle diseases of Winter include Winter dysentery, rickets and weak bones in cattle not supplemented properly with calcium, phosphorus and vitamin D, late abortion, milk fever, nervous ketosis, anoestrus. If the Lesion-Symptom Complex changes with Cold or is most marked in winter, we may deduce that the cause probably lies in one of the Water Processes, etc.

    ° Moderate winter will stimulate the wood-element.

    ° A too strong winter will weaken the wood-element.

Below is a summary of relationships between the seasons and the Channel Processes that they influence. Later, the chapter on the Back Shu Points will discuss the two homeostatic and balancing Cycles that complete Five Phase Theory.

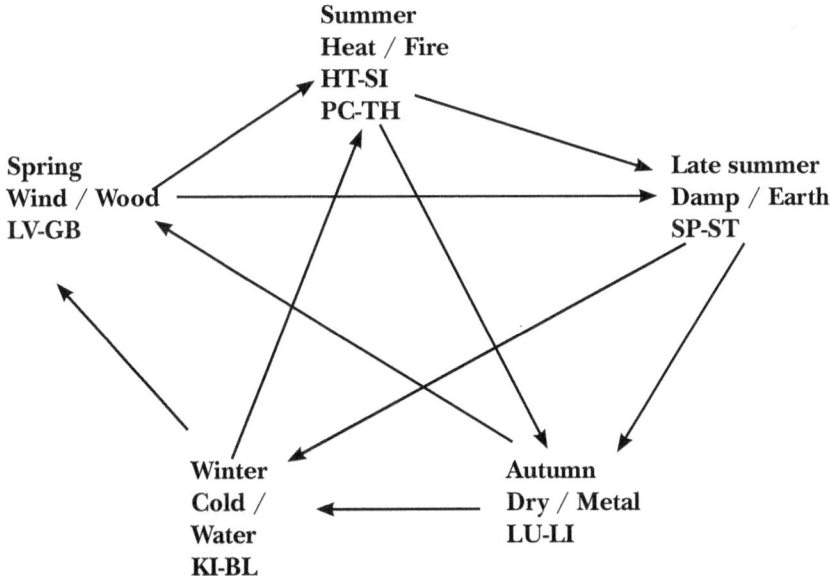

Table 32; A summary table of the correlation between the Five Phases, the seasons and the Processes.

161

CLIMATIC INFLUENCES

The weather has a major importance on the variation of Lesion-Symptom Complexes. Depending on whether the weather is normal or extreme and whether the Lesion-Symptom Complex is a manifestation of Deficiency or Excess, the influence may either improve or aggravate the Lesion-Symptom Complex in the same way as explained under the influence of the seasons (see page 32).

Extreme weather may be by itself the main cause of the disease. Extreme Cold may provoke a severe KI Deficiency, while mild Cold often improves the Lesion-Symptom Complex in KI Deficiency or aggravates the Lesion-Symptom Complex in KI Excess.

How Heat or warmth changes the Lesion-Symptom Complex depends on whether the Process Imbalance that causes the Lesion-Symptom Complex is Excess or Deficiency. Extreme Heat or warmth precipitates a Deficiency HT, while mild Heat stimulates HT in HT Deficiency.

The same relationships apply to Dampness and SP, to Wind and LV and to Dryness and LU. In this way we may not only decide where the real cause of the disease is to be found, but also if an Excess or Deficiency is damaging the organ in question.

- *Strong cold weakens the Water-element, but moderate cold strengthens it (KI-BL). This is easy to observe if we have had infection of the urinary tract. It could cause the symptoms of the disease to change to either worse or better, then we know that. If cold causes the symptoms to change, either to worse or better, then we know that the underlying cause of the disease is an energetic unbalance in the water element (KI/BL). We may conclude if the water process is in excess or deficiency if strong cold;*

    ° *Make the symptoms worse, then the process is in deficiency.*

    ° *Make the symptoms better, then the process is in excess.*

Further if moderate cold;

    ° *Make the symptoms worse, then the process is in excess.*

    ° *Make the symptoms better, then the process is in deficiency.*

The same way of thinking can be applied on all the external or internal influences as heat, wind, colours, sounds ......

OTHER BIORHYTHMS

From the viewpoint of diagnosis, we have discussed the time of day in the Chinese Qi Clock. We will now discuss other biorhythms.

Several other rhythms are important in diagnosis also. Some bodily rhythms follow the lunar rhythm, some follow the annual (solar or seasonal) rhythm and some the sunspot rhythm. If we could observe well enough over long periods, we would probably find rhythms that relate to other natural processes. From ancient times humans have observed that, like the planets, the different days have different influence on the organs. The table below shows how different days, planets and metals influence the Processes differently. For the moment, however, this area is scientific heresy.

Day	Planet	Metal	Channel-Organ
Monday	*Moon*	*Silver*	*Sex organs*
Tuesday	*Mars*	*Iron*	*GB, digestion*
Wednesday	*Mercury*	*Mercury*	*SI, digestion*
Thursday	*Jupiter*	*Tin*	*LV, metabolism*
Friday	*Venus*	*Copper*	*KI, circulation*
Saturday	*Saturn*	*Lead*	*SP, digestion*
Sunday	*Sun*	*Gold*	*HT*

Table 33

4. Direct Observation

General Comments

Direct observation refers to the ability of the therapist to observe more or less directly the causes of disease, i.e. the Processes that allow the disease to manifest.

In this connection, the clinician may observe abnormalities of body odour, movement of the different bones, movement or vibration of the vertebrae, skin colour, elasticity or temperature, respiration rate, heart rate, muscle tension, electrical resistance of the AP points, different qualities of the pulse or/and fluctuations of the spinal fluid (as detected in Cranio-Sacral therapy, see page 594). By now, we have far out-stripped the normal ability of conventional doctors or vets to observe significant clues to the causes of disease. However, immense training and sharpening of awareness is needed to develop these sensitivities. Here, I will mention the way in which German specialists diagnosing tuberculosis in the 1930s were trained. When they practised percussion, they put cottonwool into their ears so that they could only feel the vibration from the lungs. In this way, they became even better diagnosticians than those without cottonwool in their ears.

In practising Pulse Diagnosis, the investigation of scars, the mobility or vibration of the vertebrae and the reactivity of the acupoints, we have to develop a supersensitivity of the fingers; about the same sensitivity shown by a wine-connoisseur tasting the different wines and claiming to know the year and place of the grapes. If these wine-people can do this, why not a veterinarian?

Further, we may be able to get an impression of the patient by the help of more subtle methods like imagination, inspiration and intuition or other more or less undefined, psychological (parapsychological) methods. I urge readers to train themselves to develop their skills in such methods. This makes us better diagnosticians in time.

Before I describe such training, I will describe *Pulse Diagnosis* in detail. This is one of the best methods and is used widely in AP.

THE TECHNIQUE OF PULSE TAKING

Pulse-diagnosis is a very old method of diagnosing used in China for thousands of years. This method may seem incredible, non-sensical or fraudulent for the western scientific mind. It is none of these; in skilled hands, it is a powerful diagnostic method.

General Comments:

Proper pulse taking requires a proper state of mind. This mind-set is similar to a form of meditation or a state of daydreaming.

Typically, a practitioner in this state is producing mainly alpha brain-waves. There are at least three conditions that help a practitioner to achieve this meditative state, a state in which detachment or disassociation is crucial:

- *Not caring:* The practitioner must not have preconceptions of the causes; s/he must shed all interest, anxiety or desire to reach a diagnosis, to get paid at the end of the treatment, or any other mundane matters. Many find this to be the most difficult aspect of the requirements, but this state is fundamental to achieving a meditative state. Simply put, it is living in the exact moment of the pulse and of being conscious of anything else.

- *Not mind-wandering:* At the moment of the pulse taking, one should concentrate totally and exclusively on the patient. One's mental focus should exclude everything and everyone else that may try to enter one's mind or field of consciousness, such as being aware of the tempting sexuality of a most desirable animal handler, etc.

- *Not acting:* This is the state that some refer to as the state of fuzzy sight. It is similar to the moments when exhaustion begins to set in and the eyes gaze into the far distance. In this state, one finds it difficult to concentrate on other things. Therefore one does not act, or attains the state of not acting.

__Rudolf Steiner__ describes the foundation for developing the necessary state of mind like this:

Between birth and death, man, at his present evolutionary stage, lives in ordinary life through three soul states: waking, sleeping, and the state between them, dreaming. Dreaming will be briefly considered later on in this book. Here let us first consider life in its two chief alternating states — waking and sleeping. Man acquires knowledge of higher worlds if he develops a third soul state besides sleep and waking. During its waking state, the soul surrenders itself to sense-impressions and thoughts that are aroused by these impressions. During sleep, the sense-impressions cease but the soul also loses its consciousness. The experiences of the day sink into the sea of unconsciousness. Let us now imagine that the soul might be able during sleep to become conscious despite the exclusion of all sense-impressions, as is the case in deep sleep and even though the memories of the day's experiences were lacking. Would the soul, in that case, find itself in a state of nothingness? Would it be unable to have any experiences? An answer to these questions is only possible if a similar state of consciousness can actually be induced, if the soul is able to experience something even though no sense-activities and no memory of them are present in it. The soul, in regard to the ordinary outer world, would then find itself in a state similar to sleep, and yet it would not be asleep, but, as in the waking state, it would confront a real world. Such a state of consciousness can be induced if the human being can bring about the soul experiences made possible by spiritual science, and everything that this science describes concerning the worlds that lie beyond the senses is the result of research in just such a state of consciousness. In the preceding descriptions, some information has been given about higher worlds. In this chapter, as far as it is possible in this book, we shall deal with the means through which the state of consciousness necessary for this method of research is developed.

This state of consciousness resembles sleep only in a certain respect, namely, through the fact that all outer sense-activities cease with its appearance; also all thoughts are stilled that have been aroused through these sense-activities. Whereas in sleep, the soul has no power to experience anything consciously, it is to receive this power from the indicated state of consciousness. Through it, a perceptive faculty is awakened in the soul that in ordinary life is only aroused by the activities of the senses. The soul's awakening to such a higher state of consciousness may be called initiation.

The means of initiation lead from the ordinary state of waking consciousness into a soul activity through which spiritual organs of observation are employed. These organs are present in the soul in a germinal state; they must be developed. It may happen that a human being at a certain moment in the course of his life, without special preparation, makes the discovery in his soul that such higher organs have developed in him. This has come about as a sort of involuntary self-awakening. Such a human being will find that through it, his entire nature is transformed. A boundless enrichment of his soul experience occurs. He will find that there is no knowledge of the sense world that gives him such bliss, such soul satisfaction, and such inner warmth as he now experiences through the revelation of knowledge inaccessible to the physical eye. Strength and certainty of life will pour into his will from a spiritual world. There are such cases of self-initiation. They should, however, not tempt us to believe that this is the one and only way and that we should wait for such self-initiation, doing nothing to bring about initiation through proper training. Nothing need be said here about self-initiation, for it can appear without observing any kind of rules. How the human being may develop through training the organs of perception that lie embryonically in the soul will be described here. People who do not feel the least trace of an especial impulse to do something for the development of themselves may easily say, "Human life is directed by spiritual powers with whose guidance no one should attempt to interfere; we should wait patiently for the moment when such powers consider it proper to open another world to the soul." It may indeed be felt by such human beings as a sort of insolence or as an unjustified desire to interfere with the wisdom of spiritual guidance. Individuals who think thus will only arrive at a different point of view when a certain thought makes a sufficiently strong impression upon them. When they say to themselves, "Wise spiritual guidance has given me certain faculties; it did not bestow them upon me to be left unused, but to be employed. The wisdom of this guidance consists in the fact that it has placed in me the germinal elements of a higher state of consciousness. I shall understand this guidance only when I feel it obligatory that everything be revealed to the human being that can be revealed through his spiritual powers." If such a thought has made a sufficiently strong impression on the soul, the above doubts about training for a higher state of consciousness will disappear.

By combining the three qualities (not caring, not mind-wandering and not acting) one concentrates on the patient but does not interfere with its energies. Done in this way, diagnostic pulse taking is as detached and objective as possible.

Our mind may very well influence the result in our diagnostic work, just in the same way that the observer may influence the outcome in quantum physics (see page 9).

When we try to take the pulse, we should also be as relaxed as possible, without tense muscles.

We should also avoid the presence of critical observers, colleagues who are aggressive towards what we do or competitors who are jealous of our good results.

What I have observed in connection to my pulse-taking is just the same as what is described in the book, *"The Secret Life of Plants"* by **Peter Tompkins** and **Christopher Bird**, as it is necessary for the plants to react according to our feelings and states of mind. This book describes how it is possible for us to get in emotional contact with plants and how the presence of jealous or aggressive persons completely diminishes the contact described. This contact is almost the same as we must obtain in pulse-taking. The same observations were made by the French scientist **Beneviste** in his investigations on homeopathy (see page 191).

Practical Pulse-taking in Humans:

The pulse of the patient is examined by using your 2nd, 3rd and 4th finger feeling the systolic and diastolic blood pressure on three special positions over the radial artery at the wrist. These are called positions 1, 2 and 3, where 1 is nearest the wrist (over LU09), 2 is just medial to the styloid process of the radius and 3 is proximal to 2; the equal distance as 1 is distal. Begin by finding the pulses on the left radial artery.

First locate Position 2 exactly. It is found by locating the styloid process of the radius of the left hand (about one tsun proximal to the root of the thumb) with the tip of the third (middle) finger of your right hand. With your right palm in contact with the dorsal (posterior) side of the left arm of the patient, just above the left wrist, place the third finger over the tubercle of the styloid process. From this position, gently slide the third finger about 0.5 cm medially until it lies over the artery. This is Position 2. Then find Position 1 by placing the second (index) finger just distal to but right beside Position 2, at the root of the thumb. Finally, find Position 3 by placing the fourth (ring) finger proximal to Position 2, at the same distance, as the first position is situated distal to the second position.

To find the positions on the right arm, perform the same procedure with the opposite hand. Note that:

- The *superficial pulse reflects the diastolic pressure.* It is found by applying gentle pressure to the radial artery and feeling for the strength of the perceptible pulse by very superficial compression of the artery.

- The *deep pulse reflects the systolic pressure.* It is found by first occluding the radial artery and then feeling the strength of the pulse just after its first perceptible beats upon gentle release of the occluding pressure.

Each Pulse-Position (1, 2 or 3) and depth (superficial or deep) correlates with a specific process. The strength and quality of the pulse at each of these positions is a direct reflection of its health and energetic status, as follows:

Pulse-Position	Palpating finger	Left Pulse superfic.	Left Pulse deep	Right Pulse deep	Right Pulse superfic.
1 distal	2 index-f	SI	HT	LU	LI
2 styloid	3 middle-f	GB	LV	SP	ST
3 prox.	4 ring-f	BL	KI	PC	TH

Table 34

When one feels the pulse, one is actually feeling the energy of the process itself, directly.

The disharmony in the Qi balance in the organism can take on many patterns and many forms. Often the resultant expressions of Qi imbalance are complicated and misleading to novices. They may cause the practitioner to follow incorrect paths toward the origin of the disorder. The pulse, therefore, allows us to form a unique mental picture of the personal Qi of the patient in relation to his relationship with the universe and the twelve expressions of Qi manifested in the Processes. Once the diagnosis is established according to the Pulse, one can evaluate how the presenting Lesion-Symptom Complex fits according to any of the above mentioned paradigms.

PRACTICAL PULSE-TAKING IN ANIMALS:

I learned how to take the pulse in humans from my benefactor, Dr. Georg Bentze and I practised this method for years in my human clinic with very good results.

As a veterinarian I always thought about the possibility of doing this also in veterinary medicine. But how to take the pulse in animals was, for a long time, a mystery for me.

I contacted the French veterinary acupuncture society to ask if they knew how, and their secretary Dr. Moliniére told me that this question or quest also had been on his mind for several years. The French veterinary acupuncturists had even sent a delegation to China to find out if anybody was able to teach them how to perform pulse-diagnosis in animals, but it had been in vain.

Then, by sheer luck, I met Dr. Malchard in Liege, Belgium. He is a pediatrician working with pulse-diagnosis in children. One day he had observed that when the child was in contact with its mother, the pulse changed drastically. The heart-pulse of the child disappeared, and knowing that the mother was suffering from a serious heart-condition, he understood the connection. The pulse of the mother influenced the pulses of the child.

When he told me about this, I instantly understood the importance of this discovery in my search for a technique to monitor the pulse in animals. It was only to monitor the changes in the human pulse as the human was in contact with the animal.

This method I have refined over the years, and it will be explained in great detail below.

First of all, we must prepare our mind as described above under how pulse-diagnosis is made in humans. When preparing to be, or being in this state of mind, place your hand or a finger on the animal. *From this moment and during the whole procedure of taking the Pulse, nobody else should touch the animal.*

Preferably, no one else should be present in a radius of about 2 meters. In practice, however, this is seldom possible as people want to be nearby to see what is going on! So, let us say that, at the moment of pulse taking, the minimum requirement is that no one else touches the animal. (*It is sometimes quite amusing to test the owner while testing the animal, by recording the change of one special pulse while the owner moves to and from the animal. One can sometimes impress the owner by describing his or her Lesion-Symptom Complex*).

While touching the animal, the practitioner takes his/her own pulse, as a TCM practitioner would do on a human patient. When the therapist touches the animal, the therapist´s pulses change dramatically (!). This change is due to his contact with the energies of the animal. When being in contact with the animal, the therapist and the animal get a common energetic pattern. From the difference in pulse-findings before and after the contact, we may deduce the energetic balance in the animal itself.

Does this sound strange to you? This phenomenon is described by many observers up through history; by the Indians, the oriental people and by several observers from the occident. Rudolf Steiner describes how married couples get a common ethereal body after some time, and to get back to ones own ethereal body after divorce or death it takes 3 years. That is why a widow or a widower should stay single for at least 3 years.

Modern science has also shown this phenomenon recently. Scientists have shown that neuronal activity in one brain is transmitted to another brain as long as this other brain is concentrated on the other individual. This is called "Mirror neurons" or "Jumping neurons" (see page XLIX).

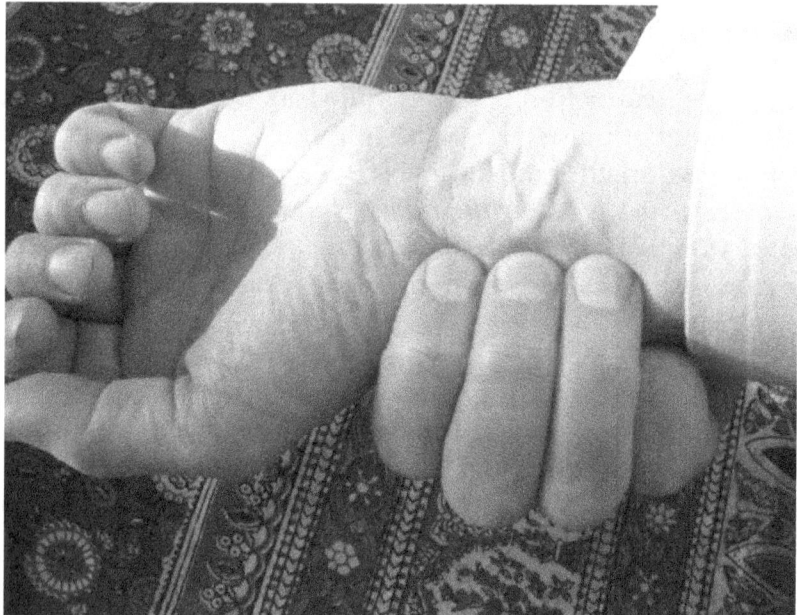

Fig. 39; Picture of how to hold the hands while taking the Chinese pulses.

I will now describe what we may expect to find in pulse-taking, and what progression we may expect:

1. TRAINING PERIOD

This period normally takes about one year. In this period, you must try to decide which of your own pulses *changes* while touching the animal. Practically, this is done by taking the pulse at your wrist, then touch the animal, and then move away from it again. This procedure is done again and again until you are sure whether your pulse changes or not while touching or not touching the animal.

Some people feel a:

- Change in rhythm, especially that the pulse gets faster.

- Change in impulse (strength), especially that the pulse gets weaker.

The "right" thing to feel is a change in strength. If the pulse grows weaker (or stronger) when touching an animal, this indicates deficient (or excess) in the correlating process.

The Neijing says that "*Some Meridians are too strong, some are too weak.*" In my experience I usually find:

- According to the Yin-processes:

    ° Deficiency in 90% of the pathological findings.

    ° Excess in 10% of the pathological findings.

- According to the Yang-processes:

    ° Deficiency in 20% of the pathological findings.

    ° Excess in 80% of the pathological findings.

When more than one pulse is "reactive" (becomes weaker or stronger), 5 element theory can be used with great success. This theory is an essential part of classical AP.

By the help of the Nogier-filters we may also be able to decide where the cause of the deficiency may be found, and also be surer that we have found the correct pulse deficiency (see page 144).

2. BEGINNERS (NOVICES)
After the training period, you may know your pulse so well that it is not necessary to move back and forth touching and not touching the animal. You may then go directly to the animal, take your pulse while in contact with it and decide which pulse is abnormal. With training you may also detect these changes in your pulse-picture at a distance from the animal, depending upon several factors that cannot be mentioned in detail here.

At this stage of your training, it is difficult to decide which Command-Point of the Meridian in question to use. It may then be opportune to just treat the Ting-point of the affected (usually weak) meridian. In my opinion, this stimulates the process in an adequate way.

3. Advanced Practitioners

After having trained for some years, you may be able to tell not only which pulse grows weaker or stronger, but also in what quality, and in which Phase (element) the pulse changes. Masters of TCM can differentiate between 28 different qualities of the pulse and make their diagnosis on that basis.

I find it more convenient to differentiate the changes according to:

- Which process is deficient (usually a Yin-process).

- Which process is in excess (usually a Yang-process).

- Which element within the pulse has changed.

- If there is any pattern in the changes of the pulses, this will indicate the use of the extra meridians (see later page 444).

- If there is any destructive energy spotted, then this energy must be wasted.

- How fast the changes occur, and how fast they fade away. This indicates the strength of the patient, and by this, also the prognosis.

Also you will by now have observed that the pulse changes according to where in the patient you focus your attention. You start the pulse-diagnosis, either you take it directly on the patient or indirectly through your own pulse, by focusing, or having your energetic center at the level of the heart, both yours and the patients. Then you move your attention inward, towards the heart of the patient, and then you feel the pulse is changing. In my opinion you then go deeper in the disease, and when you reach the patients heart you are at the deepest cause of the disease.

You may also move your center of consciousness downward (distally) in the patient, towards the Os pubis. Then you will also feel that the pulse is changing, but this time backwards in time. At the area of Solar plexus you will have the pulse as it was midway in the patients life, and when you reach Os pubis the pulse will be as it was at birth.

If you can determine all of this, you will have the complete diagnosis and treatment presented to you.

Then just use the proper therapy, which may be:

- *Acupuncture:*
    - ° Stimulation of the correct command-point of the deficient meridian.
    - ° Stimulate the right command-point of the mother-father meridians.

- *Herbal treatment:*
    - ° Give a plant that will stimulate the deficient process.
    - ° Give a plant that will stimulate the father-mother process.

- *Homeopathic treatment:*
    - ° Give a homeopathic remedy that will stimulate the deficient process.
    - ° Give a homeopathic remedy that will stimulate the father-mother process.

- *Osteopathic treatment:*
    - ° Manipulate the vertebrae related to the deficient process.

For example,

If the pulse tells you that the SP-process is weak and that there is something wrong with the Water element, you may use the Water Point of the SP Meridian (direct treatment) or the source-point or the earth-point of the LV-meridian (Ko-cycle treatment) or the fire-meridian (Shen-cycle treatment).

OTHER COMMENTS ON PULSE DIAGNOSIS:

1. The art of Pulse Diagnosis seems to be a subjective method (for me). Even if the changes we feel seem to very distinct, clear and without discussion, they may disappear or even change if we lose our concentration, our fixation or our usually correct mental state of mind. This shows that a machine is unable to detect the changes described, as a machine would be unable to detect our intention.

2. By training ourselves, the possibilities within Pulse Diagnosis seem to be without limitations (for me). This may depend more on the training than with the actual possibilities of this method, but it may equally have to do with the mental possibilities of our own mind.

3. In Pulse Diagnosis we are (I am) not able to decide on which side of the animal the problem is just in which process the unbalance originated.

4. In being concentrated in the heart area (bringing our focus to the middle chest), we (I) may more easily read the proper pulse. If we (I) move our (my) concentration further down (from the heart towards the Os pubis), the pulse changes as if we moved back in time. When I reach Os pubis, the pulse is like it was at the time of the birth of the patient. In this way, we (I) may get an impression in how the disease has changed over time.

5. The way of taking the pulse may also give us a clue of the prognosis. If we take the pulse several times just after each other on the same patient (repetitively), then we will often feel that the pulse gets stronger. This is a good prognostic sign, since by taking the pulse we "stir up" the energy. If the pulse does not become stronger, then this means that the patient is very low in energy, and that there are little reserves. This is a bad prognostic sign.

6. The advanced pulse-practitioner will also be aware of any existing *pattern* in the pulse-picture. If a pattern is to be found, then this indicates the need to use one of the *extra-meridians*.

The extra-meridians are certain channels that transfer energy from one part of the body to another (see page 444).

- **Du-channel:** All superficial pulses are strong, all deep pulses are weak (this may also be treated by the acupuncture point SP06).

- **Ren-channel:** All middle pulses are weak, both the superficial and the deep are normal. This may be felt as the pulse disappears when going from the superficial to the deep.

- **Chong-channel:** All deep pulses are strong and all superficial are weak (this condition may also be treated by using SI18).

- **Yin qiao channel:** All pulses in 1 and 2 position are weak, but the pulse in the 3 position is strong.

- **Yang qiao channel:** The pulse in the 1 position is strong, the rest are weak.

- **Dai channel:** The pulse in the 2 position is strong, the rest are weak.

- **Yin wei channel:** The pulse in the 3 position is strong, in the 2 position it is normal and in the 1 position it is weak.

- **Yang wei channel:** The pulse in the 1 position is strong, in the 2 position it is normal and in the 3 position it is weak.

*The pulse diagnosis as a way to clairvoyant observation described in connection with the anthroposophy of **Rudolf Steiner.***

Rudolf Steiners anthroposophy describes a way to obtain spiritual knowledge. This way consists of:

- *Preparation.*

- *Imagination.*

- *Inspiration.*

- *Intuition.*

In many of his lectures and books Steiner describes how this way may be followed or walked.

After using the pulse diagnosis for 29 years, I realised (2009) that the spiritual development that I had experienced through developing my skills within pulse diagnosis had clear and distinct parallels to Steiner's description of the path a spiritual disciple has to walk.
First, a short résumé of my development in pulse diagnosis.

In the beginning, the pulse observations were very fragile; I had to be newly washed, in quiet surroundings, not hungry or full, in short; in a balanced mind. After some years this became less and less important as the observations became more and more stable. After additional years, I began to literally see the etheric energy that I first detected through the pulse as if this detection gave rise to the development of spiritual sense organs. First I saw the etheric energy in and between trees, then in animals and then in humans. First the observations had its sensory center in the back of the brain, but then it started to wander. First towards the heart, then the spine, but then slowly spread out through the entire body. The observations also became enlarged, from just an intellectual observation to an immediate knowledge of the past, present and future of this special observation. Also the direction of the observation, now knowledge, also changed. In the beginning, the direction of the information streamed from the surroundings or the patient to me, but then it started to go both ways, as if the patient also received treatment at the same time as I was diagnosing. The observations also enlarged in space, as it came to also contain the astral part. This part was seen as a light flowing area together with the darker etheric energy. Then the observations started to move in time and past, present and future became one.

When I found Steiner's description of the development of Inspiration, for example in "Geisteswissenschaft im Umriss" around the pages 225 and 226, this is a close description of what I have experienced during the last 29 years. Although Steiner's description starts, it seems to me, with the development in the astral body which then spreads to the ethereal body, the description of the development of the inspiration, which takes place in the ethereal body, is identical to the development regarding the pulse diagnosis.

Pulse Diagnosis According to Dr. Paul Nogiér

Pulse-Controlled Acupuncture

Dr. Paul Nogièr began the very interesting development (or described; many M.D.´s have been famous for describing what lay-people already have found. A G.P. once told me that all important discoveries are made by lay-people, and then made known by medical doctors who "steal" their discovery) of auriculomedicine in 1954 (see page 138).

After some years, he refined the method by which the auricular points were found by the use of the RAC (or VAS) pulse (see page 140).

The Nogiér method of investigating the pulse is used more widely in the west than the "original" Chinese way.

The Nogiér method is most popular in German-speaking countries ("Kontrollierte Akupunktur") but several colleagues throughout the world use it also.

This form of Pulse Diagnosis differs from Chinese Pulse Diagnosis. Like dowsing (divining), it uses "yes/no information" to specific questions held in the clinician's mind. For example, a positive VAS-Pulse indicates if the Channel in mind is the primary Imbalanced Channel, if its Qi is Deficient or Excessive, if one's finger (or gaze) is on the most appropriate acupoint or the reactive area of a scar, etc. It can also indicate an appropriate homeopathic or herbal remedy and if one has treated the patient enough for a given session.

To use the Nogiér method of Pulse Diagnosis, the clinician palpates the quality of the pulse in a suitable artery (usually the radial, external carotid, or superficial temporal artery, see page 141). When we touch a reactive acupoint or a reactive ("toxic") area in a scar, the pulse quality changes. This reaction is called a Vascular-Autonomic Signal (VAS). This reactivity in the pulse is described under auriculomedicine, page 140.

Further Exercises in Sensitivity Training

We may exercise our abilities in sensitivity in several ways. I have during my life been advised to do such training by people as diverse as my professor in internal medicine at the veterinary highschool (Prof. Magne Aas Hansen) and my teacher in acupuncture (Dr. Georg Bentze). In several places in alternative and conventional medicine we may find chapters where the author emphasizes the need to be more sensitive to our patients than usual.

To be able to do such training, we need a certain amount of inner peace, inner tranquility. We need to obtain a certain inner state of meditative awareness, as described under the method of pulse-taking, page 165. If we obtain this inner state of alpha-waves, there are several methods to use to enhance our perception, our sensitivity or our intuition.

The percussion method was the first one taught by the professor of Internal Medicine at the Oslo Veterinary School. To exclude audible clues from differences in percussion sounds, we had to stuff our ears with cotton wool. Then we had to apply percussion over the thoracic area and learn to delineate the LU-area in animals or men by sensing the vibrations in our fingers.

The death method was one that I discovered while working in the clinic at the Oslo Veterinary School. Every day, especially on Mondays, the bodies of 5-15 dogs that had been killed by cars were examined at the School. Beside each body was a note indicating the time of death. Without knowing this, I stood at a distance of about 10 meters, trying to feel which animal had been dead the longest time, and which the shortest time. After just a few weeks I was able to tell the approximate time of death in most of the dogs.

The divining method is a simple method of dowsing to locate water pipes, or other hidden objects, using a divining instrument, such as a Y-rod, pendulum, rubbing pad, angle-irons, or even one's fingers, etc. (see page 676).

The telepathic method tries to foresee who will be next to knock on the door, or telephone, or other things like that.

The card method uses the next card in the playing-card deck instead of the next person to knock on the door.

The Eight Principles

The eight principles state that all symptoms may be divided from their appearance into Yin or Yang, and then further subdivisions according to the qualities of *inside(internal)/ outside(external), cold/hot* and *excess/deficiency* (which together with *Yin/Yang* make up 8 possible variations, a little "square" thinking if you ask me).

Well, this is a method for categorizing the symptoms to find the correct diagnosis. If you do not master the pulse, then this method may be a good substitute. Just remember to only use one needle and treat the deficient process or meridian.

The eight principles is another way or system of diagnosing disease and this system is probably the most used by acupuncturists. Therefore, although I personally don't use this system because I think that it is too symptomatically oriented, the readers should get to know it and also be able to use it if they don't find the other methods described useful for them.

When you then look at a patient, you usually start with External/Internal, then Hot/Cold, then Excess/Deficiency and then the overall summary of Yin and Yang.

- External/Internal is where the disease is presently located in the patient and is not related to the cause of disease, which may be an exterior pathogen (wind, heat, cold, damp, etc). This external pathogen can cause an external disease if the disease manifests in the skin, muscles and meridians. It can also cause an internal disease when it goes deeper into the body and affects the internal organs. For example wind cold – causes the common cold. But Cold can penetrate directly to the Spleen and cause diarrhoea. I have found that students often find this confusing and I think it is because of the terminology when we use "External pathogen" and then use External/internal classification. Perhaps we should use Exogenous pathogenic factor and external disease to avoid confusion. Once a disease is internal, then the organs are affected and the clinical signs will relate to the affected organ. This will also be the most deficient organ in the body at that time.

- Hot/Cold – This depends on how the patient feels and the symptoms, if the patient feels hot then it is most likely a hot disease. Keeping in mind the confusing symptoms of deficient heat with a yin deficiency and deficient cold with yang deficiency.

- Deficiency/Excess (empty or full) - The way I think of this is how does the patient look and what are the symptoms. If the patient is strong and is able to mount a good defence (e.g. acute high fever) then the disease is full. If the patient is weak and does not show a strong response (e.g. anaemia – blood deficiency) then this is deficient.

- Yin/Yang - At the end of the above, the Yin and Yang classification is generally a summary of the above. It is Yang if it is external hot and full and Yin if it is internal, cold and empty. The last I think is merely to give the practitioner a sort of double check if the overall picture is one of Yin or Yang or is it empty Yin or empty Yang.

Treatment is then directed to resolving the problem. If it is external then treat points to remove the pathogenic factor. If it is internal then treat the deficient organ and use points to alleviate the symptoms.

In acute disease – remove the pathogenic factor and tonify the organ.

In chronic disease – remove symptoms and tonify the organ (remove the cause if this is due to work practices, modify lifestyle, etc.).

The final treatment is to balance all the pulses. To maintain optimum health, balance the pulses each season – therefore the maintenance treatment is to tonify the deficient organ.

So, according to internal/external we classify the

1. Origin of the disease.

   - From internal:

     ° Joy.

     ° Anger.

     ° Melancholy (dryness).

     ° Sorrow (dampness).

     ° Fear.

   - From external:

     ° Wind.

     ° Heat.

     ° Dryness.

     ° Dampness.

     ° Cold.

Where the pathological symptoms are situated:

   - Situated internal:

     ° Heat

     ° Dampness

   - Situated external:

     ° ?

2. *Symptoms according to cold and warm:*
    - ° *More (too much) cold.*
    - ° *More (too much) warmth.*

3. According to deficiency and excess:
    - Deficiency (chronic):
        - ° Qi.
        - ° Yang.
        - ° Blood.
        - ° Yin.
        - ° Jing.
        - ° All the organs or processes as described under processes and 5 elements.
    - Excess (acute).

4. According to Yin/Yang
    - Is the overall disease related to Yin.
    - Is the overall disease related to Yang.

After settling on these parameters (which really is nothing more than finding the symptoms´ place in the Yin/Yang system), then we may find a treatment as dispersing wind, dispersing cold, fighting warmth and so on (see page 220).

Also, most of the Chinese plants and herbs are categorized after this pattern, except for the classifications in this book on page 558. They are classified after the five elements and the organs.

The diagnosis may then come up with such conclusions:

- Damp heat invasion from outside.
- Wind attack from outside.

- Dampness in the blood inside.

- Liver fire rising inside.

- Damp heat rising from below.

This method often gives very good results in practice, and if perfected in observation and logic, it leads to the correct deficient process. I have seen systems including also the processes and organs, so it becomes a total system which is good.

But if used only symptomatically and with many points, it gives, in my opinion, only a more or less symptomatic treatment (which often seems very effective and fast).

In my opinion, the only causal treatment is to find the true deficiency of one or more processes, either by pulse-diagnosis or by observing the symptoms, modifications and origin (as described in 8 principles).

Chapter 3

METHODS OF THERAPY

When we diagnose an illness and then proceed to treat it, we must move from a world of *knowledge,* **intuition** *and comprehension* to a world of *technique,* **intention** *and courage.*

We also move from a situation where the limit is *our own intelligence and intuition,* to a situation where we are limited by the abilities of:

- The physical body of our patient according to the anatomical situation.

- The potential of the self-healing abilities of the patient.

- Our own capability to influence the patients self healing systems by our own:

  - ° Intention.

  - ° Knowledge.

  - ° Empathy.

  - ° Devices.

  - ° Technique.

° Will.

° Courage.

We have no other possible way to go in our therapy than the possibilities that the body of the patient itself offers us. No therapy, whether conventional or alternative, can heal anything or any symptom that the bodies own abilities cannot heal itself.

Nothing on earth can make a wound heal except the ability of self-repair inherent in the body itself. What we can achieve by therapy (except for surgery, transplantation and other invasive techniques, although such procedures will not succeed unless the body has the abilities to accept or heal the operated or transplanted organs) is only what the body itself allows us to obtain. The real possibilities within therapy are none other than those that the organism has developed naturally as self-healing abilities over aeons of time.

Most Acupuncturists and Homeopaths agree that homeopathy and acupuncture work through *information* and *regulation* to/of the somatic processes. Acupuncture and homeopathy stimulate the self-healing mechanisms of the body. Many other medicines do not do that, for example, penicillin works by its own antibacterial actions that can inhibit or kill bacteria within the body as well as *in-vitro* (outside the body). This is not the case with acupuncture and homeopathy. To be of therapeutic value, they must modulate the body's homeostatic processes, i.e. they must target the body's self-healing mechanisms.

How acupuncture and homeopathy work (*how they stimulate the body's self-healing processes*) has been debated in depth through the years, and many mechanisms have been suggested. Some of these have been identified, especially in research on acupuncture. Regardless of what mechanisms have been suggested, the end result is always that the body's self-healing mechanisms must be activated.

During the years, I have observed some paradoxical anomalies between clinical results and the results from scientific investigations. Also the results between different clinics have shown a remarkable difference. This has bothered me, and the conclusion from these observations may lead to some very interesting thoughts about the working-mechanisms of many alternative therapies.

PARADOXICAL OBSERVATIONS IN ACUPUNCTURE:

1. Most veterinary acupuncturists who use AP or gold implants at the acupoints find them to be most successful and effective to treat canine hip dysplasia (HD). Clinical experience from several colleagues with overall success rates of 80-90% supports this opinion. Recently, although they used slightly different methods of implantation, three independent uncontrolled retrospective clinical studies on the effectiveness of gold implants to treat canine HD:

   A. Denmark (the late Jens Klitsgaard, 100 dogs).

   B. Norway (Are Thoresen, 50 dogs).

   C. Germany (Erhard Schulze, 68 dogs).

All of these three clinicians reported a clinical success rate of near 90%.

However, the clinical response to gold bead implantation AP to treat canine HD was evaluated also in three double-blind studies.

   D. Finland by Anna Hielm et al (1998).

   E. U.S.A. by Bebchuk et al (1998).

   F. Norway by Gry Jäger *et al* (Oslo 2003).

The dogs in these double-blinded studies showed a somewhat different reaction to the treatment compared to the dogs treated in an ordinary veterinary clinic. In Hielms study both groups of dogs (that is those treated and those not treated) showed positive results, but there was no difference between the two groups. The evaluation in her study was the owner's subjective impression. Bebchuk also treated the dogs in a double-blind study, but the evaluation was objective; it used force-plates to measure the force exerted by the dogs on the treated limbs; neither group of dogs improved, and there was no difference between the two groups. The dogs in the treatment group even tended to get worse. Gry Jäger's article will conclude (as reported at the IVAS Congress in Spietz) that there was a positive and statistical difference between the two groups, but much less than one may expect according to the results reported by Klitsgaard, Schulze and Thoresen. All three studies show the same result: gold-implantation in the hip area had little or no positive effect on the dogs. So we see that a very successful therapy in the clinic is almost without effect in a double-blind trial.

1. A good friend and colleague in Norway had good results in his acupuncture therapy in recent years. He then hired helpers, colleagues and animal-caretakers who did not believe in acupuncture. After two years he told me; "Are, I do not understand what is happening, acupuncture does not seem to work for me any more".

2. A colleague in the US said the following: "Twenty-five years ago I had great results treating just GB29, 30, and BL54 in canine hip dysplasia. If I treat just these points today, I would see very little improvement in my patients. I agree that focus and mindset is a major part in one's treatment protocol and point selection. In the treatment of hip dysplasia, you (i.e. Are) place a much higher degree of power on the use of LV03 than I do; therefore LV03 works for you but not for me. I treat many conditions for which I use only one needle, or implant only one point, but my focus is different from when I am treating hip dysplasia." We are getting back to focus and intent, the two most important factors in acupuncture. A German colleague answered to this: "Some years ago I opened the Du Mai with GB41 in about 80% of my horse patients. Today it happens about once a week. Who changed? The horses or I?"

PARADOXICAL OBSERVATIONS IN HOMEOPATHY:

1. **Beneviste's** investigations showed that the results differed when he did the trials alone versus in the presence of sceptics. He suggested that the presence of the critical persons "zeroed" the results of the investigations.

2. Many investigations have shown that homeopathy works sometimes, and sometimes not (**Coulter 1980, Linde 1997, Vaarst 1996**). Also many homeopathic studies show that results are very good in the clinic but are bad in double-blinded trials.

3. If we carefully read **Hahnemann´s** (The founder of homeopathy, see page 510)last edition of his writings [the 6. edition of "Organon der Heilkunst", finished in 1842 (the year before Hahnemann died) and published in 1921] we may find strong indications that also he was aware of the importance of the will and intention of the therapist *(although many therapists interpret the following quotes that he wanted to be sure that he did not give medication that was not correctly made).

   • In §288 (see also §289), he thus writes: "*Through the strong will of a person with positive intentions, when such a person touches the patient, yes he does not even have to touch the patient, then a sort of healing power flows over from that person to the diseased one. This kind of healing is one of the most powerful there is.*"

   • In §265 he writes that, "*The therapist must give the correct remedy to the patient **with his own hands*** (underlined by Hahnemann himself) and in his original manuscript, he has written that: "*In following this **important** principle, I have had to endure many attacks from opponents.*"

What Hahnemann describes here resembles very much my description of healing under "Anthroposophical medicine," page 592. As Hahnemann did not conduct double-blinded trials and as he did not let machines make or give his remedies, he surely could not observe that this described "power" is one of the most important factors in all healing (as Rudolf Steiner described in 1920, see page 194).

PARADOXICAL OBSERVATIONS IN BIODYNAMIC AGRICULTURE:

1. Biodynamic agriculture uses homeopathic substances called the "Remedies." As in homeopathy, Biodynamic agriculture has given paradoxical results in practical situations; some people have had good results but others not. Many farmers report good results but controlled trials have shown little or no effect.

2. In farming, I have often heard that methods or remedies that clearly work in the field totally lose their effect when submitted to double-blind investigations.

PARADOXICAL OBSERVATIONS IN OTHER AREAS OF SCIENCE:

1. **Viktor Schauberger** between the first and the second world wars conducted many interesting trials and studies in Austria on the peculiarities of water. His results amazed many scientists, and even Hitler ordered him to work for his war-machine. Later, it emerged that it was almost impossible to replicate Schauberger's results but few or none have suggested that he was cheating.

2. **Sir Jagadis Chandra Bose,** one of the most famous scientists in India, showed with his self-constructed machines that plants and metals had a soul-life of their own. The problem was that nobody could replicate his results. My interpretation of his trials is that his own psyche (intention) was so strong that it influenced his results.

3. **Professor Kröplin** from Stuttgart has shown that the patterns of crystallisations and the forms of drops falling into water was up to 48% influenced by the emotions of the scientists. This would explain the results of

many great "alternative" scientists, such as Shauberger, Bose and even Rudolf Steiner.

4. **Quantum-physics** also indicates that the observer influences the observed results; the scientists influence the outcome from a given experimental protocol and the variation between their results is unexplained. Many quantum-physicists accept this today; however, Werner Heisenberg's uncertainly-equation may explain the differences practically and theoretically. Here is a quote from *"The Tao of Physics"* by *Fritjof Capra*: "In modern physics, the question of consciousness has arisen in connection with the observation of atomic phenomena can only be understood as links in a chain of processes, the end of which lies in the consciousness of the human observer." In the words of *Eugene Wigner*: "It was not possible to formulate the laws of quantum theory in a fully consistent way without reference to consciousness." Wigner and others have argued that the explicit inclusion of human consciousness may be an essential aspect of future theories of matter.

These concepts all indicate that the qualities of the therapist may influence the outcome of a treatment or experiment, as modern quantum physics has suggested. Many serious AP books from China expressed this opinion, for example:

- *Chapter 26 of the Suwen*: "... That which differentiates craftsmen is [to observe] what is not manifested to be observed externally and that all [others] cannot observe. Therefore observing that which is obscure means seeing that which has no form and tasting that which has no flavour. *This [capacity] seems to be divine.*"

- *Scheid & Bensky*: In pre-Han China, yì (intention) was considered a pre-requisite of the knowledge and understanding required for and derived from the divination practices based on the I-jing. "*Yì is what the sages used to search profundity and study the all encompassing. As it is profound, it can penetrate throughout the purpose of the subcelestial realm. As it is all encompassing, it can penetrate throughout the affairs of the subcelestial realm. As it is divine, it is fast but never hurries; it arrives but never travels".*

- *Zhenjiu Dacheng:* "The importance of AP lies in *concentration of the mind."*

- *Guo Yuzhi:* "Needling ability rests with whether [acupuncturist] can *focus his attention on the heart and hand* during the needling."

- *Xu Yinzong: "Medicine is Yì (intention); it is in one's thoughts and deliberations."*

One can not overemphasise the power of willed, directed intention in healing. *It is very important that we activate and project our intention to heal our patients, i.e. we really want to make the treatment work and we visualise that this is happening. Late in life, Rudolf Steiner had a revelation after he had met the well known German naturopath, Marie Ritter. He realised that healing did not depend on the remedies themselves but on the awareness or intention of the therapist at the time of prescribing or administration of the remedies. Rudolf Steiner wrote: "In reality it does not depend on the **remedy** given but on the intention of the one **making** the remedy" (may be the therapist then often made the remedies themselves?) (**R. Steiner**, 1920). Even without remedies, without needles or direct treatment of any kind, **focused intention can heal**. Sometimes it can work even better than a treatment given directly.*

The conclusion that the qualities of the therapist, especially *Yì (intention),* seem to influence the outcome of a treatment may explain why homeopaths and doctors disagree, and never will agree. If the therapist's intent, formed by years of study and clinical conviction, really is the most important aspect of clinical medicine, it may explain very well why scientists and doctors (who rely on dispassionate randomised controlled trials for evidence of clinical efficiency) disagree with homeopaths and acupuncturists about the reality of their clinical results. Double-blinded studies cannot allow for the influence of *Yì (intention)*, and *must show* little difference between the treated and control groups.

These conclusions have been supported by some extraordinary interesting investigations and results done within neuroscience. There it has been shown that neuron-activity in one brain triggers likewise activity in another brain in mental contact with the first one, called Mirror neurons (see page XLIX)

Also the possibility to take the animals pulses through our own energetic system shows clearly that there is an extensive contact between two entities (see page 178).

References for the scientific oriented or critical reader:

1. *Proceedings of 22. Annual International Congress on Veterinary Acupuncture, 5-8th September 1996, Spiez, Switzerland).*

2. *Proceedings of 22. annual International Congress on Veterinary Acupuncture, 5-8th September 1996, Spiez, Switzerland).*

3. *Zeitschrift für Ganzheitliche Tiermedizin, 3/98, side 103-105.*

4. *Bebchuk et al (1998) Double-blind study to evaluate the clinical response to gold bead acupuncture as a treatment in dogs with naturally occuring hip dysplasia. Communication from Dept. of Small Animal Clinical Sciences, Michigan State University.*

5. *Hielm et al (1998) Double-blind study to evaluate the clinical response to gold bead acupuncture as a treatment in dogs with naturally occurring hip dysplasia.*

6. *Jäger, Gry: "Alternativ behandling av hofteleddsdysplasi i en hundemodell. Resultater ved stimulering med gullimplantater i akupunkturpunkter". Dette er ennu ikke publisert.*

7. *Beneviste J. Et al. (E. Davenas, F. Beauvais, J. Arnara, M. Oberbaum, B. Robinzon, A. Miadonna, A. Tedeschi, B. Pomeranz, P. Fortner, P. Belon, J. Sainte-Laudy, B. Poitevin), "Human basophil degranulation triggered by very dilute antiserum against IgE", Nature, Vol. 333, No. 6176, pp. 816-818, 30th June, 1988 C Macmillan Magazines Ltd., 1989.*

8. *Hahnemann Samuel, "Organon der Heikunst", Karl F. Haug Verlag, Heidelberh, 1992, 327 pages, page 230. ISBN 3-7760-1253-6.*

9. Coulter H., "Homeopatic Science and Modern Medicine", North Atlantic Books, 1980.

10. Linde K., Wayne B. J., Melchart D., Worku F., Wagner H., Eitel F. "Critical Review and Meta-Analysis of Serial Agitated Dilutions in Experimental Toxicology", Human & Experimental Toxicology, 1994; 13:481-92.

11. Vaarst M., "Veterinær homeopati: Baggrund, principper og anvendelse med speciell fokus på økologiske melkekvegbesetninger – et litteraturreview", Statens husdyrbrugsforsøk, Denmark, Beteraktning nr. 731, 51 sider, 1996.

12. Linde K., Clausius N., Ramirez G. et al., "Are the clinical effects of homeopathy placebo effects? A metaanalysis of placebocontrolled trials", Lancet 1997; 350 (9081): 834 - 843.

13. Kröplin B., "Welt im Tropfen", Gutesbuchverlag ISD – Universität Stuttgart, 2001, ISBN: 3-930683-64-6, 83 sider.

14. Capra F., "The Tao of Physics," Bantam Books, New York, 1975.

15. Bohm D., "Hidden Variables and the Implicate Order," Zygon, vol. 20, nr. 2, USA 1985.

16. Lawden D. F., "A Berkeleyan Model for Psychic Phenomena," Psycoenergetics, vol. 5 1983, Gordon and Breach Science Publishers Inc, England.

17. Walker E. H., "International Journal of Quantum Chem," vol. 11, 103, 1977.

18. Conti A., "Oncology in Neuroimmunomodulation, what progress has been made?" Annals of the New York Academy of Sciences, 2000, vol: 917, 68 – 83.

19. Thoresen A., „Verifizierung von Akupunkturerfolgen – Ein Diskussionsbeitrag" Zeitschrift für Ganzheitliche Tiermedizin, Nr. 1/1999, 20-21.

As we have discussed earlier, the organism and life itself have developed complex self-regulating or self-stimulating systems or methods to regulate or stimulate its fundamental Processes. Our only real ability to heal is to help these systems or methods to function better than they are. Such systems or methods are necessarily developed within the natural environment or possibilities that the organism has been living with, possibilities that were available to the organism. Such systems have been:

- The mental processes as discusses in the writings above
  - ° Of the patient:
    - Placebo (+)
    - Nocebo (-)
  - ° Of the therapist (intention):
    - White magic
    - Black magic
- The natural herbs found in the natural environment of the individual.
- The colours existing in the natural environment of the individual.
- The light, especially sunlight, stimulating specific zones of the individual.
- Points of the body stimulated by the individual itself, its fellow beings or by causal electric charges occurring in its natural environment.
- Other natural occurring phenomena which may be taken into use by the body.

Out of this, we may conclude that "natural therapy" is the only real therapy.

All of these methods are developed to balance the fundamental Processes; therefore, they are secondary to the Processes. Thus I have discussed these in a separate chapter and not combined the description of the fundamental Processes with the methods to influence them. The system of AP is not fundamental or primary. It is developed as a system to be able to balance the primary Processes.

Many different therapeutic paths can lead to the same goal. One can usefully combine various methods of therapy if one knows the relevant and compatible methods. However, conflicting therapeutic paths in the same patient can neutralise each other. Thus, severe adverse clinical results can arise if two incompatible methods are used in the same case at the same time by an inexperienced therapist. The same can happen if two therapists who are acting independently of each other treat the case.

It is therefore very important to choose *one therapeutic path* and to follow it. If we chose other simultaneous methods, they should be compatible and both follow the same energetic rationale.

I emphasise that this applies only for methods that work on the animal's vital energies. However, methods of therapy, such as conventional medicine that do not work on the animal's energetic pattern (Qi) balance, combine well with complementary treatment. I have stated many times in this book that conventional and alternative therapies can be combined, usually without difficulty. Even if the various methods of natural medicine appear to be different from each other, they are all based on the body's own physiological and energetic system.

Therapy models can generally be divided into **Substantial** and **Functional** (in the same way as the Processes are classified in the chapter about diagnosis methods).

- **Substantial disorders** (disorders of Yin Process): To treat these, use functionally (energetically) based therapies, such as AP or Zone Therapy.

    ° Stimulation of the process in deficiency.

    ° Sedating the process in excess.

- **Functional disorders** (disorders of Yang Process): To treat these, use materially (substantially) based therapies, such as spices, herbs, tinctures or pills. AP also is very effective in functional disorders.

    ° Stimulation of the process in deficiency.

    ° Sedating the process in excess.

Similarities between the different therapeutic methods

1) AGGRAVATION

Within a few days or weeks after starting therapy, a certain part (%) of all treated patients show aggravation of the symptoms.

- If I treat the primary deficiency, this part is about 40%.

- If I treat the secondary excess, the part is just 5%.

The time from treatment to the start of aggravation depends on how:

1. Effective the method is (shorter if more effective).

2. How deep seated the disease is (longer if deep seated).

3. How long it has lasted (longer if more chronic).

4. The age of the patient (longer in older patients).

The duration of the aggravation depends on how:

5. Effective the method is (shorter if more effective).

6. How deep seated the disease is (longer if deep seated).

7. How long it has lasted (longer if more chronic).

8. The age of the patient (longer in older patients).

We can understand why such an aggravation occurs due to the theory of how the healing process is initiated. The Lesion-Symptom Complex is the body's attempt to compensate for a Process Deficiency. Effective therapy works in the same way; it helps to restore the body's normal Processes; it tonifies the Deficiency (thereby sedating the Excess Processes). Therefore, the Process Imbalances in the location of the compensatory symptoms (which are of the same nature as the Deficient Process) also receive stimulation for a short period of time, because the stimulation boosts the complete Process, both in the usual organ and in its helper organs. This aggravates the symptoms for a short time.

A strange phenomenon during the aggravation is that conventional preparations that previously could suppress the symptoms eventually and suddenly lose that ability. This applies, for example, to pain that was suppressed by analgesic medication, or eczema that was suppressed by cortisone ointment. We may explain this phenomenon in two ways:

- *The initial aggravation occurs in the Process, i.e. the energetic part of the patient. Symptom suppressive medicine cannot influence the Process.*

- *The strong stimulation of the Weakest Process by complementary therapy is more efficacious than the suppressant effect of allopathic medicine on the same Process. Thus, allopathic medicine, such as high-dose cortisone, or insulin, or thyroxin, which actually suppresses the endocrine capacity to produce its own hormones, loses its usual ability to "improve" (suppress) the symptoms at this stage.*

1) Recurrence of Lesion-Symptom Complexes in Reverse Order of their Appearance

Lesion-Symptom Complexes that had presented in the earlier history of the patient often recur in the reverse order of their original appearance. For example, let us suppose that a dog had eczema, urticaria, urinary tract disorder and aggression/ sleep disorders at 1, 2, 3 and 4 years old, respectively. As the treatment progresses, these Lesion-Symptom Complexes recur in the reverse order, i.e. the most recent signs recur first and the oldest signs recur last. After each treatment session, it seems as if one is moving from Process to Process backward in time, often in accordance with the reverse Ko-Cycle. Occasionally, it may follow the reverse Sheng-Cycle. On many occasions I have noted this reverse order in detail. The last treatment usually ends when one reaches the original trauma or the earliest Lesion-Symptom Complex of the disease.

This phenomenon resembles, in many respects, our experience of psychiatry. There we also look for the initial trauma. We experience an initial aggravation when we begin to dig into the subconscious. In this case we also travel backwards within the Lesion-Symptom Complex and finally reach the trauma that initiated the disease.

That the previous Lesion-Symptom Complexes return in the reverse order can be seen in relation to the law of the "mirror relationship" of the energetic body or etheric body to the physical body. According to occult tradition, the physical- and etheric- bodies are exact mirror reflections of each other. This means that the left arm energetically corresponds to the right arm and the right ear energetically corresponds to the left ear. However, this mirror effect is relevant on all levels, making the left arm also correspond to the right leg energetically and the left shoulder correspond to the right hip.

Time can be seen as a mirror also; physical time travels from the past toward the future, while etheric time travels from the future to the past. This explains the recurrence of earlier Lesion-Symptom Complexes since they are stored in the energy body. In a more philosophical way it can also shed some light on "Deja vu" experiences, the cyclic characteristic of the phenomenon and the return of all actions (fate, Karma) which is nothing less than earlier Lesion-Symptom Complexes (actions and/or reactions) that return also as a mirror effect.

The Placebo Effect

Many sceptics claim that the clinical efficacy of complementary therapy is exclusively a placebo effect. When complementary medicine "works" they attribute its effect to misdiagnosis, spontaneous remission, or to the ***imagination of the patient,*** *or his/her belief in the treatment and desire to be healed.*

Many sceptics do not know or believe the real meaning and significance of the word "placebo." The exact meaning of the Latin word means "***I (the therapist)*** *will placate or please.*"

The emphasis in the word "placebo" and its real significance is on "***I (the therapist).***" This is a most important distinction because *the **therapist's directed will and intention** while s/he is treating a case is of paramount importance to the clinical outcome.* This is even more important in energetic (Qi-based) therapies, in which the healer's skill and intent channels his/her Qi, or cosmic Qi, is passed to the patient. This has been discussed in greater detail at page 611.

Of course, part of the clinical cure is due to psychosomatic interaction, i.e. positive motivation of the patient's psyche may partially mediate the outcome. This is used to best advantage in humans undergoing any form of therapy, conventional or complementary. Experienced vets know that gaining the animal's "trust" and "confidence" makes their task easier, and benefits the clinical outcome.

Thus, the "placebo effect" is variable in time within the same group of subjects and very variable between experiments. Its variability is due to an unpredictable mixture of three components that are, themselves, difficult to quantify:

(a) Random outcome (positive or negative) which embraces spontaneous, unwilled remission.

(b) The "therapist effect," which can be powerful even without the conscious knowledge of the patient or the therapist (see page 613).

(c) The effect of the patient's psyche (which can be positive or negative, and is what we usually address as placebo (+) or nosebo (-)).

Frequently we really get better or get completely cured by the "placebo-effect," then this form of "treatment" is not just something we imagine, but rather, is real. Positive results in most of the alternative therapies depend upon the self healing processes of the body, so whether these processes are started by the help of psychological methods should not be of importance. Whether it is the intention of the therapist, the belief of the patient, the vibration of the remedy or a combination of it all, should not be of great importance. The result is what is important!

The importance of placebo is easy to see in double blinded investigations, where there is a well defined placebo group. Group 1 do not get any medication. Group 2 gets the real medication. Group 3 gets a placebo remedy (just sugar). A common result in such an investigation is that in group 1, 7 % gets better (there are always someone that gets better). In group 2, 75 % gets better. In group 3, 44 % gets better. The placebo effect will then be 44 – 7 = 37 %, and the "real" effect from the "real" remedy will be 75 – 44 – 7 = 24 %.

We see here that the placebo effect actually is greater and more important than the remedy. Then we have to consider the number of patients that get the symptoms back when they stop taking the "real" remedy, and how many get their symptoms back when we stop the placebo or the acupuncture treatment. In reality, we will often see that the healing based on placebo is longer lasting than the healing based on the "real" remedies.

This shows that the placebo effect is more important than the "real" remedy.

Dr. Ario Conti has also shown that the changes in the brain produced by the placebo often are like the changes produced by the "real" remedy.

Chapter 4

ACUPUNCTURE

The system of meridians and acupuncture points has been developed by ourselves through the billions of years as a system of self-healing or auto- regulation, as an ECIWO-system. A Point that needs stimulation to be able to re-establish the normal balance shows tenderness, scratchiness, changed blood circulation and decreased electric resistance (Ohm) as described on page 103. These changes will lead to these points being treated more often by the individual itself, by other individuals in the group or flock and by several factors in the environment such as electric charges, colours, sounds or plants.

Of themselves, the AP Channels do not represent or are not part of the processes themselves; they are an energetic infrastructure developed to balance the processes.

In China, acupuncture is called Zhen Jiu (Zhen = needle and Jiu = Fire, or moxibustion), which means to needle and burn the points in question. The word "acupuncture" comes from the Latin "acus" (needle) and "pungere" (to puncture). Many modern interpreters of AP theory have claimed that AP is an empirical method, i.e. one based on anecdotal experience and one with little or no scientific basis for development. This theory is not correct. AP is inextricably part of Chinese culture and civilisation. We can trace the therapeutic use of needles to at least five thousand years ago, when AP was already a highly respected and organised medical method. We should remember that at the time when AP was evolving, Chinese culture and science had a knowledge base significantly ahead of that of western cultures. Also, recently we have acquired new insight into neurophysiological mechanisms that explain many of the clinical effects of this ancient Chinese method.

The Chinese were familiar with such things as the timing for the spring equinox and the fall equinox. They were also familiar with the fact that the Earth's axis is tilted on the solar level. They knew this as early as the 22nd century BC. They calculated the Earth's axis to be 22.5°. We now know that it is tilted exactly 23.27°. The accuracy of the ancient calculation is such that the greatness of the Chinese ability to observe must be admired.

The Chinese culture yielded bronze vases in the 22nd century BC. They also mixed copper and aluminium, whereas western science has known of metallic aluminium for barely 100 years. Although certain amalgams containing aluminium have been known since antiquity (alumen), metallic aluminium was not produced until 1825 here in the west. To be able to do this, we need temperatures of 1300°C. This means either that the Chinese have been able to generate these temperatures, or they have had the knowledge of the processes by which to make these alloys of which we are not familiar.

A thousand years ago, a Chinese astronomer described with great precision the development of the galaxies and the spiral galaxies. He determined that the distance between them was increasing and that the universe was expanding. This claim can be interpreted poetically and is not necessarily meant to be a scientific statement.

European scientists and philosophers were burnt at the stake only a few hundred years ago because they said that the Earth was round and circled around the Sun. An example of this is Giordano Bruno (1548-1600) who was burnt on Campo dei Fioro in Rome in the year 1600.

The ancient Chinese were also familiar with the art of printing books. They also knew that the blood circulated within the body 3500 years before William Harvey (1587-1657) made the same discovery in Europe in the year of 1628.

Over several millennia, the Chinese made very precise observations of the laws that determined changes in nature, in humans and in the universe. They put their entire comprehension and ability to observe nature into the development of a very complete and auto-regulating cosmology. They committed these laws to writing in the old Classics, such as the *Neijing*, the *Suwen* and the *Ijing*. AP evolved and derived directly from these writings. Arising from these classical texts, the total system of TCM is amazingly comprehensive. It made extensive use of herbs, spices, massage, exercise, meditation and AP. In the west, we have adopted AP widely and view it as TCM. That is a great mistake as AP is only a small part, possibly the least important part, of TCM.

Computer tomography confirmed that "Öetzi, the iceman", found in the Alps (1994), had arthrosis of the lumbar spine. He also had tattoos on, or within a few mm of classical acupoints on BL Channel in the lumbar area and others on the pelvic limb (BL60, KI07, SP06). Those points are used in AP to treat lowback pain and hip disorders [http://www.akupunktur-arzt.de/oetzi/science.htm]. From this, we may conclude that AP was known in Europe already 5300 years ago.

For more than 6000 years ago, there was a great and catastrophically draught in the area north of the Caspian Sea. This period lasted for 2000 years and lead to wanderings of the people living there to the west and north-west. Without the use of the horse, this movement would have been impossible and on horse-back, these people changed the European history for all time. They came to Europe in three great waves, just parted by a few hundred years between each, and 5000 years ago these people had influenced the greater parts of Europe and South Scandinavia. 4000 years ago also the British islands and Iberia (Spain/Portugal) was part of their sphere.

Everywhere these people came to dominate. The old gods representing fertility and female qualities (the moon-cults, Vanene) were exchanged with a war hero on horse back (Odin, the sun-cults, Æsene).

The so-called Troy castles are other signs or indications that Asian tradition and thinking was known in Europe long ago. Close to my home in the Norwegian costal town of Sandefjord is a marine peninsula called Østerøya ("East Island"). About 1000 years ago, this land was separated from the mainland. It was a real island, with a narrow straight used by the Vikings as they sailed between the two main cities of Norway at that time (Kaupanger and Tönsberg). On the southern part of the peninsula there is an area called Yxney. A part of Yxney forms a separate and smaller peninsula as an appendix to the main peninsula, the Truber headland (Truberodden). Two small fjords, the south and north Truberfjord, form this headland. Between these small fjords there is a quiet isthmus (eid), over which one can walk out to the headland of Truber. Up to the year 1800, a strange man-made stone formation was visible on this isthmus. It was a row of stones placed in a special pattern to form a labyrinth. This labyrinth has given the name to the area; as such constructions are called labyrinths of Troy, in this special case; "Truber".

Several labyrinths like the one near Sandefjord are known in Europe but especially in Scandinavia. From ancient times, these constructions have been called "Labyrinths of Troy". Variations of this name, such as Trøyenborg, Trøborg, Trelleborg, Troytown are found all over Europe. The origin of the name lies in the mighty old city of Troy. Why this name is connected with the labyrinths is uncertain but we may see some relationships if we investigate the ancient city culture of Troy.

Homer's Iliad describes in detail the fierce war between Sparta and Troy. At that time, Troy was the most western outpost of eastern philosophy and thinking, while Sparta was more western orientated. The people (read prince) of Troy had captured and imprisoned Helen, the beautiful princess of Sparta. After several years of fighting, Helen's followers set her free. They managed to conquer Troy by the help of a giant hollow wooden horse, in the belly of which they managed to get into the city. Via the wooden horse, the western way of thinking got access to the eastern philosophy. As we will see later, the constructors of the Troy castles possibly were oriental horse-warriors that rode from the east during the time of population migrations and settled in different parts of Europe, especially Scandinavia.

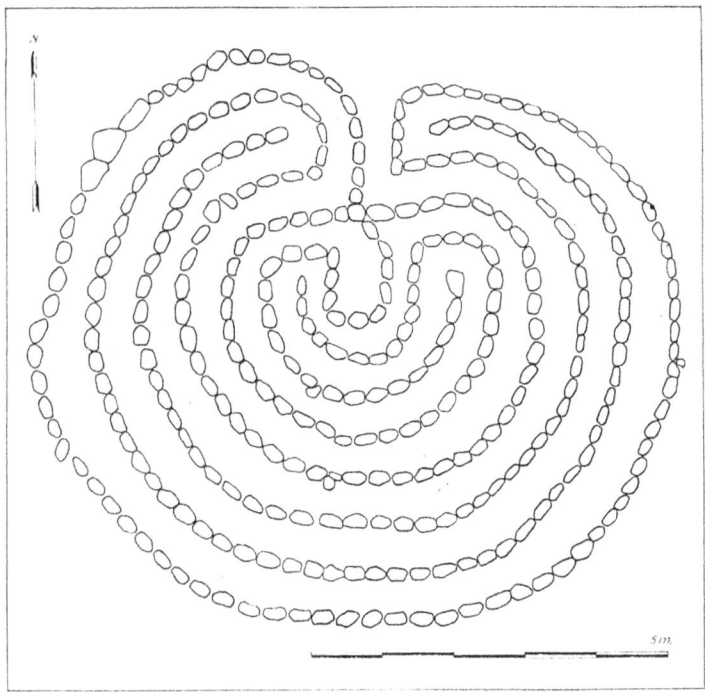

Fig 40; A Troy labyrinth found in Finnmark, North Norway

With regards to the Troy castles, there are usually myths about horses, showing that the parallel to the Iliad may be of some value, at least of some interest. Much, which has been written over the years about the Troy castles often mentions visions or myths of black horses in connection with the labyrinths. In Sandefjord, seamen tell stories about seeing a couple of black horses just before bad weather or storms. Such visions usually made the seamen return to shore. This has also happened to me once. If I had not returned at that moment, my boat would undoubtedly have been wrecked in the oncoming storm. A glowing castle has also been observed several times at the headland.

Most of the labyrinths have several other stories associated with them. These stories include the ability to warn of storms, or that a ritual held in the labyrinth would prevent wreckage and guarantee a good catch of fish, as the fishermen then would have more power over the winds and the movements of the seawater, as well as over the fish.

Most scientists are also convinced (Colin Bord, Lorens Berg) that there were rites connected to the labyrinths, rites to prepare the seamen to cope with bad weather, fish catches, or horsemen to manage and tame horses. The same scientists have also agreed on the age of these labyrinths and dated then to 1500-500 BC. As earlier mentioned, it is highly possible that the builders of these labyrinths were Asian shamans who came together with Mongolian conquerors on horseback during or before the times of the folk migrations.

Before we take a closer look at the construction of the Troy labyrinth, we should discuss the Asian view of human energetic physiology. Qi (the meridian energy) flows in a highly complex 3-dimensional network of specific Channels and Pathways throughout the body. The network of the 12 Main Channels, their pathways and organs is called the Channel-Organ System of TCM. Qi itself is 12-fold. TCM Theory held that the body and soul were 12-fold. Man stands between heaven and earth and in communication with the 12 cosmic Qi streams, or energy forces, also represented by the 12 signs of the zodiac. These streams transverse the human body in 6 levels or depths (divisions), named from the outermost layer to the deepest into the body; the Taiyang (Greater Yang), Yangming (Yang of Sunlight), Shaoyang (Lesser Yang), Taiyin (Greater Yin), Jueyin (Reverting Yin) and Shaoyin (Lesser Yin).

Qi flows in the Channels and Collaterals in a sort of "lemniscates," or 8-shape. It flows through the arms, through the body and then out in the limbs.

Qi enters the human body with or through all sense organs (smell (LU), sound (KI), sight (LV), touch (HT) and taste (SP). It enters LU, where it goes into the Channel-Organ System of the body and flows in specific streams; Qi circulation starts in the middle layer of the body (in LU, Taiyin), moves in lemniscatic form outwards in two rounds (Yangming, LI-ST) and then returns to the middle layer again (SP, Taiyin). Then Qi flows inwards to the deepest layer (HT, Shaoyin), where it gathers a lot of Qi or strength before it goes out to the exterior of the body in 2 rounds (Taiyang, SI-BL) to protect it against all influences of the Stressors. Then Qi enters the depths again in a two-round lemniscatic circle (Shaoyin, KI and Jueyin, PC), then to the exterior in two circles (Shaoyang, TH-GB). Finally Qi flows to the Interior to reach Jueyin (LV), from which it flows to LU, to begin the whole Qi cycle again.

According to the Chinese sages, it is very beneficial to meditate on these lemniscatic Qi flows throughout the body. This form of meditation is a form of Qigong; it gives power over bodily Qi and also over the Qi in nature, helping both internal and external balance, health and harmony.

Does this indicate some sort of correlation with the construction and myths of the Troy labyrinths? If we walk the paths of the labyrinth, we start in the middle layer. After that we move outwards in two turns. We head inwards in two turns almost to the centre, outwards again two turns and finally towards the absolute centre. The correlation of the labyrinth with the Asian teachings concerning the situation (paths) or construction of the Qi flow in the body and the clamed effects in "walking" or "thinking" these paths is not absolute but is amazingly coherent. These imaginations or beliefs are amazingly coherent with the beliefs of our forefathers occupied with fishing and hunting. The only difference is that our Scandinavian forefathers went physically where the Asian shamans did the exercise in their minds. It is uncertain if this knowledge was universal at the time or was discovered by our European forefathers or if Asian horse-warriors imported them before or during the times of the population migrations. However, I argue that the last possibility is the most probable.

Background History

It is probable that TCM was already in practice around 2000 BC, as the oldest of all medical books, *Neijing*, usually is believed to be written by the legendary *Yellow Emperor (2698-2598 BC)*. The first physical sample of this book, the *Neijing Suwen*, is only from circa 300 BC. This book describes the AP system in detail, as well as other medical knowledge.

Horses were very important during this time and horse-priests practised veterinary medicine from at least during the time of the *Zhou Mu Emperor (974-928 BC)*. The first book on veterinary acupuncture was written by *Sun Yang* around 630 BC. Many books on veterinary medicine were written in the period from 221 BC until 1608 AD.

One of the most famous books, called the *"Horse Classic,"* was written in 1635 by the brothers *Yu Benyuan and Yu Benheng.* This book is translated to German by Michael Heerde. There are a lot of interesting observations in this book, although I doubt several of the observations to have reference to reality. The two veterinary educated brothers describe horses with only 12 ribs and they also describe several signs that indicate that the horse will be able to live up to 90 years. This shows that we must be very critical to old Chinese observations, and not accept all old books as authorities.

In the period around Christ's birth, many books on animal diseases were published and AP use in horses was common. Around the year 1000 AD, China developed a formal veterinary education system, of which AP was a part.

Jesuit priests, who had returned from Peking in the late 16th and early 17th century, introduced human AP to Europe. Harvieu, a Jesuit, was the first to translate a book on AP into French. However, the practice of AP in Europe fell into discredit, most likely due to the Jesuit's bad training and results.

Soulie de Morant, a French diplomat who returned from Shanghai in 1927, re-introduced AP in Europe. He translated some modern Chinese books on AP into French. This work became the basis for the French AP School and is still one of the greatest European textbooks on AP today. From France, the knowledge spread to the rest of the western world.

In the 1970s, AP was given a boost after China opened its borders during the Nixon (former American president) visit. For the first time, westerners could see film and TV documentaries on operations carried out under AP analgesia.

Unfortunately, the impression that AP had merely analgesic effects has surrounded AP since that time. However, AP analgesia is only one of many therapeutic applications of AP. Other important applications are the regulation of the autonomic nervous system, metabolism and of a myriad of vital Processes (which can be reduced to the 12 main Processes that keep the body functioning, from secretion of mucus, to hair growth, to excretion of urine, etc).

In Europe, interest in veterinary AP followed its use in humans. Drs. Oswald Kothbauer (Austria), Jacques Milin (France) and Erwin Westermayer (Germany) were pioneers of veterinary AP in Europe. Interest grew in America later; American pioneers included Drs. Shelly Altman, Marvin Cain, David Jaggar, Alan Klide and Grady Young. They were founders of NAVA (National Association of Veterinary Acupuncture) in 1973. IVAS (the International Veterinary Acupuncture Society) arose out of NAVA in 1974. IVAS is the largest and most highly organised group of veterinary acupuncturists in the western world. It has members from many different countries and has held 26 international annual congresses on veterinary AP. IVAS has trained hundreds of veterinary acupuncturists in Europe, America and Australia.

In 1989, NoVAS (Nordic Veterinary Acupuncture Society), a sister organisation to IVAS, was founded. Today, NoVAS has members in all of the Nordic countries (Norway, Sweden, Denmark and Finland). NoVAS organised the 19th International World Congress of Veterinary AP in Tromsø in 1993.

The Acupuncture Method

The principle of AP is simple; one inserts thin needles into the body at specific points, the acupoints. The acupoint locations and their relationships to the Processes and clinical uses have been documented for millennia.

The stimulus produced by needling the acupoints sends its "message" to the Processes that are Deficient, Excessive or otherwise imbalanced. If the body's Channel-Organ System is intact (without too much trauma) and if the process can respond, this message induces the Process Imbalances to normalise. In western terms, provided that the homeostatic capacity can respond, the AP stimuli mobilises the body's adaptive mechanisms to assist in the resolution of the functional imbalance.

- The stimulation of the points has but one message to the process; get in balance!

In TCM, needling and moxibustion were used as effective ways to stimulate the effects of a point. However, many other ways are effective also, including point-injection, massage, warmth, cold, electromagnetic waves (microwave, chromotherapy, laser, sonotherapy, ultrasound, etc) and many other methods, including the projected Qi and Yi of the therapist, especially of a therapist trained in Qigong, but *the choice of the correct point (in fact the choice of the correct meridian is more important than which point is chosen on this special meridian) is more important than the choice of the method used to activate the effect of the point.*

When we want to treat an acupoint we should be aware of the effects it has on the process in question, and the relation of this process to the other processes.

Then we must know the laws that govern the different processes. These laws are described at page 24, but will in short be mentioned here. Two new laws, especially designed for the therapeutic use, are described in greater detail.

The Laws of Acupuncture:

- **Five Phase Law, page 25.**
- **Yin-Yang Law, page 29.**
- **Chinese Qi Clock (biorhythm), page 31.**
- **Husband-Wife Law, page 32.**
- **Deficiency law, page 33.**
- **Mirror law, page 217.**

There are also two more laws or classification-systems that many practitioners use in their practise. Personally I find very little use for these systems, but I mention them so that the reader will be aware of their existence.

- **Six divisions, page 219.**
- **Eight principles, page 220.**

1. Five Phase Law (see page 25)

This Law states that all created things (Processes) can be classified into Five Phases, or Elements. These are fundamental qualities that correspond with common experiences of the natural world. The Phases interact or influence each other directly in two ways, the Sheng Cycle and the Ko Cycle. These Cycles either support (Sheng) or control (Ko) each other.

2. Yin-Yang Law (see page 29)

The predictable interaction of Yin-Yang is the most universal law in Asia. It derives from holistic concepts in a cosmological thinking process, or world-view, used to relate all natural phenomena.

3. Biorhythms (see page 31)

We often find that the manifestations of disease (the Lesion-Symptom Complexes) change at or near specific times of the day, night, week, month or year. The Lesion-Symptom Complexes aggravate, begin, improve, or in some way or another, change at these times. These changes coincide with the biorhythms of the deficient or excessive Process.

The time of day is also important in relation to therapy. If it is possible to do so, we should preferably choose the corresponding time to treat Lesion-Symptom Complexes that relate to a specific time of day.

Two examples:

- A woman with a migraine asked me to treat her. The migraine had been present for several years; severe pain had confined her to bed at least once per week. It was difficult to find a pattern in her Lesion-Symptom Complexes, but when she told me about her first attack, the cause became clear. She remembered the first attack very well. It appeared on the beach exactly 12 noon during strong Summer Heat. It was the middle of the summer and it was a Sunday. I diagnosed HT-deficiency due to the relations to different aspects of the Fire-element. I tonified her HT-process (HT09, Ting Point of HT). One session of treatment was enough to heal her migraine.

- A horse with KI-deficiency may consequently develop joint or bone disorders. In such horses, we must stimulate KI-Process, for example by stimulating KI01. Improved KI-process automatically stimulates PC (PC is the Qi Clock successor of KI, and also the 5-Phase successor in the Ko-cycle of KI) and this helps blood circulation in the forelimbs. In contrast, aiming to stimulate blood circulation to help the forelimb, but not knowing the Laws of the processes, a novice might treat the Lesion-Symptom Complexes only. For example, s/he might stimulate PC directly by using its Ting-point (PC09). However, that intervention could *exaggerate* KI Deficiency, as stimulation of the fire element may suppress the water element, and eventually would increase the damage to the forelimb joints.

4. THE HUSBAND-WIFE LAW (SEE PAGE 32)

The interpretation of ancient Chinese calligraphy is that harmony within organisms and seasons is best preserved when the husband is stronger than the wife is. The Chinese had noted that the most harmonious households had strong husbands and somewhat weaker wives. Likewise, if summer becomes stronger (more energetic) than autumn, this creates imbalance and illness in nature and in human or animal bodies.

5. THE DEFICIENCY LAW (SEE PAGE 33)

This Law states that whenever there is an excess (painful condition, mainly in the Yang Channels), there must be a deficiency (not painful condition, mainly in the Yin Channels).

The inferior acupuncturist treats the excess, but the superior acupuncturist treats the deficiency.

The Nei Ching states that: "The normal doctor treats the thousands of symptoms (local, symptomatic treatment), the good doctor treats the underlying excess (excessive Channel), but the superior doctor treats the underlying deficiency (usually the Ko-father of the symptom-carrying meridian).

An example:

- A dressage horse had a deficiency in the Heart Channel over a long period of time. Then he began to develop sore muscles in the left leg, due to pain in the right leg. After investigating the right leg, I did find a painful muscular nod in Musculus Pectoralis Profundus, pars scapularis (the subclavius muscle). This muscle lies in the exact parthway of the LI Channel, and this Channel showed excess and pain. But the real underlying cause was the deficiency in the HT Channel, and only after treating the HT Channel, the situation resolved permanently, although the horse felt much better after treating the LI Channel. But the treatment of the LI Channel did not last permanently.

6. THE MIRROR LAW (SEE PAGE 33)

The Law of Mirror applies to all life. As explained earlier on Page 33, it applies to the recurrence of symptoms, to life-parts (the seventh 7-year period mirrors the first 7-year period and so on), to Karma, to time and also we may see this law within acupuncture. Here this "Mirror Rule" or "Rule of Opposites" applies in several ways:

- **Within the same Channel**, the last point mirrors the first point; the second last point mirrors the second point, etc. For example ST45 mirrors ST01; ST44 mirrors ST02, ST24 mirrors ST22, etc.

- **Between mirrors of the same Channel**, the last point on the left mirrors the last point on the right; the first point on the left mirrors the first point on the right, etc. For example left ST45 mirrors right ST45; left ST01 mirrors right ST01, etc.

- **Between homopolar diagonal members of a Big Channel Pair**: Processes form special homopolar pairs within the Six Levels. These are LU-SP (Taiyin), HT-KI (Shaoyin), PC-LV (Jueyin), LI-ST (Yangming), SI-BL (Taiyang) and TH-GB (Shaoyang). Homopolar diagonal members of a Big Channel Pair balance each other. For example, left LU balances right ST, and vice-versa; right SI balances left BL, and vice-versa, etc.

- **Other Mirrors**, which cannot be discussed in detail here, include the:

  1) Phase Mates: Within a Phase (Metal-LU-LI, Earth-ST-SP, Fire-HT-SI, Water-BL-KI, Fire-PC-TH, Wood-GB-LV), the Yin balances it's Yang Mate on the contralateral limb, and vice-versa. For example, left LU balances right LI, and vice-versa; right ST balances left SP, and vice versa, etc.

  2) Heteropolar diagonal Six Level Opponents (LI-LV, ST-PC, SI-SP, BL-LU, TH-KI and GB-HT) balance each other. For example, right ST balances left PC, and vice versa; left BL balances right LU, and vice versa, etc.

  3) Heteropolar ipsilateral Qi Clock Opponents (LU-BL, LI-KI, ST-PC, SP-TH, HT-GB, SI-LV) balance each other. For example, left SP balances left TH, and vice-versa; right HT balances right GB, and vice-versa.

  4) Homopolar diagonal Qi Clock Neighbours (LV-LU, SP-HT, KI-PC, LI-ST, SI-BL, TH-GB) balance each other. For example, left KI balances right PC, and vice-versa; right SI balances left BL, and vice-versa, etc.

AP therapy often uses these Mirror Relationships, especially to treat local disorders. One way to treat pain in a local area is to treat its corresponding opposite, or Mirror, area. For example, for pain in the thumb near LU11 or LU10, one may treat LU11 or LU10 on the other thumb, or SP01 or SP04 on the ipsilateral or contralateral big toe, which is on the Mirror Digit. (SP01 and SP04 are the closest exact Mirror Points of LU11 and LU10. Also LU-SP forms the same Big Channel in Taiyin). Alternatively one may treat points on the opposite end of the Channel, for example, LU01 or LU02 on the chest.

7. THE SIX DIVISIONS

The six divisions state that all symptoms may be related to one out of six levels, which are, counted from external to internal:

- Taiyang (SI and BL, *Greater Yang*).

- Yangming (LI andST, *Yang of sunlight*).

- Shauyang (TH and GB, *Lesser Yang*).

- Taiyin (LU and SP, *Greater Yin*).

- Jueyin (PC and LV, *Reverting Yin*).

- Shauyin (HT and KI, *Lesser Yin*).

The seriousness of the disease is also thought to be greater the deeper inside the disease is located.

Be aware that the circulation of Qi within these meridians is not in the same succession as their depth.

When combining both the depth and the succession of Qi-circulation (according to the Chinese clock, page 31 & 220), then we get the complicated pattern as shown in dealing with the Troy-castle at page 206.

This way of categorising the processes gives an impression of how deep or longstanding the disease has come.

In my opinion, this knowledge is important when meditating over the energy-circulation of the Meridian-Qi and when studying Qi-Gong or Tai-Qi, but in actual treatment of the deficient process, it does not really give much important information.

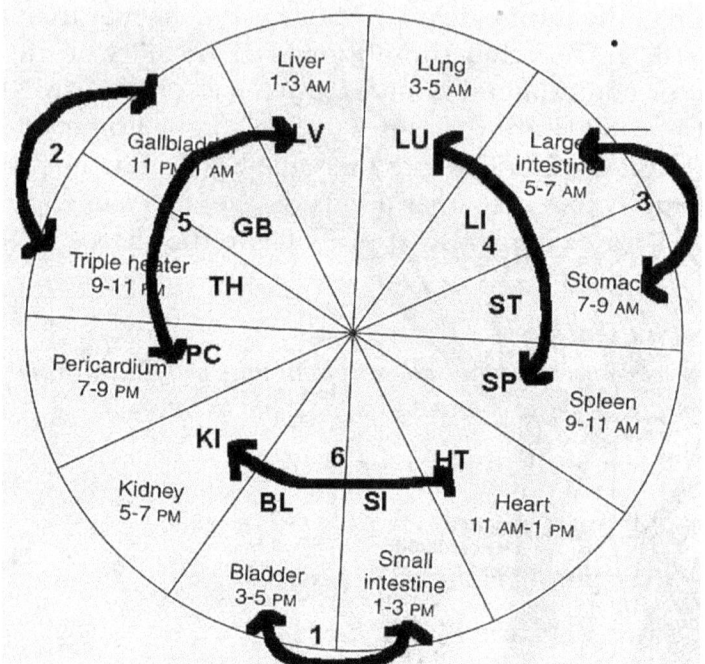

Fig 41; Illustration of the 6 divisions

8) THE EIGHT PRINCIPLES

The eight principles state that all symptoms may be divided from their appearance into Yin or Yang, and then further sub-divisions according to the qualities of **inside/outside, cold/hot** and **excess/deficiency** (which together with **Yin/Yang** make up 8 possible variations, a little "square" thinking if you ask me).

1. According to Internal/external we may classify the

   a. Origin of the disease

      • From internal:

         ° Joy: SP10, BL40, PC03, PC09, LI11.

         ° Anger: BL18, GB20, LV02, LV03, GV20.

         ° Melancholy (dryness): ?

- ° Sorrow (dampness): LI11, SP06, SP09, ST40, LU09, PC05, BL17, SP08, SP10.

- ° Fear: KI03.

- From external:

  - ° Wind: LU07, LU09, LI04, BL12, BL13, TH05, GB20, GV14, GV16.

  - ° Heat: LU10, LU11, LI01, LI04, LI11, TH05, GB20, GV14.

  - ° Dryness: LU01, LU11.

  - ° Dampness: SP03, SP06, SP09, BL20, BL21, BL22, BL23, LV13, CV06, CV12.

  - ° Cold: BL23.

b. Where the pathological symptoms are situated

- Situated internally:

  - ° Heat: LI11, GV14, GV26.

  - ° Dampness: ST40, LU09.

- Situated externally.

2. Symptoms according to cold and warm:

- More (too much) cold: treatment: ST36, CV04.

- More (too much) warmth: treatment: CV03, BL20, BL28, BL39, BL40, SP06, KI03, HT07, HT05, PC06, BL15, BL23, KI06, LI11, GV14.

3. According to deficiency and excess

- Deficiency (chronic):

  - ° General: BL20, SP03, SP06, ST36, LV13, CV12.

  - ° Qi: ST36, SP06, CV06, CV17.

  - ° Yang: GV04, GV14, GV20.

    °   Blood: ST36, BL17, BL20, CV06.

    °   Yin: SP06, CV04, HT06.

    °   Jing: CV04, CV06, GV04.

        °   All the organs or processes as described under processes and 5 elements

- Excess (acute):

    °   General: LU07, PC06, ST25.

4. According to the overall impression of Yin and Yang

    a. Yin impression

    b. Yang impression

After settling on these parameters (which really is nothing more than finding the symptoms´ place in the Yin/Yang system) then we may find a treatment as dispersing wind, dispersing cold, fighting warmth and so on. Also the Chinese plants and herbs are categorized after this pattern.

The diagnosis may then come up with such conclusions:

- Damp heat invasion from outside.

- Wind attack from outside.

- Dampness in the blood inside.

- Liver fire rising inside.

- Damp heath rising from below.

This method often gives very good results in practice, and if perfected in observation and logic, it leads to the correct deficient process. I have seen systems including also the processes and organs, so it becomes a total system which is good.

But if used only symptomatically and with many points, it gives, in my opinion, only a more or less symptomatic treatment (which often seems very effective and fast).

In my opinion, the only causal treatment is to find the true deficiency of one or more processes, either by pulse-diagnosis or by observing the symptoms, modifications and origin (as described in 8 principles).

Modern Explanations of the Mechanisms of AP

Recent studies have given us a better understanding of mechanisms by which AP has its clinical effects in accordance with concepts of western medicine and physiology. Various mechanisms have been presented to explain the effects of AP but none gives a satisfactory explanation for all of the physiological changes that AP can induce. Probably several other mechanisms, some still unknown, can explain the effects also. However, the eight main theories that, in my opinion, explain the diverse effects of AP in the best way are:

1. The *neural mechanism of effect.*

2. The *hormonal mechanism of effect.*

3. The *opiate mechanism of effect.*

4. The *ECIWO-theory.*

5. The *cellular theory.*

6. The *consciousness-theory (remembrance) of function.*

   a. *Embryonic remembrance (from the body).*

   b. *Conscious or subconscious remembrance (from the brain).*

   c. *Electro-magnetic remembrance:*

      i. *Interference.*

      ii. *Induction.*

      iii. *Resonance.*

7. The *bioelectric theory.*

8. The *intention-depending effect (outgoing intention, Qi-Gong).*

1) *Neural effects:* Stimuli from needling of the acupoints influence body functions by reflex action via the nerve receptors and neural tracts. For example, the Gate-Control Theory of Ronald Melzack and Patrick Wall explains some of the analgesic effects of AP. AP stimuli from the periphery "close gates" in the spinal cord and thalamus, thereby blocking the ascending pathways in the cord and thalamus. This prevents pain stimuli from areas related to the stimulated acupoints from reaching the cerebral cortex in the brain, i.e. the subject feels no pain from the area that otherwise would feel painful. The neural theory explains how competing neural signals from the acupoints can block pain signals from an injured area from reaching the brain.

2) *Hormonal effects:* Many research studies confirmed that AP stimulation can modulate hormonal production and release. For example, AP can influence metabolism and endocrine release in the hypophysis-hypothalamus, thyroid, adrenal, pancreas and gonads.

3) *Endogenous opioid effects:* Brain, nervous tissues and other sites in the body secrete endogenous opioid compounds, such as enkephalin, endorphin, dynorphin, etc. The physiological effects of endogenous opioids resemble those of powerful opiate drugs. Opioids influence pain perception, mood, behaviour, blood pressure, appetite, and many other bodily functions. For example, long-distance running, extreme jogging, anxiety, battle and fatal situations activate opioid mechanisms; under their influence, the person usually is unaware of (or less aware of) pain, feels euphoric and shows unusual strength. AP stimulation releases endogenous opioids in the brain and circulation. This influences various pathways in the central nervous system (CNS). Release of endogenous opioids in the brain and cord can explain some effects of AP, especially its analgesic and euphoric effects.

4) *ECIWO biological effects:* ECIWO is the acronym for E=Embryo, C=Containing, I=Information, W=Whole,

O=**O**rganism. Several scientists have written recently about ECIWO Biology. Several books (for example by Vilhelm Schjelderup, Høyskoleforlaget 1998) and three international congresses focused on ECIWO biology. Its theory is very old indeed; it stems from the ancient TCM theories on relationships between microcosms and macrocosms, but it is also very new and analogous to modern holographic theory (see page 10). The new aspect of ECIWO theory is that some scientists acknowledge this law as a fact, even a general phenomenon; it may be found at all stages in a living organism. For example, if we look at a tree, its stem represents an ECIWO System at the first level, a branch on the second level, a leaf on the third level etc. All these smaller parts contain all the information needed to build the total organism and all the systems are in internal communication (intercommunication) with the totality and also with each other. *The foundation and function of the Process and their acupoints and the diagnostic and clinical applications of these concepts depend totally on this intra- and inter- communication.*

Several books on this subject have been published lately (among others by the Norwehian doctor Dr. Vilhelm Schjeldrup, Høyskoleforlaget 1998) and as much as three world congresses on the subject have been arranged. In New Scientist of 01/17/2010 the main article is about this subject, and some scientists think that the total human organism might be a hologram of the whole cosmos.

5) *Professor Pishinger* from the University of Berlin describes the *cell,* its environment, and the reaction of the cell to the connective tissue as the most important auto-regulative mechanism in the body. We may say that a cell-based ECIWO System can influence the whole organism.

6) I will also mention, to make the picture of what we see happening in the clinic complete, a theory which is called the *theory of remembrance.* This is mostly an empiric and deductive theory, and it has two different features.

- One relating to what is called "organizing islands." Organizing islands is thought to be organizing cellular centres remaining from the foetal life. When imbalances in the processes occur, these centres may be rejuvenated or woken to life, to organize the organs or processes once again. The body will then in a way remember how it shall behave. This is not a scientific theory, though.

- We may also describe this theory as if disease develops because the mind of the patient (or the totality) in a way forget the organ or part or process in question. Such may happen if the nerves or the communication or the contact with the area is lost due to a trauma, overwork or similar conditions. When the body is then reminded about the existence of the forgotten part, process or organ, then the cooperation will be re-established, and the symptoms will disappear. The different methods of acupuncture, neural-therapy, homeopathy or the numerous forms of manipulative methods will, if they are done properly, remind the body of this missing part and the former relations to this part, so that normal relations may continue.

- All living creatures have an electromagnetic field. This field has, in many connections, proved to be of great importance (see the works of Becker page 227 and also the influence of the electromagnetic field of the earth page 672). Irregularities in this field may cause serious disease, even be the origin of disease. Inserting a metal needle or stimulation of energetic points may change this field to do its proper tasks. Such interfering may be due to:

    ° Interference of the electromagnetic field.

    ° Induction in the electromagnetic field.

    ° Resonance with the electromagnetic field.

7) *Bioelectrical Theory* attempts to merge eastern and western ways of thinking. It explains the AP effects from weak electrical currents, which penetrate to every part of organism. EEG, ECG

and EMG can detect tiny bioelectrical currents. Abnormalities in these currents can be of diagnostic value because the electrical conductivity of pathological parts of the body changes. Conduction can be improved by stimulating acupoints; non-AP stimulation, or stimulation of unrelated acupoints, or stimulation of carefully chosen non-AP points usually does not elicit these effects. AP normalises the bioelectric flows throughout the body's pathological parts. This latter way of thinking has much in common with the old way of thinking on which AP is based. Dr. Robert Becker, a US Army surgeon in the Veterans' General Hospital, New York, wrote the best explanation of this theory in "The Body Electric," His book describes 30 years of his research on the importance of effects of the body's electrical signalling system. He shows how they relate to research in medicine, AP and our own natural environment.

Becker concluded that electrical currents exist within the body as a form of slow acting "Primitive Nervous System," analogous to that of plants and invertebrate forms of animal life. This system uses a cell-to-cell signalling by direct electrical currents to control many of the body's slower-acting processes, such as those of wound-healing, tissue regeneration and growth. Becker's Bioelectrical Theory indicates that the eastern concepts of Qi, Yin and Yang are not just philosophical figures of speech; they describe measurable and comprehensible phenomena for westerners. Apart from religious and sociocultural beliefs, hard-headed westerners are reluctant to believe in phenomena that cannot be measured. Also, it has been impossible until recently to detect these weak bioelectrical currents by modern technology.

Becker became interested in bioelectricity as part of his research on tissue regeneration in US soldiers that were badly wounded in battle in the Far East. While amputating salamander tails, he discovered that a special electric pattern arose in regenerating before the amputated tail was fully regenerated. Frogs, who do not have the ability to regenerate amputated limbs, show a totally different electrical pattern. He hoped that this could lead him to a solution as to why various bone fractures do not knit again. He concluded that bone fracture healing in all types of organisms depend on the electrical pattern, much resembling his observation of salamander regeneration.

This theory was added to the previous idea of how the nervous system worked. Becker discovered the fact that there exists in all organisms a continual electric flow, which is totally unlike normal nerve impulses. (Nerve impulses are explained as an unstable threshold value and chemical transfer between synapses, and not as constant currents).

Becker was able to prove the existence of these currents related mainly to the Schwann cells, which encircle all nerve fibres (axons and dendrites). Schwann cells surround even small nerve fibres, which do not have any myelin chains. These cells create an electrical area enabling them to adapt to changes like injury, pain, or an altered state of consciousness. It also seems as if feelings can have a curing effect by modifying these currents. Professor Nordenstrøm from Sweden has also demonstrated similar electrical currents, which accompany the blood veins.

Another electric current, for example, via attached rubber electrodes, can modify or influence these weak currents in the tissues. Such methods have been used for several years (electrical medical treatment).

There are also various angles of incidences for the use of electric stimulation, amongst which are the uses of magnetic and electromagnetic fields (EMFs). Becker holds that we should be cautious with the use of such methods, due to a lack of research in this field. Possible side effects should be uncovered; therefore, the use of electromagnetic stimulation should only be used as a last resort.

We are able to develop new technology for the use of EMFs for healing because electrical fields are produced and influenced by magnetic fields. Stationary magnetic fields used to influence specific areas can, according to Becker, have a good therapeutic effect without noticeable side effects. He is contrarily concerned about the continual use of technological inventions which allow pulsating EMFs to influence the whole body. These not only accelerate certain aspects of healing but can also accelerate the growth of cancer cells. Such equipment is accessible to everyone but should be used with caution.

The earth has two types of EMF. One, the balanced background EMF, appears to interact with the currents of the organism and is essential to the regulation of biorhythms, a good immune system and life itself. The other earth field, geopathic radiation (to be discussed on page 671), has adverse effects on health and well being of animals and plants.

Becker claimed that cancer could arise only by the influence of natural causes, such as the influence of the sun, moon, stars and chance exposure to photoradiation, or natural geopathic forces, before this century. However, in this century, we have changed our electromagnetic background more than at any other time in human evolution. For example, the density of radio waves, which now surrounds us, is 100-200 times that of the natural radiation of the sun.

The large increase in cancer cases, especially amongst children, has been related to living close to high voltage electric wires. Pregnant woman working at computer terminals have a higher risk of abortion and many people who live or work exposed to EMFs complain of headaches and irritability.

Clearly, when we try to diagnose the factors that cause their diseases, we must consider the adverse effects that EMFs may have on our patients. Without widespread public demand for proper regulations for our safety, it is most unlikely that national or international authorities will legislate to reduce or ban man-made EMFs or that industry will accept such regulations. As educated citizens with power to educate others, it is our duty to inform all who will listen as to the existence and effects of these noxious energies. (See also the Appendix about the geopathic radiation, page 667).

8) *The Intention-Dependent Theory:* I will describe a theory which I have developed myself and which may explain the numerous paradoxical observations I have made through the years. These observations are described on page 641 and I will here only recapitulate the conclusions.

*The **will**, **intention**, **empathy** and **courage** of the therapist are of great importance concerning the outcome of the treatment.*

The Meridians/Channels of AP

Each of the twelve fundamental processes of the placental living organism (human and animal) has developed an intricate system of points of stimulation or energetic connections to the outer world. These points or receptors are connected by pathways through witch impulses or information may run. These pathways are called meridians. The meridians use the connective tissue surrounding the veins, arteries or nerves, and it is this connective tissue that constitutes the meridians through which the impulses travel. The connective tissue forms a network throughout the whole body including the organs and the central nervous system. In such a way will the impulses from the acupuncture points be able to stimulate multiple structures and balance several systems and processes.

For example:

- *Lung-meridian* follows: *V. cephalica humerii, V. cephalica antebrachii, A/V. radialis proximalis, A. radialis, V. (metacarpalis) palmaris medialis, V. digitalis medialis and V. coronalis phal. III.*

- *Large Intestine-meridian* follows: *A/V. coronalis phal. III, A/V. phal. II et I, ramus dors., A. mtcs dors. med., Rete carpi dors., A. collat. radialis (dist), A. carotis communis, V. jugularis., A. maxillaries, A. facialis, A. labialis maxillaris, A. incisive and A. dorsalis nasi.*

- *Stomach-meridian* follows: *A. dors. nasi, A. angularis oculi, A. malaris., V. angularis oculi, V. facialis, V. labialis maxillaris, V. labialis mandibularis, V. masseterica, V. temporalis superficialis, V. jugularis (A. carotis communis), A/V. iliolumbalis, (A/)V. tibialis cran., (A/)V. dorsalis pedis, Rete tarsi dors., (A/)V. mtts. dorsalis media, (A/) V. dorsalis phal. I et II and (A/) V. coronalis phal. III.*

- **Spleen-meridian** follows: *A/V. coronalis phal. III, A. et V. digitalis med., A/V. mtts. plant. prof. med., A. mtts. dors. med, Rete malleolus med., A/V. tibialis caudalis, A/V. popliteus, A/V. genus desc., A/V. femoralis, A/V. epigastrica caudalis, V. thoracica externa* and *A/V. thoracodorsalis.*

- **Heart-meridian** follows: *A. mediana, A. prof.antebrachii, A. palmaris lat., A. mtcp. palm. prof. lat., A/V. digit. lat.* and *A/V. coronalis phal. III.*

- **Small Intestine-meridian** follows: *A/V. coronalis phal. III, A. mtcs. dors. lat., A. collateralis ulnaris, A. collateralis ulnaris, A/V. subscapularis, A/V. circumfl. scap., A/V. cerv.prof., A/V. vertebralis, A/V. transversa faciei, A/V. temporalis superfic.,* and *A/V. auricularis magna.*

- **Bladder-meridian** follows: *A/V. angularis oculi, A. vertebralis, A/V. obturatoria, A/V. femoris caud. ramus asc., A/V. gluteus cran., A/V. gluteus caud., A. et V. vertebralis, A. et V. intercostalis, A. et V. lumbalis, A. et V. gluteus caud., A/V. femoris caud. ascend., A/V. tarsica recurrens, A/V. tarsica lat., A/V. mtts. plant. supf. lat., A/V. digit. lat.* and *A/V. coronalis phal. III.*

- **Kidney-meridian** follows: *A/V. torica phal. III, A/V. digitalis med., A/V. mtts. plant. supf. med., A/V.. tarsica med., A/V. tibialis caud., A/V. recurrens tib., Rete malleolus med., A/V. recurrens tib., A/V. caud. femoris Ramus desc., A/V. obturatoria* and *A/V: pudendalis int.*

- **Pericardium-meridian** follows: *A. thoracica ext., A/V. brachialis, A/V. mediana, A/V. mtcp. palm. supf., A/V. digitalis med.* and *A/V. torica phal. III.*

- **Trippel-heather-meridian** follows: *A/V. coronalis phal. III, A/V. dorsalis phal.I, Rete carpi dors., A/V. interosseus dors., A/V. interosseus recurrens, A/V. profunda brachii, A/V. circumflex. hum. caud., A/V. vertebralis, A/V. occipitalis ramus desc., A/V. auricularis magna, A/V. auricul. rostr., A/V. supraorbit.* and *A/V. auric. rostr.*

- **Gall Bladder-meridian** follows: *A/V. temporalis supf., A/V. supraorb., A/V. occipitalis and A/V. cervicalis supf. (asc.).*

- **Liver-meridian** follows: *A/V. coronalis phal. III, V. digit. med., V. mtts. dors. med., V. saphena, A/V. femoralis, A/V. iliaca ext., A/V. femoralis prof. and A/V. pudenda ext.,*

Many studies have tried to establish the real nature of these Channels. Are they just imaginary lines, like the meridians of the earth, or have they a physiological and anatomical reality? If they are real, it must be possible to show either:

a) Functional structures/lines linking points with similar action.

b) A sort of current or Qi-flow through these structures/ lines.

Some studies and observations have concluded that the Channels are not just some theoretical lines:

1. Injected radioactive isotopes in the acupoints gave a marked increase in the radioactivity along the Channel, rather than in all directions around the injected points (lecture by Prof. Pekka Pöntinen).

2. If we hold a tuning fork (or apply a sound signal) on an acupoint, we can induce and record an increased sound resonance along the Channel, rather than in all directions around the injected points (personal information by Dr. Dominique Giniaux).

3. Treatment of an acupoint sometimes causes piloerection (rising of the hairs) along the Channel, rather than in all directions around the injected points (my own experience in equine clinical work).

4. Human patients also report Propagated Channel Sensation (PCS), a strong feeling of paraesthesia, as if something "moves along" the Channel, rather than in all directions around the injected points (my own clinical experience).

We cannot claim that the Channels conduct some sort of current nor any kind of measurable impulses as nerves do. My impression of this concept is that the Channels are more like wave-conductors. It is also possible to regard them as channels that hold constant or varying static electrical potentials (Björn Nordenstrøm, Sweden) or a system of wave or static- governed communication using the connective tissue around the nerves and blood vessels as their transport route.

The energy in the meridians, called Qi, is provided from the fundamental processes, but do also have their own sources like external radiation, light and sounds. The energy of the fundamental processes (Jing or ethereal energy) is often quite similar to the energy (Qi) in the meridians, but not necessarily. The energy in the process may be in deficiency, while the Qi in the meridian may be in excess. That is why the skin areas transversed by the meridian may show eczema due to an excess while the "mother process" inside the body may be in deficiency. That is also why the Ting-points may show deficiency (they are strictly meridian-situated points) while the Shu-point may show excess (they are more connected to the organs themselves due to their connection to the spinal nerves) and the process itself may show still another state of energy. So, the pulse-diagnosis (which shows the state of the process) may be different from the Ting-point diagnosis (which shows the energy in the meridian) which may be different from the Shu-point diagnosis (which shows the energy in the organ) and all these three may be different from other forms of diagnosis which may show different layers of the energy that constitute the whole of the organism.

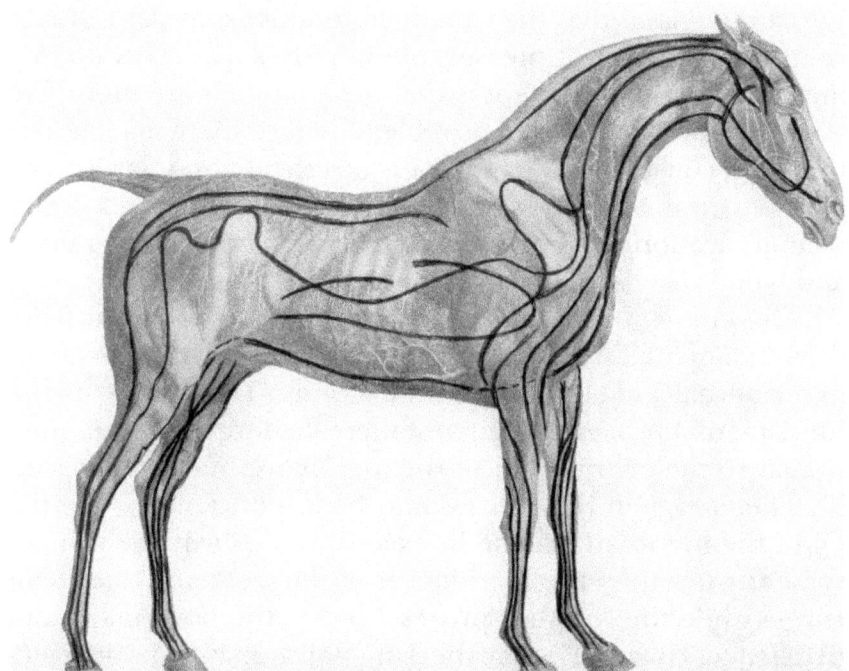

Fig 42; Illustration of the meridians in the horse

In Chinese concepts the meridians are energetic pathways nourishing the whole body. They consider them much more fundamental than I do, and not only as a means to regulate the processes.

In Chinese thought the Meridians or Channels (I take KI as an example) relate to:

- Its physical organ (kidney);

- Its known western functions;

- Its TCM functions;

- Its TCM Five Phase Relationships or Correspondences [Water Phase, winter, salt, fear, bones/teeth/marrow/ brain, ears/hearing, etc.];

- KI Channel, i.e. the complex Channel Organ System with its Vessel Network and Processes of its:

º Channel (KI, Foot Shaoyin Channel), both superficial branches that carry the acupoints and its deep branches that link to its physical organ;

º *Luo* (Collateral or Connecting Branch) that links it to its paired Phase Mate Channel (BL, Foot Taiyang Channel);

º *Relationship to its Qi Linked Channels* (the Channel that precedes and follows it in the diurnal Qi Cycle; *SI* precedes KI and *BL* follows KI;

º *Links to the Extraordinary Vessels* (for example KI links to the Yinqiaomai Yin Heel Vessel)

Discussion of the main internal organs and their TCM relationships and functions is intricately related to TCM concepts of the **JingLuoMai (Channels, Collaterals and Extraordinary Vessels)**. The **JingLuo** are pathways that circulate the Qi and Blood throughout the body. The main TCM Processes of the JingLuo are to transport Qi and Blood, regulate Yin-Yang and the Interior and Exterior, resist pathogens, reflect (manifest) symptoms and signs, transmit DeQi (needling sensation) and regulate Deficiency and Excess states. The JingLuo pertain to the ZangFu interiorly and extend over the body exteriorly forming a network and linking the tissues and organs into an organic whole.

The *Jing* (Channels), which constitute the 12 main trunks, run longitudinally and interiorly within the body.

The *Luo* (Collaterals), which are connecting branches for the Channels and run transversely and superficially from the Channels.

The *8 Mai* (Extraordinary Vessels) act as Qi reservoirs connected to the 12 Main Channels.

• *Dumai* (Governing Vessel, GV) runs in the dorsal midline; it governs all the Yang Channels.

• *Renmai* (Conception Vessel, CV) runs in the ventral midline. Ren means fostering and responsibility; it is responsible for all the Yin Channels.

- *Chongmai* (Vital Passage Vessel) regulates the flow of Qi and Blood in the 12 Main Channels; it is called "the Sea of the 12 Main Channels."

- *Daimai* (Girdle Vessel) goes around the waist, binding up all the Channels.

- *Yangqiaomai* (Yang Heel Vessel) starts from below the external malleolus.

- *Yinqiaomai* (Yin Heel Vessel) starts from below the internal malleolus.

- *Yangweimai* (Yang Connecting Vessel) connects and networks the Exterior Yang of the body.

- *Yinweimai* (Yin Connecting Vessel) connects and networks the Interior Yin of the body.

Thus, the *JingLuoMai* system is a 3-dimensional Qi network that includes the *12 Jing* (Main Channels), *8 Mai* (Extraordinary Vessels) and *15 Luo* (Collaterals). Chapter 33 of *Miraculous Pivot* says "The 12 Main Channels connect internally with the ZangFu and externally with the joints, limbs and other bodily superficial tissues." The Channels and Collaterals are distributed both interiorly and exteriorly over the body, transporting Qi and Blood to nourish the ZangFu, skin, muscles, tendons and bones. Normal functioning of various organs is thus ensured and a relative equilibrium maintained. Chapter 10 of *Miraculous Pivot* says "So important are the JingLuo which determine life and death in the treatment of all diseases and the regulation of deficiency and excess states that one must gain a thorough understanding of them. Indeed, the importance of studying the theory of Channels and Collaterals cannot be overemphasised."

The Acupoints

Each of the 12 Main Channels (+ two of the extra meridians) has a line of well defined acupoints along its superficial pathway. These points are situated where the blood-vessels or the nerves make unusual or unexpected changes in their partway. Either where they form a loop, anastomose with other vessels, break through different facies, go through muscles or surface in other ways. This may be seen especially in connection with the KI-points just above the tarsus. When we look up the pathway of the arteries in an anatomical book, we may see an accurate resemblance between the meridian-points and the arteries. We may especially find the points where the arteries form anastamosis or split up into many smaller vessels. That is why many of the acupoints are situated just above or below the joints (the commandpoints) or in areas of greater blood-circulation or sensitivity (the Ting-points). It is often enough to look at an anatomical atlas to know where the points are located just by where the arteries behave as described.

Although the points have *individual, generalised and local effects,* all points along a Channel have many common traits that relate to their effect on the functions of that Channel. Also, 2 of the 8 Extraordinary Vessels, the Dumai-GV and Renmai-CV, have their own specific acupoints. Altogether, there are 361 documented points in total along these 14 Channels in humans:

LU	LI	ST	SP	HT	SI	BL	KI	PC	TH	GB	LV	GV	CV	Total
11	20	45	21	9	19	67	27	9	23	44	14	28	24	**361**

Table 35

The Chinese names, English translations and locations of all those points are on the WWW, in the paper "*Acupoint Codes, Names, Translations and Locations,*" at: http://homepage.tinet.ie/~progers/ptc.htm.

There are also many documented Ear points, Scalp Points, etc. Overall, there are circa 2000 documented acupoints. However, in accordance with the principles of the hologram, or of the macrocosm in the microcosm, there may be millions of points as yet undiscovered.

SYSTEMATIC DESCRIPTION OF THE DIFFERENT GROUPS OF POINTS.

2. The Command Points

- *Jing-well or the Ting-points;* is the very point where the Qi either enter or leave the meridian. Here it also changes from Yin to Yang or from Yang to Yin. In needling this point it is possible to drain or fill up the meridian, and the Ting-point is thus very suitable in treating excesses or deficiencies. In deficiencies, the symptoms this point may treat belong to the wood element. Several writers claim that this point belongs to the metal element in Yang meridians, but that is only because an excess of Qi usually shows up in the Yang meridians and leads to painful symptoms. Draining the meridian takes away the pain, and as metal = pain, many think that this point belongs to the metal element in Yang meridians. This is not so, at least not if we diagnose and treat *according to deficiencies.* In this book, and especially in horses, I use the Ting-point as belonging to the *wood*-element, and according to the old Chinese books, these points are used in problems with pressure under the heart, liver problems and in problems with the "zang," the yin-organs (which point to their connection to the wood-element).

- *Ying-spring points;* is where the Qi flows quietly to the superficial part of the skin. Ying means "source." In my opinion, as I think that all Ting-points belong to the wood element, all Ying-points should belong to the Fire-element. This is also found in the old writings where these points are used to cure symptoms related to heat and heart-pathogens. They are used to dissolve heat in all the "zangfu" (internal organs) and in the meridians. They are also capable of dissolving excess of pathogenic factors and stagnant Qi in the meridians.

- *Shu-stream points;* is where the energy (Qi) of the meridian flourishes. Shu means to transport. In horses (and also in dogs and in my opinion, also in humans) they belong to the *earth*-element. According to the old Chinese, they are used (in all meridians, both the Yin and the Yang) for symptoms of "heaviness," of pain in the joints and in spleen-problems (symptoms that come and go like in malaria).

- *Jing-river points*; is where the Qi flows or streams through. Jing means to pass. They are connected to the *metal*-element. According to the old Chinese, they were used for coughing, problems with respiration, could and fever; LU-pathogens. They are used for the problems mentioned above and for diseases that change the voice of the patient, for problems of the tendons, muscles and the joints. Also for painful conditions.

- *He-sea points*; where the energy dived deeper into the body. He means to join. In horses (and in my opinion, in all animals and even in humans as long as we relate the symptoms to states of deficiency) these points belong to the water element and they are situated just above the carpus and the tarsus. According to the old Chinese, these points are used in symptoms of "Qi going the opposite direction" and in diarrhoea. Also in KI-pathogens, diseases in the ST, and in problems due to irregular meals (like in Spleen problems). The He-sea points are very important in treatment of all problems in the abdomen.

- *Yuan-source points;* are points that belong to the command-points as it commands the meridian and does not act only as a local point. It has no connection to the elements, and stimulation of a source-point stimulates the whole meridian in a non specific manner.

Command Point	Key energetic functions
Fire Point	Commands, or influence the Fire Aspects of the Processes represented by that Channel
Earth Point	Commands, or influence the Earth Aspects of the Processes represented by that Channel

Metal Point	Commands, or influence the Metal Aspects of the processes represented by that Channel
Water Point	Commands, or influence the Water Aspects of the Processes represented by that Channel
Wood Point	Commands, or influence the Wood Aspects of the Processes represented by that Channel
Horary (Own Phase) Point	Is the name of the elemental point that correlates with the element of the meridian itself. It is used like the other elemental points.

Table 36

3. Xi-cleft Points

Xi means to divide, to open or to make a crack or a hole. This is where Qi and Blood, flowing superficial in the meridians, intermingle and dives deeper into the body.

These points are used in acute diseases and in acute pain and also in problems with the blood.

Xi-cleft points on the 12 main meridians;

LU06	BL63	LI07	KI05	ST34	PC04	SP08	TH07	HT06	GB36	SI06	LV06

Table 37

4. Yuan-source Points

Each and every one of the 12 main meridians have one or more of the "source"-points; points that stimulate the whole meridian without the connection to any of the elements. Here Qi emerges to the superficial skin and makes a superficial whirl of energy.

In humans it is one source-point in every meridian as follow;

LU09	BL64	KI03	ST42	PC07	SP03	TH04	HT07	GB40	SI04	LV03

Table 38

In the yin-meridians, the yuan-source point is the same as the shu-stream point. In the yang-meridians, the yuan-source point is a separate point situated between the shu-stream and the jing-river points.

240

5. Luo-Points

Every one of the 12 main meridians has a luo-connection, that is a connective channel, between the each Yin/Yang meridian pair. Additionally, there are 3 more luo-connecting points; CV 15, GV 1 and SP 21 (the great lo-point). These points are used to treat;

- When there is energetic imbalance between a Yin/Yang pair (LU/LI, SP/ST, KI/BL and so on).

- When there is a problem in the area where the lo-meridian passes.

- When there is a psycho-emotional problem.

There is a special method or protocol of treatment called "host and guest," which consists of treating the yuan-source point of the meridian that has the least energy, and the luo-point of the paired meridian that has the most energy.

1. Back-Shu Points

The 12 back-shu points of the 12 zangfu (organs) are situated on the BL-meridian along the spine, in humans 1.5 cun, in dogs 2 cun and in horses 3 cun from the midline. Shu means to transport.

The points are situated more or less in the same anatomical area where the organs that they represent are situated.

BL 13 – lung	BL 21 – stomach
BL 14 – pericardium	BL 22 – trippel heather
BL 15 – heart	BL 23 – kidney
BL 16 – GV	BL 24 – Sea of Qi
BL 17 – diaphragm	BL 25 – large intestine
BL 18 – liver	BL 26 – gate of the Source
BL 19 – gall bladder	BL 27 – small intestine
BL 20 – spleen	BL 28 – urinary bladder

Table 39

According to the old Chinese, the back-shu points are used especially when cold, deficiency and wind are etiologic factors in the development of the symptoms. In modern times, many practitioners use these points in all cases, in both cold and warm symptoms, in excess and in deficiency.

7. Mu-Points or the Alarm-Points

There are 12 Mu points placed on the chest and the abdomen, close to their respective zang or fu organ. Only 3 of them are situated on the meridian that relate to their respective zang or fu.

LU01 – lung, LU	CV03 – urinary bladder, BL
ST25 - large intestine, LI	GB25 – kidney, KI
CV12 – stomach, ST	CV17 – pericardium, PC
LV13 – spleen, SP	CV05 – trippel heather, TH
CV14 – heart, HT	GB24 – gall bladder, GB
CV04 – small intestine, SI	LV14 – liver, LV

Table 40, Mu or Alarm points

Mu means to gather together, and the Mu points are where the energy (Qi) from the zangfu gathers and concentrates on the abdominal side of the body. Except the 3 points that are situated on their respective meridians (LU 1, LV 14, GB 24), the Mu points stimulate the organs to which they are related and not the meridians.

The Mu points, just as the back-shu points, may be used diagnostically as they become tender in problems of their respective functions (Mu for the organs and Shu for the meridians/organs).

8. Master-Points

LI04 – Face and mouth
LU07 – Head and neck
PC06 – Chest and abdomen
BL40 – Back and hip
ST36 – Abdomen and the intestines
SP06 –Abdomen and the urinogenitals

Table 41

These points may be used to treat problems in the related areas.

9. Hui-Points (the meeting points)

BL 11 – bones	CV 17 – Qi
BL 12 – wind and lungs	LU 9 – veins and arteries
BL 17 – blood and diaphragm	CV 12 - Fu; Yang organs
GB 34 – tendons	LV 13 - Zang; Yin organs
GB 39 – marrow	ST 40 – mucus

Table 42

10. Window of the Sky-Points

This is a group of 10 points, where all but two are situated around the neck and throat. The word "sky" refers to the head, and the word "sky" is found in all the names of all these points.

The use of these points are in;

- *Hypo- or hyper-thyroxin, throat problems, swelling of the throat.*

- *Coughing, astma.*

- *Vomiting.*

- *Headace and dissiness.*

- *Heat in the head, redness of the face or eyes.*

- *Sudden onset of symptoms.*

- *Problems of the sensory organs.*

- *Mental and emotional problems.*

ST09	CV22	LI18	GV16	TH16	SI17	GB09(?)	SI16	LU03	BL10	PC01

Table 43

THE EFFECT OF THE ACUPOINTS

1. Every point has a *local effect.* This applies to all acupoints on or out of the Channels.

2. Many points also have a *distant effect* or *Channel effect* that travels proximally and distally along its Channel. Examples include points on the limbs to treat disorders on the head (GB44, or BL67, or ST44) to treat disorders of the eye; TH05, or LI04 to treat disorders of the ear, or points on the head to treat disorders on the other end of the Channel (GV20 to treat prolapsed rectum; Earpoints to treat disorders in the limb joints).

3. *Generalised effects: Master Points* have generalised effects as well as local and distant effects. Examples include *immunomodulation* and *general analgesic effects* from Master Points *LI04, LI11, ST36, SP06, LV03, GB34 or GV14. PC06*, (Master Point of the chest, heart, lungs and stomach) is very effective to treat *nausea and vomiting.*

4. Some points have *specific effects*, for example *BL02* (*"Valium Point."* see page 344) which acts to calm nervous or aggressive animals.

5. A special group of points have a related *Channel effect*, i.e. they have powerful effects on the *Channel-Organ System of the same name.* This group is mainly the

    (a) *Back Shu Points.*
    (b) *Front Mu Points.*
    (c) *Distal Ting Points*, which also belong to point 5, below.
    (d) *Source Points* and *Xi-cleft Points.*

6. *The 66 Command Points* (at or below the elbow and stifle in humans and in dogs, at or below the carpus and tarsus in horses) influence the organism in a very powerful way. They affect the Channels on which they are placed, the other Channels according to the Five Phases and its rules, as well as the related Processes. Thus, each

Channel has 5 points, a Fire Point, Earth Point, Metal Point, Water Point and a Wood Point.

THE PLACEMENT OF THE ACUPUNCTURE-POINTS IN ANIMALS RELATED TO HUMANS:

To be able to understand that the location of points in every species is different and unique we have to consider the reason why we have acupuncture points at all; why the points are present in the first place.

They exist with the only purpose to help the "owner" to regulate and stimulate the deficient process or sedate the processes in excess. To do so, they are situated just where they have the greatest chance to be selectively stimulated, either by environmental factors, by the owner himself or by his companions or partners.

As every species or individual have a different shape, lifestyle, social life, eating habits and use different food, plants and herbs for survival, these points or stimuli-receptors have to be developed and placed differently and also have different functions. Just think about the difference between humans and horses in relation to the access of the breast area, stomach area, legs and other body parts. The possible use of the belly in humans as a means for treatment is enormous in relation to the belly of a horse. The same goes for the chest. So the points that the horse may have on the abdomen must have been redefined or of less importance during the millions of years. As a result of this we find many less points and also many less important points on the abdomen of the horse. Also, as the legs have been retracted into the body, the important points have been developed further down on the horse's legs.

Many writers of textbooks or creators of point atlases do not take the mentioned factors into consideration but more or less translate the human point-locations and functions to animals. That is why Annica Nygren Thoresen DVM (my x-wife) and I have created an entirely new acupuncture-point atlas for the horse. We have detected and tried all the available points in

the horse and mapped them out. This atlas has more points on the legs and fewer on the abdomen as in humans, as explained above.

To use only the transpositional points may give fairly good results, as all the placental animals do have a common off-spring, and by such also do have a large number of common points, or at least do have a body-remembrance of the different point locations.

In order to get a better grasp of this and understand what I mean with the concept of "Body-remembrance," we must re-capitulate the doctrine of evolution and the evolution of the *equine embryo*. The horse has evolved from a five-toed animal to the one-toed animal familiar to us today. This evolution is also evident in the horse's foetal development. As a tiny foetus, the horse has five toes, which, during the span of 11 months of pregnancy, two disappear, two minimise to form the splints, and only the third toe evolves to become the real leg. This development happens gradually and smoothly of course. The transference of LU Channel, for example, from finger 1 to 2 (as we later will see that it is in dogs today) and then finger 3 (as we later will see that it is in horses today) happened gradually. Therefore, during the stage of five toes in pregnancy, the horse foetus has a LU Channel on digit 1, but as that digit disappears gradually, the Channel moves to digit 2, and finally, ends up at digit 3. Therefore, we still find LU11 on the canine dewclaw (the vestige of digit 1) and on digit 2 (the innermost large fore-toe of a dog). In horses, we then find LU11 today in three locations:

(a) Above the chestnut (representing the terminus of digit 1);

(b) Below the inner splint bone (representing the terminus of digit 2);

(c) In the posteromedial coronary band (digit 3, the equine LU Ting Point, as used today).

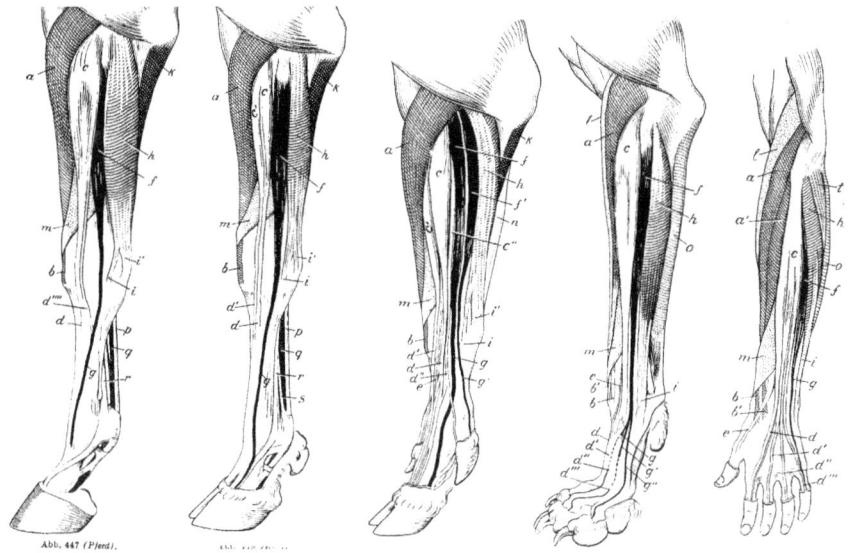

Fig 43; Development of the limbs

In horses and dogs (all animals really), the points that have moved to the most developed toes are the most effective points.

> *__In dogs__ the LU points on human digit 1 (the thumb) and SP and LV points on toe 1 (big toe) have moved 1 digit laterally. Also, the LI points on the radial side of human digit 2 have moved to the ulnar side of digit 2. The ST points on the lateral side of digit 2 also have moved to digit 3 (one laterally).*

> *__In horses__, all human finger points have moved over to the third finger or toe. Also, the most proximal Command Points, which in humans and dogs are placed near the elbow or stifle, are placed directly above the carpus and tarsus.*

It is also important to note that in human Chinese TCM, the effect of all Ting-points of the Yin Meridians is related to the Wood Element. All the Ting-points of the Yang Meridians are related to the Metal Element. This rule is sprung from the effects as seen by the Chinese practitioners when dealing with the excessive symptoms of the body. Deficiencies are usually found in the Yin meridians while excesses are usually found in the Yang meridians. Therefore, the Chinese have observed that in Yin meridian deficiencies the Ting-point has cured symptoms relating to the Wood element. In Yang meridian, the Chinese have observed that needling a Ting-point relieves pain and therefore they have related the point to the metal element (metal = pain). But as the Ting-points are one of the best fitted points to drain Qi, the Chinese have observed that the Ting-point has cured symptoms of pain and then related the point to the Metal element. But if the point is needled in a deficiency, it cures symptoms related to Wood-element, and in my opinion this is the true relation of the Ting-point.

Also, as we now know, all excesses are almost always due to an underlying deficiency. This indicates that when we observe a Metal excess it is really a Wood deficiency according to the Ko-cycle as described on page 61.

I have thus found that all Ting-points relate to the Wood element when we deal with or think in the concept of deficiency. ***So, in all animals* I have seen that all Ting-points are related to the Wood Element.** *(This I have also seen in humans, but as I don't want to bring up this discussion here, I will let it be for the time being).*

I want to retain for animals the same alphanumeric coding system that is used for human acupoints, but the differences in horses are so major that it is difficult to fit the changed locations, effects and relations in the same table as human points. So, I have made a separate table for the equine points below the carpus and the tarsus and put this new table after the main table. Here the elemental points and the source-points are described and named after their elemental relation, for example as "Equine LU-metal point."

Also, the source-points, which in humans are situated over important joints, are found in horses over the joint-cavities of the carpus, the tarsus and all the fetlock joints. A source-point is a special point that stimulates the whole meridian without belonging to a special element. To understand the quality of such a point, look at the energy circulation on page LVIII. Where the energy "streams" cross and is being changed into another element the elemental relation is, for a short moment, dissolved. This is why several of the source-points in humans are related to earth-element because in such a death of the elemental relation, the earth element is active (earth = death). So in horses I have found more than one source-point in all the meridians.

The work with the placement of the equine points started when I and my x-wife Annica prepared for the teaching in acupuncture of our students at SSHH, "*Scandinavian School of Holistic Horse therapy.*" I realised that the existing materials on point location and effects in the horse did not correlate with my clinical experience.

Qi is energy, which, according to the Chinese medicine, flows through the body following certain paths or channels, here called meridians. The Chinese also state that the flow of the Qi depends on the circulation of the Blood. To treat Qi stagnation, it is necessary to stimulate the blood circulation first. The description of the pathways of the meridians, both superficially and deep, shows an intimate relation to the blood vessels.

After reading several articles on "BCEC, Biologically Closed Electric Circuits," by Dr. Björn E. W. Nordenström, M.D., we are convinced that meridian-Qi is equivalent to electromagnetic energy. Dr. Björn E. W. Nordenström, M.D. has shown that such electric flow may create entirely new structures as fibrous membranes, organ capsules and different forms of channels. Electric current created by the ionic flow in the blood vessels, the lymph vessels and in the interstitial channels, the fascias, creates an electromagnetic field; Qi.

When the vessels branches, it usually happens in a ~90⁰ angle and it often form "loops." These may act as revitalizing transformers for both the ionic current and the electromagnetic field.

As the oriental medicine already has mapped out the exact location of the human points and meridians, it appeared obvious to first investigate along which structures these meridians travel, and what characterises the spot where the points are located.

This led us to a thorough study of the human anatomy. It very soon became obvious to us that the meridians follow the blood vessels and that the acupuncture points are located where the vessels branch, make anastomoses or form loops.

We transferred this *system* to the horse. We located the pathways of the equine vessels and meridians. The active structures where acupuncture points are expected to be found were correlated to the ancient equine points from China, the possible transpositional locations of the west and the empirical points found by western and eastern equine practitioners.

This work led us to the following conclusion: that the command points of the horse are placed differently than in humans; they are situated between the coronary band and the carpus/tarsus.

Our findings of the nature of the command points differ from what is usually taught. According to classic Chinese medicine as cited in *Classic of Difficulties* och *Compilation of Acupuncture and Moxibustion* by Liao Run-hong, the Qing-dynasty, the elemental relations of the command points are as follows;

- *Jing-Well* ("Ting-points," situated at the coronary band) "for fullness under the heart," Liver pathogen. Usually in Yin-meridians this point is related to wood, in Yang meridians to metal.

- *Ying-Spring* (just under the fetlock) "for heat in the body," Heart pathogen. Usually in Yin-meridians this point is related to fire, in Yang meridians to water.

- *Shu-Stream* (just proximal to the fetlock) "for heaviness of the body," Spleen pathogen. Usually in Yin-meridians this point is related to earth, in Yang meridians to wood.

- *Jing-River* (just distal to the carpus/hock) "for dyspnoea, cough, chills and fever," Lung pathogen. Usually in Yin-meridians this point is related to metal, in Yang meridians to wood.

- *He-Sea* (just proximal to the carpus/hock) "diaorrhoea, counterflow Qi," Kidney pathogen. Usually in Yin-meridians this point is related to water, in Yang merid-ians to fire.

This old system correlates perfectly with our opinion. We sus-pect that the change of the Ting-points in Yang-meridians to metal is due to the fact that most modern or contemporary treatments with acupuncture are based on the draining of excesses (pain) of the Yang meridians. Pain is related to the metal element; then the most draining point is related to the metal element. But, in dealing with deficiencies, the symptoms treated by the Ting-point relates to the wood element in all meridians.

GENERAL EFFECTS OF THE COMMAND POINTS.
It is important to understand clearly that the Command Points do not influence the *organs directly*; they influence mainly the fundamental Processes. It is far too easy for us to associate the bodily Processes exclusively to specific organs. In humans, we associate ST with the "storage and ripening" of food. We have particular acupoints that influence ST, for example the Back Shu Point BL21. It is directly behind the last rib. BL21 is said to influence ST, which is really only partially true. It really in-fluences the ST Processes of "storing and ripening" food. That this Process, amongst other things, relates to ST is something, which for humans, happens to be right in our present stage of evolution on this earth. However, the function "storing and ripening" of food in horses relates much more to LI than to ST. This is because LI in horses has taken over most of these func-tions from ST, i.e. LI is the horse's "main stomach." "Storing and Ripening" are Earth Processes and Earth Points, especially those of LI, ST and SP [the equine Earth Points, plus LI11, ST36 and SP Earth Point (SP03)] influence them.

The Command Points do not necessarily influence the or-gans. Their organ-effect is secondary because the Processes underpin the organs. In previous prehistoric eras, other or-gans and their related acupoints served those Fundamental

Processes. In some species today, certain organs have different effects and relationships than those classically assigned to the 12 main organs in human TCM. In birds, pelicans for example, the beak has taken over parts of the function of ST, and ST Points have an effect on the beak in this case.

NOTE:

About the description of the placement of points in general:

In the description of many of the points, we will use the symbol '. For example the position of a point may be described as: 5' below LU05 (elbow), 7' above LU09 (wrist) (LU06). The symbol ' is read "cun" or "*køn,*" and this is an important measure within acupuncture. It is in:

- Animals the distance between the cranial and the caudal border of the last rib.

- Humans the width of the interphalangeal joint of the thumb. The width of the sum of the fingers 2-5 is 3 cun.

The Channels of AP and their most important acupoints

LU (Lung Hand Taiyin) Channel uses the connective tissue around *V. cephalica humerii, V. cephalica antebrachii, A/V. radialis proximalis, A. radialis, V. (metacarpalis) palmaris medialis, V. digitalis medialis and V. coronalis phal. III.* as the main pathways for carrying its impulses:

Anatomically it begins:

In horses:
The deep path of the Lung-meridian:

- begins in the middle Jiao, in the area of the Stomach (ST),

- travels caudally to connect with the Large Intestine (LI),

- Turns in a cranial direction and passes the upper part of the Stomach, Cardia, traverses the diaphragm and penetrates the Lungs (LU),

- continues to the area of the throat,

- Turns again and travels towards the shoulder joint and surfaces at LU01.

The superficial path of the Lung meridian:

- begins at LU01; *V. cephalica* parts from *V. jugularis,* medial to the shoulderjoint,

- travels dorsomedially to the triangular space between Mm. Pectoralis descendens, brachiocephalicus and cutaneous colli, at LU02,

- Follows the lateral aspect of *V. cephalica humerii* to LU05 (situated in the elbow crease, lateral to the tendon of M. biceps brachialis), and passes dorsal to *V. cephalica antebrachii* and Os radius along the upper ¼ of the forearm (antebrachus).

- continues along the medial side of the radius and the carpus; *A/V. radialis prox., A/V radialis,*

- travels along the groove between the interosseus and the deep digital flexor tendon; *V. (metacarpalis) palmaris medialis,*

- Follows the medial border of the deep digital flexor tendon; *V. digitalis medialis,* and ends at the coronary band, dorsal to the medial cartilage of the distal phalanx, about 90^0 medial to the tip of the toe; *V. coronalis phal. III.*

In dogs LU01 is situated in the triangular area between Musculus brachiocephalicus, Musculus sternomandibularis and Musculus pectoralis descendens. From LU01, the Channel descends the posteromedial side of the forelimb and ends at the bottom of the inside of the paw, hoof or claw. In horses, LU11 is at the medial side of the coronary band. In dogs, it is at the medial side of the second toe. The rest of the channel pathway is the same as in the horse.

In humans LU01 (near the coracoid process in the lateral part of the first intercostal space). The channel travels down the anterior midline of the biceps to the centre of the elbow crease (LU05, at the radial side of the biceps tendon), passes to the carpal (wrist) crease (LU09, at the radial edge of the radial artery), on to the thenar eminence of the thumb, to end at LU11, at the radial side of the nail-root of the thumb. The rest of the channel pathway is the same as in the horse.

Phase	Metal		Earth		Fire		Water		Fire		Wood
Yin Channel	LU[1]		SP[4]	>>	HT[1]		KI[4]	>>	PC[1]		LV[4]
	‖		‖		‖		‖		‖		‖
Yang Channel	LI[2]	>>	ST[3]		SI[2]	>>	BL[3]		TH[2]	>>	GB[3]
Limb	Hand		Foot		Hand		Foot		Hand		Foot

(‖ and >>) mean that Qi Flow sequence is LU-LI-ST-SP, etc;
‖ = Yin-Yang Phase Mates (Partners);
[1] Qi flow from chest to hand; [2] Qi flow from hand to face; [3]
Qi flow from face to foot; [4] Qi flow from foot to chest

Table 44

All energy that the body needs, come from food, air, smell, sounds, light, taste or sight. This energy is integrated in the processes, and a part of it is used for the function of the meridian system. This energy enters the meridian energy-circulation via LU01. LU Qi also comes from the Qi that ends its Diurnal Qi Cycle in LV. LU Qi flows into (connects with) LI Channel, its Yang Mate in Metal/Air. As in the case of all the other Yin Channels in animals, LU Channel is much more important than its paired Yang Channel (LI).

LU-LI, the Yin-Yang Couple in Metal/Air, regulate all gaseous exchanges; they are also important in gaseous excretion, including belching and flatus. Human athletes who receive stimulation of LU Channel before a race have increased stamina and oxygen intake. Racehorses clearly respond in this way also, but some countries ban this practice under their Anti-doping Regulations. LU Points often give very effective but transient protection to "bleeders". Most bleeders bleed in the right lung and show reactivity in the reflex areas for LU on the right side. Right-sided shoulder pain or spasm often disappears after stimulation of LU, SP, Diaphragm and Blood Points on the right side (especially the reactive Ting Points +/- LU09). The Bleeder Symptom Complex includes epistaxis and/or lung haemorrhage, a history of recurring respiratory infection, coughing, rhinitis and forelimb lameness. Typically, bleeders run well in the first half of the race but "fade" towards the finish, or are "exhausted" after the race. Severe cases may show emphysema. Dusty bedding, dry dusty food and dusty paddocks in dry windy spells exaggerate LU Process Imbalance. One can seldom attain full cure in such cases. However, one can reduce the severity of the symptoms greatly (and often help a good horse to win) by treating LU in the days before each race. For bleeders and horses with chronic respiratory disorders, regular treatment of LU Process Imbalance and, where possible, elimination of dust are necessary to keep these disorders at bay.

Since the skin "breathes" (excretes gas and body odour), it may be considered as a part of the lung system; LU is important for dry eczema. This is especially important in dogs, which seem to have more frequent LU disorders than other animals.

Therefore, dogs suffer from dry eczema more often than other species. This may relate to the scarcity of sweat glands in dog skin and their need to pant heavily to control their body temperature in hot weather. In humans, mouth breathing and increased bronchial contact with pollen and dust, are known to aggravate respiratory disorders, especially asthma. Elbow joint arthrosis in dogs also responds to treatment via LU Channel. In accordance with the Chinese Qi Clock, around 0400h is the best time of day to treat LU Channel.

The energy in the lung meridian (Qi) may, as for the lung-process itself, be in:

- *Excess*

- *Deficiency*

Particular for the meridian the energy may also be in:

- *Destructive*

- *Blocked*

Excess show itself rather seldom as pain, as this is a Yin meridian, and Yin meridians seldom show excesses as pain (contrary to Yang-meridians which often show excesses as painful points or areas). An excess in the lung-meridian, although very seldom, may be the result of a deficiency in the heart- or pericardium-processes. An excess in the lung meridian usually passes without observation or unpleasant symptoms.

Deficiency is a much more common and serious pathological finding than excess. Such a deficiency show itself in the same way as described under the lung-process on page 66. In addition we may find skin-changes in the form of eczema along the lung-meridian.

A deficiency in the lung meridian is often the cause of an excess in the gall-bladder meridian, and pain along this meridian may be the result.

This pain is often the symptoms we are confronted with in our daily practise.

Destructivity show itself as in all animals as particular vis-cious symptoms of the skin, erosions and wounds (see more about destructive energy on page XXXIV).

Blockage of the lung-meridian is caused by a trauma on the structures of connective tissue that lead the impulses travelling through this meridian. Such a trauma will not hurt or destroy the energy of the process itself, but hinder the Qi-flow in the meridian. This is why the pulse in such a case shows absolutely good health for the process, but the acupuncture points may show dis-balance. Such a disbalance shows excess above the trauma, and deficiency below the trauma.

LU 01	Zhongfu (Central Treasury)
	Mu-Alarm Point of LU:
	In horses: In M. pectoralis descendens, just medial to the shoulder joint, 1 cun distal and lateral to LU02.
	In dogs: LU01 is situated in the triangular area between Musculus brachiocephalicus, Musculus sternomandibularis and Musculus pectoralis descendens.
	In humans: it is near the coracoid process in lateral part of intercostal space 1.
	Effect: It is here where Qi enters the LU Channel, and by this the entire Channel-system. Qi arrives here from the whole body (food, air, senses, sound and feelings). An injury here (or at the first rib, damaging the stellate ganglion) would decrease the Qi level within the whole Channel. As LU Channel is the start of the whole Qi Cycle, such an injury can reduce the total Qi level within the body. LU01 treatment helps animals that are lazy and powerless. A man presented his 6-year old Schnauzer who had been totally drained of energy after stepping on a sharp object the previous autumn. It preferred to lie around, ate only when it was hungry and seemed to have no desire to do anything. On closer examination, I discovered that the object had torn the skin at LU01. I then treated the wounded area and when he returned with the dog 4 weeks later, it was unrecognisable. It had become rejuvenated, regained its desire for attention and loved to go for walks. It had also regained its enormous appetite.

LU 02	**YUNMEN** (Cloud Door) *In horses:* it is situated in the triangular space between M. pectoralis descendens, M. brachiocephalicus and M. cutaneous colli. *Effect;* Similar to LU01, although not so strong effect.
LU 05	**Chize (Cubit - 12', Elbow - Marsh)** **Water Point of LU** (*in horses the main elemental functions are moved down to a point at the carpus called Waterpoint*)**:** *In horses:* in the elbow crease, lateral to the tendon of M. biceps brachii. Most easily found with the elbow bent 90⁰. *(For the Water-point of the horse, see the special commandpoints of the horse, page 262).* *In dogs:* it is at radial edge of biceps tendon in elbow crease, lateral to the tendon. *In humans:* it is at radial edge of biceps tendon in elbow crease, lateral to the tendon. *Effect:* It helps the respiratory system, trachea, bronchi, lung, cough, asthma and pneumonia. It is a Local Point for the elbow. It helps especially lung edema, swelling within the body in general and particularly along LU Channel, lung edema and fluid inflammation, bronchitis with excess mucus, rapidly growing sores and all disorders along LU Channel that relate to Water-type states. (In cases where mucus gravitates into the lungs one can use the Earth Point instead of this Water Point).
LU 06	**Kongzui (Collection Orifice)** **Xi Point of LU:** *In horses:* cranial to the V. cephalica and the radius, in a small depression just palmar of M. extensor carpi radialis, where M. pectoralis transversus attaches to the lower limb. *In dogs:* it is 5 cun below LU05 (elbow), 7 cun above LU09 (wrist) close to Vens cephalica. *In humans* it is 5 cun below LU05 (elbow), 7 cun above LU09 (wrist), close to Vens cephalica. *Effect:* It helps in acute pneumonia and lung hemorrhage. Some trotters with lung hemorrhage were cured after just one treatment at LU06. In most cases, improvement is short lived. Therefore, bleeders should be treated every 1-4 month to retain the effect.

	It also disperses and descends Lung Qi, ameliorates acute conditions; acute cough, bronchospasm and asthma of any aetiology.
LU 06-2	**Extra point in horses** *Location;* At the mediopalmar aspect of the radius, 4 cun proximal to the antebrachiocarpal joint, at the level of the proximal border of the chestnut.
LU 07	**Lieque (Broken Sequence)** **Luo Point of LU and Masterpoint for the head and neck: It connects LU Channel with its Phase Mate, the LI Channel. It also is an activation point (confluent point) for Ren Mai (CV).** *In horses:* 1.5 cun proximal to the medial distal Tuberositas radii, at the mediopalmar aspect of the radius. *In dogs:* it is above radial styloid process, 1.5 cun above distal carpal (wrist) crease. *In humans:* it is above radial styloid process, 1.5 cun above distal carpal (wrist) crease. *Effect:* It helps asthma, bronchi, carpus, cough, forehead, frontal sinuses, head, headache, lung, occiput, ovary, PID, pneumonia, respiratory system, sinusitis, temple, trachea and vertex. In my practise I also use this point when I am satisfied with the results obtained with the treatment; it stabilises the results. It releases the exterior and expels wind; influenza type of symptoms. Supports the descending function of the Lung, coughing up phlegm, vomiting of foamy, watery saliva. It benefits the head and neck; painful conditions, wind, and it is the Luo-connecting point with LI, which ascends to the head. It opens and regulates the CV, conception vessel; urogenital problems. It regulates the water passages; a wide range of urinary disorders and problems with the carpus.
LU 08	**Jingqu (Channel Ditch)** **Water-point in horses and Metal/Air Point in dogs (and in humans) where it also is a Qi Clock (Horary) Point of LU.** *In horses:* Palmar to, and at the level of the medial distal Tuberositas radii, in a small depression 1 cun proximal to LU09. *In dogs:* it is 1 cun above distal carpal (wrist) crease, on radial edge of radial artery. *In humans:* it is 1 cun above distal carpal (wrist) crease, on radial edge of radial artery.

	Effect: In horses it is a local point for the carpus, influences edema and circulatory conditions locally and along the course of the meridian, and generally in the body when the LU is in excess or deficiency. Pulmonary edema (as a water-point in horses). It helps in sweating disorders and all respiratory infections. In dogs, as LU is a Metal Channel, LU08 (the Metal/Air Point) is especially relevant to lung diseases, such as coughing, chronic bronchitis and increased mucus production in the bronchi. Descends lung Qi and ameliorates cough and bronchospasm.
LU 09	**Taiyuan (Supreme Abyss)** **Source-point and influencial point for the vessels.** **(Shu-Stream, Yuan-Source and Earth point in Humans)** *In horses:* At the mediopalmar aspect of the thoracic limb, at the level of the antebrachiocarpal joint, just distal and palmar to the medial distal Tuberositas radii. (*For the horse´ earth-point and the other source-point(s), see the special command-points of the horse page 262*). *In dogs:* it is at the distal wrist crease, at radial edge of radial artery. *In humans:* it is at the distal wrist crease, at radial edge of radial artery. *Effect:* As a Source Point, it commands Yuan Qi in LU, and as Earth is the Mother of Metal, LU09 is the source of Metal Qi in LU also. It can treat LU Qi Deficiency. It helps asthma, coughing and pain in the chest area, weak resistance and weak stamina. Stimulation of LU09 shortens the recovery time of painful ulcers and inflammation along LU Channel. Just at this point I have had very good results with gold-implants in elbow-arthrosis in dogs.
LU 10	**Yuji (Fish Border)** **Metal point in horses and fire point in dogs** *(and in humans).* *In horses:* Just distal to the carpus, palmar to the head of Os metacarpale II. *In dogs:* it is situated at the caudo-medial area of the metacarpal pad (together with a similar point at the cranio-medial aspect of the metacarpal pad). *In humans*, it is at the centre of palmar edge of metacarpal 1.

	Effect: In horses, as LU10 is just under the fetlock joint and related to metal, it is very useful in all painful conditions of this joint. In dogs it will alleviate all circulatory disorders, which arise as locally cold or warm regions along LU Channel. LU10 also influences reduced blood circulation between the right side of the atlas and occiput. Trotting horses that trot with a pull on the right rein often respond when treated at this point. It also helps the throat, pharynx, tonsil, larynx, voice, cough, fever and sweating disorders.
LU 11	**Shaoshang (Lesser Shang)** **Jing-well (Ting) and Wood Point of LU and Emergency Point:** ***In horses:*** At the coronary band, dorsal to the medial cartilage of the distal phalanx, ~ 90^0 medial to the tip of the toe. ***In dogs***, it is at the medial side (abaxial) of the claw of toe 2. We must here remember that this point in humans is at the level of the nail-root, but in dogs all Ting-points are a little further back, a few mm behind the visible nail-root (see picture page 394). ***In humans:*** it is 0.1 cun from posterior edge of nail-root of finger 1 (thumb), radial side. ***Effect:*** It helps all tendons and muscles, particularly those near LU Channel. It helps eczema along LU Channel, exhausted ("worn out") lungs and respiratory haemorrhage, chronic respiratory infection and coughing. It also helps the pharynx, throat, tonsil, larynx and voice. It also helps in emergencies, first aid and sweating disorders. This point also helps sholder pain due to a LU Meridian Deficiency, tensions along the right side of the neck and pain between the right Atlas and the right Occiput. Also in both light and severe asthma this point proves to be very effective. In humans I have used it in cases of chlaustrophobia, and good effect has been obtained.

Table 45

The special commandpoints in the horse are as follows:

S O U R C E carpus	*Location;* At the medial aspect of the carpus, at the level of the intercarpal joint, directly distal to LU09. *Effect;* Stimulates the meridian.
E A R T H LU-E	*Location;* Just proximal to the medial fetlock, in a small depression between the deep digital flexor tendon and Os metacarpale II. *Effect;* Helps in asthma, cough and pain connected to the lung area. Local point for the fetlock-joint, and especially effective in symptoms of degeneration of the fetlock joint, the joints along the meridian, other tissues along the meridian and also in the entire body as long as the energy in the LU-meridian is in excess or deficiency. It can treat LU Qi Deficiency. It helps asthma, coughing and pain in the chest area, weak resistance and weak stamina. Stimulation of LU09 shortens the recovery time of painful ulcers and inflammation along LU Channel. In horses it is also a local point for the fetlock, and is especially effective in degenerative processes in the fetlock joint.
S O U R C E fetlock	*Location;* At the mediopalmar aspect of the fetlock, at the level of the metacarpophalangeal joint. **Effect:** Stimulates the meridian.
F I R E LU-F	*Location;* At the medial aspect of the fetlock, in a small depression between the deep flexor tendon and the first phalanx. *Effect;* All lung disorders characterised by fever and heat. Circulatory problems along the LU-meridian, and in the area between the right wing of Atlas and Os occipitalis. Disorders of the throat; pharyngitis, tonsillitis, laryngitis, the voice and cough. Fever and profuse sweating.

Table 46

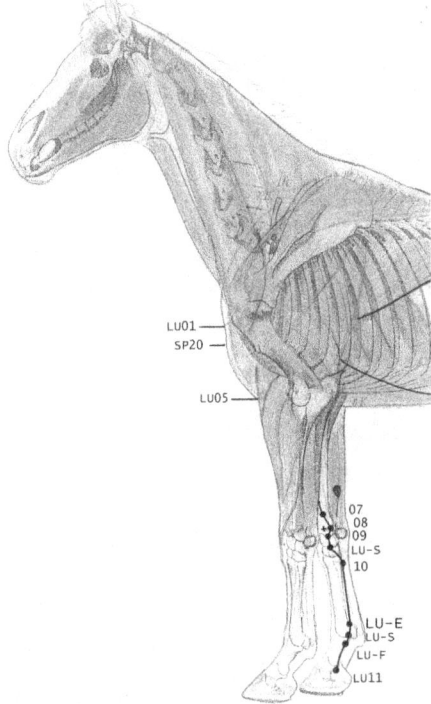

Figure 44: the most important points on the LU-Channel in horses.

LI (Large Intestine Hand Yangming) Channel uses the connective tissue around *A/V. coronalis phal. III, A/V. phal. II et I, ramus dors., A. mtcs dors. med., Rete carpi dors., A. collat. radialis (dist), A. carotis communis, V. jugularis., A. maxillaries, A. facialis, A. labialis maxillaris, A. incisive and A. dorsalis nasi.* as the main pathways for carrying its impulses:

Anatomically:

In horses the superficial path of the LI-meridian:

- Begins at the coronary band, ~ 55⁰ medial of the tip of the toe; *A/V. coronalis phal. III,*

- Ascends along the dorsomedial aspect of the phalanges; *A/V. phal. II et I, ramus dors.,*

- Continues at the dorsal aspect of the second (medial) metacarpal bone; *A. mtcs. dors. med.,*

- passes the carpus at the dorsal aspect, medial to the tendon of M. extensor carpi radialis; *Rete carpi dorsalis,*

- crosses over to the lateral aspect proximal to the carpus, and ascends between M. ext. carpi radialis and M. ext. digitorum communis; *A. collateralis radialis (dist),* to the cranial aspect the elbow joint,

- continues along the ventral border of the lateral head of M. triceps brachii,

- travels along M. brachiocephalicus to the point of the shoulder, LI15,

- Crosses over to the neck and ascends between the ventral and the dorsal part of M. brachiocephalicus (M. brachiocephalicus and M. omotransversarius); *A. carotis communis* and *V. jugularis.*

- At the level of the ventral border of the mandible (Os mandibularis) the meridian turns towards the head, passes along the medial side of the mandible and emerges just in front of M. masseter following *A. maxillaris* and then *A. facialis,*

- travels dorsally along the cranial border of M. masseter to Crista facialis, makes a 90^0-turn and continues rostrally, following *A. labialis maxillaris,* curves under the nostrils at GV26; *A. incisiva,* and ends in LI20, 3.5 cun caudal to the upper border of the nostrils; *anastomosis between A. incisive and A. dorsalis nasi.*

The deep path of the LI - meridian;

1. At LI16 a deep branch travels via SI12 to GV14, where it meets with the other five yang meridians.

2. From GV14 it travels, via ST12, into the thorax and penetrates the Lungs before it travels further down through the diaphragm to connect with the Large Intestine, LI.

3. From the large intestine it descends to ST37; the lower He-sea point of the Large Intestine meridian.

In dogs *it begins in LI01 at the lateral side (axial) of the nail-root of foretoe 2. It then ascends from LI01, along the medial side of the meta-carpal area, passing LI04 to turn laterally across to the laterocaudal side of the carpus. From here, it ascends to the lateral edge of the elbow crease (LI11), to the anterolateral point of the shoulder (LI15), to the lateral neck, near the larynx (LI18). From here it ascends the face, to cross the philtrum at GV26 and end on the contralateral side at LI20, beside the nasal wing.*

In humans LI01 is situated at the abaxial nail-root (the lateral side) of the thumb. It then follows the same way as described under the dog/horse.

Phase	Metal		Earth		Fire		Water		Fire		Wood
Yin Channel	LU[1]		SP[4]	>>	HT[1]		KI[4]	>>	PC[1]		LV[4]
	‖		‖		‖		‖		‖		‖
Yang Channel	LI[2]	>>	ST[3]		SI[2]	>>	BL[3]		TH[2]	>>	GB[3]
Limb	Hand		Foot		Hand		Foot		Hand		Foot

(‖ and >>) mean that Qi Flow sequence is LU-LI-ST-SP, etc;
‖ = Yin-Yang Phase Mates (Partners);
[1] Qi flow from chest to hand; [2] Qi flow from hand to face; [3]
Qi flow from face to foot; [4] Qi flow from foot to chest

Table 47

LI Qi comes from LU Channel, its Yin Mate in Metal/Air, and flows into (connects with) ST Channel. It also comes from parts of the food, strong tastes of the food and sunlight shining directly into the rectum, especially in the morning (my uncle, a farmer, used to do that). LU-LI, the Yin-Yang Couple in Metal/Air, regulate all gaseous exchanges; they are also important in gaseous excretion, including belching and flatus. In contrast to LU, LI Channel does not have as many applications in animals as in humans. For humans it is a very relevant Meridian.

It has three main areas of function:

- Shoulder muscles

- Nose / nasal passage / sinuses

- LI activity / defecation / treatment of colic

LI Channel is more important in humans who subject themselves to a sedentary, overeating, rigid or regimented, cold, stressed and sad life. With animals, however this is not the case. Many LI Points can stimulate a dog's sense of smell. LI Channel is the main depository of Qi; its functioning is crusial to an ample supply of Qi to the body. In accordance with the Chinese Qi Clock, around 0600h is the best time of day to treat LI Channel.

LI Source Point (LI04) regulates the entire Yuanqi (Source Qi) of the body. In constipation there is often a loss of tone in the large intestine (LI Deficiency); this allows susceptibility to parasitism. Tonification of the Earth Point (LI11) is indicated in these cases. Tonifying both LI04 and the Wood Point (LI03) can treat constipation due to an absence of colonic mucus secretion (also an outcome of LI Deficiency). Sedation of the Water Point (LI02), or LI03 is effective in spastic constipation (LI Excess or Full).

Daily stimulation of LI04, a technique forbidden to use when treating other points with therapeutic indication, helps even a balanced organism.

Note the following:

- *Because of its path and its connections to LU and ST Channels, LI is the **Main Channel** used to treat diseases of the nose, throat and sinuses (paranasal and frontal).*

- ***LI** (superficial Pulse-Position 1, right radial artery) is the **Wife of SI** (superficial Pulse-Position 1, left radial artery). One should not stimulate LI unless SI has ample Qi.*

- ***HT and PC control LI** (via the Ko Cycle). In cases of colon cancer (see page 466 & 473), one should treat HT and PC Channels.*

- **KI** *governs the* **last part of LI** (distal colon, rectum and anus). *One should consider stimulating SP (Earth controls Water in the Ko Cycle), or a combination of the Dumai + Renmai in cases of cancer of the distal colon (see page 466 & 473).*

The energy in the large intestine meridian (Qi) may, as for the large intestine-process itself, be in:

- *Excess*

- *Deficiency*

Particular for the meridian the energy may also be :

- *Destructive*

- *Blocked*

Excess show itself usually as pain, as this is a Yang meridian, and Yang meridians usually show excesses as pain (contrary to Ying-meridians which often show excesses just as an elevated and positive function of the process). An excess in the Large Intestine-meridian may be the result of a deficiency in the Heart- or Pericardium-processes.

Deficiency in a Yang meridian is much more seldom as it is in a Yin meridian. Often symptoms arising from Yang-meridians are due to excesses, but of course deficiencies are also found. A deficiency may express itself as underfunction of the associated organ, as underfunction in the associated muscles and in the skin-area transversed by the meridian, as described at page 68. In the large intestine meridian this may result in stagnation of the large intestine and obstipation, dysfunction of the Mm. brachiocephalicus and omotransversarius or skin changes along the path of the meridian.

A deficiency in the Large Intestine meridian is often the cause of an excess in the Gall-Bladder meridian, and pain along this meridian may be the result. This pain is often the symptoms we see most easily.

Destructivity show itself as in all animals as particular vicious symptoms of the skin, erosions and wounds (see more about destructive energy on page XXXIV).

Blockage of the large intestine-meridian may be caused by a trauma on the structures of connective tissue that lead the impulses travelling through this meridian. Such a trauma will not hurt or destroy the energy of the process itself, but hinder the Qi-flow in the meridian. This is why the pulse in such a case shows absolutely good health for the process, but the acupuncture points may show dis-balance. This disbalance shows excess above the trauma, and deficienct below the trauma.

LI01	Shangyang (Shang Yang)
	Ting and Wood Point of LI in horses and dogs **(Jing-Well and described as a Metal point in Humans)** *In horses*, At the coronary band, ~ 55° medial of the tip of the toe. *In dogs* LI01 is on the lateral side (axially) of toe 2, which is situated on the medial side of the front paw (*not* the dewclaw, which is now a vestigial digit). *In humans*, it is on 0.1 cun from posterior edge of nail-root of finger 2, radial (abaxial) side. *Effect:* As a Ting Point, it functions both locally, along LI Channel and as one of the commandpoints it influences the whole body. This means that it stimulates the Wood Element of the LI Meridian. This means all symptoms that are related to the wood-element (like muscular and growth-related problems) *along or in connection with the LI-meridian*. In horses LI01 helps spastic neck muscles greatly. In the horse it also helps the muscles of the sholder and lower neck. LI01 also has a profound effect on the mucus membranes. This is an example of the Mirror Effects of AP, i.e. a point at one position on (say the end of) a Channel influences the parts and functions at the mirror-position (say the other end) of the same Channel. Therefore, LI01 helps to increase resistance to diseases of the nose, throat, main lymph glands and dizziness. It also helps fever and lymphadenopathy. It also helps sight. It also helps horses with "toed in" feet. LI01 as well as LU11 forces the action outward. It also helps the metacarpus, hand, palm, finger, lips, oral muscles, gums and teeth.

LI02	**Erjian (Second Space)**
	Fire Point of LI in horses and dogs *(Si Guan; extra point according to Van den Bosch/Guray)* **(Ying-Spring and Water point in Humans)**
	In horses, Just distal to the fetlock, in a small depression dorsal to the medial tendon of interosseus to the digital extensor tendon.
	In dogs, it is situated at the lateral aspect of the second toe (the same toe as described under LI01), just distal to the junction of Phalanx proximalis digiti II and Metecarpale II.
	In humans, it is on the hand-dorsum, proximal end of the 2nd finger on the radial side.
	Effect: Since all Fire Phase Points near joints help warm conditions (twists, sprains and so on), LI02 helps to a large degree trauma of the nearests joints.
	It also helps rhinitis, pharyngitis and diarrhea.
LI03	**LI03 Sanjian (Third Space)**
	Earth Point of LI in the horse and the dog **(Shu-Stream and Wood point in Humans)**
	In horses: Just proximal to the fetlock, in a small depression at the dorsomedial aspect of Os metacarpus III (cannon bone), at an angle of ~55° medially to the cranial-caudal axis of the leg.
	In dogs it is on the paw-dorsum, distal end of 2nd metacarpal, radial side, between metacarpale II and III.
	In humans, it is on the hand-dorsum, distal end of 2nd metacarpal, radial side, between metacarpale I and II.
	Effect: In both dogs and horses this point can be treated after operations or injection of the forelimb, or various wounds or trauma in the same area, or also all along the LI Meridian. It helps the repair and contraction of the wounds. This point also helps the eyes, and in movement of the horse`s front leg it helps horses with "toed in" feet. LI03, like LI01, forces the action outward. It also helps the metacarpus, hand, palm, finger, lips, oral muscles, gums and teeth.

LI04	LI04 Hegu (Union Valley)
	Master Point for the Upper Body, Immunostimulant Point, Analgesic Point and Emergency Point in all species. **Source Point of LI in dogs** *(and humans)*. *In horses,* At the proximal medial aspect of Os metacarpale III (cannon bone), just dorsal to the head of Os metacarpale II, 1.5 cun distal to the carpometacarpal joint. *In dogs:* Some people locate canine LI04 in exactly the same place as in humans. They put it in the notch between the dewclaw (metacarpal 1) and metacarpal 2 (which today represents the innermost toe) on the medial side of the forepaw. This is a mistake, because the dewclaw usually is atrophied (which means that the energy has more or less withdrawn). Also, if LI04 were positioned here, LU11 and LU10 would have to be on the same atrophied dewclaw. An atrophied or absent claw shows that Qi is about to retreat from the claw. Therefore LU Channel has migrated to the medial side of toe 2, while LI Channel has migrated to the lateral side of toe 2. (See the account given for the development and transposition of points from humans to dogs and horses page 191). Thus, in contrast to its human location (between metacarpals 1-2), the *correct location of LI04 in dogs is between the upper heads of metacarpals 2-3.* *In humans,* it is on the hand-dorsum, between metacarpals 1-2, midway down 2nd metacarpal. LI04 is of extraordinary importance in dogs. *Effect:* It is a very important Command Point but is not a Phase Point. It is the most important Source Point; it strengthens the Yuan (Source, Ancestral) Qi Processes of LI but also regulates the Yuanqi throughout the body. It is sometimes called the Kaada Point, after Dr. Birger Kaada. His research showed that LI04 increased microcirculation in lemmings, increased human athletic performance, increased physical resistance and had a general analgesic effect. As it decreases pain, it must be viewed as a "**Doping Point**". (See also section on AP and endurance page 487). Through its endorphin-releasing effect, LI04 has an analgesic effect on the eyes, nose, mouth, throat and face. It helps jaw disorders and toothache (excellent in teething disorders in infants). Also, it helps disorders along LI Channel, headache, pain in the eye, teeth, arm, spasm, colic and intestinal disorders, constipation and can activate the uterus in

	parturition. It is very important in nasal disorders; it is important for dogs, as many dogs have anosmia, eczema, sores or altered pigmentation on the snout. I have seen many dogs with sores and depigmentation on the snout being healed with regular treatment of LI04, amongst other points. As a **Master Point for the Upper Body**, it has wide effects. It helps emergencies, first aid, head, brain, meninges and their functions and parts, addictions, mind, psyche, convulsions and epilepsy. Especially the different parts of the mouth. It also helps some **abdominal and general functions**: inappetance, indigestion, nausea, vomiting. It is a forbidden point in pregnancy (may cause abortion), but may be used in other obstetrical disorders. In humans and in dogs this is also a very good point for gold-implants. In all my life I have suffered from a severe morning diarrhea, but after I implanted a gold piece on myself in 1999, I have been totally cured from this condition.
LI05	**Yangxi (Yang Ravine)** **Source-point in horses** **Water Point in dogs** **(Jing-river and Fire-point in humans)** *In horses* At the dorsal aspect of the carpus, at the level of the antebrachiocarpal joint, at the medial side of the tendon of M. extensor carpi radialis. *In dogs* it is in the 'snuff box' at wrist, between tendons of extensor pollucis brevis and longus muscles. *In humans*, it is in the 'snuff box' at wrist, between tendons of extensor pollucis brevis and longus muscles. *Effect:* In horses it stimulates the entire meridian, and is a local point for carpus. In dogs it helps common disorders accompanied by water-signs – especially "floating" symptoms.
LI06	**Pianli (Veering Passageway)** **Luo Point of LI** (*It connects LI Channel with its Phase Mate, LU Channel*) *In horses* 3 cun proximal to the lateral distal Tuberositas radii, between M. extensor carpi radialis and M. extensor digitorum communis.

	In dogs it is at the same place as in humans. *In humans*, it is 3 cun above LI05 ("snuff box"), 9 cun below LI11 (lateral end of elbow crease). *Effect:* It helps when there is excess of energy in the LI Meridian, and a deficiency of energy in the LU Meridian. Possible symptoms of such a condition might be diarrhea getting better with work (worst in the morning, morning diarrhea) comined with a lack of energy in the breath.
LI07	**Wenliu (Warm Dwelling)** **Xi Point of LI** *In horses* 1.5 cun proximal to LI06, between M. extensor carpi radialis and M. extensor digitorum communis. *In dogs* it is 10 cun above LI05 ("snuff box"), 2 cun below LI11 (lateral end of elbow crease). *In humans* and it is 10 cun above LI05 ("snuff box"), 2 cun below LI11 (lateral end of elbow crease). *Effect:* It helps the mouth, and also acute conditions along the entire meridian. Xi-points are always for acute conditions along the meridian. In humans it helps acne.
LI10 **(-1 in** **horses)**	**Shousanli (Forearm Three Li)** **Immunostimulant Point** *In horses* 2 cun distal to LI11, in M. extensor carpi radialis (see this point below). *In dogs* it is aproximately one sixth the distance from the elbow joint to the carpal joint, between Musculus extensor carpi radiale and Musculus brachioradiale. *In humans*, it is 10 cun above LI05 ('snuff box'), 2 cun below LI11 (lateral end of elbow crease). *Effect:* It is one of the main immunostimulant points in humans, dogs and horses (all species?). It is most important and very often used, especially in cases with a reduced immune system, allergy, chronic infections, drowsiness and general weakness. I have used LI10 especially on chronic cough, chronic rhinitis and pharyngitis, as well as in chronic diarrhea, food allergy, allergic asthma, hypersensitivity to hay dust (remember to soak dusty food), and in chronically swollen

	lymph glands in the forelimb and throat. It also helps the thoracic limb, arm, humerus, elbow, forearm, radius, ulna, salivation, salivary glands and esophagus. This point should be combined with GV (Du-mo) 14 (page 432).
LI 10-2 (for horses)	*In horses:* 1 cun distal to LI11, in M. ext. carpi radialis. *Effect:* ~ LI10-1
LI11	**Quchi (Bend Pool)** **In horses it is an immunstimulating point** **In dogs it is a Water point and Tonification Point** **(in humans it is an earth-point)** *In horses* At the lateral end of the transverse cubital (elbow) crease, in M. extensor carpi radialis, at the level of the lateral humeral epikondyl. Easier to find with the elbow flexed 90°. *In dogs* it is at the lateral end elbow crease, midway from biceps brachii tendon to lateral epicondyle of humerus when the elbow is flexed to 90°. *In humans* is at the lateral end elbow crease, midway from biceps brachii tendon to lateral epicondyle of humerus when the elbow is flexed to 90°. *Effect:* It is a key **Immunostimulant Point,** and is as important as LI04. It helps all changes within LI-process related to the Water Phase. It also stimulates the muscles in the shoulder area, stimulates the immune system related to the air passages and counteracts the build up of mucus in the throat. Also it counteracts pain, calcification in the elbow joint, stomach pain, diarrhea, eczema and vomiting. It also helps emergencies, brain, meninges and their functions and parts, mouth, teeth and nose. It also helps in the lower abdomen.
LI15	**Jianyu (Shoulder Bone)** **Meeting point (confluent point) of the LI and Yang Qiau mai** *In horses* In a small depression just cranial to the palpable part of Tuberculum majus (humerus), at the level of the shoulder joint. *In dogs,* as they have no clavicle (clavicula), the point is situated between the greater tubercle of humerus and acromion. *In humans,* it is in the anterior hole at anterior edge acromioclavicular joint.

	Effect: It is a very important point for the shoulder area and helps shoulder arthralgia. It also helps arthritis in joints along the superficial path of LI Channel, paralysed nerves, brain, meninges and their functions and parts, convulsions, CVA, paralysis, hemiplegia, polio, tetanus, amnesia; neck stiffness and thyroid disorders; thoracic limb, shoulder, scapula, clavicle, axilla, arm and humerus.
LI16	**Jugu (Great Bone)** **Meeting point (confluent point) of the LI and Yang Qiau mai** *In horses:* In the groove between the ventral M. brachiocephalicus and M. omotransversarius, where the muscle traverses from the shoulder area to the neck area, 5 cun cranio-dorsal to LI15. *In dogs* and horses it is situated just above LI15, about 2 cun (which in horses is about 6 cm), on the cranial border of scapula. *In humans*, it is in a hollow between scapular spine and acromial end of clavicle. *Effect:* It helps shoulder arthralgia.
LI18 **(18-1** **for** **horses)**	**Futu (Protuberance Assistant)** **Window of the sky-point** *In humans*, it is 3 cun lateral to center of the laryngeal prominence, between the heads of sternocleidomastoid muscle. *In dogs:* Most colleges place the point more towards the head, in horses all the way up to the ventral border of the mandible. *In horses:* At the level of the ventral border of the mandibula, in the groove between the ventral part of M. brachiocephalicus and M. omotransversarius. *Effect:* It helps a loose soft palate; treat also CV23 in this case. It also helps the throat, larynx, pharynx, tonsil, voice, thyroid and parathyroid. LI18 (-1) belongs to a group of points known as the **"Windows of the Sky"** or **"Celestial Windows"**. This group includes **LI18-1, LI18-2, ST09-1, ST09-2, SI16-1, SI16-2, TH16-1 and TH16-2**, all of which lie close together on Yang Channels on the lateral side of the neck. Any muscular or vertebral blockage in this area of the neck can act as a "bottleneck" to obstruct the free movement or transportation of Qi to and from the head. Wounds, bite-marks or scars in the area can

	have the same adverse effect. Complications can arise easily due to Channel trauma or blockage in this area. Experts in the martial arts know that a heavy blow, or application of pressure to this area may cause unconsciousness or temporary paralysis. **"Windows of the Sky" Points** are used to release Qi Obstruction in the neck and head, especially for disorders of the "Windows of the Head" (eyes, ears, mouth and throat). Reactivity and/or treatment at one or more of these points is/are important in "wobbler" in horses and for imbalances (dizziness) in dogs. In dogs this area is often injured by senseless use of leashes. One can imagine that all the jerking in this area could lead to a hindrance for the dog. These points, especially ST09, are used to treat disorders, such as headaches, that aggravate after work. Aggravation of a disorder after work indicates a state of pre-existing Deficient Qi. **NOTE: Symptoms that improve through work (activity in all Processes) indicate Excess. Symptoms that aggravate indicate Deficiency.**
LI 18-2 (for horses)	**Window of the sky-point** *In horses :* In the groove between the ventral part of M. brachiocephalicus and M. omotransversarius, at the level of the intervertebral space of the 4th and 5th cervical vertebra. Erwin Westermayer places it in front of the 6th cervical vertebrae. I think it is more in front of the joint between the 5th and the 6th vertebrae, more in the middle of the neck (throught), between the head (caudal part of the mandible) and the shoulder (margo cranialis). *Effect :* opens the pathways between the head and the body, between the heaven and the earth.
LI19	**Kouheliao (Grain Bone-Orifice)** *In horses:* Lateral to GV26, below the lateral border of the nostrils. *In dogs:* Lateral to GV26, below the lateral border of the nostrils. *In humans*, it is 0.5 cun lateral to GV26. *Effect:* It helps the nose, olfaction and nasal sinuses.

LI20	Yingxiang (Welcome Fragrance)
	Meeting-point for the LI- and ST-meridians
	In horses: 3.5 cun caudal to the upper border of the nostril, in a small depression close to Vena dorsalis nasii. *In dogs:* it is latero-caudal to the nasal wing. *In humans:* it is lateral to the nasal wing, in the nasolabial groove.
	Effect: Opens the nasal passages. Expels wind and clears heat from the face; headache, sinusitis, nasal discharge. In China humans with biliary ascariasis, are treated with a needle from LI20 through to ST02 with strong manipulation. In horses there is an ECIWO-system in the face. Maybe this is also the case in humans, so that the needle passes the liver area between LI20 and ST02?

Table 48

The special commandpoints in the horse are as follows:

S O U R C E fetlock	*Location;* At the dorsolateral aspect of the fetlock, at the level of the metacarpophalangeal joint. *Effect;* Stimulates the meridian.
D A B A I	*Location:* In a small depression on Os metacarpus III, midway between LI03 and LI04.
M E T A L LI-M	*Location;* 1 cun proximal to LI04, between the head of Os metacarpale II and the tuberositas on Os metacarpale III. *Effect;* Influences painful conditions locally, along the course of the meridian and generally in the body when LI is in deficiency or excess.

W **A** **T** **E** **R** **LI-W**	*Location;* Proximal to LI05, at the level of the medial distal Tuberositas radii, proximal to the tendon of M. extensor carpi obliquus, and medial to the tendon of M. extensor carpi radialis. *Effect;* Influences all types of symptoms related to the Water element like exsudative, dripping, bleeding and swelling, locally and along the course of the meridian and generally in the body when LI is in excess or deficiency. Helps rhinitis (nasal discharge), pharyngitis with mucus production and watery diarrhea.

Table 49

To differentiate nasal and pulmonary epistaxis, it is important to confirm the source of the blood:

Blood source	*Key differential features* *Note: Fiberoptic endoscopy helps definitive diagnosis of the source of the blood.*
Lung	*Usually occurs as hemorrhage from* **both nostrils;** *the blood is* **bright red** *and* **foaming.** *As taught by Marvin Cain, bleeders (horses with LU-haemorrhage) usually show sensitivity to pressure palpation of* **LU-related Back Shu Points** *in the "Lung Triangle" behind the scapula, especially on BL13-BL17 and the outer BL Line as far as the diaphragm (BL42 to 46).*
Nose	*Usually is* **unilateral;** *the blood is* **dark red** *and* **does not foam.**

Table 50

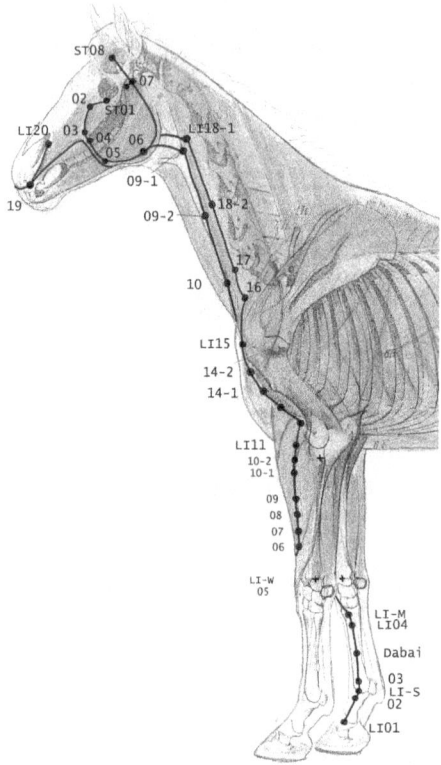

Figure 45; The most important points on the LI Channel in horses.

ST (Stomach Foot Yangming) Channel uses the connective tissue around *A. dors. nasi, A. angularis oculi, A. malaris., V. angularis oculi, V. facialis, V. labialis maxillaris, V. labialis mandibularis, V. masseterica, V. temporalis superficialis, V. jugularis (A. carotis communis), A/V. iliolumbalis, (A/)V. tibialis cran., (A/)V. dorsalis pedis, Rete tarsi dors., (A/)V. mtts. dorsalis media, (A/) V. dorsalis phal. I et II and (A/) V. coronalis phal. III.* as the main pathways for carrying its impulses:

Anatomically it begins:

In horses the superficial path of the ST meridian:

- Begins in the depth at LI20, caudal to the nostrils, and ascends towards the medial canthus of the eye, where it meets with BL01; *A. dorsalis nasi* and *A. angularis oculi*.

- Travels laterally along the infraorbital ridge to ST01, directly under the pupil, between the eyeball and the cheekbone; *A. malaris.*

- From the eye the meridian curves rostrally, with a dorsal convexity; *V. angularis oculi,* to the rostral end of Crista facialis, from where it continues ventrally, along the rostral border of M. masseter; *V. facialis.*

- At the level of Crista facialis it gives off two branches:

    ° One along the upper lip to meet with GV26; *V. labialis maxillaries.*

    ° One along the lower lip to meet with CV24; *V. labialis mandibularis.*

- At ST05 the meridian turns caudally in M. masseter, along the ventral border of the mandibula, *V. masseterica,* and further along the caudal border in direction of the TM-joint to ST07, where it turns directly dorsally to ST08 in M. temporalis; *V. temporalis superficialis,* and continues to reach GV24.

- The main meridian turns towards the throat, from the caudal border of the mandible, and travels along the ventral part of M. brachiocephalicus to the chest area; *V. jugularis (/A. carotis communis),* at ST12,

- Continues 2 cun lateral to the ventral midline, along the chest and the abdomen, to the cranial border of the pelvis at ST30.

- From the inguinal region the meridian travels laterally to ST31, cranial to the hip joint, between M. tensor fasciae latae and M. gluteus superficialis; *A. et V. iliolumbalis,*

- Continues at first cranioventrally on the lateral aspect of the thigh, and then distally to the lateral part of the patella and the stifle joint,

- Follows the dorsal midline of the pelvic limb; *(A/)V. tibialis cran.,* passes the hock at the dorsal aspect; *(A/)V.*

dorsalis pedis; Rete tarsi dors., continues along the dorsal aspect of the metatarsus III (cannon bone); *(A/) V. mtts. dors. media,*

- Along the dorsal midline of the phalanges; *(A/) V. dors. phal. I et II,*

- To end at the coronary band, ST45, at the dorsal midline; *(A/) V. coronalis phal. III.*

The deep paths of the ST- meridian;

1) One branch travels from ST12, situated in the chest, to GV14, and further caudally through the diaphragm, contacts CV13 and CV12 to enter the Stomach, ST, and connect with the Spleen, SP.
2) Another branch begins in the pyloric orifice of the Stomach, and travels within the abdomen to meet the main meridian at ST30.

3) One branch starts at ST42 and ends in SP01, at the medial aspect of the coronary band, where it links with the SP-meridian.

In dogs it begins at ST01, under the eye. It runs to ST04 lateral to the oral canthus, around the edge of the mandible to the point of the jaw (ST06), temporomandibular joint (ST07) and temple (ST08). From ST06, a branch runs down the neck along the upper part of the jugular groove, crosses the groove and continues at the ventral border of musculus Sternocleidomastoideus to ST11 at the thoracic inlet, to ST12, 4 cun lateral to CV Line. From here, it descends the thorax 4 cun from CV Line following the mammary line, to ST18 (5th intercostal space, below nipple). From here it runs to ST19 (2 cun lateral to CV14), and descends in a line 2 cun lateral to CV Line between the ascending KI and SP Channels to the pelvic brim (ST30). From ST30, it runs distally along the anterolateral side of the thigh, to the lateral side of the patellar tendon (ST35), to the anterior side of the ankle (ST41), to end at ST45, at the lateral edge of the nail-root of toe 3.

In humans begins at ST01, under the eye in humans, horses and dogs (all species). It runs to ST04 lateral to the oral canthus, around the edge of the mandible to the point of the jaw (ST06), temporomandibular joint (ST07) and temple (ST08). From ST06, a branch runs down the neck along the upper part of the jugular groove, crosses the groove and continues at the ventral border of musculus Sternocleidomastoideus to ST11 at the thoracic inlet, to ST12, above the clavicle (in humans), 4 cun lateral to CV Line. From here, it descends the thorax 4 cun from CV Line, through the nipple (ST17), to ST18 (5th intercostal space, below nipple). From here it runs to ST19 (2 cun lateral to CV14), and descends in a line 2 cun lateral to CV Line between the ascending KI and SP Channels to the pelvic brim (ST30). From ST30, it runs distally along the anterolateral side of the thigh, to the lateral side of the patellar tendon (ST35), to the anterior side of the ankle (ST41), to end at ST45, at the lateral edge of the nail-root of toe 2.

Phase	Metal		Earth		Fire		Water		Fire		Wood
Yin Channel	LU[(1)]		SP[(4)]	>>	HT[(1)]		KI[(4)]	>>	PC[(1)]		LV[(4)]
	||		||		||		||		||		||
Yang Channel	LI[(2)]	>>	ST[(3)]		SI[(2)]	>>	BL[(3)]		TH[(2)]	>>	GB[(3)]
Limb	Hand		Foot		Hand		Foot		Hand		Foot

(\|\| and >>) mean that Qi Flow sequence is LU-LI-ST-SP, etc;
\|\| = Yin-Yang Phase Mates (Partners);
[(1)] Qi flow from chest to hand; [(2)] Qi flow from hand to face;
[(3)] Qi flow from face to foot; [(4)] Qi flow from foot to chest

Table 51

ST Qi comes from LI Channel and flows into (connects with) SP Channel, its Yin Mate in Earth. Like the LI Channel (actually all Yang-channels), ST Channel is also more relevant in humans than in animals. The reason why it is of greater importance to humans than animals probably relates to the modern human lifestyle, and the fact that humans are more mental beings than animals (as described in the section on LI Channel, page 263).

After the stomach has completed its digestive Process, the purified Qi derived from the digesta is sent to SP through the internal pathways of TH. The stomach has three sections corresponding to each of the Three Heaters, and an individual ST Point controls each part (see page 382). Then the Qi continues upwards where it enters the channel circulation through LU01.

Today's stressful lifestyle is a main cause of human gastric ulcers. However, gastric ulcers are also important in animals, especially those farmed intensively; such practices put animals under great amounts of stress and pain. They are very common in thoroughbred foals and racehorses. In cattle, ST Channel relates strongly with the udder and the "four stomachs". Apart from its importance in the development of rumen acidosis and abomasal ulcers, it relates to the reticulum and omasum also.

In horses, ST Channel is important for the action of the muscles that drive the hindlimbs forward. This function is very important in horses; restricted action of these muscles can shorten the stride by 10 cm. If ST points are reactive, their effective treatment can restore stride length by up to 10 cm. In contrast, AP at non-reactive ST points may still increase the pace by 5 cm. Treatment of ST Channel can regulate other irregularities in horses also.

In dogs, ST Channel is important in relation to mastitis and mammary tumours, as it runs exactly along the teats. The mammary glands or teats in all mammals develop along the pathway of ST Channel.

ST Channel has some of the most important "Doping Points" (hypo-algesic points). These may of course have a positive therapeutic effect on for example birth and disorders involving chronic pain, but simple hypo-algesia is usually considered to be inferior therapy. Expanding pains, contractions and postpartum hemorrhage usually respond very well to ST points, for example, ST36. Facial (trigeminal nerve) pain also responds well to stimulation of several points on ST Channel.

In accordance with the Chinese Qi Clock, around 0800h is the best time of day to treat ST Channel.

The location of ST30 (close to (beneath) the pelvic brim) emphasises the importance of ST in the production of Nutrient Qi. The Chongmai, Renmai (Conception Vessel, CV) and Dumai (Governing Vessel, GV) all begin at ST30 (Qichong, Qi Thoroughfare). As all three of these Vessels are Seas of Blood and Qi, it becomes clear why this concept is valid. According to the Neijing, "when ST Qi is in harmony, the five Yin organs are at peace. In ST Excess, the pulse is full, mouth and lips are dry and there is pain and swelling in the armpits and the face is hot. You must disperse ST". However, in ST Deficiency, the pulse is empty; abdominal pain and intestinal borborygmus occur and the eyes and face appear empty. In this case one must tonify ST.

Note: In humans, the *Source Point* of all the *Yin organs* is the third most distal point (LU11, SP03, HT07, KI03, PC07, LV03). It is also the *Earth Point*; it derives from the Earth Phase. Therefore the Earth ST Channel is intricately involved in the energetics of all the Yin Organs in TCM.

The energy in the stomach meridian (Qi) may, as for the stomach-process itself may be in:

- *Excess*

- *Deficiency*

Particular for the meridian the energy may also be:

- *Destructive*

- *Blocked*

Excess show itself usually as pain, as this is a Yang meridian, and Yang meridians usually show excesses as pain (contrary to Ying-meridians which often show excesses just as an elevated and positive function of the process). Excess in the Stomach-meridian may be the result of a deficiency in the liver process. Such excess may often be the result of irritation and grief as well as long standing stress.

Deficiency in a Yang meridian is much more seldom as it is in a Yin meridian. Often symptoms arising from Yang-meridians are due to excesses, but of course deficiencies are also found. A deficiency may express itself as underfunction of the associated organ, as underfunction in the associated muscles and in the skin-area transversed by the meridian, as described at page 70. In the stomach meridian this may result in stagnation of the stomach and a feeling of fullness, dysfunction of the M. quadriceps or skin changes along the path of the meridian.

A deficiency in the stomach meridian is often the cause of excess in the bladder or kidney process, and pain along the bladder-meridian may be the result. This pain is often the symptoms we see most easily.

Destructivity shows itself as in all animals as particular vicious symptoms of the skin, erosions and wounds (see more about destructive energy on page XXXIV).

Blockage of the Stomach-meridian is caused by a trauma on the structures of connective tissue that lead the impulses travelling through this meridian. Such a trauma will not hurt or destroy the energy of the process itself, but hinder the Qi-flow in the meridian. This is why the pulse in such a case shows absolutely good health for the process, but the acupuncture points may show dis-balance. This disbalance shows excess above the trauma, and deficienct below the trauma.

ST 01	**Chengqi (Contain Tears)**
	Meeting point of the ST meridian with the Yang Qiao mai and CV
	In horses: it is deep in the eye-socket, between the eye and infraorbital ridge, at midpoint of the ridge, directly under mid-pupil. When needling ST01, do not penetrate the eyeball; it is important to use a long needle and to push the eyeball upwards, away from the needle. Animals need very good restraint for the procedure to be safe.
	In dogs: it is deep in the eye-socket, between the eye and infraorbital ridge, at midpoint of the ridge, directly under mid-pupil. When needling ST01, do not penetrate the eyeball; it is important to use a long needle and to push the eyeball upwards, away from the needle. Animals need very good restraint for the procedure to be safe.
	In humans: it is deep in the eye-socket, between the eye and infraorbital ridge, at midpoint of the ridge, directly under mid-pupil. When needling ST01, do not penetrate the eyeball.
	Effect: It helps general eye disorders, sinusitis under the eye, sight and night blindness. It has a marked stimulating action on the pastern and coffin joint of horses.
ST 02	**Sibai (Four Whites)**
	In horses: Rostrodorsal to ST01, in a wide V made by the V. angularis oculi dorsalis.
	In dogs: it is somewhat dorsal to the infraorbital foramen, below ST01.
	In humans, it is in the infraorbital foramen just below ST01.
	Effect: It helps the face, cheek; eye, eyelid, sight; nose, nasal sinuses, olfaction; maxilla, mandible and upper teeth. It has a marked effect on the sinuses and the eye. I have found a marked stimulating effect on the tarsus of horses.

ST 03	**Juliao (Great Bone-Orifice)** **Meeting point of the ST meridian with the Yang Qiao mai** *In horses:* At the level of the dorsal border and the rostral end of Crista facialis, where V. lateralis nasi meets with V. facialis. *In dogs:* it is just where the vena lateralis nasi leaves vena angularis oculi. *In humans:* it is below mid-pupil, level with inferior edge of nasal wing. *Effect:* It helps the face, cheek, maxilla, mandible, lips, oral muscles, gums, teeth and nose (see LI04 and LI20 also).
ST 04	**Dicang (Earth Granary)** **Meeting point of the ST- and LI meridians with the CV and the Yang Qiao mai. Kai Guan; extra point according to Van den Bosch/Guray** *In horses:* At the level of the rostral end of Crista facialis, just ventral to its ventral border. *In dogs:* dogs and horses it is below mid-pupil, in groove lateral to oral canthus. *In humans:* dogs and horses it is below mid-pupil, in groove lateral to oral canthus. *Effect:* It helps the brain and meninges, and their functions and parts (convulsions, CVA, hemiplegia, paralysis, polio, tetanus, amnesia) and face (cheek, mouth, oral muscles, maxilla, mandible, chin). It also helps the lips and hemorrhage through the gums and can thereby be used in gum infections (pyorrhea) and non-healing wounds (wounds from sharp teeth. ***Don't forget to check the teeth!, see page 450).***
ST 05	**Daying (Great Reception)** *In horses:* 1 cun dorsal to the ventral border of Os mandibularis, in a small depression just cranial to M. masseter. *In dogs:* is behind facial artery at anterior edge of masseter muscle above inferior edge of mandible. *In humans:* is behind facial artery at anterior edge of masseter muscle above inferior edge of mandible.

	Effect: Helps the brain and meninges and their functions and parts (convulsions, CVA, hemiplegia, paralysis, polio, tetanus, amnesia) and the face (cheek, mouth, lips, oral muscles, tongue, speech, gums, teeth, chin, maxilla, mandible, masseter, temporo-mandibular joint). It is used especially in facial pain (trigeminal neuralgia) and facial paralysis and to relax the masseter muscles in lockjaw (trismus) in tetanus in all species. I have also used this point very effectively in salivary calculi (stones).
ST 06	**Jiache (Jaw Chariot, Jawbone)** *In horses:* In M. masseter, midway along and 1 cun dorsal to the ventral border of the mandible. *In dogs:* ST06 is in masseter muscle, 1 cun on a line from angle of jaw to nasal wing. *In humans:* ST06 is in masseter muscle, 1 cun on a line from angle of jaw to nasal wing. *Effect:* help the brain and meninges and their functions and parts (convulsions, CVA, hemiplegia, paralysis, polio, tetanus, amnesia) and the face (cheek, mouth, lips, oral muscles, tongue, speech, gums, teeth, chin, maxilla, mandible, masseter, temporo-mandibular joint). It is used especially in facial pain (trigeminal neuralgia) and facial paralysis and to relax the masseter muscles in lockjaw (trismus) in tetanus in all species. I have also used this point very effectively in salivary calculi (stones).
ST 07 (in horses **ST07-1 and ST07-2)**	**Xiaguan (Below the Joint)** **Meeting point of the ST- and GB meridians** *In horses:* In a small depression just cranial to the mandibular condyle, ventral to Proc. zygomaticus, 2 points close to each other, 0.5 cun apart. *In dogs:* in a hollow below zygomatic arch, anterior to condyloid process of mandible. *In humans:* in a hollow below zygomatic arch, anterior to condyloid process of mandible. *Effect:* It helps the face (cheek, lips, oral muscles, gums, teeth, maxilla, mandible, masseter, temporomandibular joint), especially in facial pain (trigeminal neuralgia) and facial paralysis of all species.

ST 08	Touwei (Head´s binding) **Meeting point of the ST- and GB meridians with the Yang Wei mai** *In horses:* In the dorsal part of Fossa temporales, on a dorsal line from ST07-1. *In dogs:* In the dorsal part of Fossa temporales. *In humans:* 0,5 cun within the anterior hairline at the corner of the forehead, 4,5 cun lateral to the Du Channel. *Effect:* Eliminates wind and alleviates pain; headache and migraine in humans.
ST 09 (In horses ST09-1)	**Renying (Man's Prognosis)** **Meeting point between the ST- and GB-meridians, Point of the Window of the Sky, Point of the Sea of Qi** *In horses:* At the ventral aspect of M. brachiocephalicus, at the level of the ventral border of Os mandibularis. *In dogs:* lateral to the laryngeal prominence, behind the carotid artery. *In humans:* lateral to the laryngeal prominence, behind the carotid artery. *Effect:* helps blood circulation, blood pressure and the parathyroid / thyroid. It is one of the important **"Windows of the Sky" Points** (see LI18). I obtained good results from ST09 in many dogs and horses that presented with ataxia, dizziness and unsteadiness.
ST 09-2	**Extrapoint in horses** *In horses:* At the ventral aspect of M. brachiocephalicus, at the level of the intervertebral space between the 4th and 5th cervical vertebrae. Erwin Westermayer and Andreas Roesti place it further down, just in front of the 6th cervical vertebrae. Here they also place LI18. *Effect:* It is one of the important **"Windows of the Sky" Points** (see LI18). I obtained good results from ST09 in many dogs and horses that presented with ataxia, dizziness and unsteadiness.

ST 10	**Shuitu (Water Prominence)**
	In horses: At the ventral aspect of M. brachiocephalicus, 3 cun cranial to the border between the shoulder and the neck, 3 cun caudoventral to ST09-2. *In dogs:* it is just cranial of LI15, just in front of the shoulder joint, and just dorsal to the jugular groove. *In humans*, it is midway from ST09 to ST11. *Effect:* It helps asthma and in a restricted forward motion of the **forelimb**. Dr. *Marvin Cain reports that ST10 [plus BL21 and BL36-BL38 (the local stifle points)], may be sensitive in ipsilateral stifle disorders in horses.* *Marvin also describes an **Immune Point** near the jugular groove between ST10 and ST11. He combines it with BL20, BL18, LV13 and the three special points that lie in a triangle dorsal to the external angle of the ilium (called the herpes triangle by Dr. Marvin Cain) to treat **immunocompromised horses**, especially those with the **Equine Herpes Syndrome**. Marvin often injects those points with Vitamin B12 +/- Echinacea, or with autogenous blood from the jugular vein. He claims excellent results within 24-72 hours after this treatment.*
ST 11	**Qishe (Qi Abode)**
	In horses: 2 cun ventral to ST10, at the cranial aspect of M. brachiocephalicus. *In dogs:* it is about 6 cun directly caudal to ST10. *In humans*, it is just dorsal to the jugular groove, on the superior edge of the medial end of the clavicle, between the heads of sternocleidomastoid muscle. *Effect:* In problems with the throat.
ST 21	**Liangmen (Beam Gate)**
	In horses: On the abdomen, 2 cun lateral to the midline, at the level of CV12 (midway between the umbilicus and the xiphoid process. *In dogs:* 2 cun lateral to CV12 (midway between CV08 and the sternoxiphoid junction. *In humans:* 2 cun lateral to CV12 (midway between CV08 and the sternoxiphoid junction.

	Effect: It relates especially to ST and digestion. It helps gastritis, colic, diarrhea and inappetance.
ST 25	**Tianshu (Heavenly Pivot)** **Front-Mu (alarm) Point of LI** *In horses:* On the abdomen, 2 cun lateral to the umbilicus. *In dogs:* 2 cun lateral to the navel (CV08). *In humans:* 2 cun lateral to the navel (CV08). *Effect:* It relates especially to LI and digestion. It helps the abdomen and its organs and functions: pain, colic or spasm in abdomen and its organs; gastrointestinal tract (stomach, duodenum, small intestine, appendix, cecum, colon, rectum, constipation, diarrhea, dysentery, inappetance, indigestion, nausea, vomiting, peritonitis). It also helps the back and ovary; edema, ascites, allergy, allergic shock, and vasomotor allergy.
ST 27	**Daju (Great Gigantic)** *In horses:* it is 3 cunlateral and 3 cun caudal to the navel. *In dogs:* it is 2 cun lateral to CV05, 2 cun below CV08. *In humans:* it is 2 cun lateral to CV05, 2 cun below CV08. *Effect:* It stimulates the ovary and testicle (ovulation and sperm production).
ST 30	**Qichong (Qi Surging)** **Starting point of the Chongmai (Extraordinary Vessel, see page 444)** *In horses:* it is just cranial to the inguinal ring (near the pelvic brim) (not on the drawing). *In dogs* it is just cranial to the inguinal ring (near the pelvic brim) (not on the drawing). *In humans* it is 2 cun lateral to CV02, 5 cun below CV08, just above the pubis. *Effect:* It stimulates the general Yin Qi and thus resembles SP06 somewhat. It helps male and female urogenital and reproductive disorders, ureter; fallopian tube, ovary, uterus, cervix, vagina, vulva, clitoris; penis and testicle. It also helps the groin, inguinal area, perineum and patella.

ST 34	**Liangqiu (Beam Hill)** **Xi Point of ST:** *In horses:* The length of the patella, ~ 3 cun, proximal to the proximal and lateral edge of the patella. *In dogs* it is directly proximolateral to the patella, right beside the tendon that is inserted on the top of the patella. *In humans,* it is 2 cun above superior edge of patella on a line from the lateral edge of the patella to the anterior superior iliac spine. *Effect:* It stimulates the stifle, especially in younger horses that show pain or inflammation here. It also helps all acute states along ST Channel.
ST 35	**Dubi** (Calf's Nose), also called **Waixiyan** (Outer Knee Eye) *In horses:* Just distal to the patella, in a depression between the middle and the lateral patellar ligaments. It can be blistered, using a local subcutaneous injection of a mild irritant. *In dogs:* it is just below the patella, in a hollow lateral to the patellar tendon with knee flexed. *In humans* it is just below the patella, in a hollow lateral to the patellar tendon with knee flexed. *Effect:* It helps chronic stifle disorders. It is often used with the point directly opposite on the medial side of the patellar tendon, **Neixiyan** (Inner Knee Eye).
ST 36	**Zusanli (Leg Three Li)** **Not a command-point in horses (*in horses the main elemental functions are moved down to a point above the tarsus called Waterpoint*).** **Water-elemental point in dogs.** **Earth-elemental point in humans.** **Master Point of the Abdomen, Master Point of Thorax and Stimulation Point of the Upper Heater (LU, HT, PC), Respiration and Circulation, Immunostimulant Point, Analgesic Point and Emergency Point:** *In horses:* 1.5 cun below Tuberositas tibiae, on the cranial midline of the leg, 1 cun lateral to Crista tibiae.

In dogs: it is 1 cun lateral to the anterior tibial crest, 3 cun below the patella, on the Musculus tibilais cranialis.
In humans: it is 1 cun lateral to the anterior tibial crest, 3 cun below the patella, on the Musculus tibilais cranialis.

Effect: It is one of the most important points in AP. In Chinese, a Li is a unit of distance, or a division. Zusanli was named when soldiers, in the civil war of ancient China, discovered that by stimulating ST36 they were able to walk through three more Li (3 Li = 1 mile). They knew that fact from before, but in wartime just this property becomes so much more important, that a change of name is appropriate.
It also helps the abdomen, epigastrium, hypochondrium, periumbilical area and its organs and functions, spasm in abdomen or its organs. Also urogenital disorders, libido, female and male reproduction [forbidden point in pregnancy (may cause abortion)], lowback- and lumbar- area, sacrum, pelvis and perineum. It also helps in emergencies and first aid, hearing and blood circulation. It also helps the skin and hair, immunity and allergy. It is the first choice in disorders of the stifle area and patella.
ST36 is noted for its analgesic effects, general pain control and tonic effects in exhaustion and chronic disease.
ST36 stimulates more or less all the muscles, and has a revitalising and pain relieving effect by the release of "endorphins". Endorphins are opium resembling substances which can be released from the nervous system and which elevate pain, increase desire feelings and endurance (see also page 487). Therefore, it must be considered a **Doping Point.**
ST36 is especially interesting in cribbing, or windsucking in horses. "Windsuckers" don't really swallow air but many owners think they do. People also think that horses get colic from air ingestion but the truth is the reverse! Horses often crib because they have stomach pain and they can relieve some of that pain by cribbing. In order to ingest air, they place their incisor teeth in the corner of their manger, create a low pressure in the pharynx and that somewhat compresses the air. This air creates a high pressure, which somewhat reduces pain elsewhere (maybe by the release of endorphins). In my practise, about 60% of cribbers suck wind to suppress pain within the digestive organs. In these cases, cribbing disappears for some days after stimulation of ST36. Disappearance of the symptoms shows that

	the cribbing is due to pain and that elimination of the pain can cure the cribbing. In the other 40% of the horses, cribbing that does not cease after needling ST36 has probably become a deep-seated vice. Even expert acupuncturists find such intractable habits hard to cure.
ST 37	**Shangjuxu (Upper Great Hollow)** **Lower Uniting Point of LI and Master Point of Upper Abdomen and Stimulation Point of the Middle Heater (ST, SP, SI, GB, LV) Digestion and Extraction:** *In horses:* 1.5 cun distal to ST36. *In dogs:* 1 cun lateral to anterior tibial crest, 6 cun below ST35 and 3 cun below ST36. *In humans:* 1 cun lateral to anterior tibial crest, 6 cun below ST35 and 3 cun below ST36. *Effect:* Wide range of intestinal disorders; diarrhea due to cold, damp, deficiency, damp-heat. Regulates ST and SP; located close to the ST36. Benefits the digestion and absorption from the intestines. May be used instead of TH02, since both points stimulate the blood-circulation in the middle and upper part of the body.
ST 38	**Tiaokou (Lines opening)** *In horses:* 1 cun distal to ST37, at the cranial aspect of the leg, midway between the femorotibial joint and the lateral malleolus. It is easy to find if we measure the distance between the lower point of the Patella and the upper edge of the hock, and exactly midway between these two points we find ST38. *In dogs:* This point is situated directly 2 cun below ST37. It is easier to find if we measure the distance between the lower point of the Patella and the upper edge of the hock, and exactly midway between these two points we find ST38. *In humans:* This point is situated directly 2 cun below ST37. It is easier to find if we measure the distance between the lower point of the Patella and the upper edge of the hock, and exactly midway between these two points we find ST38. *Effect: it* is a special point for ipsilateral shoulder problems.

| ST 39 | **Xiajuxu (Lower Great Hollow)**

Lower Uniting Point of SI and Master Point of Lower Abdomen and Stimulation Point of the Lower Heater (LI, BL, KI), Elimination and Reproduction:

In horses: 1 cun distal to ST38. It is easier to find if we measure the distance between the lower point of the Patella and the upper edge of the hock, and exactly 1 cun below the midway between these two points we find ST39.
In dogs: it is 1 cun lateral to anterior tibial crest, 9 cun below ST35 or 3 cun below ST37.
In humans: it is 1 cun lateral to anterior tibial crest, 9 cun below ST35 or 3 cun below ST37 and 1 cun below ST38.

Effect: It can be used for pain in the lower abdomen. Moves SI Qi and transforms stagnation; severe pain of the lower/caudal abdomen that radiates to the lumbar region, chronic diarrhea. Regulates and harmonizes the intestines and clears damp-heat; diarrhea with pus and blood in the stools. Stimulates blood circulation in the lower leg. |
| ST 40 | **Fenglong (Bountiful Bulge)**

Luo Point of ST (connects ST Channel with its Phase Mate, SP Channel).
Influential point for phlegm.

In horses: 1 cun lateral to ST38; 1 cun lateral to the dorsal midline of the pelvic limb, midway between the femorotibial joint and the lateral malleolus.
In dogs: it is 1 cun laterally to ST38.
In humans: it is 1 cun laterally to ST38.

Effect: helps gastric hyperacidity, or *stomach ulcers* (then it should be combined with SP03) and shoulder pain. It also helps the respiratory system, trachea, lung, bronchi, asthma, cough, pneumonia, salivation and salivary glands. Transform phlegm and dampness in the whole body. |

ST 41	Jiexi (Divide Ravine)
	Water Point of ST in horses **Fire point in humans** *In horses:* At the level of a line just proximal to the lateral malleolus, 1/3 cun lateral to the cranial midline of the pelvic limb. *In dogs:* is at the junction of foot-dorsum and leg, centre of the cruciate ligament, between tendons of extensor digitorum (tibialis cranialis and extensor digitalis longus. *In humans:* is at the junction of foot-dorsum and leg, centre of the cruciate ligament, between tendons of extensor digitorum (tibialis cranialis and extensor digitalis longus. *Effect:* The point helps, apart from the elemental actions, also infections in the throat. Also, it helps general disorders in the Achilles, heel, metatarsus, tarsus and foot.
ST 42	**Chongyang (Surging Yang)** **Metal point in horses** **Source Point in humans** *In horses:* Just distal to the hock, on the dorsal midline of the pelvic limb. *In dogs:* it is on the foot-dorsum, on the hump between metatarsals 2-3 and cuneiform bone, near dorsalis pedis artery. *In humans:* it is on the foot-dorsum, on the hump between metatarsals 2-3 and cuneiform bone, near dorsalis pedis artery. *Effect:* Influences painful conditions locally and along the course of the meridian and generally in the body when the ST is in excess or deficiency.
ST 43	**Xiangu (Sunken Valley)** **Earth Point in horses and dogs** **Wood point in humans** *In horses:* Just proximal to the fetlock, on the dorsal midline of the pelvic limb.

	In dogs: it is between metatarsal 3 and 4, *In humans:* it is on foot-dorsum, in a hollow below union of metatarsals 2-3. *Effect:* it may be used as a comman point which is related to the Earth Phase. ST43 also helps the salivary glands and salivation. In horses it is used in degenerative lesions in the fetlock joint.
ST 44	**Neiting (Inner Court)** **Fire Point in horses and dogs** **Water point in humans** *In horses:* Just distal to the fetlock, on the dorsal midline. *In dogs:* it is between metatarsal 3 and 4, in the web distal to the lower heads of metatarsal bones 3-4. *In humans:* it is on foot-dorsum, in web between toes 2-3, in a hole lateral and distal to metatarsophalangeal joint 2. *Effect:* It helps joint disorders generally and in fetlock disorders especially. In both humans, dogs and horses it also helps the forehead; frontal sinuses; gums; larynx; lips; mandible; maxilla; mouth; oral muscles; pharynx; throat; tonsil; teeth; voice.
ST 45	**Lidui (Severe Mouth)** **Ting-point, Wood Point of ST in horses and dogs** **Metal point in humans** *In horses:* it is in the coronary band of the hindfoot, at exact cranial point. *In dogs:* it is on the lateral aspect (axially) of **toe 3** (the dewclaw, which may be absent from the inner side of the foot, is toe 1). *In humans:* it is 0.1 cun from posterior edge of nail-root of toe 2, lateral side. *Effect:* As all Ting Points are related to the Wood Phase, ST45 is a Wood Point. As a Wood Point it is especially effective against muscular pain and spasm along the entire Channel, and may also be used in the aftermath of painful gas colic. It may be used on "Wood" disorders along ST Channel and on Wood

disorders in general which are related to the Earth Phase (ST-meridian). As this sounds complicated, I will give an example. Wood disorders mean disorders of the muscles, or symptoms characterised by growth. The relation to the Earth Phase is characterised in that the disorder disconnects itself from the whole and gives itself over to the powers of gravitation, in which decomposition arises. Typically, this combination of events manifests as wounds that proliferate as granulating ulcers, scar overgrowth or proud flesh (necrotic tissue), or that disintegrate on the surface. In both dogs and horses ST45 especially stimulates the quadriceps muscle, a muscle that makes it possible to stretch the hindleg forward. This is especially important for competition horses; stimulation of ST45 can add 5-10 cm to the horse´s stride. It also contains within itself an even smaller point, belonging to the ECIWO System of the equine coronary band; this smaller ECIWO-ST45 stimulates the hindfetlock joint (see page 134).

Table 52

The special commandpoints in the horse are as follows:

S **O** **U** **R** **C** **E** **tarsus**	*In horses:* At the dorsolateral aspect of the hock, just lateral to the dorsal midline of the pelvic limb. *Effect;* Stimulates the meridian.
S **O** **U** **R** **C** **E** **fetlock**	*In horses:* On the dorsal midline, at the level of the metatarsophalangeal joint. *Effect; Stimulates the meridian.*

Table 53

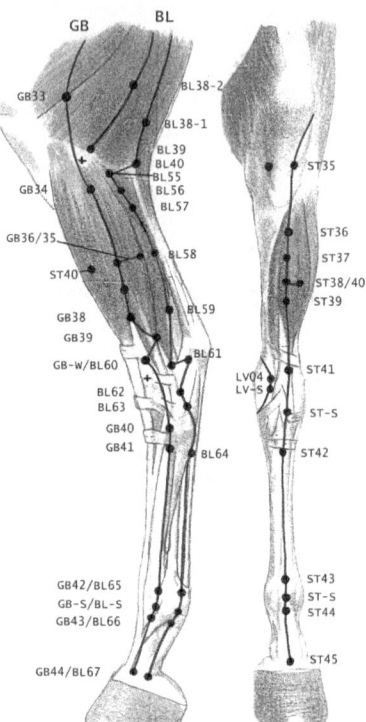

Figure 46; The most important points on the ST Channel in the horse.

SP (Spleen/Pancreas Foot Taiyin) Channel uses the connective tissue around *A/V. coronalis phal. III, A. et V. digitalis med. och A/V. mtts. plant. prof. med. A. mtts. dors. med, Rete malleolus med., A/V. tibialis caudalis, A/V. popliteus. A/V. genus desc., A/V. femoralis, A/V. epigastrica caudalis, V. thoracica externa and A/V. thoracodorsalis* as the main pathways for carrying its impulses:

Anatomically it begins:

In horses:

The superficial path of the SP meridian:

- Begins at the coronary band of the pelvic limb, just dorsal to the medial cartilage of the distal phalanx, $\sim 90^0$ medial to the tip of the toe; *A/V. coronalis phal. III,*

- Ascends along the deep digital flexor tendon to the distal part of the head of Os metatarsale II; *A/V. mtts. plant. prof. med.*

- Here the meridian turns slightly towards dorsal; *A. mtts. dors. med.*, at SP05, located just distal and dorsal to the medial malleolus; *Rete malleolus med.*,

- Continues along the caudomedial border of the tibia; *A/V. tibialis caudalis*, passes the stifle joint at the caudal aspect; *A/V. popliteus.*

- Travels towards the patella, and continues proximally to the inguinal region; *A/V. femoralis.*

- Traverses directly over to the abdomen; *A/V. epigastrica caudalis*, follows the lateral border of M. rectus abdominis,

- Intersects with the Conception vessel at CV03, CV04 and CV10, before it enters the Spleen and contacts the Stomach.

- The meridian emerges again at the caudal border of M. pectoralis ascendens, where this muscle crosses the lateral border of M. rectus abdominis, and follows this muscle along with *V. thoracica externa*, until the first rib,

- Makes a sharp turn and follows the ventral border of M. latissimus dorsi; *A/V. thoracodorsalis*, until it reaches the 11th intercostal space, at SP21, where the superficial path of the SP-meridian ends.

The deep path of the SP - meridian has two branches:

1. One deep branch begins in the Spleen and passes through the diaphragm, travels along the esophagus and ends at the ventral side of the tongue.

2. Another branch begins in the Stomach, traverses the diaphragm and ends in the Heart.

In dogs: it begins at SP01, on the medial side of the nail-root of the hindtoe 2. It ascends the medial side of the metatarsus, tarsus, leg, stifle and thigh. It ascends the abdomen 4 cun from CV Line to SP16 (4 cun lateral to navel), and then ascends the thorax 6 cun from CV Line to SP20 (6 cun from CV Line, in intercostal space 2) and then descends to end at SP21, 6 cun below axilla, on mid-axillary line, in intercostal space 7, midway from axilla to tip of rib 12, midway from the shoulder-joint and the head (not tip) of the second last rib.

In humans begins at SP01, at the medial nail-root of toe 1 (big toe).

It ascends the medial side of the metatarsus, tarsus, leg, stifle and thigh. It ascends the abdomen 4 cun from CV Line to SP16 (4 cun lateral to navel), and then ascends the thorax 6 cun from CV Line to SP20 (6 cun from CV Line, in intercostal space 2) and then descends to end at SP21 (6 cun below axilla, on mid-axillary line, in intercostal space 6, midway from axilla to tip of rib 11).

Phase	Metal		Earth		Fire		Water		Fire		Wood
Yin Channel	LU[1]		SP[4]	>>	HT[1]		KI[4]	>>	PC[1]		LV[4]
	‖		‖		‖		‖		‖		‖
Yang Channel	LI[2]	>>	ST[3]		SI[2]	>>	BL[3]		TH[2]	>>	GB[3]
Limb	Hand		Foot		Hand		Foot		Hand		Foot

(‖ and >>) mean that Qi Flow sequence is LU-LI-ST-SP, etc;
‖ = Yin-Yang Phase Mates (Partners);
[1] Qi flow from chest to hand; [2] Qi flow from hand to face; [3] Qi flow from face to foot; [4] Qi flow from foot to chest

Table 54

SP Qi comes from ST Channel, its Yang Mate in Earth, and flows into (connects with) HT Channel. As in the case of all the other Yin Channels in animals, SP Channel is much more important than its paired Yang Channel (ST). SP has many important Qi Processes that are very similar to those of the Liver. Its superficial pathway is also nearly parallel with the LV Channel. In the Husband-Wife Law of TCM, SP is the Wife of LV, which is the Husband of SP (deep Pulse Position 2 on the right and left radial artery, respectively; see page 169).

As I have already stated, SP and LV have many functions in common. Both are very important for the:

- *Digestion;* SP controls the rhythmic part of digestion, LV controls more the material part of the digestion ("the kitchen" of the body). Eating irregularly, or a sudden or total change of diet, completely drains SP Qi, whereas eating unhealthily drains LV Qi. Colic is most often related to LV and/or SP. (However, the cause of colic can also derive from any of the abdominal or pelvic organs, for example SI and LI, gas formation, GB, KI, the uterus, etc).

- *Blood:* SP controls the venous system, the blood returning to the heart after delivering nutrients to the tissues. Also SP "keeps the blood in the vessels"; hemorrhage and bruising occur easily in SP Deficiency. LV controls blood circulation in the long muscles of the back and hip (gluteal) area. Therefore, LV is responsible for azoturia (Monday Morning Disease),

- *Muscles and tendons:* SP usually is responsible for the deeper tendons and muscles, LV for the more superficial ones. I have seen whole trotting stables suffer with pain in the deep muscles of the hip (especially musculus Iliopsoas) because the diet was changed too hastily. This can come from something as basic as a change in the source of hay. If the fodder has been insufficient, the superficial muscles will suffer (especially musculus Gluteus). Therefore it is important to find out if we should improve feed quality, or feed more regularly.

- *Immune system:* Both the Spleen and the Liver as organs and SP and LV (as Channels, representatives for the processes) are involved in most allergies, resistance against infection, viruses and cancer.

Because of the close association of SP and LV, it is important to ensure that LV is in proper Qi order before stimulating SP. If you master the puls-diagnosis this is easy, if not; always treat the Liver before you treat the Spleen.

In SP Deficiency, the hair coat often loses its sheen. Some dog owners have noted this. Often, prior to an event or show, they stimulate their pet's spleen, creating a shinier coat effect. They do this by giving small doses of arsenic, a drug that stimulates SP {1% potassium arsenate, at approximately 1 drop/3 kg liveweight daily for 30 days}. Excessive doses induce the same symptoms as SP colic or stomach pain that improves on bending forward.

SP Channel also has another strange function: SP Deficiency usually arises if a general Process Imbalance exists in *any of the other Channels for >1 year*. If we find a SP Deficiency (not connected to the Lesion-complex) as well as a Process Imbalance (connected to the Lesion-complex) in the Channel(s) related to the disease, we may conclude that the disease has lasted for >1 year.

Also, SP Channel is also the only one that almost always is Deficient in cancer. In old European tradition SP relates to the planet Saturn, which again was related to metallic lead and to death. This is now understandable as regards the relation of SP to chronic and deadly diseases. In accordance with the Chinese Qi Clock, around 1000h is the best time of day to treat SP Channel.

Soulie de Morant says that the left SP Channel acts more on the pancreas, while the right SP Channel acts more on SP functions, such as purifying blood and intellectual accomplishments. Therefore, it is better to treat SP01 and SP04 on the right side when using them to help concentration, for example when taking examinations.

The energy in the spleen meridian (Qi) may, as for the spleen-process itself, be in:

- *Excess*

- *Deficiency*

Particular for the meridian the energy may also be:

- *Destructive*

- *Blocked*

Excess show itself rather seldom as pain, as this is a Yin merid-ian, and Yin meridians seldom show excesses as pain (contrary to Yang-meridians which often show excesses as painful points or areas). An excess in the Spleen-meridian, although very sel-dom, may be the result of a deficiency in the liver-process. An excess in the Spleen meridian usually passes without observa-tion or unpleasant symptoms.

Deficiency is a much more common and serious pathologi-cal finding than excess. Such a deficiency show itself in the same way as described under the spleen-process on page 72. In addition we may find skin-changes in the form of eczema along the Spleen-meridian.

A deficiency in the Spleen meridian is often the cause of an excess in the Bladder meridian, and pain along this meridian may be the result.

This pain is often the symptoms we are confronted with in our dayly practise.

Destructivity show itself as in all animals as particular vicious symptoms of the skin, erosions and wounds (see more about destructive energy on page XXXIV).

Blockage of the Spleen-meridian is caused by a trauma on the structures of connective tissue that lead the impulses travel-ling through this meridian. Such a trauma will not hurt or de-stroy the energy of the process itself, but hinder the Qi-flow in the meridian. This is why the pulse in such a case shows abso-lutely good health for the process, but the acupuncture points may show dis-balance. This disbalance shows excess above the trauma, and deficienct below the trauma.

SP 01	**Yinbai (Hidden White)**
	Ting, Wood Point in all species
	In horses: it is at the medial side of the coronary band of the hindlimb, ~ 90° medial of ST45 and ~ 35° plantar to LV01.
	In dogs: it is at the medial aspect of hindtoe 2, just in the joint between phalanx distalis and phalanx media.
	In humans: it is 0.1 cun from posterior edge of nail-root of toe 1 (big toe), medial side.
	Effect: As a Command Point, it may be used in local disorders, disorders along SP Channel and of the spleen and SP function. As a Ting Point of the Yin Earth Phase it may be used in general disorders of the Earth Phase in the whole organism, when the symptoms show signs of Wood (because it is a Wood Point). SP01 may be used for decreased production of synovial fluid in the fetlock, disorders with the superficial and deep flexor tendon, the medial suspensory ligament or splint in horses and in pain of the surrounding area. It is used also in generalised muscular disorders along the pathway of SP Channel, especially in the deeper muscles of the hips and the psoas muscles. Horses and dogs with SP Deficiency often walk in a particular way, moving the hip under the body. Such a gait is easy to see and one can diagnose SP Deficiency from that sign, just by looking at the animal from a distance. SP01 acts generally on all deeper layers of muscles. It is useful also in chronically affected animals with poor appetite, emaciation and dull hair that have lost their sheen, especially in cases with chronic diarrhea, polyps and hemorrhage. It may also be used in chronic uterine hemorrhage, especially when combined with SP06. SP01 also has a special affinity with the cervix and uterus.
SP 02	**Dadu (Great Metropolis)**
	Fire Point
	In horses: it is just under the hindfetlock at its medial aspect.
	In dogs: at the medial side of toe 2, at the proximal area of phalanx proximalis.
	In humans: at the medial side of the proximal phalanx of toe 1.

	Effect: As a Fire Point, it may be used especially in infections and other circumstances related to "Fiery" or Hot Syndromes. It helps Hot conditions in the hindlimb fetlock and generally in Lesion-Symptom Complexes characterised by temperature changes along SP Channel. For a Hot phlegmon (local edema), we should use SP02 because Heat indicates a Yang state, for which we should use a Yin Point. For a Cold phlegmon (local edema), a Yang Point on ST Channel is preferable. In humans SP02 is often used in sweating disorders and in febrile states related to digestive symptoms.
SP 03	**Taibai (Supreme White)** **Earth and Horary point in horses and dogs** **Source Point of SP in humans** *In horses:* Just proximal to the fetlock, at the level of the dorsal border of the medial proximal sesamoid bone, in a small depression on the large metatarsal bone. *In dogs:* it is at the medial and distal part of metatarsal II. *In humans:* it is at medial side of distal end of metatarsal I. *Effect:* It is a very important point for the entire Channel, especially in degenerative changes. It has a strong local effect on the fetlock, especially in degenerative changes of the joint. Such changes usually manifest as a painful joint without heat or swelling. Such symptoms may also come from calcification, in which case SP03 also may be used. As well as its local effects and effects along SP Channel, SP03 helps all degenerative processes in the body. Examples of this include atrophy, anemia and other instances where tissues regress in size. (*In humans SP03 (as a sourse point) is often used in combination with ST40 (as a Lo-point) in stomach-ulcers in the so called "House-guest", which is about transferring energy from the ST to the SP when there is too much energy in the ST-meridian and too little energy in the SP*).

SP 04	**Gongsun (Yellow Emperor)** **Luo-Connecting point** *(It connects SP Channel with its Phase Mate, ST Channel)* **Confluent point of the Chong mai** *In horses:* Just distal and plantar to the base of the second metatarsal bone. *In dogs:* it is at medial, anterior internal edge of metatarsal II, 1 cun proximal to the metatarsophalangeal joint. *In humans:* it is at medial, anterior internal edge of metatarsal 1, 1 cun proximal to the metatarsophalangeal joint. *Effect:* This point is used when there is too much energy in the SP-meridian (the Luo Points opens up a meridian and lets the energy pass out of the meridian, usually to the mate), and too little in the ST-meridian [in which the Source Point must be used (the Source Point leads energy to the meridian) (the opposite as described for humans above, under point SP03)]. It helps salivation, salivary glands; stomach, Duodenum, inappetance, indigestion, nausea, vomiting, disorders of pregnancy, testicle pain and pain in the 1. toe in humans and the 2. toe in dogs.
SP 05	**Shangqiu (Shang Hill).** **Source point in horses** **(Jing-River and Metal point in dogs and in humans)** *In horses:* At the junction of straight lines drawn along the distal and dorsal borders of the medial malleolus, just under the hock-joint. *In dogs:* it is in a hollow below and anterior to the distal and medial malleolus of tibia. *In humans:* it is in a hollow below and anterior to the distal and medial malleolus of tibia. *Effect:* As a source-point it is important for the entire meridian in horses. In dogs and humans it is effective especially in painful states and when the symptoms have a certain Metal/Air(Gas) Relationship in their degenerative tendency. An example on this may be gas gangrene. It also helps the patella, tarsus, metatarsus and toe.

SP 06	Sanyinjiao (Three Yins Meeting)

Meeting Point of the 3 Foot Yin Channels (LV, SP and KI), Master Point for the Urogenital Tract and Lower Abdomen and an important (the most) Immunostimulant Point:

In horses: On the medial aspect of the pelvic limb, just caudal to the tibia, where the V. saphena, and the Liver meridian crosses the caudal border of the tibia, approximately 5 cun proximal to the medial malleolus, on a line that ascends the exact midline of the medial aspect of the back leg upwards from the tarsus. Just where this line meet the saphenous vein, the first big vein that transverses the leg from anterodistally to posteroproximally; just distal to the vein, is SP06.

In dogs: it is just behind the tibia, just distal to where musculus popliteus and musculus flexor digitorum superficialis separate.

In humans: it is at the posterior edge of tibia, 3 cun above medial malleolus.

Effect: SP06 is one of the most important acupoint as it **stimulates all Yin Channels**. It is excellent when all the Yin Channels are weaker than the Yang Channels, not only the 3 Yin Channels of the hindlimb but also the Yin Channels on the forelimb. **It is indicated in a general Yin Deficiency** by Pulse Diagnosis, or other diagnostic methods. A general Yin Deficiency is mainly the result of stress, and in the same way as the cause of the immune deficiency. In this way SP06 is an important **Immunostimulant Point**.

NOTE: Diseases that are precipitated by stress may manifest in Lesion-Symptom Complexes of several different systems. A stress-related symptom may occur as:

- Qi Stagnation in ST Channel, such as gastritis (treat ST40);
- HT Deficiency and decreased circulation (treat HT09);
- Weakening of the immune system leading to many infections (treat SP06);
- Weakening of the nervous processes of the entire body (treat SP21 and SI18).

It helps recurrent or chronic (in fact also acute) infections like throat infections, urinary infections etc. It should also be used when we vaccinate an animal or child. In vaccinating, the immune system is heavily stressed and several negative results may follow. I have several times seen an aggravation of allergies, growth of different tumours and other negative immunomediated

	disorders. Vaccines seem to weaken the immune system and many studies support this claim (Steve Tobin, USA; see also the chapter on AP and vaccines, page 631). [In my practise I have seen many cases of cancer and immunomediated diseases manifesting within weeks after the administration of vaccines]. In immunomediated diseases like allergy, cancer and chronic infections, I usually postpone vaccination until the immune system is re-established, that is when all Yin-meridians are full of Qi (diagnosed by pulse, see page 176). Even then, the effect of the vaccine improves if SP06 is stimulated when the vaccine is injected. It is important to note that the immune system of all mammals is bilateral. By this I mean that the right and left immune system are two independent entities. This is easily found by Pulse Diagnosis, but also conventional medicine has shown this. Professor Pishinger from Berlin found that blood tests from the left and the right jugular vein show distinct different results in analysing values concerning the immune system. Therefore, it is important which SP06 point we stimulate. Sometimes the right one is the correct point to stimulate, some times the left one. If we do not master the art of Pulse Diagnosis, or do not have time to wait for the results of the blood tests from each side (remember the immune system can be weakened on both sides), I recommend that we treat both points. As **Master Point for the urogenital and lower abdominal organs**, it helps the abdomen and its organs and functions, spasm in abdomen or its organs, male and female genitalia, disorders of pregnancy, problems before, during and after parturition, hypoglycemia and hyperglycemia, inguinal area and groin.
SP 08	**Diji (Earth's Crux)** **Xi Point of SP** *In horses:* 1 cun proximal to SP07 and 3 cun proximal to SP06, on the caudomedial border of the tibia, caudal to V. saphena. *In dogs:* it is at the medial leg, between tibia and gastrocnemius muscle, 6 cun below the patella, 3' below SP09. *In humans:* it is at the medial leg, between tibia and gastrocnemius muscle, 6 cun below the patella, 3 cun below SP09.
	Effect: This point is where the Qi and blood, which have been flowing superficially from the Ting-point, gather and plunge more deeply. It is used for treatment of acute conditions.

SP 09	**Yinlingquan (Yin Mound Spring)** **SP Water Point in dogs** *and humans* *In horses:* On the medial side of the lower leg, on the caudal border of the tibia, 2 cun below the femorotibial joint. *In dogs:* it is at inferior edge of medial condyle of tibia, 3 cun below the patella, between the tibia and the gastrocnemius muscle, 1 cun anterior to LV07. *In humans:* it is at inferior edge of medial condyle of tibia, 3 cun below the patella, between the tibia and the gastrocnemius muscle, 1 cun anterior to LV07. *Effect:* SP is an Earth Channel and Earth controls Water. However, as the dry earth needs water to bloom, SP needs Water to show its plenitude. Therefore, SP09 is very important for the Water Phase of SP functions in doga and in humans. In horses and dogs this point is difficult to needle, but it is easy to treat this point with the Dermojet (see page 458). In horses, as a not command-point, it helps the abdomen, constipation and diarrhea, urinary tract and functions, ischemia of extremities, gangrene, stifle, patella and the popliteal area.
SP 10	**Xuehai (Blood Sea)** **Allergy Point, Blood Point and Master Point of Lower Abdomen (LI, BL, KI), Elimination and Reproduction:** *In horses:* Caudal to the medial femoral trochlea, between Mm. vastus medialis and sartorius. *In dogs:* it is 2 cun above the medial superior edge of patella, on the bulge of quadriceps femoris muscle, knee flexed. *In humans:* it is 2 cun above the medial superior edge of patella, on the bulge of quadriceps femoris muscle, knee flexed. *Effect:* It helps allergy, Blood, hemorrhage, thymus, vasomotor disorders, female genitalia and reproduction.
SP 15	**Daheng (Great Horizontal)** **Meeting point of the SP meridian with the Yin Wei mai** *In In horses:* On the abdomen, 4 cun lateral to the umbilicus, on the lateral border of M. rectus abdominis.

	In dogs: it is in the nipple line, 4 cun lateral to CV08 (the navel). *In humans:* it is in the nipple line, 4 cun lateral to CV08 (the navel). *Effect:* It has similar effects to ST25, especially on the small intestine, appendix, cecum, colon and rectum.
SP 21	**Dabao (Great Embracement)** **The Great Luo Point (Luo Point of all the Luo Points):** *In horses:* In the 11th intercostal space, 8 cun lateral to the dorsal midline. *In dogs:* it is 6 cun below the axilla, on mid-axillary line, or in intercostal space 6, midway from the axilla to the tip of rib 11. *In humans:* it is 6 cun below the axilla, on mid-axillary line, or in intercostal space 6, midway from the axilla to the tip of rib 11. *Effect:* this point is the main Luo Point of the whole body. This means that SP21 opens communication from one side of the body with the other (from the ipsilateral to the contralateral side). It is stimulated on the Excess side. The symptoms of this special situation are many; usually all symptoms are unilateral. Remember to stimulate SP21 on the side that improves with work. It markedly influences the entire body. It has an opposite, or better expressed, mirror effect of SP06, in that it stimulates all Yang Channels (SP06 stimulates all Yin Channels). It helps the lower chest, ribs, hypochondrium; respiration disorders, lung; pleura; mammary disorders; pelvic limb and weak joints.

Table 55

The special commandpoints in the horse are as follows:

S O U R C E fetlock	*Location;* On the medial aspect of the fetlock, at the level of the metatarsophalangeal joint. *Effect;* Stimulates the meridian.

M **E** **T** **A** **L**	***Location***; Distal to the hock, just dorsal to the base of the second metatarsal bone. ***Effect***; Influences painful conditions locally and along the course of the meridian, and generally in the body when the Spleen is in excess or deficiency. Local point of the hock.
W **A** **T** **E** **R**	***Location***; Just proximal to the hock, on the medial side, between the tibia and the tendon of M. flex. digit. longus, along a transverse line 0.5 cun proximal to the medial malleolus. ***Effect***; Local point of the hock. Influences conditions characterised by the water element, locally and along the course of the meridian, and generally in the body when the Spleen is in excess or deficiency. Edema.

Table 56

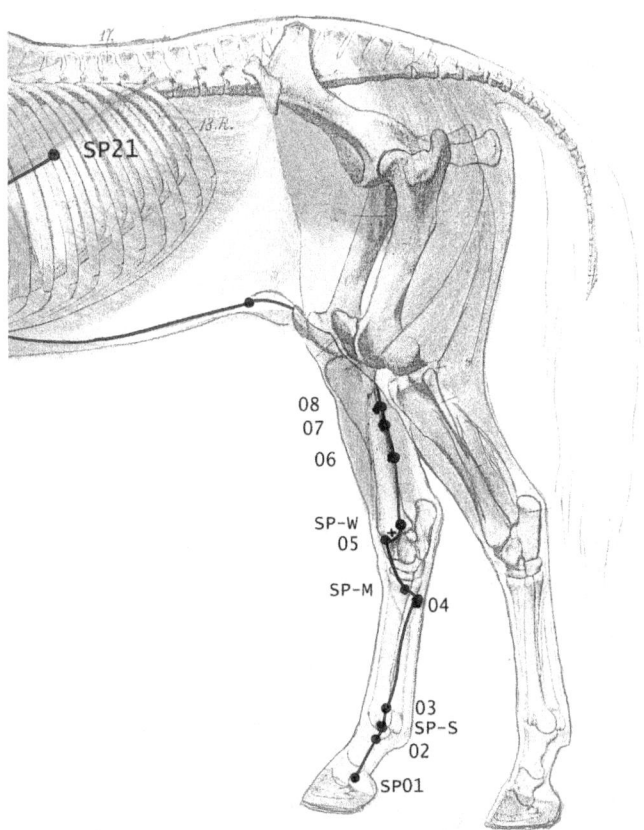

Figure 47; The most important points on the SP Channel in horses.

HT (Heart, Hand Shaoyin) Channel uses the connective tissue around *A. mediana, A. prof.antebrachii, A. palmaris lat., A. mtcp. palm. prof. lat., A/V. digit. lat. and A/V. coronalis phal. III.* as the main pathways for carrying its impulses.

Anatomically it begins:

In horses
The deep path of the Heart meridian has 3 branches:
1. The first branch begins in the depth, within the heart itself, and travels caudally through the diaphragm to connect with the Small Intestine.

2. One branch starts in the heart, travels cranially along the esophagus, across the cheek and ends in the area around the eyes.

3. Another branch starts in the heart, travels directly to the lungs, and surfaces in the axilla at HT01.

The superficial path of the Heart meridian:

- Travels from HT01 in the axilla, distally on the medial aspect of the thoracic limb, between M. flexor carpi ulnaris and M. flexor carpi radialis, passing the chestnut on its caudal border; *A. mediana, branch of; A. prof. Antebrachii,*

- Passes Os accessories on its medial side and turns to the lateral aspect of the leg; *A. palmaris lat.*

- Continues distally on the palmar side of Os metacarpale IV; *A. mtcs. palm. prof. lat.,*

- Passes the fetlock on the lateral border of the deep digital flexor tendon; *A/V. digit. lat.,*

- To end at the coronary band, just dorsal to the lateral cartilage of the distal phalanx, ~ 90° lateral to the tip of the toe; *A. coronalis phal. III.*

In dogs the meridian starts at HT01 in the axilla. It descends the medial side of the arm to HT03 (at the medial end of the elbow crease). From here, it descends the ulnar side of the palmar side of the forearm to HT07 (on radial side of flexor carpi ulnaris, between the ulna and pisiform on the carpal (wrist) crease). From here, it runs to HT08 (between metacarpal bones 4-5 on the palm), to end at HT09, at the radial side of the claw-root of the 5th claw.

In humans HT01 is located in the axilla. It descends the medial side of the arm to HT03 (at the medial end of the elbow crease). From here, it descends the ulnar side of the palmar side of the forearm to HT07 (on radial side of flexor carpi ulnaris, between the ulna and pisiform on the carpal (wrist) crease). From here, it runs to HT08 (between metacarpal bones 4-5 on the palm), to end at HT09, at the radial side of the nail-root of the little (5th) finger.

Phase	Metal		Earth		Fire		Water		Fire		Wood
Yin Channel	LU[1]		SP[4]	>>	HT[1]		KI[4]	>>	PC[1]		LV[4]
	‖		‖		‖		‖		‖		‖
Yang Channel	LI[2]	>>	ST[3]		SI[2]	>>	BL[3]		TH[2]	>>	GB[3]
Limb	Hand		Foot		Hand		Foot		Hand		Foot

(‖ and >>) mean that Qi Flow sequence is LU-LI-ST-SP, etc; |
| = Yin-Yang Phase Mates (Partners);
[1] Qi flow from chest to hand; [2] Qi flow from hand to face; [3]
Qi flow from face to foot; [4] Qi flow from foot to chest

Table 57

HT Qi comes from SP and flows into (connects with) SI Channel, its Yang Mate in Fire. As in the case of all the other Yin Channels in animals, HT Channel is much more important than its paired Yang Channel (SI). HT Channel relates to the heart and thus to the whole blood circulation of the entire body. All Lesion-Symptom Complexes or changes related to blood circulation can therefore come from a Process Imbalance in HT Channel.

Here we will discuss some heretical ideas about what propels the blood. The human heart has an output effect power of approximately 1.7 W. This is far too little to force such a great volume as 5 l through all the vessels and arterioles of the body. Also, during bypass operations (when the heart is taken out of the circulation), the blood moves **faster** *than if the heart was in the circulation (personal communication with Dr. Wollf, MD, Germany). It is true that death occurs or that the patient usually faints when the heart stops but this fact shows that the heart drives the blood as little as the hose pipe drives the water. As a kink in a hose pipe stops water flow, an obstructed blood vessel restricts blood flow. This shows that other forces govern the movement of the blood and that the heart just adds rhythmical force and regulates the flow. I will leave unanswered the question of whether these forces depend on the rhythmical movements in the blood vessels, or if the blood itself has a genuine ability to move like the white blood cells. However, it is this total blood circulation we refer to when we talk about HT Process.*

Lesion-Symptom Complexes can, as mentioned earlier, manifest differently in different species. Reduced blood circulation (both regional and local) usually occur in bovine mastitis. Reduced blood circulation (regional and general) in calves can manifest as diarrhea, whereas, in horses (local, regional and general), it usually manifests as joint-pain or arthralgia.

Lesion-Symptom Complexes that originate from HT Channel usually show a specific characteristic; they occur in many locations, especially when the symptom manifests as a joint-related lameness. One week the left forefetlock may be sore, the next week it may be the right tarsus. In diarrhea of neonatal animals, we usually see variable symptoms: green, yellow, profuse diarrhea, and sometimes constipation. In relation to dogs and cats, the symptoms are even more diverse than in horses and cows. This relates to the fact that dogs and cats are not as specialised (they have multiple purposes) as horses and cows and can thereby display a much greater variation in Lesion-Symptom Complexes. Then Lesion-Symptom Complexes such as rheumatism, arthritis, eczema and chronic inflammation can arise due to a Process Imbalance in HT Channel.

HT Channel also relates to obvious psychic symptoms. A Process Imbalance in HT often induces depression, sadness, apathy (lack of motivation) and dissatisfaction. After treatment of HT, owners often comment that the horse or dog has become high spirited, happy, playful and satisfied, and looks rejuvenated, like it was 2 or 3 years ago.

One can expect some success in treating functional heart disorders, such as rhythm defects and circulatory disorders. One also may have some success even in anatomical disorders that cause systolic murmur, such as valve defects, or rather the effects of such defects, as I assume that the anatomical defects remain unchanged. Homeopathic remedies, especially gold, also can influence HT Channel and homeopathy combines well with AP. (See the relationship between homeopathy and AP, page 546). In accordance with the Chinese Qi Clock, around noon (1200h) is the best time of day to treat HT Channel. (See also biorhythms page 31).

The energy in the heart meridian (Qi) may, as for the heart-process itself be in:

- *Excess*

- *Deficiency*

Particular for the meridian the energy may also be:

- *Destructive*

- *Blocked*

Excess show itself rather seldom as pain, as this is a Yin meridian, and Yin meridians seldom show excesses as pain (contrary to Yang-meridians which often show excesses as painful points or areas). An excess in the Heart-meridian, although very seldom, may be the result of a deficiency in the Kidney-process. An excess in the Heart meridian usually passes without observation or unpleasant symptoms.

Deficiency is a much more common and serious pathological finding than excess. Such a deficiency show itself in the same way as described under the heart-process on page 75. In addition we may find skin-changes in the form of eczema along the Heart-meridian.

A deficiency in the Heart meridian will often lead to an excess of the Large Intestine- or Bladder-meridian, and pain along these meridians may be the result.

This pain is often the symptoms we are confronted with in our daily practise.

Destructivity show itself as in all animals as particular vicious symptoms of the skin, erosions and wounds (see more about destructive energy on page XXXIV).

Blockage of the Heart-meridian is caused by a trauma on the structures of connective tissue that lead the impulses travelling through this meridian. Such a trauma will not hurt or destroy the energy of the process itself, but hinder the Qi-flow in the meridian. This is why the pulse in such a case shows absolutely good health for the process, but the acupuncture points may show dis-balance. This disbalance shows excess above the trauma, and deficienct below the trauma.

HT 01	Jiquan (Highest Spring)
	In horses: In the axilla, 1 cun proximal to HT02, 2 cun proximal to HT03. *In dogs:* it is deep in the centre of axilla, medial to axillary artery. *In humans:* it is deep in the centre of axilla, medial to axillary artery. *Effect:* It is the Entry Point of Qi to HT Channel (uppermost source). HT01 increases Qi in the whole Channel, just as HT07 (HT07 is in some sources labelled as the Sedation Point; but it seems to me that no point is really a genuine sedation point. A point may have a sedative effect if the meridian it

	controls has too much energy, but if it has too little energy the point acts as a stimulating point. The traditional sedating point has only a controlling effect). HT01 may also be labelled as a Source Point, as all of the initial points on Channels, i.e. point 1 on any Channel acts like a Source Point. Also, HT01 is a distant Alarm Point for HT (CV14 is the classic HT Mu Point), which means that if HT01 is painful to the touch, if there is something wrong with the heart organ itself.
HT 03	**Shaohai (Lesser Sea)** **Water Point of HT in humans** *In horses:* At the medial end of the transverse cubital crease, at the meeting point between M. pectoralis transversus, M. flexor carpi radialis and M. flexor carpi ulnaris. *In dogs:* it is midway between condylus mediale and the tendon of musculus biceps brachii. *In humans:* it is medial to the elbow joint, at medial end of elbow crease, with elbow flexed. *Effect:* It "**Boosts Qi and Blood**". It helps laziness, amnesia; throat and teeth, neck, thoracic limb, leg pains; ischemia of extremities, gangrene and lymphadenopathy.
HT 04 (-1 for hors-es)	**Lingdao (Spirit Pathway)** **Metal Point of HT in humans** *In horses:* In M. flexor carpi ulnaris, at the proximal, caudal corner of the chestnut. *In dogs:* it is 1.5 cun above the distal wrist crease, on ulnar side of flexor carpi ulnaris muscle. *In humans:* it is 1.5 cun above the distal wrist crease, on ulnar side of flexor carpi ulnaris muscle. *Effect:* It is important for painful states in the carpus of both horses and dogs.
HT 04 (-2 for hors-es)	**Extrapoint in horses** *Location;* In M. flexor carpi ulnaris, at the distal, caudal corner of the chestnut.

HT 05	**Tongli (Connecting Li)**
	Luo Point of HT: It connects HT Channel with its Phase Mate, SI Channel.
	In horses: Directly distal to the chestnut, in the groove between M. flexor carpi radialis and M. flexor carpi ulnaris.
	In dogs: it is 1 cun above distal carpus (wrist) crease, on ulnar side of flexor carpi ulnaris muscle.
	In humans: it is 1 cun above distal carpus (wrist) crease, on ulnar side of flexor carpi ulnaris muscle.
	Effect: It helps the heart and pericardium and in speech and tongue disorders.
HT 06	**Yinxi (Yin Cleft)**
	Xi Point of HT:
	In horses: 1 cun distal to HT-W, at the level of the medial distal Tuberositas radii, between the tendons of M. flex. carpi ulnaris and M. flex. digit. superficialis.
	In dogs: it is 0.5 cun above distal (carpal) wrist crease, on ulnar side of flexor carpi ulnaris muscle.
	In humans: it is 0.5 cun above distal (carpal) wrist crease, on ulnar side of flexor carpi ulnaris muscle.
	Effect: It helps acute diseases. It helps states that place an acute strain on the circulation or heart such as sunstroke, shock and acute HT disorders. It also helps chills and sweating disorders.
HT 07	**Shenmen (Shen-Spirit Gate)**
	Source-point in horses
	Earth and Source Point in dogs and humans
	Master Point of the Upper Body in all species
	In horses: On the mediopalmar aspect of the forearm, at the level of the antebrachiocarpal joint, 0.5 cun distal to HT06, on the medial side of Os accessorius.

	In dogs: it is on the wrist crease, on radial side of flexor carpi ulnaris, between the ulna and pisiform. *In humans:* it is on the wrist crease, on radial side of flexor carpi ulnaris, between the ulna and pisiform. *Effect:* It is the most important point on HT Channel, with the possible exception of the Ting-point, HT09. Its name indicates that it has strong psychic effects. Its sedative effect is somewhat like BL02, only it is stronger and more long lasting, and it helps the circulation It also helps the suspensory ligament and the flexor tendons. Its Earth Phase action helps chronic states such as stagnant swellings of the fetlock (Earth relates to long lasting states). Also, it counteracts pain in the upper body, possibly via the endorphin mechanism. It helps the mind, psyche, amnesia; back, thoracic organs and functions, heart, pericardium, blood circulation, blood pressure; forearm, radius and ulna.
HT 08	**Shaofu (Lesser Mansion)** **Earth point in horses, fire point in dogs** **(Ying-Spring and Fire point in Humans)** *Qian Chan Wan; extra point according to Van den Bosch/Guray* *In horses:* Just proximal and dorsal to the lateral proximal sesamoid bone, in a depression between the lateral tendon of the interosseus and the deep digital flexor tendon. *In dogs:* it is at the caudo-lateral aspect of the metacarpal pad. *In humans:* it is in the palm, between metacarpals 4-5, where finger 5 touches when fist clenched. *Effect:* As a command Point, it influences all states within the body where earth- or circulatory changes dominate the symptoms.
HT 09	**Shaochong (Lesser Surge)** **Ting-, Wood- and Tonification Point of HT:** *In horses:* At the coronary band, just dorsal to the lateral cartilage of the distal phalanx of the front leg, ~ 90^0 lateral to the tip of the toe. It can be punctured both from the back and from the side.

In dogs: it is 0.1 cun from the posterior edge of nail-root of finger 5, axial side (a little more proximal than in humans, at the junction between phalanx I and II).

In humans: it is 0.1 cun from the posterior edge of nail-root of finger 5, axial side.

Effect: Because it is a Wood Point, HT09 has special relevance for the muscles and "warm" growth states (a "growth state" is when the symptoms show growth of the tissues). An example of this can be warm muscles-knots. It also works in states where there is too little joint fluid production, especially if there is heat or inflammation in the joint, or it is dried up. The joint needs "fluids". It is used after operations and joint injections that have led to infected and swollen joints. HT09 also has surprising effects on the heart organ itself. I have noted that use (stimulation) of HT09 often completely eliminated pathological sounds over the heart. I was asked to treat a colt with serious heart disorders and profound fatigue. It was very weakened and had strong pathological sounds over the heart. Two colleagues were present and they became angry with me for even attempting something like this. They thought that I should at least not charge anything for so hopeless an attempt. Since this stable was far from where I live, I asked the two vets to drop by the following week to check on the colt. This they did, and after one of them had listened and admitted that the heart sounded normal (and actually the colt had no more symptoms of fatigue), the other vet refused to listen (in reference to Galileo Galilei). The colt was better for at least a year and I have not heard anything from the owner in several years. HT09 also helps amnesia.

Table 58

The special commandpoints in the horse are as follows:

W A T E R	*Location*; Proximal to Os accessories, at the caudomedial aspect of the forearm, between the tendons of M. flexor carpi ulnaris and M. flex. digit. superficialis, caudal to the PC-Water point and 1 cun proximal to the medial distal Tuberositas radii. *Effect*; Influences conditions caracterised by "watery" symptoms locally and along the course of the meridian, and generally in the body when the Heart is in excess or deficiency. Local problems of the carpus, related to the production of synovia and blood circulation in the area.
M E T A L	*Location*; Just distal to the carpus, on the lateropalmar aspect, between the two digital flexor tendons. *Effect*; Influences painful conditions locally and along the course of the meridian, and generally in the body when the Heart is in excess or deficiency.
S O U R C E fetlock	*Location*; On the lateral aspect of the fetlock, at the level of the metacarpophalangeal joint, palmar to the A/V. digitalis. *Effect;* Stimulates the meridian.
E A R T H	*Location:* Just over the fetlock, on the lateral aspect *Effect:* Stimulates the meridian in an earth-like way
F I R E	*Location*; Just distal to the fetlock, dorsal to the lateral border of the deep digital flexor tendon. **Effect**; Influences circulatory and heat related conditions locally and along the course of the meridian, and generally in the body when the Heart is in excess or deficiency. Fire point on a fire meridian; Horary point.

Table 59

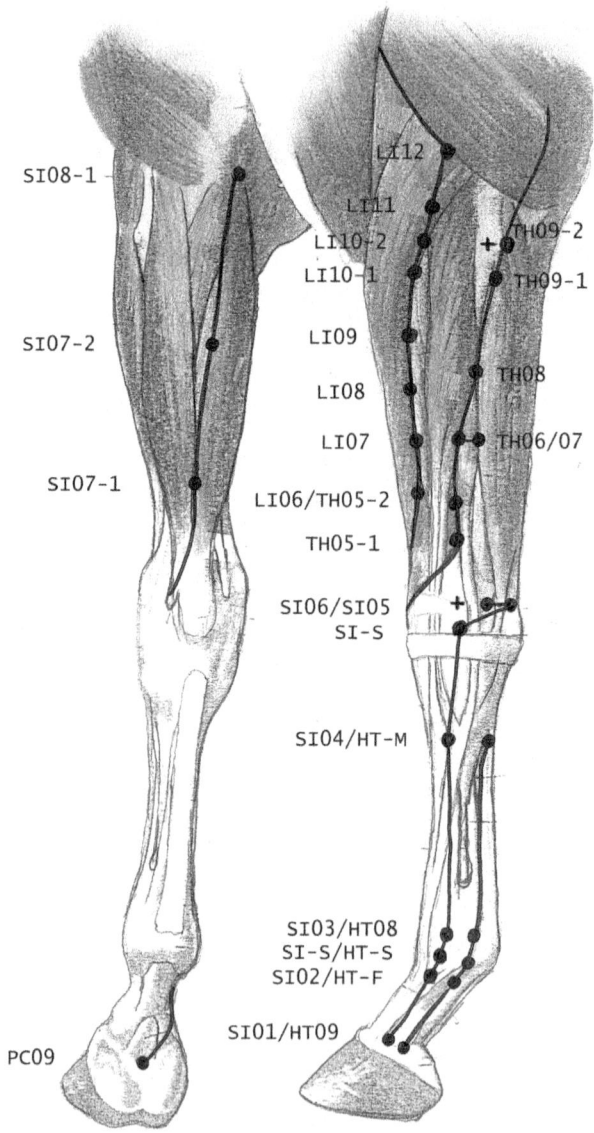

SI08-1

LI12

LI11

LI10-2 ✛ TH09-2

LI10-1 TH09-1

SI07-2 LI09

LI08 TH08

LI07 TH06/07

SI07-1 LI06/TH05-2

TH05-1

SI06/SI05
SI-S ✛

SI04/HT-M

SI03/HT08
SI-S/HT-S
SI02/HT-F

SI01/HT09

PC09

*Figure 48, Some of the most important points
on the HT/SI/LI/TH meridians in the horse*

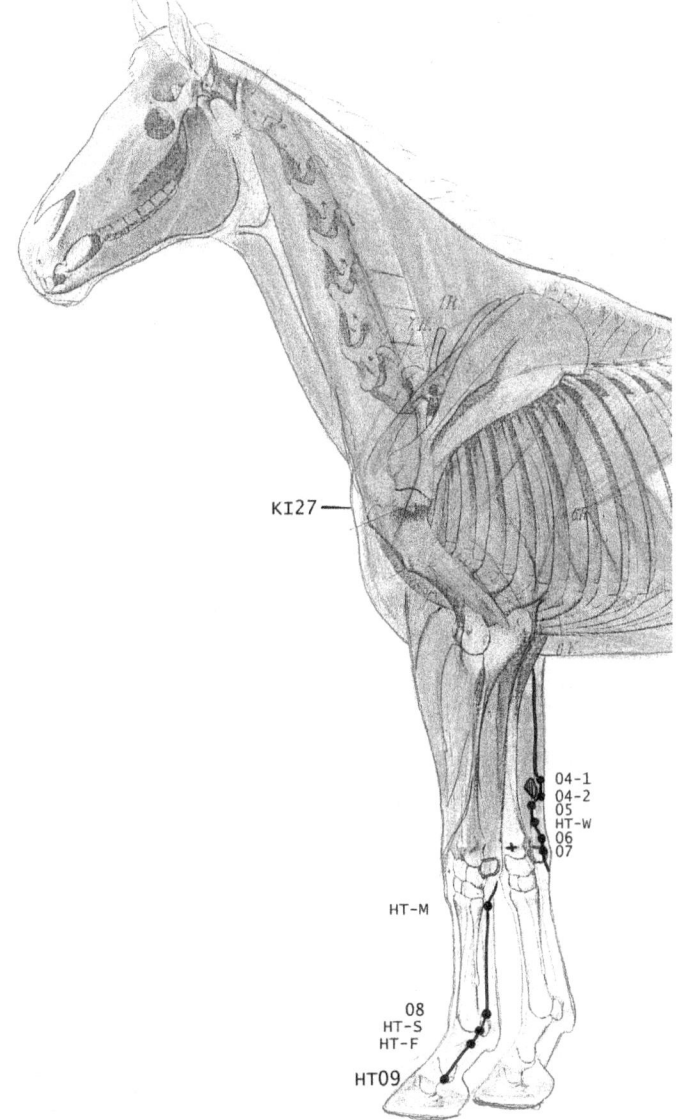

KI27

04-1
04-2
05
HT-W
06
07

HT-M

08
HT-S
HT-F

HT09

Figure 49; Some of the more important points on the HT Channels in the horse.

SI (Small Intestine, Hand Taiyang) Channel uses the connective tissue around *A/V. coronalis phal. III, A. mtcs. dors. lat., A. collateralis ulnaris, A. collateralis ulnaris, A/V. subscapularis, A/V. circumfl. scap., A/V. cerv.prof., A/V. cerv. prof. och A/V. vertebralis, A/V. transversa faciei, A/V. temporalis superfic. A/V. tempor.*

superfic., A/V. auricularis magna., A/V. auricularis magna. as the main pathways for carrying its impulses:

Anatomically it begins:

IN HORSES
The superficial path of the Small Intestine meridian:

- Begins at the coronary band on the thoracic limb, ~ 55⁰ lateral to the tip of the toe; *A/V. coronalis phal. III,*

- Ascends along the dorsolateral aspect of the phalanges and dorsal to Os metacarpale IV; *A. mtcs. dors. lat.*

- Follows the tendon of M. ulnaris lateralis towards caudal; a branch of *A. collateralis ulnaris,*

- Continues along the caudal side of the frontleg, between M. ulnaris lateralis and M. flexor carpi rad., and further proximally between M. flex. carpi uln. and M. flex. digit. prof., reaching the medial side of the elbow; *A. collateralis ulnaris,*

- Travels along the caudal border of the medial epicondyle of the humerus and traverses the M. triceps brachii, (intersects LI14), to the caudal part of the shoulder joint,

- Follows the caudal border of the scapula; *A/V. subscapularis,* to the area of the caudal angle of the scapula; *A/V. circumfl. scap.,*

- zig-zags cranially over the scapula,

- Ascends along the neck, dorsal to the cervical vertebrae as far as the second cervical vertebra, C2; *A/V. cerv.prof.,*

- Crosses the cervical column between the C2 and C3; anastomoses between *A/V. cerv. prof.* and *A. et V. vertebralis,*

- Crosses the cheek along the ventral border of Crista facialis; *A/V. transversa faciei,* SI18,

- Sends a branch to the medial canthus of the eye, where it meets with the Bladder meridian, at BL01.

- Another branch travels from the caudal border of the mandible to the lateral canthus of the eye, where it meets with the Gall Bladder meridian, at GB01; branches from *A/V. temporalis superfic.*

- The meridian continues dorsally and medially to the ear where it intersects with the Gall Bladder meridian again, at GB11, and with the Triple Heater meridian, at TH20 and TH22; branches of *A/V. tempor.superfic.* and *A/V. auricularis magna,* enters the ear at SI19, rostroventral to the base of the ear; *A/V. auricularis magna.*

The deep path of the Small Intestine meridian has the following branches:

1. One branch from SI14 and SI15 to GV14, intersects with the Bladder meridian at BL11,

   - descends via ST12 and connects with the Heart, travels along the esophagus,

   - intersects the Conception vessel at CV17 and passes through the diaphragm to the Stomach,

   - Intersects the Conception vessel again at CV13 and CV12 and enters the Small Intestine.

2. Another branch descends from the Small Intestine, to ST39, the lower he-sea point of the Small Intestine.

In dogs begins at SI01, on the ulnar edge (abaxial, lateral) of the nail root of the 5th claw. It travels along the ulnar edge of the little finger and hand, up the ulnar side of the forearm to SI08 (between the medial epicondyle of humerus and olecranon of the ulna). From here it ascends the back of the arm to SI09 (1 cun above the posterior axillary crease), to zigzag over the scapular spine to SI15, 2' lateral to GV14. From here it runs through SI16 and SI17 on the lateral neck, to the face (SI18, under the zygomatic bone, to end at SI19 in front of the ear.

In humans begins at SI01, on the ulnar edge (abaxial, lateral) of the nail root of the little finger (5th finger). It travels along the ulnar edge of the little finger and hand, up the ulnar side of the forearm to SI08 (between the medial epicondyle of humerus and olecranon of the ulna; the 'funny bone' point). From here it ascends the back of the arm to SI09 (1 cun above the posterior axillary crease), to zigzag over the scapular spine to SI15, 2 cun lateral to GV14. From here it runs through SI16 and SI17 on the lateral neck, to the face (SI18, under the zygomatic bone, to end at SI19 in front of the ear.

Phase	Metal		Earth		Fire		Water		Fire		Wood
Yin Channel	LU(1)		SP(4)	>>	HT(1)		KI(4)	>>	PC(1)		LV(4)
	||		||		||		||		||		||
Yang Channel	LI(2)	>>	ST(3)		SI(2)	>>	BL(3)		TH(2)	>>	GB(3)
Limb	Hand		Foot		Hand		Foot		Hand		Foot

(\|\| and >>) mean that Qi Flow sequence is LU-LI-ST-SP, etc;
\|\| = Yin-Yang Phase Mates (Partners);
(1) Qi flow from chest to hand; (2) Qi flow from hand to face; (3)
Qi flow from face to foot; (4) Qi flow from foot to chest

Table 60

SI Qi comes from HT, its Yin Mate in Fire, and flows into (connects with) BL Channel. Anatomically, SI is comprised of jejunum, ileum and duodenum, and controls the decomposition of and absorption of food. Since HT and SI Channels connect and belong to the Fire Phase, SI Channel also has great influence on the circulation, especially the blood circulation in the digestive tract, the lumbar area and the neck. Patients with a strongly decresed absorption of foodstuffs from the intestines, often have a deficiency in the SI-meridian or Process.

In my practice I often see that a deficient Process SI Channel often arises together with a deficient Process in SP Channel. SP is mainly important for venous circulation in the digestive tract, especially in the intestines. In a weakness of the venous circuit in the digestive tract, this can influence the arterial circuit adversely and vice versa. This is why a deficiency in SP and SI often manifests similar pathology.

In calves we often find an imbalance in SI Channel related to diarrhea. In horses we find SI Channel more related to disorders on the left side of the neck (LU Channel reacts to disorders on the right side). In humans we usually find SI Deficiency in cases of chronic diarrhea, as in patients with Celiac Disease and Crohn's Disease. In accordance with the Chinese Qi Clock, around 1400h is the best time of day to treat SI Channel.

The energy in the Small Intestine Meridian (Qi) may, as for the small intestine-process itself, be in:

- *Excess*

- *Deficiency*

Particular for the meridian the energy may also be:

- *Destructive*

- *Blocked*

Excess show itself usually as pain, as this is a Yang meridian, and Yang meridians usually show excesses as pain (contrary to Ying-meridians which often show excesses just as an elevated and positive function of the process). An excess in the Small Intestine-meridian may be the result of a deficiency in the Kidney-process.

Deficiency in a Yang meridian is much more seldom as it is in a Yin meridian, exept for the Small Intestine- and the Triple Heater-meridians. A deficiency expresses itself as underfunction of the associated organ, as underfunction in the associated muscles and in the skin-area transversed by the meridian, as described on page 79. In the Small Intestine meridian this may result in a decreased function of the small intestine, and a marked decrease in the absorption of food-stuffs from the intestines and a marked weight loss. Also a dysfunction of the Mm. supraspinatus, infraspinatus, trapetzius, deltiodeus and triceps, also in the depth Musculus teres major, and/or skin changes along the path of the meridian see page 323.

A deficiency of the Small Intestine meridian mat also cause an excess in the Bladder- or/and Large Intestine-meridians, and pain along these meridians may be the result. This pain is often the symptoms we see most easily.

Destructivity show itself as in all animals as particular vicious symptoms of the skin, erosions and wounds (see more about destructive energy on page XXXIV).

Blockage of the Small Intestine-meridian is caused by a trauma on the structures of connective tissue that lead the impulses travelling through this meridian. Such a trauma will not hurt or destroy the energy of the process itself, but hinder the Qi-flow in the meridian. This is why the pulse in such a case shows absolutely good health for the process, but the acupuncture points may show dis-balance. This disbalance shows excess above the trauma, and deficienct below the trauma.

SI 01	**Shaoze (Lesser Marsh)**
	Ting point in horses and dogs, as well as a Wood point (Jing-Well and Metal point in Humans)
	In horses: At the coronary band of the thoracic limb, ~ 55⁰ lateral to the tip of the toe.
	In dogs: it is 0.1 cun from posterior edge of nail-root of the 5th claw on the front leg, ulnar side.
	In humans: it is 0.1 cun from posterior edge of nail-root of finger 5, ulnar side.
	Effect: This point has a marked effect on the lateral muscles of the front leg, and treatment of this point may cause the front leg to move quite a few cm more laterally in races. This point is also very effective in many cases of emaciation (cahexia), thin and seemingly malnutritioned animals. The owner reports that the horse or dog has ample food, but "it don't put weight on". After treating this point just once, I am often presented to quite a different animal after just a few weeks.
	Also, SI01 helps pain along SI Channel, the left shoulder and the left side of the neck, and also locally. It also helps pain and inflammation of the mucus membranes, and has a special affinity to the mammary gland.

SI 02	**Qiangu (Front Valley)**
	Fire point in horses and dogs **(Human Ying-spring and Water point)** **Si Guan; extra point according to Van den Bosch/Guray** *In horses:* Just distal to the fetlock joint, in a small depression dorsal to the lateral tendon of interrosseus to the extensor digital tendon. *In dogs:* it is at the ulnar (lateral) side of metacarpophalangeal joint of the 5th foretoe, the most lateral. *In humans:* it is at the ulnar (lateral) side of metacarpophalangeal joint of the 5th finger. Clears heat especially from the exterior; nose, eyes and ears; redness of the eyes, congested nose, and from the Lung and throat; cough, pharyngitis, fever.
SI 03	**Houxi (Back Xi-Cleft (Ravine))** **Earth point** **(Shu-stream and Wood point in Humans)** **Confluent point for GV** *In horses:* Just proximal to the fetlock, in a small depression on the dorsolateral aspect of the large metacarpal bone. *In dogs:* it is at the junction of the hand dorsum and palm, at the ulnar edge of the hand, proximal to the distal head of the 5th metacarpal bone. *In humans:* it is at the junction of the hand dorsum and palm, at the ulnar edge of the hand, proximal to the distal head of the 5th metacarpal bone. *Effect:* As an *Earth Point*, it thus influences "degenerative states" in the entire organism, somewhat like the SP-meridian itself (Earth-meridian). As the wife of the wood-element, it also helps muscular disorders. This action on both degenerative and muscular problems may be very marked sometimes. An English setter had got his right forelimb completely destroyed and crushed under the wheel of a car, broken in several places and the limb had healed (grown) together in a position where the limb was twisted outwards 45° and the dog had chronic and continuous pain. I just treated SI03 and was on my way out of

	the treatment room when a yell from the owner called me back. The paw was literally twisting itself back to normal position and stopped only 5° out of normal alignment. After this one treatment the dog could run in the mountains for several hours without getting tired, as he had done before. The GV runs in the dorsal midline along the spine. Stimulation of SI03 (together with BL62) activates this meridian, and thus increases blood circulation along the spine. This is very important in all spinal or paraspinal problems. Dogs may often develop severe pain along the spine, and the body will then try to eliminate this pain by hindering the movement of the spinal joints. The best way to do this is by calcification. This condition is called spondylosis. Spondylosis itself does not cause pain, the calcification is a response to the pain and unstability of the spine, and the following calcification is just a response to this pain and lack of stability. If the calcification becomes severe, this may lead to further problems like invalidity. SI03/BL62 may be used alone in this syndrome, as it takes away the pain. When the pain is gone, there will be no need for further calcifications, and the whole condition is relieved. This also applies in calcification and pain in the neck and cervical spine. It also helps the vertex, occiput, thoracic limb, hand, palm, metacarpus, finger; infections (cholera, herpes, malaria, rubella, TB, typhoid, typhus, varicella etc) and sweating disorders. *SI03 + BL62* is a classical combination for disorders mediated by the spine or GV, including bilaterally symmetrical skin disorders or pain in both forelimbs and / or both hindlimbs. The combination (treat SI03 before BL62) activates GV and the entire spine. It markedly improves the Lesion-Symptom Complexes after a few weeks.
SI 04	**Wangu (Wrist Bone)** **Metal point** **(Yuan-Source point in Humans)** *In horses:* On the dorsolateral aspect of the large metacarpal bone, just distal to the carpus, dorsal to the tendon of M. extensor digit. lat. *In dogs:* it is between metacarpal 5 and the hamate bone (the 4th carpal bone), radial side. *In humans:* it is between metacarpal 5 and the hamate bone (the 4th carpal bone), radial side. *Effect:* It helps the carpus, metacarpus, hand, palm and finger,

SI 05	**Yanggu (Yang Valley)** **Water point in horses** **Metal Point in dogs** **(Jing-River and Fire point in Humans)** *In horses:* Just proximal to Os accessorius, between the two tendons of insertion of M. ulnaris lateralis. *In dogs:* it is at ulnar side of ulnocarpal joint, between ulnar styloid and triquetal bone (the "ulnar carpal bone"). *In humans:* it is at ulnar side of ulnocarpal joint, between ulnar styloid and triquetal bone (the "ulnar carpal bone"). *Effect:* It helps salivation, salivary glands and upper teeth. As a command-Point it helps conditions along the entire meridian.
SI 06	**Yanglao (Nursing the Aged)** **Xi Point of SI:** *In horses:* At the level of the lateral distal Tuberositas radii, just cranial to SI05, immediately caudal to the tendon of M. ext. digit. lateralis. *In dogs:* it is on forearm-dorsum, in bony cleft on radial side of ulnar styloid, above the distal head of ulna. *In humans:* it is on forearm-dorsum, in bony cleft on radial side of ulnar styloid, above the distal head of ulna. *Effect:* It helps the coccyx, and all acute situations.
SI 07 **(-1 in horses)**	**Zhizheng (Branch to the Correct)** **Luo Point of SI** *(It connects SI Channel with its Phase Mate, HT Channel)* *In horses:* On the caudal midline of the thoracic limb, at the level of the distal border of the chestnut, between Mm. ulnaris lateralis and flexor carpi ulnaris. *In dogs:* it is situated on the lateral aspect of the forelimb about half way between the carpus and the cubital fossa, on the cranial edge of musculus ulnaris lateralis. *In humans:* it is on forearm-dorsum, on the radial side of the ulna, 5 cun above SI05 (carpus, wrist), 7 cun below SI08 (elbow).

	Effect: It helps the chin, elbow and finger. It connect the SI with the HT, and if it is used it opens the gates of the SI meridian so that a surplus of energy in this meridian may flow over to the HT meridian. If we also needle the source-point of the HT-meridian (HT07) it further helps the flow of energy from SI to HT.
SI 07-2	**Extra point in horses** *Location;* 4 cun proximal to SI07-1, on the caudal midline of the thoracic limb, between Mm. flexor carpi ulnaris and flexor digit. prof.
SI 08 **(-1 in horses)**	**Xiaohai (Small Sea)** **Local point in horses, Water Point in dogs** *(He-Sea and Earth point in Humans)* *In horses:* In the most caudal part of the medial side of the forearm, on the borderline between Mm. pectoralis transversus and flexor carpi ulnaris. *In dogs:* it is between the medial epicondyle of the humerus and olecranon of the ulna. *In humans:* it is between the medial epicondyle of the humerus and olecranon of the ulna (the 'funny bone' point). *Effect:* It has a marked effect on the whole area from the groin to the back of the head. It stimulates blood circulation in this area. It also helps the forearm, radius and ulna.
SI 08-2	**Extra point in horses** *Location;* 1.5 cun proximal to SI08-1.
SI 09	**Jianzhen (Shoulder True)** *In horses:* In the long head of M. triceps brachii, on the caudal border of M. deltoideus, at the level of Tuberculum majus. *In dogs:* it is just behind the humerus, about half way between the olecranon and the shoulder joint. *In humans:* it is 1 cun above the top of the posterior axillary crease.

	Effect: It helps especially Hot Syndromes in the scapula, shoulder, clavicle, axilla, arm and humerus.
SI 10	**Naoshu (Upper Arm Shu)** **Meeting point of the SI and BL meridians with the Yang Qiao and Yang Wei mai** *In horses:* In a small depression in M. deltoideus, on the caudal border of the scapula, at the level of the ventral end of Spina scapulae. *In dogs:* directly above SI09, in a depression inferior and lateral to the scapular spine. *In humans:* This point is situated directly above SI09, in a depression inferior and lateral to the scapular spine. *Effect*; Shoulder problems.
SI 11 (-1 in hors-es)	**Tianzong (Heavenly Gathering)** *In horses:* On the scapula, close to the caudal angle, between the thoracic part of M. trapezius, M. deltoideus and M. latissimus dorsi. *In dogs:* it is in center of the scapula, in the infraspinatus muscle, 1/3 the distance from the scapular spine to the inferior angle of the scapula. *In humans:* it is in center of the scapula, in the infraspinatus muscle, 1/3 the distance from the scapular spine to the inferior angle of the scapula. *Effect:* It helps with pain when the forelimb is moved backwards. It also helps the shoulder, scapula, clavicle, arm and humerus; mammary disorders, mastopathy and milk disorders.
SI 11-2	**Extra point in horses** **Bo Lan; according to Van den Bosch/Guray** *Location*; 2 cun ventral to SI11-1.

SI 12	**Bingfeng (Grasping the Wind)** **Meeting point between the SI, LI, TH and GB meridians** *In horses:* In a small depression cranial to and at the level of Tuber spinae scapulae, between M. supraspinatus and M. subclavius. *In dogs:* In the centre of the suprascapular fossa, directly above SI11. *In humans:* In the centre of the suprascapular fossa, directly above SI11. When the arm is lifted it is at the site of the depression. *Effect;* Expels wind; painful conditions in the shoulder and scapula.
SI 16 (-1 for hors- es)	**Tianchuang (Heavenly Window)** **Window of the sky point** *In horses:* In M. brachiocephalicus, at the level of the ventral border of the mandibula, ventral to and between the second and third cervical vertebrae, dorsal to LI18-1. *In dogs:* just behind vertebrae C4, which is about in the middle of the neck. *In humans:* at the posterior edge of the sternocleidomastoid muscle, level with CV23 (just above the laryngeal prominence). *Effect:* It is one of the "**Windows of the Sky**" Points (see LI18). It helps infections in the throat and lungs and in disorders in the cervical spine and neck.
SI 16-2	**Extra point in horses** *Location;* In M. splenius, just dorsal to the intervertebral space between the 4th and 5th cervical vertebrae. *Effect;* Similar to SI16-1.

SI 18	Quanliao (Cheek Bone Hole)
	Meeting point between the SI and TH meridians
	In horses: Ventral to the facial crest, on an oblique line towards rostral and ventral, from the lateral canthus of the eye.
	In dogs: just where the vertical line touching the lateral canthus of the eye crosses the horizontal line touching the distal aspect of the nose.
	In humans: just where the vertical line touching the lateral canthus of the eye crosses the horizontal line touching the distal aspect of the nose.
	Effect: This point stimulates ***all the Yang-meridians,*** and may be used when all the Yang-meridians are (show) Deficient (in pulse-diagnosis). A special section of the "Worn Out (Exhaustion) syndromes" is that all Yang meridians are depleted. (Another section is when all the Yin-meridians are depleted (SP06). Still another is when both the Yin- and the Yang-meridians are depleted (LU01).) This point is very useful in all such cases.
SI 19	**Tinggong (Hearing Palace)**
	Meeting point between the SI, TH and GB meridians
	In horses. In a depression, just rostroventrally to the base of the ear, directly ventral to GB02.
	In dogs: in a hole between ear tragus and temporomandibular joint, with the mouth slightly open.
	In humans: in a hole between ear tragus and temporomandibular joint, with the mouth slightly open.
	Effect: It helps disorders in the ear, Eustachian tube, hearing, masseter, mastoid, Meniere's disease and temporomandibular joint.

Table 61

The special commandpoints in the horse are as follows:

S O U R C E fetlock	*Location;* At the level of the metacarpophalangeal joint, dorsolaterally. *Effect;* Stimulates the meridian.
S O U R C E carpus	*Location;* On the lateral aspect of the carpus, at the level of the antebrachiocarpal joint, palmar to the tendon of M. ext. digit. communis. *Effect;* Stimulates the meridian.

Table 62

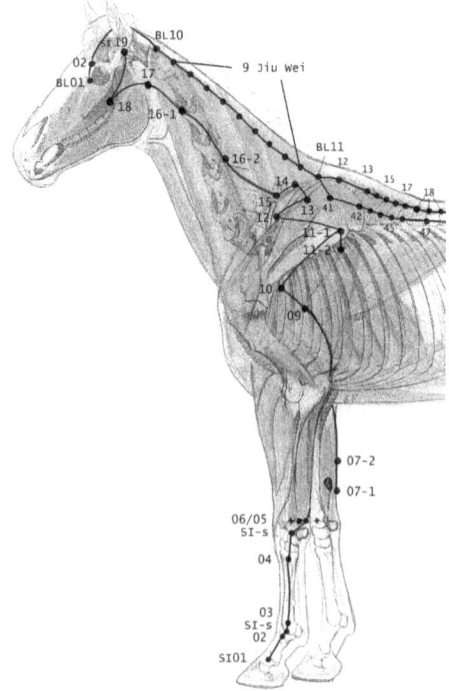

Figure 50; some of the most important points on the SI/BL-meridians in the horse.

BL (Bladder, Foot Taiyang) Channel uses the connective tissue around *A/V. angularis oculi, A. vertebralis, A/V. obturatoria, A/V. femoris caud. ramus asc., A/V. obturatoria. , A/V. gluteus cran.* och *A/V. gluteus caud., A. et V. vertebralis, A. et V. intercostalis, A. et V. Lumbalis, A. et V. gluteus caud., A/V. femoris caud. ascend.* och *A/V. tarsica recurrens, A/V. tarsica lat. A/V. mtts. plant. supf. lat., A/V. digit. lat., A/V. coronalis phal. III.* as the main pathways for carrying its impulses:

Anatomically it begins:

In horses:
The superficial path of the Bladder meridian:

- Begins at the medial canthus of the eye, at BL01; *A/V. angularis oculi,* and travels dorsocaudally along the forehead, where it contacts:

    ° GB15, GV24 and GV20.

- A branch is sent to the temporal area, medial to the ear, where it connects with the Gall Bladder meridian.

- The meridian travels caudally on the dorsal aspect of the neck and splits into two branches.

- The inner (medial) branch curves around the dorsal aspect of the scapular cartilage and continues 3 cun lateral to and along the dorsal midline.

- At the level of the 4th sacral foramen, the meridian turns cranial and medial to the first sacral foramen, at BL31,

- Travels caudally along the sacrum and the first coccygeal vertebrae until it reaches the muscular groove between M. biceps femoris and M. semitendinosus, *A/V. obturatoria,*

- Continues along the muscular groove to the popliteal fossa of the knee, BL40; *A/V. femoris caud. ramus asc.,* and anastomoses with *A/V. obturatoria.*

- The outer (lateral) branch travels, parallel to the inner branch, from to scapular cartilage, 5 cun lateral to the dorsal midline, to the gluteal region; A/V. *gluteus cran.* and A/V. *gluteus caud.*,

- Here it intersects with GB30, caudal and dorsal to the hip joint, and descends along M. biceps femoris, to meet with the inner branch at BL40.

- Along the neck, back and croup the Bladder points are located where the dorsal and lateral branches of A/V. *vertebralis*, A/V. *intercostalis* and A/V. *lumbalis*, as well as the spinal nerves emerge.

- A small branch leaves the main meridian just above the popliteal fossa, and travels between the medial and the caudal head of M. biceps femoris to the caudal part of the stifle joint, BL39.

- The meridian continues just cranial to the Achilles tendon; A/V. *femoris caud. ascend.* and A/V. *tarsica recurrens*,

- Continues lateral to Os calcaneus; A/V. *tarsica lat.*

- And plantar to the base of the fourth metatarsal bone, along the flexor tendons; A/V. *metatarsale plant. supf. lat.*,

- Follows the lateral border of the deep digital flexor tendon; A/V. *digit. lat.*,

- Ends at the coronary band, just dorsal to the lateral cartilage of the third phalanx, ~90° lateral to the tip of the toe; A/V.*coronalis phal. III.*

The deep path of the Bladder meridian:

1. One branch is sent from the area of GV20 to the brain, meets the Governing vessel at GV17 and then surfaces (to continue caudally along the dorsal part of the neck), BL10; A. *vertebralis*.

2. Another branch leaves the inner (medial) part of the meridian, in the lumbar area and penetrates deep into

the interior to connect with the Kidneys and link with the Bladder.

In dogs and in humans the meridian begins at BL01 in the medial canthus of the eye. It travels over the head to BL10 (medial and caudal to GB20, behind the occiput). Here, it splits into two lines, the inner line 1.5 cun, and the outer line 3 cun, from GV Line. Both lines run parallel down the paravertebral area from the neck to the sacrum. They continue down the posterolateral side of the thigh, to unite at BL40 in the center of the popliteal fossa. From here, one path of the deep BL-meridian runs upwards again to unite with the Bladder, and the superficial parth of the BL Channel runs as one line down the posterior midline of the leg to BL57 (midway from BL40 to the calcaneus), and then curves laterally to BL60 (level with the lateral malleolus of the tibia, between the malleolus and the Achilles tendon). From here it runs on the lateral side of the tarsus and metatarsus, to end at BL67 on the lateral side (abaxial) of the nailbed of the 5th toe (little toe).

Phase	Metal		Earth		Fire		Water		Fire		Wood
Yin Channel	LU(1)		SP(4)	>>	HT(1)		KI(4)	>>	PC(1)		LV(4)
	‖		‖		‖		‖		‖		‖
Yang Channel	LI(2)	>>	ST(3)		SI(2)	>>	BL(3)		TH(2)	>>	GB(3)
Limb	Hand		Foot		Hand		Foot		Hand		Foot

(‖ and >>) mean that Qi Flow sequence is LU-LI-ST-SP, etc;
‖ = Yin-Yang Phase Mates (Partners);
(1) Qi flow from chest to hand; (2) Qi flow from hand to face; (3) Qi flow from face to foot; (4) Qi flow from foot to chest

Table 63

BL Qi comes from SI and flows into (connects with) KI Channel, its Yin Mate in Water. BL-KI, the Yin-Yang Couple in Water, regulate all bodily water and fluids (together with the HT, PC, LV, LI, TH and SI). They are especially important in *fluid excretion*, including urine, sperms, ova and genital fluids.

BL Channel has 67 points in humans, the most points of any Channel. As there are 1 or 2 BL Points between each pair of vertebrae, dogs have at least 70 points and horses have at least 74 points. However, to avoid systematic problems caused by the variation of BL Point numbers between different species, we will consider only the transposition (in dogs) or partly transposition (in horses) of the 67 human points in all animals.

The Back Shu Points are Diagnostic Points that lie bilaterally and parallel to the spine along the inner pathway of BL Channel from the thorax to the sacrum. Each point relates to a different Channel or Process. When there is a Process Imbalance, usually Excess in a Channel, its related Back Shu Point usually becomes tender or hypersensitive. Thus, evaluation for pain or tenderness at the Back Shu Points can give a valid diagnosis of the Imbalanced Channel. (See the Back Shu Point method page 107). Reactivity at the Diagnostic Points indicates Process Imbalances in the related Channels; there may be nothing with BL Channel itself, unless the Back Shu of BL itself is reactive.

Some BL Points also have a special action on the psyche or emotions. They lie outside of the Back Shu Points for the 5 Yin Organs. These special "Spirit Points" are:

Shu Point	Organ	Spirit	Emotion influenced	Spirit Point	Translation
BL13	LU	Po	Grief, sadness	BL42-Pohu	Spirit Door
BL15	HT	Shen	Joy, excitement	BL44-Shentang	Spirit Hall
BL18	LV	Hun	Anger, envy, courage	BL47-Hunmen	Soul Gate
BL20	SP	Yi	Worry, obsession	BL49-Zhishe	Reflection Abode
BL23	KI	Zhi	Fear, terror, willpower	BL52-Zhishi	Will Chamber

Table 64

Thus, BL Channel is the most psychic Channel in its physiological manifestations. Consider how anguish, fear and other psychic states manifest. Severe fright or terror weaken Water (BL-KI) and may cause immediate involuntary urination and defecation (KI controls the "Lower Orifices"). Cold also precipitates a Weakest Process in BL-KI, causing similar psychic effects - we must pee often when we go out in cold weather in winter (below -10^{0}C). This last simple fact shows that BL-KI relate to the Water Phase. BL Channel therefore reacts to Cold and Cold Damp. Pain along BL Channel usually predominates most in winter.

BL Qi Deficiency often leads to bed wetting, lumbalgia, pain in the legs, damp (moist, sweaty) feet and headache. Many teenage and adult males who wet their beds have suffered mental, physical or sexual abuse as children. The abuser was often their father or an older brother or a close male relative. This abuse can cause subconscious Fear, which is the Internal Cause of KI Deficiency. Recognition (and elimination) of this fear cures many of these cases quickly, except where the mental trauma is severe.

In relation to the Process, however, BL has a more important, energetic function; it transfers Qi to KI. Though BL follows or is "downstream from" KI in anatomy and physiology, BL precedes or is "upstream of" KI in the Qi Clock, the 24 hour cycle of Qi (energy) flow through the Channel system.

Since BL is one of the most psychic Channels, Process Imbalances in BL Channel occur most often in humans and not so frequently in animals (remember that pain in the diagnostic points of the bladder-meridian do not indicate that the BL is imbalanced (except for BL28 which is the BL shu-point)!). Animals, especially dogs, show Process Imbalances (deficiency) in KI more often than in BL. Old dogs usually die from KI Deficiency. My geriatric dog practice centres mostly on keeping these old kidneys functional. In accordance with the Chinese Qi Clock, around 1600h is the best time of day to treat BL Channel.

The energy in the Bladder meridian (Qi) may, as for the Bladder-process itself be in:

- *Excess*

- *Deficiency*

Particular for the meridian the energy may also be:

- *Destructive*

- *Blocked*

Excess show itself usually as pain, as this is a Yang meridian, and Yang meridians usually show excesses as pain (contrary to Ying-meridians which often show excesses just as an elevated and positive function of the process). An excess in the bladder-meridian may be the result of a deficiency in the Heart, Pericardium or Spleen-processes.

Deficiency in a Yang meridian is much more seldom as it is in a Yin meridian. Often symptoms arising from Yang-meridians are due to excesses, but of course deficiencies are also found. A deficiency may express itself as underfunction of the associated organ, as underfunction in the associated muscles and in the skin-area transversed by the meridian. In the Bladder meridian this may result in stagnation of the urine in the bladder, dysfunction of the M. longissimus or skin changes along the path of the meridian, as described on page 80.

A deficiency in the Bladder meridian is often the cause of an excess in the Trippel Heather- or Small Intestine meridian, and pain along these meridians may be the result. This pain is often the symptoms we see most easily.

Destructivity show itself as in all animals as particular vicious symptoms of the skin, erosions and wounds (see more about destructive energy on page XXXIV).

Blockage of the Bladder-meridian is caused by a trauma on the structures of connective tissue that lead the impulses travelling through this meridian. Such a trauma will not hurt or destroy the energy of the process itself, but hinder the Qi-flow in the meridian. This is why the pulse in such a case shows absolutely good health for the process, but the acupuncture points may show dis-balance. This disbalance shows excess above the trauma, and deficienct below the trauma.

BL 01	**Jingming (Eye-Pupil Bright)**

Meeting point between the BL, SI, ST, GB and TH meridians with the GV, Yin Qiao and Yang Qiao mai

In horses: Just rostromedial to the medial canthus of the eye.
In dogs: Just rostromedial to the medial canthus of the eye.
In humans: Just rostromedial to the medial canthus of the eye.

When needling here, it is important to deflect the eye, and not to penetrate the eyeball.

Effect: Its main use is to help the eye, eyelid and sight. It is very effective to free obstructed tear ducts, a disorder I earlier thought was impossible to "cure". Several owners of Bichon Frise dogs asked me if there was anything to do with this disorder, and I thought not. Then one day an owner demanded that I try; just to please him I stimulated BL01 bilaterally with my Dermojet. I sent the patient home and thought no more about it. About a year later, the owner phoned me to say that the dog had been totally cured for one year, but now the Lesion-Symptom Complex was beginning to reappear. Since then, I have used BL01 to treat many dogs for obstruction of the tear ducts, and it usually works very well. It also helps cataract and glaucoma. I usually inject a little vitamin B12 at BL01. BL01 has also a very interesting effect on the uterus, especially with cows; it can correct foetal malposition (and dystocia). In the near-parturient cow, needling BL01 (plus BL67, BL62 and BL02) influences the uterus, causing the unborn calf to react - it tries to move its body into a normal presentation position for birth. GV03 contracts the uterus, while BL62 relaxes the upper third, so that the calf can correct its position. BL01 has an even more potent effect if we stimulate it directly in the calf with the help of the fingers or a device called the "eye hook". Then we may feel the calf struggling really hard to normalise its position for birth.

BL 02	**Zanzhu (Bamboo Gathering)** **"Valium Point":** *In horses:* Proximal to BL01, at the medial end of the eyebrow. *In dogs:* Proximal to BL01, at the medial end of the eyebrow. *In humans:* Proximal to BL01, at the medial end of the eyebrow. *Effect:* This "Special Action" Point ("Valium Point") can be used to calm nervous or aggressive animals (effect much like HT07). After AP at BL02, many horses that have been afraid of shiny or moving objects, etc., have lost their fear to a great extent, and aggressive dogs have lost their aggression (especially when the aggression was caused by fear, as it often is). However, the main uses of BL02 are to help the eye, eyelid, sight, face, cheek, forehead, frontal sinuses, head, forehead, vertex, occiput, temple, headache and sinusitis.
BL 10	**Tianzhu (Heavenly Pillar)** **Diagnostic Point for the contralateral stifle in horses** **Point of the Window of the Sky** *In horses:* Dorsal to Atlas, in a depression at the level of Foramen alare, in M. splenius. *In dogs:* at the lateral edge of trapezius muscle. *In humans:* at the lateral edge of trapezius muscle, on the natural hairline of the occiput. *Effect:* It is a **Diagnostic Point for the contralateral stifle in horses** (See ST10 in relation to its use as a **Diagnostic Point for the ipsilateral stifle**). Because it is near (medial and caudal to) GB20 (Fengchi - Wind Pool), BL10 helps disorders of Wind and Wood. It also helps arteriosclerosis, blood vessels, cervical spine, forehead, skin and hair, head, headache, ischemia, neck, occiput, esophagus, parathyroid, sinusitis, spinal cord, temple, thyroid and vertex. Headache.

BL 11	**Dashu (Great Shuttle)** **Hui-Influential point of Bones** **Meeting point of the BL, SI, TH and GB meridians and the GV** **Point of the Sea of Blood** *In horses:* Just cranial to the scapular cartilage, 3 cun lateral to the dorsal midline. *In dogs:* just in front of the scapula, 2 cun lateral to the midline. *In humans:* 1.5 cun lateral to GV13, level with T1-T2 space. *Effect:* It helps bones, joints, spinal cord, scapula, shoulder, clavicle, patella, trachea and pleura.
BL 12	**Fengmen (Wind Gate)** **Meeting point between the BL meridian and the GV** **Hui-Influential point of Wind and Trachea** *In horses:* The most proximal point dorsal to the scapular cartilage, 2 cun lateral to the midline. *In dogs:* it is 1.5 cun from GV Line, level with T2-T3 space. *In humans:* it is 1.5 cun from GV Line, level with T2-T3 space. *Effect:* It helps Wind diseases, and the respiratory system, trachea, bronchi, lung, asthma, cough, chills and pneumonia.
BL 13-BL 30	These are the **Back Shu Points** that were discussed earlier (page 108). They are used diagnostically when there is a Process Imbalance (dysfunction in their related Channel-Organ System). They are described in detail for horses and dogs (see page 111 & 109).

BL 31-BL 34	**Baliao (Four Holes)** - the 4 sacral foramina
	meeting points of the BL and GB meridians
	BL31 Shangliao (Upper Bone-Hole)- sacral foramen 1 **BL32 Ciliao (Second Bone-Hole)** - sacral foramen 2 **BL33 Zhongliao (Central Bone-Hole)** - sacral foramen 3 **BL34 Xialiao (Lower Bone-Hole)** - sacral foramen 4
	In all species, BL31-BL34 are over the 4 sacral foramina, midway between GV Line and BL27-BL30, respectively, i.e. 1,5 cun in horses and 0.75 cun in dogs and humans from GV Line, on medial edge of each sacral foramen.
	Effect: All of these sacral points influence disorders of defecation and urination. They may be used also in disorders at parturition, especially during labour, and in prolapse of the uterus or rectum. BL31-BL34 may also be very effective in disorders of the sacroiliac joint and the area behind the joint (both sides of the sacrum). Horses can seriously traumatise this area when they roll in a stable that is too small, hit the wall and then must twist to stand up. **Such trauma is very common**. I diagnose such trauma by listening to the sound of my fist hitting both sides of the sacrum. The traumatised side gives us a more dull sound. Also we should look for concave scratches on the wall of the stable! The horseshoes make the marks during the struggle. The Lesion-Symptom Complex for this disorder is very diffuse but manifests as pain, spasm and tenderness in the area. To heal this pain, it might also be necessary to correct with a simple chiropractic manipulation (see page 584)
BL 35 **(-1 in horses)**	**Huiyang (Meeting of Yang)**
	In horses: At the dorsal end of the muscular groove between M. biceps femoris and M. semitendinosus. *In dogs:* it is 0.5 cun lateral to GV01. *In humans:* it is 0.5 cun lateral to GV01.
	Effect: It helps pain in the coccyx.

BL 35-2	**Extra point in horses** **Xie Qi; according to Van den Bosch/Guray** *Location;* In the muscular groove between M. biceps femoris and M. semitendinosus, at the level of GV01. *Effect;* Impaired tail mobility.
BL 36-BL 38	**Local Diagnostic Points for:** **BL36: the hip** **BL37: the stifle** **BL38: the hock** **BL36:** 3 cun below the prominence of Tuber ischii, in the muscular groove between Mm. biceps femoris and semitendinosus. **BL37:** In the muscular groove, between Mm. biceps femoris and semitendinosus, 3 cun distal to BL36. **BL38-1:** In the muscular groove, between Mm. biceps femoris and semitendinosus, 2 cun proximal to BL40. **BL38-2:** In the muscular groove, between M. biceps femoris medial and caudal heads, 2 cun proximal to BL39. In horses and dogs these points are on the posterior thigh, between the tuber ischii and the stifle, in the groove between the musculus biceps femoris and musculus semitendinosus. In stifle and tarsal joint disorders, one may palpate muscular knots or nodules in the groove between these two muscles (in my experience these knots are more in the medial area of of this groove, at the lateral side of musculus biceps femoris rather than on the medial side of musculus semitendinosus). In my experience, finding such lumps is a better diagnostic aid to stifle or tarsal disorders than flexion tests on those joints (at least without local anesthesia). They also help the dorsolumbar-, lowback-, lumbar-, lumbosacral-, sacroiliac- area, sacrum, coccyx, buttock, thigh and femur.

BL 39	**Weiyang (Bend Yang)**
	Lower He-Sea Point of TH and Diagnostic Point for the equine tarsus and ovary
	In horses: At the lateral aspect of the stifle, at level with and just caudal to, the femoro-tibial joint, between the middle and the caudal heads of M. Biceps femoris.
	In dogs: lateral to BL40, at the bottom of the same groove as BL36-BL38.
	In humans: on lateral side of popliteal crease, lateral to BL40, on medial side of biceps femoris tendon.
	Effect: This is a very interesting and special point. As we will see later, TH Channel, and its Shu and Mu Points (BL22 and CV05) relate also to the ovary and reproduction. BL39 relates clearly to the **equine tarsus and ovaries** (and testicles). It is tender to palpation in equine tarsal disorders, especially if there is pain in the joint, and in degenerative disorders in the hocks. It is a Diagnostic Point for the ovary in mares (possibly also in other female animals and in women). A tender reaction (sensitivity) at BL39 may arise in painful or degenerative changes in the ovary. To see if the mare is ready for mating, a stallion bites her at BL39. If she kicks, he knows that she is not receptive and he leaves her alone. It is very interesting that mares with ovarian disorders often move with short hindlimb movements, called "hocky". A tender reaction at BL39 may arise in painful or degenerative changes in the testicle also.
BL 40	**Weizhong (Bend Centre)** (coded BL54 in older textbooks)
	Local point in horses **Earth point in dogs and humans** **Master Point of the Back**
	In horses: In the centre of the popliteal fossa, between Mm. biceps femoris and semitendinosus.
	In dogs: In the centre of the popliteal fossa, between Mm. biceps femoris and semitendinosus.
	In humans: In the centre of the popliteal fossa, between Mm. biceps femoris and semitendinosus.

	Effect: Because of its broad effect, BL40 is indicated in all degenerative states in the genital area and the urinary apparatus. It is effective in BL disorders, prostatitis, sciatica and the dorsal muscles of the hip area and back (longissimus dorsi muscle). BL40 has a marked effect on the entire genital area. To treat prostate disorders, the effect is much better if the patient drinks a cup of cooked poplar (branch) every day. Other main uses include allergy, vasomotor allergy, fever and chills; disorders with the thoracic spine and back, flank and waist, dorsolumbar-, lowback-, lumbar-; lumbosacral- and sacroiliac-area, sacrum and coccyx, pelvis, pelvic limb (hip, buttock, thigh, femur, stifle, patella, popliteal area, leg, calf, tibia, fibula, Achilles area and heel), skin and hair.
BL 41-BL 54	The **outer branch of BL Channel** runs from **BL41-BL52** (6 cun in horses, 4 cun in dogs and 3 cun in humans lateral to GV Line (and in the same vertebral segment as) BL12-BL23, respectively. **BL53 and BL54** lie 6 cun lateral to GV Line, 3 cun lateral to BL28 and BL30, respectively. Points BL41-BL54 have similar uses to their segmental partners on the inner branch. **BL42, BL44, BL47, BL49 and BL53 are the Spirit Points**. They are in horses 3 cun, and for dogs 2 cun and for humans 1.5 cun outside BL13 (LU), BL15 (HT), BL18 (LV), BL20 (SP) and BL23 (KI), respectively. They House the Spirit or Emotional Faculty of **LU, HT, LV, SP, KI**, respectively, i.e. the **Po, Shen, Hun, Yi and Zhi**. They are used to treat spiritual / emotional disorders of their related organs.
BL 57	**Chengshan (Support Mountain)** **In horses:** 1 cun distal to BL56, 2.5 cun distal to BL40. **In dogs:** 5 cun below BL40, 5 cun above superior edge of calcaneus, midway from BL40 to the heel. **In humans:** 8 cun below BL40, 8 cun above superior edge of calcaneus, midway from BL40 to the heel. **Effect:** It is It helps the anus (tenesmus, prolapse, hemorrhoids), lowback-, lumbar-, lumbosacral- and sacroiliac- area, sacrum and pelvic limb, especially the leg and calf, Achilles area, heel, tarsus, metatarsus and foot. It is an important point for muscle cramps in racing dogs.

BL 58	**Feiyang (Taking Flight)** **Luo Point of BL** *In horses:* Midway between the femoro-tibial joint and the lateral malleolus, cranial to the Achilles tendon, at the same level as GB35, GB36 and ST40. *In dogs:* Midway between the femoro-tibial joint and the lateral malleolus, cranial to the Achilles tendon, at the same level as GB35, GB36 and ST40. *In humans:* it is 9 cun below BL40, 1 cun lateral to BL57, 7 cun directly above BL60, on the posterior edge of the fibula, at the lateral edge of the gastrocnemius muscle. *Effect:* It connects BL Channel with its Phase Mate, KI Channel. In humans,
BL 59	**Fuyang (Instep Yang)** **Xi-Cleft point of Yang Qiao mai** *In horses:* 3 cun proximal to BL60, cranial to the Achilles tendon, on the caudal border of M. flexor digit. prof.. *In dogs:* Proximal to BL60, cranial to the Achilles tendon, on the caudal border of M. flexor digit. prof.. *In humans:* It is 3 cun above BL60. *Effect:* It helps the tarsus, metatarsus, salivation and salivary glands. Also it helps all acute conditions.
BL 60	**Kunlun (Kunlun Mountains)** **Water point in horses and in dogs** **(Jing-river and Fire point in humans)** *In horses:* At the caudolateral aspect of the tibia, just proximal to the lateral malleolus. *In dogs:* level with the lateral malleolus of the tibia, between the bone and the Achilles tendon, directly opposite KI03. *In humans:* level with the lateral malleolus of the tibia, between the bone and the Achilles tendon, directly opposite KI03.

	Effect: It helps tarsal disorders, sciatica and pain in the genital area. It helps also the head, back, spinal cord, Achilles area and heel, tarsus, metatarsus, foot and toe. It also helps parturition and lymphadenopathy. It is a forbidden point in pregnancy, as it may cause abortion.
BL 61	**Pucan (Subservient Visitor)** **Meeting point of the BL meridian with the Yang Qiao mai** *In horses:* In a small depression on the lateral side of the calcaneum, caudal to BL60. *In dogs:* In a small depression on the lateral side of the calcaneum, caudal to BL60. *In humans:* , it is 1.5 cun below BL60. *Effect:* It helps the Achilles and heel.
BL 62	**Shenmai (Extending Vessel)** **Confluent point (activation) of the Yang Qiao mai** **Source point** *In horses:* 0.5 cun distal to a horizontal line tangential to the distal border of the lateral malleolus, in a small depression plantar to the tendon of M. extensor digit. lat. *In dogs:* in a hollow below the lateral malleolus. *In humans:* in a hollow below the lateral malleolus. *Effect:* It enhances blood circulation in the leg, and helps the tibia, fibula and lower part of the hindlimb. **Combination of SI03/BL62** enhances circulation along the spine all the way to the head. This combination is effective in spondylosis and the patient usually improves within a few weeks. BL62 also relaxes the upper third of the uterus and may be used in foetal malposition and to assist parturition. It also helps sore heels in horses, in fetlock infections and in cold feet in humans. As it stimulates blood circulation along the spine and relaxes the uterus, the mechanism for both effects may be the same.

BL 63	**Jinmen (Metal Gate)**
	Xi-Cleft point
	Meeting point of the BL meridian with the Yang Wei mai
	In horses: In a depression proximal to the base of the fourth metatarsal bone and dorsal to the long plantar ligament. *In dogs:* it is in a hole behind tuberosity of metatarsal 5, anteroinferior to BL62. *In humans:* it is in a hole behind tuberosity of metatarsal 5, anteroinferior to BL62.
	Effect: Modererates acute conditions. Relaxes tendons and muscles, activates the meridian and alleviates pain.
BL 64	**Jinggu (Capital Bone)**
	Metal point in horses and in dogs
	(Yuan-Source point in humans and dogs)
	In horses: Plantar to the base of the fourth metatarsal bone. *In dogs:* it is at posterior inferior edge of the tuberosity of metatarsal 5. *In humans:* it is at posterior inferior edge of the tuberosity of metatarsal 5.
	Effect: Because of its position, it has a special effect on the tarsus. It helps degenerative tarsal disorders and wear and tear or pain in this joint. Also, BL64 may help in pain in the upper lateral suspensory ligament. In horses that have restricted medial movements of the hindlimb, it helps to convey it outwards. In such cases it is very helpful to combine BL64, BL65, BL67 and GB44. This is relevant if the horse brushes its other hindleg in a race. It also helps the brain and meninges.
BL 65	**Shugu (Bundle Bone)**
	Earth point in horses and dogs
	(Shu-Stream and Wood point in humans)
	In horses: Just proximal to the fetlock and the laterala proxoimal sesamoid bone, between the deep digital flexor tendon and the lateral tendon of the interrosseus.

	In dogs: at the posterior lateral edge of the head of canine metatarsal 5. *In humans:* at the posterior lateral edge of the head of human metatarsal 5. *Effect:* helps painful states of this area. As an earth point, it has special relevance to muscles and tendons, and is relevant to degenerative conditions in the area and along the meridian. It also helps the occiput. In horses that have restricted medial movements of the hindlimb, it helps to convey it outwards. In such cases it is very helpful to combine BL64, BL65, BL67 and GB44. This is relevant if the horse brushes its other hindleg in a race.
BL 66	**BL66 Zutonggu (Foot Connecting Passage)** **Fire point in horses and in dogs** **(Ying-Spring and Water point in humans)** *In horses:* Just distal to the fetlock, on the dorsolateral border of the deep flexor tendon. *In dogs:* in the hole anterior and inferior to metatarsophalangeal joint. *In humans:* in the hole anterior and inferior to metatarsophalangeal joint 5. *Effect:* Because it is a Fire Point in the horse, it is of special relevance for infection of the joint and synovial fluid in the fetlock of the hindlimbs, especially in warm (hot) conditions. As with all Command Points, it helps the whole Channel, especially all the Fiery Processes of the body. Examples of uses of BL66 are all warm cystitis, general swellings, swellings in the back muscles and frequent urination due to psychic reasons. Also, it helps especially the eye and poor sight.
BL 67	**Zhiyin (Reaching Yin, Extremity of Yin)** **Ting, Wood Point of BL in the horse and dog** **(Ting and Metal Point in humans)** *In horses:* At the coronary band on the pelvic limb, just dorsal to the lateral cartilage of the distal phalanx, ~ 90⁰ lateral to the tip of the toe.

In dogs: it is 0.1 cun from posterior edge of nail-root of little toe, lateral side.

In humans: it is 0.1 cun from posterior edge of nail-root of little toe, lateral side.

Effect: Since it is the Ting Point, it influences both the Channel and its Process, especially in relation to painful and / or muscular disorders. One can see the influence of BL67 on the whole BL Channel in cases of muscular backpain in horses. Such cases often have many tender Back Shu Points and general soreness. When BL67 is used, all tenderness and pain can disappear within minutes. In horses that have restricted medial movements of the hindlimb, it helps to convey it outwards. In such cases it is very helpful to combine BL64, BL65, BL67 and GB44. This is relevant if the horse brushes its other hindleg in a race. BL67 also is very effective in lumbago and sciatica. It also helps problems before, during and after parturition; disorders of pregnancy; forbidden point in pregnancy (may cause abortion).

Table 65

The special commandpoints in the horse are as follows:

S O U R C E fetlock	*Location;* Just distal to the lateral proximal sesamoid bone, at the level of the metatarsophalangeal joint, plantar to A/V. digitalis lat.. *Effect;* Stimulates the meridian.

Table 66

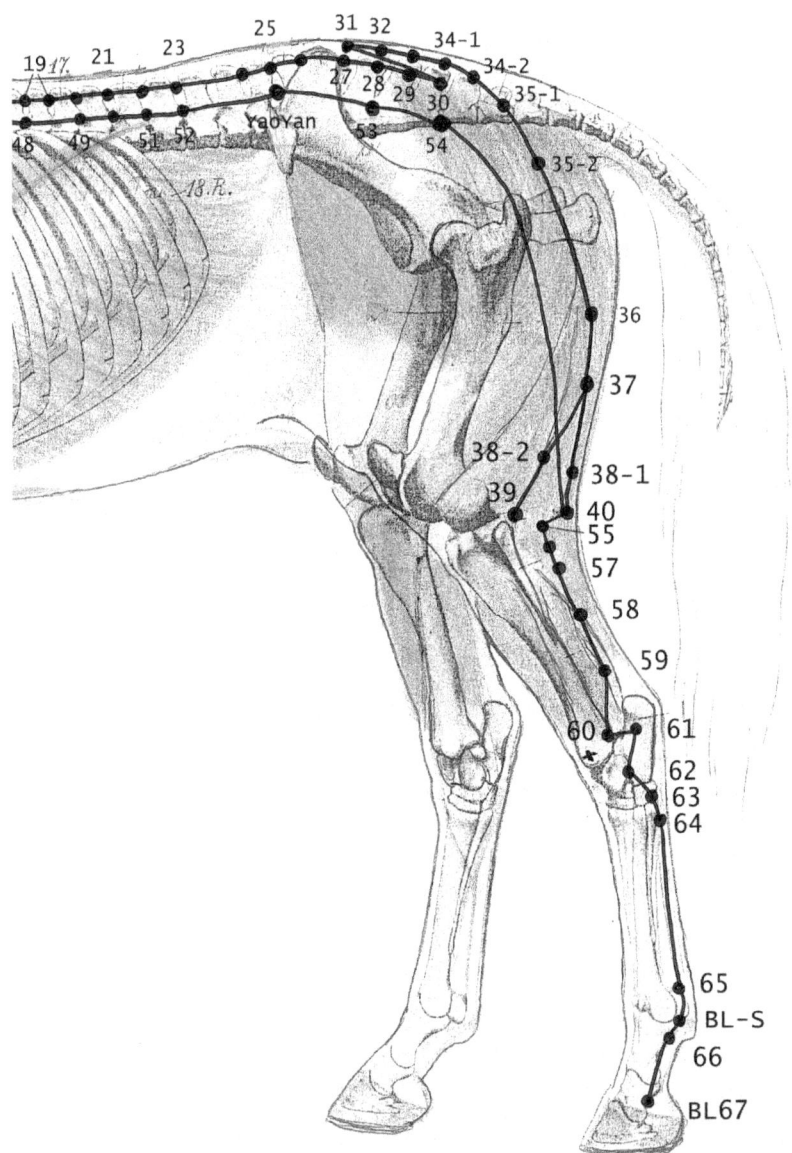

Figure 51; Diagram of the most important points on the BL Channel in the horse.

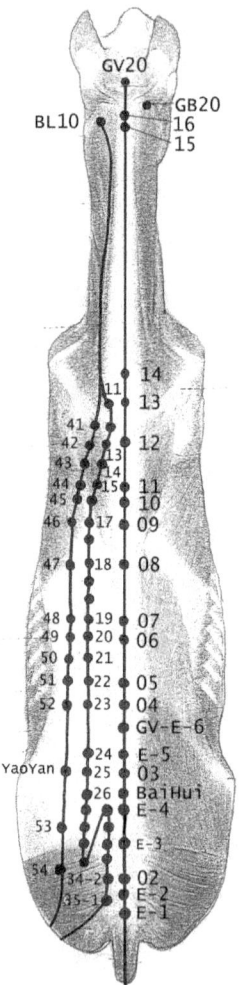

Figure 52; some of the most important points on the BL-meridian in the horse

KI (Kidney, Foot Shaoyin) Channel uses the connective tissue around *A/V. torica phal. III, A/V. digitalis med., A/V.. mtts. plant. supf. med., A/V.. tarsica med., A/V. tibialis caud., A/V. recurrens tib., Rete malleolus med., A/V. recurrens tib., A/V. caud. femoris Ramus desc., A/V. obturatoria, A/V: pudendalis int.* as the main pathways for carrying its impulses:

Anatomically it begins:

IN HORSES:
The superficial path of the KI-meridian:

- Begins in the depression between the bulbs of the heel of the pelvic limb, KI01; *A/V. torica phal. III,*

- Ascends along the medial caudal border of the deep flexor tendon; *A/V. digitalis med.,*

- Follows the deep flexor tendon; *A/V. mtts. plant. supf. med.,* and *A/V. tarsica med.,* to KI03 at the caudomedial aspect of the tibia, just proximal to the medial malleolus,

- Sends a branch up to SP06, *A/V. tibialis caud.,*

- Ascends from KI03 towards the cranial border of the Achilles tendon, KI04, where it makes a turn; *A/V. recurrens tib.,*

- And descends distal and plantar to the medial malleolus; *Rete malleolus med.,*

- Turns again and ascends along M. flexor digit. prof.; *A/V. recurrens tib.* and *A/V. caud. femoris ramus desc.,* to the medial aspect of the popliteal crease,

- Continues along the caudomedial aspect of the thigh; *A/V. obturatoria,*

- To the anus; *A/V. pudendalis int.,* where it intersects with the Governing vessel at GV01.

- At GV01 the meridian dives into the depth of the body (see the deep branch nr. 1) and emerges at the cranial border of the pubic bone, where the superficial path continues along Linea alba, 1 cun lateral to the ventral the midline of the abdomen and chest to the Manubrium, where the it ends at KI27.

The deep path of the KI-meridian has 3 branches:

1. One branch enters the body at GV01, travels through the spine, enters the Kidneys and contacts the Bladder, CV03, CV 04 and CV07, before it emerges at the cranial border of the pubic bone (see above).

2. Another branch starts in the Kidneys, travels cranially through the Liver and diaphragm, enters the Lungs and ascends along the trachea to end at the root of the tongue.

3. The third branch starts in the Lung, travels to the Heart and disperses in the chest and connects with the Pericardium meridian and CV17.

In dogs: it begins at KI01 which is under the main hindlimb pad, or at the medial side of the 5th toe. From KI01, it curves up along the caudo-medial side of the deep flexor tendon, along the caudo-medial side of the tarsus, leg, stifle and thigh, to the groin in much the same way as described under horses. Travelling 0.5 cun from CV Line, it ascends the ventral abdomen from KI11 on the pelvic brim, to KI16 (lateral to the navel), to KI21 (lateral to the xiphoid). From here, it ascends the thorax 2 cun lateral to CV Line, to end at KI27, 2 cun from CV Line.

In humans: it begins at KI01 on the sole of the foot, just proximal to the distal heads of metatarsal bones 2-3 in humans. Some sources say that it begins at the medial (axial) aspect of the 5th toe. From KI01, it curves up along the caudo-medial side of the deep flexor tendon, along the caudo-medial side of the tarsus, leg, stifle and thigh, to the groin. Travelling 0.5 cun from CV Line, it ascends the ventral abdomen from KI11 on the pelvic brim, to KI16 (lateral to the navel), to KI21 (lateral to the xiphoid). From here, it ascends the thorax 2 cun lateral to CV Line, to end at KI27, 2 cun from CV Line, just below the clavicle.

Phase	Metal		Earth		Fire		Water		Fire		Wood
Yin Channel	LU[(1)]		SP[(4)]	>>	HT[(1)]		KI[(4)]	>>	PC[(1)]		LV[(4)]
	‖		‖		‖		‖		‖		‖
Yang Channel	LI[(2)]	>>	ST[(3)]		SI[(2)]	>>	BL[(3)]		TH[(2)]	>>	GB[(3)]
Limb	Hand		Foot		Hand		Foot		Hand		Foot

(‖ and >>) mean that Qi Flow sequence is LU-LI-ST-SP, etc;
‖ = Yin-Yang Phase Mates (Partners);
[(1)] Qi flow from chest to hand; [(2)] Qi flow from hand to face; [(3)]
Qi flow from face to foot; [(4)] Qi flow from foot to chest

Table 65

KI Qi comes from BL Channel, its Yin Mate in Water, and flows into (connects with) PC Channel. As applies to all the other Yin Channels in animals, KI Channel is much more important than its paired Yang Channel (BL). BL-KI, the Yang-Yin Couple in Water are significant (together with HT, PC, SI, LV, SP) in regulating water and many of the bodily fluids, especially the excretions and the lymph. They are also important in fluid excretion, including urine and genital fluids, semen, sperm and ova. Often, most bones, joints, back and back joints and their disorders are associated with a Process Imbalance in KI.

KI01 and KI02 are two important acupoints <u>to stimulate</u> the Channel. This reduces salivation, sweating and diarrhea, just like a stimulation of the sympathetic function of the splancnic nerve would do. This shows, what I say several places in this book, that there are no genuine sedation-points. But, as all of the commandpoints do have a commanding or controlling (as the father) function via the Ko-cycle, and as the Ko-cycle is a regulating cycle, all commandpoints may act as a sedating point if the function in question is in excess. If the function in question is in deficiency, then the controlling point will act as a stimulating point. The reason why so many practitioners consider certain points as sedation points is the exaggerated attention that excesses have, and the lack of diagnostic attention on the deficiencies of the organism.

KI Imbalance often causes mastitis in cows and diarrhea in calves. In dogs it can cause Lesion-Symptom Complexes of calcification in the back, hips and joints, and backpain. Also eczema, especially wet eczema, hair growth, anal function and psychic stability depends on KI Channel. KI is very important with regards to the metabolism of phosphorus and calcium. KI function also includes adrenal function, and the adrenal is involved in mineral-, glucose- and water metabolism. KI Imbalance may cause pathological bony deposits, such as in osteoarthritis and spondylosis. This is relevant to joint and skeletal development and general growth pains and growth soreness (related to the bone structure). Some are also related to the muscles and tendons, and thus react on LV and GB. KI Imbalance also may cause calcification of smooth muscle, arteries and brain. Therefore, widely varying Lesion-Symptom Complexes almost always react positively to treatment of KI Points.

KI Deficiency is most often found in horses in their second or third winter. During this period KI should be treated by Tonification to get the best possible joint development.

KI is of special importance in dogs. While humans usually develop geriatric HT or LU disorders in old age, dogs usually develop KI disorders. Geriatric practice in dogs usually involves maintaining good KI function. There are 5 ways in which we may help such old animals with KI Deficiency:

1. *Give AP treatment at relevant KI Points, such as KI03 (Earth-Source Point), KI07 (Metal-Tonification Point), BL23 (KI Shu Point) or GB25 (KI Mu Point).*

2. *Give KI-tonifying herbs, such as Equisetum arvense or Chamomilla.*

3. *Change the diet to low protein, with a lot of cooked vegetables.*

4. *Reduce the salt content of the feed.*

5. *Warm KI by using a **woollen** blanket or waistcoat over the lumbar area.*

In this way, old, tired and sick dogs with KI Deficiency may be rejuvenated. After KI Processes are helped to perform their normal duties, such old dogs may have 3-4 years of good life ahead of them.

In accordance with the Chinese Qi Clock, around 1800h is the best time of day to treat KI Channel.

The energy in the lung meridian (Qi) may, as for the lung-process itself be in:

- *Excess*

- *Deficiency*

Particular for the meridian the energy may also be in:

- *Destructive*

- *Blocked*

Excess show itself rather seldom as pain, as this is a Yin meridian, and Yin meridians seldom show excesses as pain (contrary to Yang-meridians which often show excesses as painful points or areas). An excess in the Kidney-meridian, although very seldom, may be the result of a deficiency in the Heart, Pericardium or Spleen-processes. An excess in the Kidney meridian usually passes without observation or unpleasant symptoms.

Deficiency is a much more common and serious pathological finding than excess. Such a deficiency show itself in the same way as described under the Kidney-process on page 81. In addition we may find skin-changes in the form of excema along the Kidney-meridian.

A deficiency in the Kidney meridian is often the cause of an excess in the Trippel Heather- or Small Intestine meridians, and pain along these meridians may be the result.

This pain is often the symptoms we are confronted with in our dayly practise.

Destructivity show itself as in all animals as particular vicious symptoms of the skin, erosions and wounds (see more about destructive energy on page XXXIV).

Blockage of the Kidney-meridian is caused by a trauma on the structures of connective tissue that lead the impulses travelling through this meridian. Such a trauma will not hurt or destroy the energy of the process itself, but hinder the Qi-flow in the meridian. This is why the pulse in such a case shows absolutely good health for the process, but the acupuncture points may show dis-balance. This disbalance shows excess above the trauma, and deficiency below the trauma.

KI01	Yongquan (Gushing Spring)
	Ting, Wood Point of KI and Emergency Point
	In horses: In the central depression between the bulbs of the heel of the pelvic limb.
	In dogs: In dogs it has two possibilities of placement: it is directly behind or under the solar pad of the hindlimb, between the distal heads of metatarsal bones 2-3. it is at the medial side of the 5th toe of the hind-leg.
	In humans: it is on foot-sole, in a hollow between distal ends of metatarsals 2-3, between the pads of toes 1, 2 and the pads of toes 3, 4 and 5. It is easier to find when the toes are curled.
	Effect: As a Command Point, it stimulates the whole Channel and all growth anomalies (by this I mean the attributes, characteristics, aspect or "colors" of the symptoms) related to KI Process (for example: leg tumors, bone-cancer, exostoses if the KI-meridian is in deficiency). Since KI is especially relevant to bone structure, KI01 is especially important in relation to development (growth) of bones and joints. It is effective against calcification throughout the body. This shows that KI Channel governs the Process of bone growth, while individual KI Points decide the nature of the symptoms. An important Process of KI Channel is to govern bone, but the different points have different actions on the bones. For example, the Wood Point regulates *growth* in the bones; the Fire Point regulates *blood circulation* in bone, etc. This is what I mean by saying that the Command Point relates to the modifications of the symptom. Although KI01 relates to the Wood Phase, it has relatively little to do with tendons and muscles. As a Local Point, KI01 helps tendon disorders (deep and superficial digital flexor tendons) and disorders in the fetlock area. It also helps the vertex, emergencies, brain, meninges, nervous disorders, convulsions, epilepsy, tetanus, blood circulation, blood pressure, allergy and vasomotor allergy.

KI02	Rangu (Blazing Valley)
	Source point in horses **Ying-Spring and Fire point in dogs (and in humans)** *In horses:* Proximal and plantar to the base of the second metatarsal bone, just distal to the chestnut. *In dogs:* it is situated at the caudolateral border in the middle of the metatarsale II. *In humans:* it is in a hollow at the inferior edge of the navicular tuberosity, on medial side of foot. *Effect:* It is especially important for "Hot Bone" (arthritis and periostitis with pain and Heat). As a Local Point, it is effective in fetlock arthritis. It also helps diabetes mellitus, hypoglycemia and hyperglycemia and disorders of the pancreas.
KI03	Taixi (Supreme Ravine)
	Water point in horses **Earth- and Source point in dogs** **(Yuan-Source, Shu-Stream and Earth point in humans)** *In horses:* In a small depression at the medioplantar aspect of the tibia, just proximal to the medial malleolus. *In dogs:* it is level with the medial malleolus of the tibia, between the bone and the Achilles tendon, directly opposite BL60. *In humans:* it is level with the medial malleolus of the tibia, between the bone and the Achilles tendon, directly opposite BL60. *Effect:* It helps disorders of the urogenital organs and functions (including male infertility and spermatopathy, kidney and upper ureter) and the pelvic limb, (special the Achilles area, heel, tarsus, metatarsus and foot). It is also a Local Point for the flexor tendons. KI03 increases the reactivity of the ovary (and testicle). It stimulates ovulation generally, especially during or just after estrus (one of my patients got pregnant during menses after stimulation of this point together with BL23). Stimulation of KI03 can induce a quicker ovulation. Because of this ability we are also able to induce abortion through KI03, which in this aspect is diametrically opposed to LV03 in effect. KI03 is unsurpassed in helping growth pains in all species. Many

	dog owners have tried AP as a last possibility before opting for euthanasia for their dogs due to unbearable growing pains. Often the pain has disappeared the day after treatment is given and euthanasia is avoided. Growth pain treatment is 90% effective (should be combined with LV03).
KI04	**Dazhong (Great Goblet)** **Luo Point of KI** *In horses:* Cranial to the Achilles tendon, at the caudal border of M. flex. digit. prof., 2.5 cun proximal to KI05. *In dogs:* it is posteroinferior to KI03, above the calcaneus, anterior to the Achilles. *In humans:* it is posteroinferior to KI03, above the calcaneus, anterior to the Achilles. *Effect:* It connects KI Channel with its Phase Mate, BL Channel. It also helps the Achilles and heel.
KI05	**Shuiquan (Water Spring)** **Xi Point of KI** *In horses:* Just distal to the insertion of the Achilles tendon into the calcaneum. *In dogs:* it is 1 cun below KI04, at medial edge of calcaneus. *In humans:* it is 1 cun below KI04, at medial edge of calcaneus. *Effect:* Moderates acute conditions. Regulates Chong mai and Conception vessel.
KI06	**Zhaohai (Shining Sea)** **Confluent point of the Yin Qiao mai** *In horses:* 2 cun distal and plantar to the medial malleolus. *In dogs:* it is just under the medial malleolus. *In humans:* it is in a hollow 1 cun below inferior edge of medial malleolus. *Effect:* It helps postpartum disorders of the uterus, cervix and vagina; it also helps the tarsus and metatarsus. It is especially important to stimulate blood circulation in the leg and the foot. These points I often use in cases of sore heels in horses.

	When combined with SI03/BL62, it also is very effective in treating spondylosis and other disorders of the spine. After a few treatments at these 3 points, at an interval of a few weeks between treatments, dogs that could barely walk because of pain began to act like puppies again. I have witnessed this many times and have observed that the effect of this treatment is also, like growth-pain treatment, more than 90% effective. Regulates Yin Qiao mai; swelling, redness and pain of the throat. It also regulates the lower jiao; indicated in gynecological problems post partum. Stimulates the general circulation in the entire pelvic limb; dermatitis of the pastern. Important distal point in the treatment of constipation.
KI07	**Fuliu (Recover Flow)** **Local point in horses** **Metal point in dogs** *(Jing-River and Metal point in humans)* *In horses:* 1.5 cun proximal to KI04, cranial to the Achilles tendon, on the caudal border of the M. flex. digit. prof.. *In dogs:* it is 2 cun above the posterior side of medial malleolus, on the anterior edge of calcaneal tendon. *In humans:* it is 2 cun above the posterior side of medial malleolus, on the anterior edge of calcaneal tendon. *Effect:* it helps against ascites, edema, sweating disorders, disorders of the ureter, spinal cord, libido, penis, urethra, erectile dysfunction and impotence. Stimulation of KI07 helps tarsal pain and generally all pain along KI Channel.
KI08	**Jiaoxin (Intersection Reach)** **Xi-Cleft point of theYin Qiao mai** *In horses:* 1 cun proximal and cranial to KI07, ~45°. *In dogs:* it is just behind the medial edge of tibia, anterior to KI07. *In humans:* it is just behind the medial edge of tibia, 2 cun above the medial malleolus, anterior to KI07. *Effect:* In humans, It helps the spinal cord and testicle.

KI10	Yingu (Yin Valley)
	Local point in horses **Water point in dogs** **(He-Sea and Water point in humans)**
	In horses: At the medial end of the popliteal crease, between the tendons of M. semimembranosus and M. gracilis. *In dogs:* At the medial end of the popliteal crease, between the tendons of M. semimembranosus and M. gracilis. *In humans:* At the medial end of the popliteal crease, between the tendons of M. semimembranosus and M. gracilis.
	Effect: It helps the production of synovia in general and especially the joint fluid in the tarsus.
KI27	**Shufu Shu (Transporting Point Mansion)**
	In horses: 1 cun lateral to the cartilage of the manubrium, on the same horisontal line as ST13 and LU02. *In dogs:* it is medial to LU01 (at a line here we have at the midline CV22, then going lateral KI27, ST13 and LU01). *In humans:* it is 2 cun lateral to CV21, just below the clavicle, in a hole between it and rib 1.
	Effect: It helps especially in bronchial and tracheal infections that result in copius mucus. According to Dr. Westermayer this point deals with mucus of the respiratory tract.

Table 66

The special commandpoints in the horse are as follows:

F **I** **R** **E**	*Location;* Just distal to the medial proximal sesamoid bone, plantar to A/V. digitalis med.. *Effect;* Influences circulatory and heat related conditions locally and along the course of the meridian, and generally in the body when the Kidneys are in deficiency (or excess).

S **O** **U** **R** **C** **E** fetlock	*Location*; At the level of the metatarsophalangeal joint, plantar to A/V. digitalis med. *Effect*; Stimulates the meridian.
E **A** **R** **T** **H**	**Hou Chan Wan; extra point according to Van den Bosch/Guray** *Location*; Just proximal to the medial proximal sesamoide bone, plantar to A/V digitalis med. *Effect*; Influences degenerative conditions locally and along the course of the meridian, and generally in the body when the Kidneys are in deficiency (or excess).
M **E** **T** **A** **L**	*Location*; Just distal to the hock, plantar to the base of the second metatarsal bone, between the deep and superficial digital flexor tendons. *Effect*; Influences painful conditions locally and along the course of the meridian, and generally in the body when the Kidneys are in defiency (or excess).

Table 68

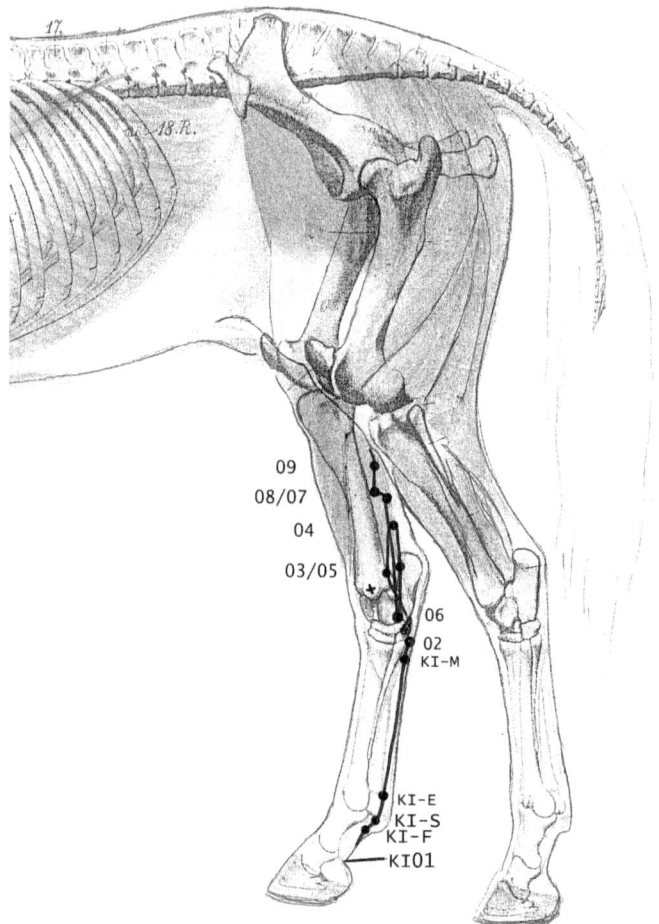

Figure 53; Illustration of the most important points on the KI Channel in the horse.

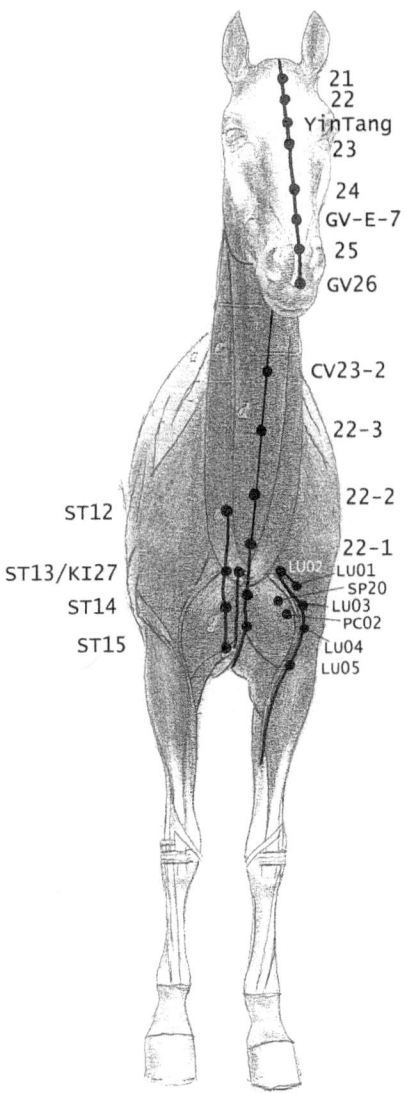

Figure 54; Illustration of the most important points on the KI Channel in the horse.

PC (Pericardium / Heart Constrictor, Hand Jueyin) Channel

uses the connective tissue around *A. thoracica ext.*, *A/V. brachialis*, *A/V. mediana*, *A/V. mtcp. palm. supf.*, *A/V. digitalis med. and A/V. torica phal. III.* as the main pathways for carrying its impulses:

369

Anatomically it begins:

IN HORSES:
The superficial path of the Pericardium meridian:

- Begins in the fifth intercostal space, at PC01, medial to the elbow; *A. thoracica ext.,*

- Arches over the axilla to the medial aspect of the upper arm; *A/V. axillaris,*

- Continues between the Heart and Lung meridians to the cubital crease of the elbow; *A/V. brachialis,*

- Descends in M. flexor carpi radialis, cranial to the chestnut; *A/V. mediana,*

- Passes the carpus on the palmar side of *V. cephalica,*

- Follows the digital flexor tendons; *A/V. mtcp. palm. supf.,*

- Passes the fetlock at the mediopalmar aspect; *A/V. digitalis med.,*

- Ends in the depression between the bulbs of the heel; *A/V. torica phal. III.*

The deep path of the Pericardium meridian has two branches:

1. One branch begins in the center of the chest, connects with the Pericardium, travels through the diaphragm to the abdomen and passes through the upper, middle and lower jiao.

2. The other branch travels from the center of the chest to surface in the 5th intercostal space, at PC01.

In dogs: the meridian begins at PC01, medial to the elbow. It descends along the anteromedial side of the front leg to the centre of the elbow crease (PC03, at the ulnar side of the biceps tendon). From here, it descends on the palmar surface of the front leg, following the course of the median nerve between the radius and the ulna, to PC06 (2 cun above wrist crease), to PC07 (center of the carpal (wrist) crease). From here, it goes to PC08 (under the pad), to end at PC09, at the medfial tip of the third claw. Some practitioners claim that the meridian ends beneath the claw pad in dogs, but I am sure it goes all the way out to the toes.

In humans begins at PC01, in humans 1 cun lateral to the nipple in the 4th intercostal space. It descends along the anteromedial side of the arm to the centre of the elbow crease (PC03, at the ulnar side of the biceps tendon). From here, it descends on the palmar surface of the forearm, following the course of the median nerve between the radius and the ulna, to PC06 (2 cun above wrist crease), to PC07 (center of the carpal (wrist) crease). From here, it goes to PC08 (in the palm), to end at PC09, at the tip of the middle finger (digit 3).

Phase	Metal		Earth		Fire		Water		Fire		Wood
Yin Channel	LU[(1)]		SP[(4)]	>>	HT[(1)]		KI[(4)]	>>	PC[(1)]		LV[(4)]
	‖		‖		‖		‖		‖		‖
Yang Channel	LI[(2)]	>>	ST[(3)]		SI[(2)]	>>	BL[(3)]		TH[(2)]	>>	GB[(3)]
Limb	Hand		Foot		Hand		Foot		Hand		Foot

(‖ *and* >>) *mean that Qi Flow sequence is LU-LI-ST-SP, etc;* ‖ = *Yin-Yang Phase Mates (Partners);*

[(1)] *Qi flow from chest to hand;* [(2)] *Qi flow from hand to face;* [(3)] *Qi flow from face to foot;* [(4)] *Qi flow from foot to chest*

Table 68

PC Qi comes from KI and flows into (connects with) TH Channel, its Yang Mate in Fire. In contrast to the other Yin Channels in animals, PC channel is less important than its paired Yang Channel (TH). PC is not in itself connected or related to a special organ. PC functions relate to the blood circulation, much like HT Channel. In humans it has many psychic relations, especially related to sexuality, sexual hormones and manic behaviour. These symptoms can be hard to observe in animals. In clinical veterinary medicine I have found most effect in cows with nymphomania, cysts in the ovary and uterus and in forelimb flexor tendon disorders in horses.

In horses PC Channel is important in disorders of the flexor tendons of the foreleg. Stimulation of any PC Point is of great value in chronic and acute tendinitis of the flexor tendons of the foreleg and may reduce treatment duration by many weeks.

In TCM, PC Channel is significant for libido, production of sperm, ovulation and for menstrual hemorrhage. In accordance with the Chinese Qi Clock, around 2000h is the best time of day to treat PC Channel.

The energy in the Pericardium meridian (Qi) may, as for the Pericardium-process itself be in:

- *Excess*

- *Deficiency*

Particular for the meridian the energy may also be:

- *Destructive*

- *Blocked*

Excess show itself rather seldom as pain, as this is a Yin meridian, and Yin meridians seldom show excesses as pain (contrary to Yang-meridians which often show excesses as painful points or areas). An excess in the Pericardium-meridian, although very seldom, may be the result of a deficiency in the Kidney-process. An excess in the Pericardium meridian usually passes without observation or unpleasant symptoms.

Deficiency is a much more common and serious pathological finding than excess. Such a deficiency show itself in the same way as described under the Pericardium-process on page 84. In addition we may find skin-changes in the form of eczema along the Pericardium-meridian.

A deficiency in the Pericardium meridian is often the cause of an excess in the Bladder- or Large Intestine meridians, and pain along these meridians may be the result.

This pain is often the symptoms we are confronted with in our dayly practise.

Destructivity show itself as in all animals as particular vicious symptoms of the skin, erosions and wounds (see more about destructive energy on page XXXIV).

Blockage of the Pericardium-meridian is caused by a trauma on the structures of connective tissue that lead the impulses travelling through this meridian. Such a trauma will not hurt or destroy the energy of the process itself, but hinder the Qi-flow in the meridian. This is why the pulse in such a case shows absolutely good health for the process, but the acupuncture points may show dis-balance. This disbalance shows excess above the trauma, and deficiency below the trauma.

PC 01	**Tianchi (Heavenly Pool)** **Meeting point of the PC, GB, LV and TH meridians** **Point of the Window of the Sky** *In horses:* In the 5th intercostal space, 5 cun lateral to the ventral midline, medial to the elbow. Westermayer describes the point as situated just behind the humerus, 3 cun below the shoulder joint. *In dogs:* it is 1 cun lateral to ST17, in intercostal space 4. *In humans:* it is 1 cun lateral to the nipple (ST17), in intercostal space 4. *Effect:* It helps the axilla and lymphadenopathy.
PC 02	**Tianquan (Heavenly Spring)** *In horses:* In M. pectoralis desc., medial to V. cephalica (the Lung meridian), 2 cun ventral to LU01. *In dogs:* it is 2 cun below the anterior end of axillary crease, between the two heads of the biceps brachii muscle. *In humans:* it is 2 cun below the anterior end of axillary crease, between the two heads of the biceps brachii muscle. *Effect:* In humans, It helps the axilla and arm.
PC 03 (-1 in hors-es)	**Quze (Bend Marsh)** **In horses a local point** **In dogs a Water point** *(He-Sea and Water point in humans)* *In horses:* Medial to the tendon of M. biceps brachii, medial and distal to LU05.

	In dogs: it is behind and beside the elbow, slightly medial to the bicipital tendon. *In humans:* it is in the elbow crease, at the ulnar side of biceps brachii tendon. *Effect:* It is a Local Point for the tendons in this area. It also helps pain in the chest, humerus, arm, elbow, forearm, radius; ulna and stomach.
PC 03-2 (in hors-es)	**Extra point in horses** *Location;* In the intersection of M. pectoralis transversus, M. flex. carpi radialis and Os radius, caudal to V. saphena.
PC 04	**Ximen (Cleft-Xi Gate)** **Xi Point of PC** *In horses:* 6.5 cun proximal to the antebrachiocarpal joint, 2.5 cun proximal to the chestnut, in M. flex. carpi radialis. *In dogs:* it is 7 cun below PC03 (ulnar side of biceps brachii tendon at elbow crease), 5 cun above PC09 (wrist). *In humans:* it is 7 cun below PC03 (ulnar side of biceps brachii tendon at elbow crease), 5 cun above PC09 (wrist). *Effect:* In humans, It helps the heart and pericardium.
PC 05	**Jianshi (Intermediary Courier)** **Local point in horses** **Metal Point in dogs** **(Jing-River and Metal point in humans)** *In horses:* 4 cun proximal to the antebrachiocarpal joint, at the level of the proximal and cranial corner of the chestnut. *In dogs:* it is 3 cun above PC09, between tendons of palmaris longus and flexor carpi radialis muscles. *In humans:* it is 3 cun above PC09, between tendons of palmaris longus and flexor carpi radialis muscles. *Effect:* It helps hot states with pain in the chest area. It also helps the axilla, heart and pericardium; fever and infections (cholera, herpes, malaria, rubella, TB, typhoid, typhus, varicella etc).

PC 06	**PC06 Neiguan (Inner Pass)** **Luo Point of PC** **Meeting Point of the Yinweimai** **Master Point of the Chest/Abdomen)** **Analgesic Point and Emergency Point** *In horses:* At the level of the distal and cranial corner of the chestnut. As the radius and ulna are fused, the needle can be inserted at TH05 and advanced to PC06 at the opposite side of the limb, just behind the bones. *In dogs:* it is 2 cun above PC09, between tendons of palmaris longus and flexor carpi radialis muscles, directly opposite TH05. As the gap between the radius and ulna can be narrow, it is easier to needle PC06 by inserting the needle between the bones at TH05, and advancing it all the way through the limb. *In humans:* it is 2 cun above PC09, between tendons of palmaris longus and flexor carpi radialis muscles, directly opposite TH05. *Effect:* It connects PC Channel with its Phase Mate, TH Channel. It has very wide clinical uses: Emergencies and first aid including convulsions, epilepsy, heart attack and tetanus. Also in troubles of the mind and psyche. Blood circulation, flushes, sweats. PC06 also helps the forearm. It helps the abdomen, menorrhalgia, dysmenorrhea, disorders of pregnancy and menopausal disorders. Like ST36, PC06 helps pain and has tonic effects in chronic disease and in infections (cholera, herpes, malaria, rubella, TB, typhoid, typhus, varicella etc). PC06 has some Functions similar to PC03. When combined with TH05 (Luo Point of TH, its Phase Mate), PC06 regulates many imbalances in sexual hormones. In humans this combination is especially important in female menopausal disorders. PC06 is also the Meeting Point ("switch") of the Yinweimai (an Extraordinary Vessel), which transports Qi from the caudoventral part of the animal to the craniodorsal area. PC06 can also be used in windsucking and the associated restlessness and signs of pain.
PC 07	**Daling (Great Mound)** **Earth and Source Point in horses, dogs and humans** *In horses:* Just distal to Os accessorius, palmar to V. cephalica. *In dogs:* it is caudal to the tendon of the flexor carpi radialis and proximal tip of the radial carpal bone (according to John Limehouse).

	In humans: it is at the palmar carpal (wrist) crease, between tendons of palmaris longus and flexor carpi radialis muscles. *Effect:* It acts like HT07 on the functions of the heart, pericardium and Shen. It also helps the thoracic limb, carpus, metacarpus, hand, palm and finger.
PC 08	**Laogong (Work Palace)** **Earth point in horses** **Fire and Horary Point in dogs** **(Ying-Spring and Fire point in humans)** *In horses:* Proximal to the medial proximal sesamoid bone, between the deep and superficial digital flexor tendons, palmar to A/V. digitalis med. *In dogs:* it is between metacarpals 2-3, only that the metacarpal pad covers this area. The point in dogs is reached best by needling the pad from behind. *In humans:* it is between metacarpals 2-3, where finger 3 touches when the fist is clenched. *Effect:* It helps the mouth, metacarpus, hand and palm. It is important for the fetlock and tendons in this area. It helps circulatory disturbances in tendons and joints.
PC 09	**Zhongchong (Central Hub)** **Wood Point and Ting point** **Emergency Point** *In horses:* In the depression between the bulbs of the heel, on the thoracic limbs. *In dogs:* it is medial of the claw (at the junction between phalanx I and II) at the third toe (digiti III) of the front leg. Some practitioners claim that PC09 is beneath the palmar pad in dogs. However, I am sure it goes all the way out to the medial side of the nail of foretoe 3. *In humans:* it is in center of tip of finger 3 (some texts: 0.1' from posterior edge of nail-root, radial edge). *Effect:* As a PC Command Point, it influences all circulatory Processes within the body, particularly those related to the Wood Phase, for example, swellings (= growth = Wood) caused

by a change in circulation. Especially in horses PC09 has a very important local effect on the flexor tendons, the suspensory, the fetlock joint, the navicular bone and the sesamoid bone. It also helps the fetlock in chronic and acute infections, as well as in cases of Heat, swelling, pain and reduced function. In tendon disorders, treatment of PC09 should be combined with two weeks of rest and a cast if necessary. It also helps emergencies, allergic shock, fever, allergy and vasomotor allergy.	

Table 69

The special commandpoints in the horse are as follows:

W A T E R	*Location*; At the level of the medial distal Tuberositas radii, caudal to V. saphena. *Effect*; Influences edema and watery conditions locally and along the course of the meridian, and generally in the body when the Pericardium is in excess or deficiency.
M E T A L	*Location*; Just distal to the carpus, at the mediopalmar aspect, between the deep and superficial digital flexor tendons. *Effect*; Influences painful conditions locally and along the course of the meridian, and generally in the body when the Pericardium is in excess or deficiency.
S O U R C E Fetlock	*Location*; At the level of the metacarpophalangeal joint, palmar to A/V. digitalis med. *Effect*; Stimulates the meridian.
F I R E	*Location*; Just distal to medial proximal sesamoid bone, at the mediocaudal border of the deep digital flexor tendon. *Effect*; *Influences heat related and circulatory conditions locally and along the course of the meridian, and generally in the body when the Pericardium is in excess or deficiency.*

Table 70

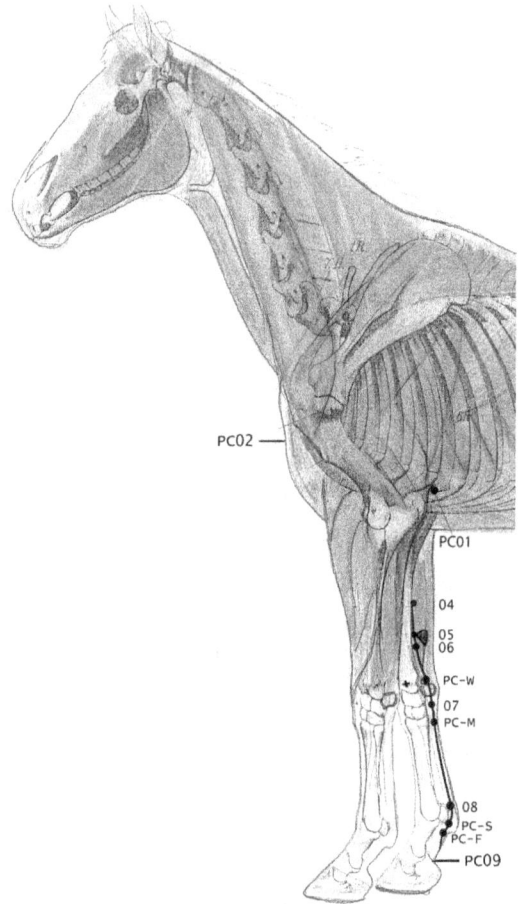

PC02

PC01

04

05
06

PC–W

07
PC–M

08
PC–S
PC–F

PC09

*Figure 55; Illustration of some of the most important points
on the PC Channel in the horse.*

TH (Triple Heater, Hand Shaoyang) Channel uses the
connective tissue around *A/V. coronalis phal. III, A/V. dorsalis
phal.I, Rete carpi dors., Rete carpi dors., A/V. interosseus dors., A/V.
interosseus recurrens, A/V. profunda brachii, A/V. circumflex. hum.
caud., A/V. vertebralis, A/V. vertebralis och A/V. occipitalis ramus
desc., A/V. auricularis magna, A/V. auricul. rostr., A/V. supraorbit.,*

A/V. auric. Rostr. as the main pathways for carrying its impulses:

Anatomically it begins:

In horses
The superficial path of the Triple Heater meridian:

- Begins at the dorsal aspect of the coronary band of the thoracic limb; *A/V. coronalis phal. III,*

- Ascends along the tendon of M. extensor digit. communis (the dorsal midline of the leg), to the carpus; *A/V. dorsalis phal.I, Rete carpi dors.,*

- Passes the carpus between the tendons of M. ext. digit. comm. and M. ext. carpi rad.,; *Rete carpi dors,*

- Turns over to the lateral side, between M. ext. digit. comm. and M. ext. digit. lat.; *A/V. interosseus dors.,*

- Ascends along the lateral aspect of the ulna and olecranon; *A/V. interosseus recurrens.,*

- Continues towards cranial along the dorsal border of the lateral head of M. triceps brachiis; *A/V. profunda brachii,* to the lateral aspect of the shoulder joint; *A/V. circumflex. hum. caud.*

- From the depth and CV17 a branch emerges at ST12 and ascends along the cervical vertebrae; *A/V. vertebralis,* to the wing of Atlas, TH16; anastomoses between *A/V. vertebralis* and *A/V. occipitalis ramus desc.,*

- Curves towards the head ventral to the ear, at TH17,

- Circles behind the ear,; *A/V. auricularis magna,*

- Contacts several of the local Gall Bladder points,

- Descends along the chin and contacts SI18,

- Ascends again to the area under the eye.

- One branch enters the ear and reemerges cranial to the ear and contacts SI19 and GB03,

- Travels just dorsal to the condylar process of the mandible; *A/V. auricul. rostr.*,

- Ends at the lateral end of the eyebrow, TH23, and links with GB01; *A/V. supraorbit., A/V. auric. rostr.*

The deep path of the Triple Heater meridian:

- Travels dorsally from the shoulder area and makes contact with SI12, BL11 and GV14,

- Turns towards ventral and intersects with GB21,

- continues ventrally to ST12, and enters the chest and disperses at the level of CV17,

- Connects with the Pericardium and travels through the diaphragm to the abdomen via CV12, linking the upper, middle and lower jiao.

In dogs TH01 is at the outside nail root of toe 4 (2nd outermost) on the forelimb. The Channel ascends from TH01, along the cranial side until it passes the carpus. The Channel then passes to the lateral side of the foreleg, turning more and more caudal. It reaches the caudal aspect to the olecranon and shoulder. It ascends the lateral neck and throat, to end after making a trip around the ear, at the lateral edge or end of "the eyebrow".

In humans begins on the ulnar (lateral, abaxial) side of the nail root of finger 4 (ring finger). It ascends along the dorsal side of the hand to TH04 (on the ulnar side of the dorsal wrist crease), to TH05 (2' above dorsal wrist crease, between radius and ulna, directly opposite PC06), to TH10 (1 cun above the olecranon). From here, it ascends the back of the arm to TH14 (posterolateral point of shoulder), to TH16 (dorsal to larynx), to TH17 (under root of ear). From here, it skirts upwards and around the back of the ear, to end at TH23, 1 cun lateral to the eyebrow.

Phase	Metal		Earth		Fire		Water		Fire		Wood
Yin Channel	LU[(1)]		SP[(4)]	>>	HT[(1)]		KI[(4)]	>>	PC[(1)]		LV[(4)]
	‖		‖		‖		‖		‖		‖
Yang Channel	LI[(2)]	>>	ST[(3)]		SI[(2)]	>>	BL[(3)]		TH[(2)]	>>	GB[(3)]
Limb	Hand		Foot		Hand		Foot		Hand		Foot

(‖ and >>) mean that Qi Flow sequence is LU-LI-ST-SP, etc;
‖ = Yin-Yang Phase Mates (Partners);
[(1)] Qi flow from chest to hand; [(2)] Qi flow from hand to face; [(3)]
Qi flow from face to foot; [(4)] Qi flow from foot to chest

Table 71

In TCM, TH precedes (is "upstream of") GB in the Qi Clock, the diurnal Qi-flow Cycle through the Channel system. Therefore TH transfers Qi to GB Channel and regulates it; tonification of TH strengthens GB and *vice-versa*, and both belong to the same Six Energy Level, the Shaoyang (see page 220).

The Neijing states that whatever you can do by stimulation of all the other Processes by the help of AP, you can do by stimulating the TH Channel alone. TH Qi comes from PC, its Yin Mate in Fire, and flows into (connects with) GB Channel. In animals, TH Channel is more important than PC Channel. TH Channel relates especially to metabolism, blood circulation (especially important for the quality of the claw, hoof and nails). It also relates to synovial fluid production in the fetlock and carpus and for the circulation in the respiratory tract mucus membranes. Good local microcirculation is vital to good local immunity and resistance to infection in the sinuses, nose, throat, trachea, and esophagus, digestive and urogenital tract. In young children, a Process Imbalance in TH Channel is almost always responsible for middle ear disorders. Treatment of TH Channel in >90% of cases eliminates otitis media infection in children within 1-3 treatments.

In diagnosing different kinds of allergy, I usually find either a Yin Deficiency or a TH-deficiency as the cause of the allergy. It seems to me that the Yin Deficiency is connected to an immunodeficiency and an elevation of circulating IgG, while the

TH Deficiency is restricted to only this meridian and an elevation of IgE in the mucosal membranes. Thus, there are two different ways of treating allergies, eighter TH04 or SP06.

In dogs, treatment of TH Channel drastically improves chronic infection of the outer ear. In horses, which seldom develop ear infections or sinusitis, TH Channel is important for the forelimb extensor tendons, hoof quality, the fetlock and the carpus. In contrast to humans, TH-related metabolic imbalances occur much less than in humans. In accordance with the Chinese Qi Clock, around 2200h is the best time of day to treat TH Channel.

TH has three parts, called the Three Heaters (Jiao, Burners or Burning Spaces). Each Heater dominates specific Organs. Thus, each Heater has a specific sphere of influence. Specific Master acupoints influence each of the three Heaters and their Processes. Also, ST Channel has unique points for the Processes within the three parts of the TH system.

This TH concept also has specific relationships with ST Channel. These relationships are:

	UPPER HEATER	MIDDLE HEATER	LOWER HEATER
Location	Thorax	Upper abdomen	Lower abdomen
Processes influenced	LU, HT, PC	ST, SP, SI, GB, LV	LI, BL, KI
Sphere of influence	Respiration and circulation	Digestion and extraction	Elimination and reproduction
Master Points	CV17	CV12	SP10
Master ST Points	ST36	ST37	ST39
ST Channel relationships	Esophagus, cardia and upper third of ST Channel	Stomach body and middle third of ST Channel	Pylorus and lower third of ST Channel

Table 72

Soulie de Morant discussed French experiments that showed the effect of TH on the nervous system. For example, sedating TH at its Earth Point (TH10) has a powerful effect on the sympathetic nervous system and is useful for agitated or tense patients. TH10 also acts on the internal organs and can reduce high blood pressure caused by nervous tension. In contrast, tonifying TH at its Wood Point (TH03) can stimulate the sympathetic nervous system in patients with neurasthenia, apathy or Qi Deficiency.

TH (Fire) normally controls LU (Metal) via the Ko Cycle. In TH Deficiency, control of Metal is lost and the Metal Process may show Excess. Thus, a Process Imbalance in TH may manifest in Lesion-Symptom Complexes that include LU Excess, chilliness, congestion and swelling in the mid section of the body. Other symptoms of severe TH imbalance (Deficiency or Excess) include tinnitus, urinary dysfunction, weakness of the extremities and a feeling of exasperation.

The External Stressor of Heat Invasion of TH manifests as fullness in the thorax, thirst and swelling of the pharynx.

Lesion-Symptom Complexes of a Process Imbalance in each of the Three Heaters are unique. For example, Upper Heater Deficiency may induce dull thinking, due to deprivation of energy to the brain. Other symptoms may include tinnitus, a despondent expression and darkening of the eyes. In contrast, Middle Heater Deficiency can manifest as irregular stool formation and intestinal damage. A Process Imbalance in the Lower Heater may manifest as paresis and arrhythmia.

The energy in the TH meridian (Qi) may, as for the TH-process itself, be in:

- *Excess*

- *Deficiency*

Particular for the meridian the energy may also be in:

- *Destructivity*

- *Blocced*

Excess show itself usually as pain, as this is a Yang meridian, and Yang meridians usually show excesses as pain (contrary to Ying-meridians which often show excesses just as an elevated and positive function of the process). An excess in the TH-meridian may be the result of a deficiency in the Kidney-process.

Deficiency in a Yang meridian is much more seldom as it is in a Yin meridian. Often symptoms arising from Yang-meridians are due to excesses, but of course deficiencies are also found. A deficiency may express itself as underfunction of the associated organ, as underfunction in the associated muscles and in the skin-area transversed by the meridian. In the TH-meridian this may result in changes of the hormonal system or other changes as described on page 86-87, or skin changes along the path of the meridian.

A deficiency in the TH-meridian is often the cause of an excess in the Bladder- or Large Intestine meridians, and pain along these meridians may be the result. This pain is often the symptoms we see most easily.

Destructivity show itself as in all animals as particular vicious symptoms of the skin, erosions and wounds (see more about destructive energy on page XXXIV).

Blockage of the TH-meridian is caused by a trauma on the structures of connective tissue that lead the impulses travelling through this meridian. Such a trauma will not hurt or destroy the energy of the process itself, but hinder the Qi-flow in the meridian. This is why the pulse in such a case shows absolutely good health for the process, but the acupuncture points may show dis-balance. This disbalance shows excess above the trauma, and deficienct below the trauma.

| TH 01 | **Guanchong (Passage Hub-Thoroughfare)**

Ting point and Wood point in horses and dogs
(Jing-Well and Metall point in Humans)

In horses: On the dorsal midline of the coronary band, of the thoracic limb. Many authors put this point a little lateral to the exact midline. This is wrong. Probably this mistake has come from the fact that the ECIWO-point of the carpus lies a little lateral to the midline, and in carpal problems the point seems to be a little lateral. Marvin Cain asked me once if I had noticed that the TH-Ting-point seems to move laterally in older horses. Of course they don't move, but as older horses have many more problems with the carpus than yonger horses, the point then gives the illusion of moving, as it increasingly merges with the ECIWO-point mentioned.
In dogs: it is at the posterior edge of the nail-root of the 4th claw, ulnar side.
In humans: it is 0.1 cun from posterior edge of the nail-root of the 4th finger, ulnar side.

Effect: It is important in fetlock joint disorders in all species; it stimulates the blood circulation to joints and hooves. It also helps the carpus. It is to be applied in all cases of ear disorders, furunculosis (purulent infections) in the forepaws, eczema on the forelimb and in all kinds of hearing disorders. It influences and stabilises hormones and helps hormonal disturbances and heat disorders (disorders of the estrous cycle). It also counteracts hypersensitivity and contact allergies (over sensitivity) as well as red eyes and sore throats. I have treated many bank clerks with nickel allergy and dentists with different kinds of allergies to dental amalgams with just this one point. |
| TH 02 | **Yiemen (Humour Gate)**

Fire point in horses and in dogs
(Ying-Spring and Water point in Humans)

In horses: Just distal to the fetlock, on the dorsal midline.
In dogs: it is at the paw dorsum, in the web between claw 4 and 5.
In humans: it is at the hand dorsum, in the web between fingers 4-5. |

	Effect: It helps swollen joints, reduced circulation within sexual organs, ovarian cysts and in reduced production of joint fluid in the forefetlock.
TH 03	**Zhongzhu (Central Islet)** **Earth point in horses and in dogs** **(Shu-Stream and Wood point in Humans)** *In horses:* Just proximal to the fetlock, on the dorsal midline. *In dogs:* it is 1 cun proximal to TH02, at paw-dorsum, between metacarpals 4-5. *In humans:* it is 1 cun proximal to TH02, at hand-dorsum, between metacarpals 4-5. *Effect:* In horses and dogs, where it is related to the Earth element, it is of special importance to degenerative states in the area (fetlock) and along the entire meridian. TH03 also helps the extensor tendons and movement of the forelimb. It also helps the temple, mastoid, ear, Eustachian tube, hearing and Meniere's disease; metacarpus, hand and palm. In humans, where it "is thought" to be a Wood (= growth, movement) Point, it is especially important to new formations, scar tissue, excess bone (callus, periostitis) and other "overgrowth" states in area of the point or along the whole meridian.
TH 04	**TH04 Yangchi (Yang Pool)** **Source Point** *In horses:* At the level of the antebrachiocarpal joint, between the tendons of Mm. ext. digit. commun. and ext. carpi radialis. *In dogs:* it is at the center of the dorsal carpal (wrist) crease, at the ulnar side of the common digital extensor. *In humans:* it is at the center of the dorsal carpal (wrist) crease, at the ulnar side of the common digital extensor. *Effect:* It is a Local Point for the carpus, but also is very important for ear disorders and infections in the outer ear, especially in long-eared dogs. Many dogs have such infections. On presentation in the clinic, dogs with irritated and painful

	ears often are apprehensive. Having learned from experience of their complaint, they try to avoid any contact with the ear. A few treatments at TH04 generally give a clear improvement, so that the dog usually allows inspection of their ears without showing signs of discomfort. It is usual, but not always necessary, to cleanse the ear during this treatment. It also helps the thoracic limb, fingers and chills. **Recipe for a very effective remedy to clean the ears** # 500 ml 60% alcohol solution 8 g Peru balm Iodine until cognac-coloured 6 g acetylsalicylic acid plus possibly 10 g of a local anaesthetic, such as 100% Lidocaine-powder. #
TH 05 (-1 in hors-es)	**Waiguan (Outer Pass)** **Luo Point of TH and Meeting Point of the Yangweimai Analgesic Point** *In horses:* 2 cun proximal to the lateral distal Tuberositas radii, between the tendons of Mm. extensor digit. communis et lateralis.. *In dogs:* In all species it is on the dorsolateral forearm 2 cun above the carpus, directly opposite PC06. In dogs, as the gap between the radius and ulna can be narrow, it is easier to needle PC06 by inserting the needle between the bones at TH05, and advancing it all the way through the limb. *In humans:* it is on the dorsolateral forearm 2 cun above the carpus, directly opposite PC06. *Effect:* It connects TH Channel with its Phase Mate, PC Channel. In horses, as the radius and ulna are fused, the needle can be inserted at TH05 and advanced to PC06 at the opposite side of the limb, just behind the bones. Like TH04, TH05 is important in ear disorders. It also helps the temple, mastoid, Eustachian tube, Meniere's disease and hearing; the neck and thoracic limb. It is used as an analgesic point in general pain control, and to restore motor power to the thoracic limb and tongue (speech) in hemiplegia or paralysis

	after trauma, polio or CVA. It helps bones and joints, mammary disorders, mastopathy and milk disorders, and anovulation. Used together with PC06, it is of great value in controlling menopausal problems in women. This is also useful in pseudo-pregnancy and other hormonal problems in all species.
TH 05-2 (in hors-es)	**Extra point in horses** *Location;* 3 cun proximal to the lateral distal Tuberositas radii. *Effect;* Same as for TH05-01.
TH 06	**Zhigou (Branch Ditch)** **Metal point in horses and in dogs** **Fire and Horary Point in humans** *In horses:* 5 cun proximal of the lateral distal Tuberositas radii, between Mm. ext.digit. communis et lateralis. *In dogs:* it is on the forearm-dorsum, 3 cun above wrist crease, between radius and ulna. *In humans.* it is on the forearm-dorsum, 3 cun above wrist crease, between radius and ulna. *Effect:* In horses and dogs, where it is a Metal Point, it reacts to painful conditions along the meridian or just locally. Like TH05 this point also has a special affinity to the sexual hormones and when treated together with PC06 it often eliminates menopausal disorders in women and in pseudopregnancy in bitches. It also helps disorders in the thorax, chest, ribs and sternum, arm, humerus and gastrointestinal tract (constipation, diarrhoea, dysentery).
TH 07	**Huizong (Convergence and Gathering)** **Xi Point of TH** *In horses:* Caudal to TH06, between Mm. ext. digit. lat. and ulnaris lat. *In dogs:* it is a little lateral to the midline of the forearm dorsum, midway between the elbow-joint and the carpal-joint (in humans it is much closer to the carpus, where both TH06 and TH07 lie 3/12 of the way from the carpus to the elbow).

	In humans: it is on the forearm-dorsum, 3 cun above the wrist crease, on the ulnar side of TH06. *Effect:* Indicated in all acute situations.
TH 08	**Sanyangluo (Three Yang Connection)** **Analgesic Point** *In horses:* 2 cun proximal to TH06, 7 cun proximal to the lateral distal Tuberositas radii. *In dogs:* it is approximately 4 cun below the elbow, just behind the radius, on the lateral side of the forearm. *In humans:* it is on the forearm-dorsum, 4 cun above the carpal (wrist) crease, between radius and ulna. *Effect:* It helps the arm, humerus and lower teeth. It is an important point for analgesia.
TH 09	**Sidu (Four Rivers)** In humans, it is on the forearm-dorsum, 5 cun below olecranon, between radius and ulna. In dogs and horses it is approximately 3 cun below the elbow, just behind the radius, on the lateral side of the forearm. It helps the forearm, radius and ulna.
TH 10	**Tianjing (Heavenly Well)** **Local point in horses** **Water point in dogs** **(He-Sea and Earth point in Humans)** *In horses:* In a depression 1 cun craniodorsal to Tuber olecranii, on the dorsal border of the lateral head of the M. triceps brachii. *In dogs:* it is in a hollow 1 cun above and behind the tip of the olecranon when the elbow is slightly flexed. *In humans:* it is in a hollow 1 cun above and behind the tip of the olecranon when the elbow is slightly flexed. *Effect:* In all species, it helps chronic carpitis and elbow disorders, especially degenerative ones. It also helps coughs and pain in the upper forearm.

TH 13	**Naohui (Shoulders meeting)** **Meeting point of the Sanjiao meridian and the Yang Wei mai** *In horses:* 6 cun craniodorsal to TH10, in a depression caudal to the shoulder joint. *In dogs:* on the line between TH10 and TH14, ¾ of the way between TH10 and TH14. *In humans:* this points are situated on the line between TH10 and TH14 (see below), TH 11 is ¼ of the way, TH12 is midway and TH13 ¾ of the way between TH10 and TH14. *Effect:* helps the axilla and arm.
TH 14	**TH14 Jianliao (Shoulder Bone-Orifice)** *In horses:* In a depression lateral to the shoulder joint, on a continued line along the scapular spine. *In dogs:* it is on the line of the scapular spine, as it crosses the shoulder joint. *In humans:* it is behind the shoulder joint, in a hole between acromion and proximal head of humerus, about 1 cun behind LI15. *Effect:* It helps the clavicle, scapula and shoulder.
TH 15	**Tianliao (Heavenly Bone-Orifice)** **Meeting point of the TH and GB meridians and the Yang Wei mai** *In horses:* Immediately in front of the cranial border of the M. subclavius, at the level of C7 (7th cervical vertebrae), dorsal to its transverse process. *In dogs:* it is situated in the bottom of the angle made by the scapula and the lower neck. *In humans:* it is midway from GV14 to the tip of acromion, 1 cun posterior inferior to GB21. *Effect:* It helps neck, scapular and shoulder disorders in horses and dogs.

TH 16 (-1 in horses)	**Tianyou (Heavenly Window)**
	Diagnostic Point for Ovary/Testicle **Point of the Window of the Sky** *In horses:* Over the transverse foramen of atlas (first cervical vertebrae, C1). *In dogs:* it is just above the axis (second cervical vertebrae, C2). *In humans:* it is posteroinferior to the mastoid process, at the posterior edge of the sternocleidomastoid muscle, level with the angle of the mandible, level with SI17 and BL10. *Effect:* In horses, this point is often sensitive in Process Imbalances of TH Channel and in ovarian and testicular disorders. It helps neck pain. It is one of the **"Windows of the Sky" Points** (see also TH16-2, LI18-1 and LI18-2).
TH 16-2	**Extra point in horses (and possible in dogs too)** **Point of the Window of the Sky** *Location;* At the level of C4 (4th cervical vertebrae), dorsal to its transverse process. *Effect;* Regulates the flow of qi and blood between the head and body; benefits the head and sense organs.
TH 17	**TH17 Yifeng (Shielded from Wind)** **Meeting point of the TH and GB meridians** *In horses:* In a depression ventral to the ear, between Processus jugularis and Processus condylaris of the mandibula. *In dogs:* it is situated above the atlas, on the wings, behind the ears. *In humans:* it is in a hollow between the mastoid process and mandible, covered by the earlobe. *Effect:* It helps neck pain and ear disorders. It is a point used to calm a nervous or difficult animal. It also helps the face, cheek, tongue, speech, mandible, masseter, temporomandibular joint, mastoid, Eustachian tube, Meniere's disease and hearing.

TH 21	**Ermen (Ear Gate)**
	In horses: Rostral to the ear, just dorsal to Crista temporalis and SI19.
	In dogs: it is ventral to the rostral border of the ear, about 2 cun under the ventral end of the ear.
	In humans: it is just anterior to the supratragic notch, in a hole formed when mouth opened, about 1 cun above SI19.
	Effect: It helps the ear, hearing, Eustachian tube, masseter, mastoid, Meniere's disease and temporomandibular joint.
TH 23	**Sizhukong (Silk Bamboo) Orifice**
	In horses: In a depression at the lateral end of the eyebrow.
	In dogs: In a depression at the lateral end of the eyebrow.
	In humans: In a depression at the lateral end of the eyebrow.
	Effect: It is a Local Point to help the eye, sight and temple.

Table 73

The special commandpoints in the horse are as follows:

S O U R C E fetlock	*Location;* At the level of the metacarpophalangeal joint, on the dorsal midline. *Effect;* Stimulates the meridian.
M E T A L	*Location;* Just distal to the carpus, between the metacarpal tuberosity and the tendon of M. extensor digit. communis. *Effect;* Influences painful conditions locally and along the course of the meridian, and generally in the body when the Triple Heater is in excess or deficiency.
W A T E R	*Location;* 0.5 cun proximal to the carpus, at the craniolateral aspect, medial to the tendon of the M. ext. digit. commun. *Effect;* Influences problems with edema and disturbed venous circulation locally and along the course of the meridian, and generally in the body when the Triple Heater is in excess or deficiency.

Table 74

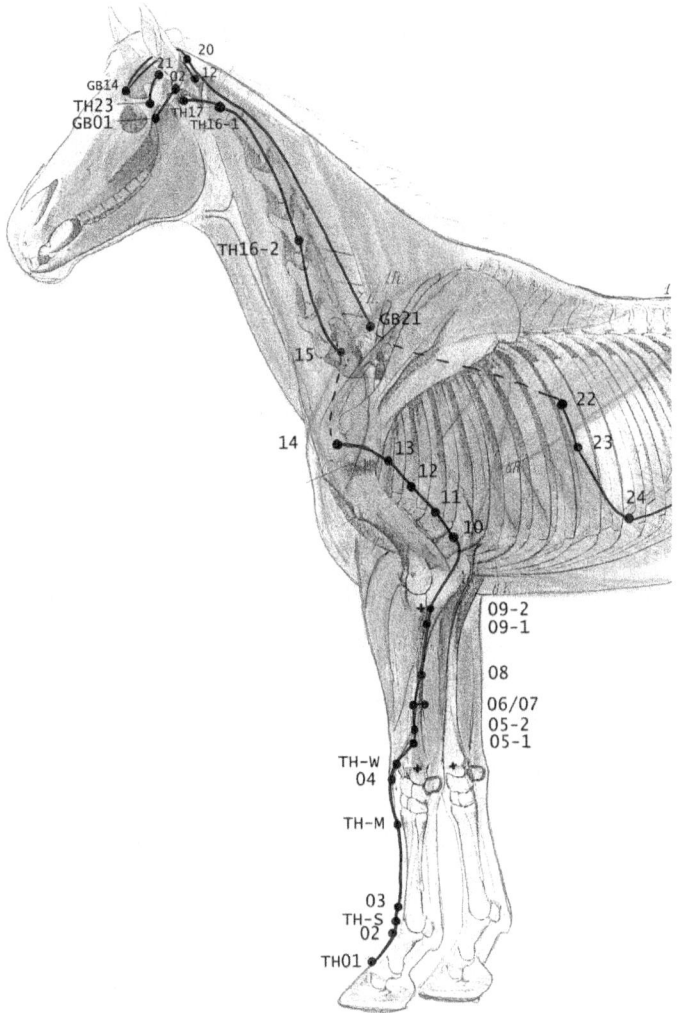

*Figure 56; Diagram of some of the most important points
on the TH Channel in the horse.*

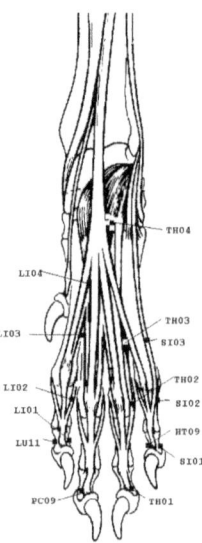

DIAGRAM OF THE MOST IMPORTANT POINTS ON
THE DORSAL SIDE OF THE DOGS PAW.

*Figure 57; Diagram of some of the most important points
on the front paw of the dog.*

GB (Gallbladder, Foot Shaoyang Channel) uses the connective tissue around *A/V. temporalis supf., A/V. supraorb., A/V.
occipitalis, A/V. cervicalis supf. (asc.)* as the main pathways for
carrying its impulses:

Anatomically it begins:

IN HORSES
The Superficial Path of the Gall Bladder Meridian:

- Begins near the outer canthus of the eye, at GB01, in a
  depression just ventral to Processus zygomaticus; *A/V.
  temporalis supf.* and anastomoses with *A/V. supraorb.*.

- Travels towards the caudal part of the TMJ and rostral part of the base of the ear.

- Curves caudally and medially around the ear to Processus mastoideus.

- Curves back again, rostrally and medially, to the supra-orbital region.

- Ascends and curves across the temporal fossa to the caudal part of Crista nuchae; at GB20; *A/V. occipitalis.*

- Crosses the neck and emerges at GB21, in M. subclavius, halfway between GV14 and the point of the shoulder; *A/V. cervicalis supf. (asc.).*

- From GB21 it passes dorsally to intersect with BL11 and SI12, then ventrally to ST12.

- Travels medial to the scapula and along the lateral costal area through GB22, GB23 and GB24.

- Contacts the Liver at LV13.

- Continues to the hip joint to rejoin with the deep branch at GB30.

- United as one, the meridian descends along the lateral aspect of the thigh and knee; *A/V. circumflexa femoris med., A/V. genus lat.*

- Travels along the lateral aspect of the lower leg, between the Mm. extensor digit. longus et lat.; *A/V. tibialis cranialis (A/V. fibularis).*

- Passes the hock on the dorsolateral side; *A/V. dorsalis pedis.*

- Follows the dorsolateral surface of Mt III; *A. mtts. dors. III`.*

- Passes the phalanges on the dorsolateral side; *dorsal branch of the proximal and middle phalanx arteries/veins.*

- Ends at the coronary band, ~ 55^0 dorsolateral to the tip of the toe; *A/V. coronalis phal. III.*

The Deep Path of the Gall Bladder Meridian:

1. One branch emerges behind the ear and enters the ear at TH17.

    *   Reemerges in front of the ear and travels via SI19 and ST07 to the outer canthus of the eye.

    *   Passes ventrally in the masseter muscle to near ST05.

    *   Crosses the Triple Heater meridian and ascends to the infraorbital area and meets with BL01.

    *   Passes close to ST06 on its way to the neck, where it intersects ST09-1 and meets the main meridian at ST12.

    *   Enters the chest and meets with the Pericardium meridian at PC01.

    *   Passes through the diaphragm, contacts the Liver and connects with the Gall Bladder.

    *   Continues along the inside of the ribs to the inguinal region.

    *   Encircles the genitals.

    *   Enters deeply again and travels to the sacral area where it meets the Bladder meridian at the four points of the sacral foramina and the Governing vessel at GV01.

    *   Emerges dorsal to the hip joint at GB30 to meet with the superficial path.

2. At GB40 a second branch leaves the main meridian and passes plantarad through the vascular canal of the tarsus; *A/V. tarsica perforans,* travels distally to the medial side, deep to the interosseus, to meet the Liver meridian at LV01 at the coronary band.

In dogs it begins at GB01, at the lateral canthus of the eye. It passes over the head to GB20 (caudal to the occipital process, over the atlas). In my opinion the Channel also expresses itself in the growth of the horns of cows. Then it passes down the lateral side of the neck to GB21 (midway from GV14 to the point of shoulder), down the mid-axillary line to GB25 (tip of last rib), to GB30 (behind the great trochanter of the femur). Then it descends the lateral thigh to GB34 (between the upper heads of the fibula and tibia) to GB40 (anteroinferior to lateral malleolus, in hollow lateral to extensor digitorum longus tendon). From here it runs in the dorsum of the paw between metatarsals 4-5 to end at GB44, at the lateral claw-root of the 4th toe.

In humans it begins at GB01, at the lateral canthus of the eye. It passes over the head to GB20 (caudal to the occipital process, over the atlas). Then it passes down the lateral side of the neck to GB21 (midway from GV14 to the point of shoulder) down the mid-axillary line to GB25 (tip of last rib) to GB30 (behind the great trochanter of the femur). Then it descends the lateral thigh to GB34 (between the upper heads of the fibula and tibia) to GB40 (anteroinferior to lateral malleolus, in hollow lateral to extensor digitorum longus tendon). From here it runs in the dorsum of the foot, between metatarsals 4-5 to end at GB44, at the lateral nail root of the 4th toe.

Phase	Metal		Earth		Fire		Water		Fire		Wood
Yin Channel	LU[1]		SP[4]	>>	HT[1]		KI[4]	>>	PC[1]		LV[4]
	‖		‖		‖		‖		‖		‖
Yang Channel	LI[2]	>>	ST[3]		SI[2]	>>	BL[3]		TH[2]	>>	GB[3]
Limb	Hand		Foot		Hand		Foot		Hand		Foot

(‖ and >>) mean that Qi Flow sequence is LU-LI-ST-SP, etc;
‖ = Yin-Yang Phase Mates (Partners);
[1] Qi flow from chest to hand; [2] Qi flow from hand to face; [3]
Qi flow from face to foot; [4] Qi flow from foot to chest

Table 75

GB Qi comes from TH Channel and flows into (connects with) LV Channel, its Yin Mate in Wood. Although horses have no physical gallbladder, like other species they have biliary function and a GB Channel and its functions. This shows that the Processes in the organism are universal and independent of special mammalian-like organs to carry out their duty (as in plants, where just the cells carry out the functions of the processes and actually no organs are present, life is still maintained, and all the processes are functioning). However, if the Process is linked to a special organ, then of course the process is dependent on this organ to carry out its duty. We cannot remove the Gall bladder if such an organ already is developed.

The GB Channel helps to control the functions of this process in the organism. The GB Process, as well as the GB Channel, is actually quite important for horses, more so than in both humans and dogs.

As mentioned earlier, the Fundamental Processes are not only present in the organ in question, but also manifest themselves throughout the entire organism. They are usually concentrated in the so-called organ. If this organ does not exist in a particular species, its related Functions are delegated to be shared by other Organs or tissues (dispersed even more throughout the body). Just think about the plants. They have a few ordinary organs, nevertheless, they maintain all of the Fundamental Processes needed for life. Life would be impossible without all the 12 Processes. For example, after splenectomy, the rest of the digestive system must compensate for the SP Processes. Although horses have no GB, the functions of GB are maintained by the rest of the body, and the properties of GB are seen clearly in the free gallop and movements of horses.

GB precedes LV in the Chinese Qi Clock Cycle, which maps how the peak-activity of the different Processes change from time to time. It also shows how Qi wanders. Therefore GB regulates and provides Qi to LV Channel. Tonification of GB strengthens LV and vice versa.

GB Channel travels along the entire side of the animal from the head to the hindleg, and has an influence on all muscles through which it passes. It is of special importance to the insertion of the tensor fascia lata muscle on the hip (tuber coxae), the outside of the stifle, tarsus and neck. Horses that dislike or show lameness on turning or bending usually have GB Channel disorders (excess = pain). GB also is important in colic, especially in children. Gallstones can be treated successfully through GB Channel points. In accordance with the Chinese Qi Clock, around midnight (2400h) is the best time of day to treat GB Channel.

The energy in the GB meridian (Qi) may, as for the lung-process itself, be in:

- *Excess*

- *Deficiency*

Particular for the meridian the energy may also be in:

- *Destructivity*

- *Blocked*

Excess shows itself usually as pain as this is a Yang meridian, and Yang meridians usually show excesses as pain (contrary to Ying-meridians which often show excesses just as an elevated and positive function of the process). An excess in the GB-meridian may be the result of a deficiency in the Lung process.

Deficiency in a Yang meridian is much more seldom as it is in a Yin meridian. Often symptoms arising from Yang-meridians are due to excesses, but of course deficiencies are also found. A deficiency may express itself as under-function of the associated organ, as under-function in the associated muscles and in the skin area transversed by the meridian, as described on page 89. In the GB meridian this may result in underfunction of all the muscles along the side of the animal or human or skin changes along the path of the meridian.

A deficiency in the GB meridian is often the cause of an excess in the Stomach meridian, and pain and cancer along this meridian may be the result. This pain is often the symptom we see most easily.

Destructivity shows itself, as in all animals, as particular viscious symptoms of the skin, erosions, pain, migrain and wounds (see more about destructive energy on page XXXIV).

Blockage of the GB-meridian is caused by a trauma on the structures of connective tissue that lead the impulses travelling through this meridian. Such a trauma will not hurt or destroy the energy of the process itself, but hinders the Qi-flow in the meridian. This is why the pulse in such a case shows absolutely good health for the process, but the acupuncture points may show disbalance. This disbalance shows excess above the trauma, and deficienct below the trauma.

GB 01	**Tongziliao Pupil (in the) Bone-Orifice** **Meeting Point of the GB, SI and TH Meridians** *In Horses:* Lateral to the lateral canthus of the eye, in a depression just ventral to Processus zygomaticus. *In Dogs:* Lateral to the lateral canthus of the eye, in a depression just ventral to Processus zygomaticus. *In Humans:* It is in a hole lateral to the orbit, lateral to lateral canthus the of eye. *Effect:* It helps the forehead, frontal sinuses, eye, eyelid, sight; face, cheek, headache and migraine.
GB 02	**Tinghui (Hearing Convergence)** *In horses:* At the caudal border of the condyloid process of the mandible, directly below SI19. *In dogs:* It is at the posterior edge of condyloid process of the mandible, anterior to the intertragic notch, in a hole when the mouth is open. *In humans:* It is at the posterior edge of condyloid process of the mandible, anterior to the intertragic notch, in a hole when the mouth is open. *Effect:* It helps the mastoid, ear, hearing, Eustachian tube, Meniere's disease, temporomandibular joint and masseter.

GB 12	**Wangu (Mastoid Process)** **Meeting Point of the GB and BL Meridians** *In horses:* 3 cun lateral to the dorsal midline, between the cranial border of the wing of Atlas and Processus jugularis, 1.5 cun lateral to GB20. *In dogs:* In a depression posterior and inferior to the mastoid process. *In humans:* In a depression posterior and inferior to the mastoid process. *Effect:* Eliminates interior and exterior wind. Worth a try in head shakers. Calms the spirit.
GB 14	**Yangbai (Yang White)** **Meeting point of the GB, TH, ST and LI meridians and with the Yang Wei mai** *In horses:* Above the pupil, just caudal and dorsal to the supraorbital foramen, at the level of the frontal crest. *In dogs:* Above the pupil, just caudal and dorsal to the supraorbital foramen, at the level of the frontal crest. *In humans:* It is directly above mid-pupil, one inch above the center of the eyebrow. *Effect:* It helps the forehead, frontal sinuses, eye, eyelid, sight, face, cheek, headache and migraine.
GB 20	**Fengchi (Wind Pool)** **Master Point for Wood / Wind disorders** **Meeting point of the GB and TH meridians with the Yang Wei and Yang Qiao mai** *In horses:* 1 cun caudal to the nuchal crest in M. obliquus capitis cran., 1.5 cun lateral to the dorsal midline. *In dogs:* It is in the muscle, over the wing of the atlas. *In humans:* It is in a hole between the trapezius and sternocleidomastoid muscles, below occipital process, lateral to BL10 and level with GV16.

	Effect: It helps mainly in first aid in headache, sinusitis, skin and hair, brain, meninges and its functions, eye, Meniere's disease, hearing, neck and cervical spine and vasomotor allergy. It helps tremendously with stiffness or soreness in the neck region in relation to throat infections or injuries to the atlas (neck vertebra C1). GB20 is especially effective in influenza.
GB 21	**Jianjing (Shoulder Well).** **Meeting point of the GB, TH and ST meridians with theYang Wei mai** *In horses:* In the M. subclavius, halfway between GV14 and the point of the shoulder. *In dogs:* It is just in front of the scapula, caudodorsal of the 6th cervical vertebrae, just in front of TH15. *In humans:* It is at the highest point of the trapezius muscle, midway from tip of acromion to the C7 vertebrae. *Effect:* In humans, as well as in animals, it helps neck and shoulder disorders. It helps the neck, cervical spine, blood vessels, arteriosclerosis, vasomotor disorders, ischaemia, mammary disorders, mastopathy, milk disorders, menopausal disorders, flushes and sweats.
GB 24	**GB24 Riyue (Sun and Moon)** **Front-Mu point** **Meeting point of the GB and SP Meridians with the Yang Wei mai** *In horses:* In the 10th intercostal space, on a line between the point of shoulder and the stifle joint. *In dogs:* It is in the angle where the 7th and the 8th rib meets the sternum, in intercostal space 7. *In humans:* It is directly below the nipple (intercostal space 4), in intercostal space 7. *Effect:* In humans, It helps the diaphragm; gallbladder and bileduct (inflammation, calculi, obstruction etc).

GB 25 (-1 in hors- es)	Jingmen (Capital Gate)
	Mu Point of KI and Diagnostic Point for KI, Ovary/Testicle
	In horses: At the most caudal aspect of the last rib. *In dogs:* At the most caudal aspect of the last rib. *In humans:* It is on the lateral abdomen, just at the tip of the last (12th) rib.
	Effect: It is a Diagnostic Point (with BL23) for ovarian disorders in horses. It helps the kidney and upper ureter, ovary, PID and chills.
GB 25-2	*Extrapoint in horses*
	Location: 8 cun lateral to the dorsal midline, lateral to BL23, on the dorsal border of the last (18th) rib.
	Effekt; Similar to GB25-1.
GB 26	**Daimai (Girdling Vessel)** **Meeting point of the GB Meridian with the Dai mai**
	In horses: 4 cun caudoventral to LV13, at the level of the umbilicus and the fold of the flank. *In dogs:* Just under the Tuber coxae. *(It is erroneously called ST30 by many veterinary colleagues.)* *In humans:* It is on the mid-axillary line, level with CV08.
	Effect: It relaxes the muscles around the stifle and relieves pain in the biceps femoris muscle. The action is similar to that of GB27 but it has a somewhat more local effect on the muscles near and related to the stifle. It also helps the female genitalia and reproduction, anovulation and leucorrhoea.
GB 27	**Wushu (Fifth Pivot)** **Meeting point of the GB Meridian with the Dai mai**
	In horses: Just dorsal and caudal to the dorsal prominence of the Tuber coxae. *In dogs:* It is just in front of the tuber coxae. *(It is mistakenly called SP13 by many veterinary colleagues.)* *In humans:* It is anterior to the anterosuperior iliac spine, level with CV04, which is three inches below CV08.

	Effect: It activates Yangweimai, an Extraordinary Vessel that acts like a Qi reservoir to vitalise all the muscles of the equine hindquarter, so that the animal gets a sudden abundance of power (Qi). Therefore, Marvin Cain calls GB27 a "Performance Point." Regulates the Dai mai. It also helps retracted testicle (at least in Humans, worth trying). Relaxes the gluteal muscles.
GB 28 (-1 in hors- es)	**Weidao (Linking Path)** **Meeting point of the GB Meridian with the Dai mai** *In horses:* Directly cranial and ventral to the middle part of the Tuber coxae. *In dogs:* Directly cranial and ventral to the middle part of the Tuber coxae. *In humans:* It is anteroinferior to the anterior superior iliac spine, 0.5' anterioinferior to GB27. *Effect:* It greatly relaxes the hip (gluteal) muscles.
GB 28-2	*Extra Point in Horses* *Location:* Ventral and slightly caudal to the ventral part of Tuber coxae, in a depression in the M. tensor fasciae latae.
GB 29	**Juliao (Squatting Bone-Orifice)** **Meeting Point of the GB Meridian with the Yang Qiao mai** *In horses:* In M. gluteus supf., cranial to the hip joint, one third of the distance between the cranial part of Trochanter major and the dorsal midline, ~8 cun lateral to the dorsal midline. *In dogs:* It is in front of the hip joint *(the joint must be palpated exactly).* *In humans:* It is midway from anterior superior iliac spine to great trochanter of the femur, on the iliac side. *Effect:* It is a very important point to treat hip dysplasia (HD) in dogs. In HD cases, one often implants little pieces of gold wire at **GB29, GB30 and BL54**. These points are all situated around and near the hip joint.

GB 30	**Huantiao (Ring of Jumping (Hip Joint))** **Meeting Point of the GB and BL Meridians** ***In horses:*** In M. biceps femoris, caudal to the hip joint, one third of the distance between Trochanter major and the sacro-coccygeal hiatus, ~8 cun lateral to the dorsal midline. ***In dogs:*** In M. biceps femoris, caudal to the hip joint, one third of the distance between Trochanter major and the sacro-coccygeal hiatus. ***In humans:*** It is behind the head of the femur, 1/3 of the way from the greater trochanter to the sacrococcygeal space. ***Effect:*** It is one of the main points to treat hip dysplasia in dogs. It also helps the brain, meninges and their functions and parts. Also the waist, flank and dorsolumbar area.
GB 31	**Fengshi (Wind Market)** ***In horses:*** On the lateral aspect of the thigh, just proximal to Trochanter tertius, between the Mm. gluteus supf. and biceps femoris. ***In dogs:*** On the lateral aspect of the thigh, just proximal to Trochanter tertius, between the Mm. gluteus supf. and biceps femoris. ***In humans:*** It is seven inches above the popliteal crease, just behind the femur, where finger 3 touches the lateral thigh when the arms are relaxed fully. ***Effect:*** It helps the entire pelvic limb, hip, thigh, femur, stifle and popliteal area, tarsus, especially pain and swelling in these areas.
GB 33	**Xiyangguan (Knee Yang Joint)** In all species, it is in a hole above the lateral condyle of the femur, three inches above GB34. It helps the patella.
GB 34	**Yanglingquan (Yang Mound Spring)** **Hui-Influential point of Sinews in all species** **Water point in dogs** **(He-Sea and Earth point in Humans)** ***In horses:*** Distal to the stifle joint, in a depression cranial and distal to the head of the fibula.

	In dogs: It is between the fibula and tibia, in a hole anterior inferior to the proximal head of fibula. *In humans:* It is between the fibula and tibia, in a hole anterior inferior to the proximal head of the fibula. *Effect:* As it has general analgesic effects, it is classed as a "**Doping Point.**" As a **Master Point**, it helps many body functions, especially the brain and meninges, thorax, abdomen, back and hip. GB34 also is a point for analgesia and pain control. It helps muscle, soft tissues, tendon, bones and joints and improves blood circulation in gangrene or ischaemia of the extremities. At my clinic I have several times seen this point normalise several blood values of different kinds, such as the red count and increase the blood haemoglobin content. It can be tried as a way to enliven lethargic animals.
GB 35	**Yangjiao (Yang Intersection)** **Xi-Cleft point of the Yang Wei mai** *In horses:* On the lateral aspect of the lower leg, midway between the lateral condyle of the tibia and the tip of the lateral malleolus, in the M. extensor digit. lat., 1 cun caudal to GB36. (*On a transverse line of the lower leg, we find ST38, ST40, GB36, GB35 and BL58.*). *In dogs:* On the lateral aspect of the lower leg, midway between the lateral condyle of the tibia and the tip of the lateral malleolus, in the M. extensor digit. lat.. *In humans:* It is seven inches above the lateral malleolus, behind the fibula, nine inches below the inferior edge of the patella, one inch behind GB36. *Effect:* It helps the leg, fibula and tibia.
GB 36	**Waiqiu (Outer Hill)** **Xi Point of GB** *In horses:* On the lateral aspect of the lower leg, midway between the lateral condyle of the tibia and the tip of the lateral malleolus, between the Mm. extensor digit. longus et lateralis, 1 cun cranial to GB35.

	In dogs: On the lateral aspect of the lower leg, midway between the lateral condyle of the tibia and the tip of the lateral malleolus, between the Mm. extensor digit. longus et lateralis. *In humans:* It is seven inches above the lateral malleolus, anterior to the fibula, nine inches below the inferior edge of patella, one inch anterior to GB35. *Effect:* In humans, horses and dogs It helps the leg, fibula and tibia.
GB 37	**Guangming (Light Bright)** **Luo Point of GB** *In horses:* On the lateral aspect of the lower leg, 1.5 cun distal to GB36, between the Mm. extensor digit. longus et lateralis. *In dogs:* On the lateral aspect of the lower leg, 1.5 cun distal to GB36, between the Mm. extensor digit. longus et lateralis. *In humans:* It is five inches above lateral malleolus, anterior to fibula, eleven inches below the inferior edge of the patella. *Effect:* It connects GB Channel with its Phase Mate, LV Channel. It helps the eyes, leg, fibula and tibia.
GB 38	**Yangfu (Yang Assistance)** **Local Point in Horses** **Analgesic Point** **Metal Point in Dogs** **(Jing-River and Fire point in Humans)** *In horses:* On the lateral aspect of the lower leg, 3 cun proximal to the tip of the lateral malleolus, between the Mm. extensor digit. longus et lateralis. *In dogs:* It is four inches above the lateral malleolus, anterior to the fibula. *In humans:* It is four inches above the lateral malleolus, anterior to the fibula, twelve inches below inferior edge of the patella. *Effect:* It has general hypoalgesic effects. It helps muscles that are painful, and helps pain along the entire Channel. It greatly helps headaches and the shoulder, axilla, salivary glands and salivation.

GB 39	**Xuanzhong (Suspended Bell)** **Hui-Influential Point for Marrow** *In horses:* 2 cun proximal to the tip of the lateral malleolus, on the caudal border of M. extensor digit. lateralis. *In dogs:* 2 cun proximal to the tip of the lateral malleolus, on the caudal border of M. extensor digit. lateralis. *In humans:* It is in a hole three inches above the tip of the lateral malleolus, between posterior edge of the fibula and tendons of peroneus longus and brevis muscles. *Effect:* It helps CVA, paralysis, hemiplegia and polio; the neck and cervical spine, waist, flank and pelvic limb (hip, leg, calf, tarsus, metatarsus and foot). It also helps lymphadenopathy.
GB 40	**Qiuxu (Hill Ruins)** **Source Point of GB** *In horses:* On the lateral aspect of the hock, on the plantar border of the M. extensor digit.lat. tendon, at the level of the vascular canal (canalis tarsi), 1 cun directly proximal to GB41. *In dogs:* It is anteroinferior to the lateral malleolus, in a hole lateral to the extensor digitorum longus tendon. *In humans:* It is anteroinferior to the lateral malleolus, in a hole lateral to the extensor digitorum longus tendon. *Effect:* It helps the gallbladder and bileduct (inflammation, calculi, obstruction etc); axilla, waist, flank, tarsus and metatarsus.
GB 41	**Zulinqi (Foot Overlooking Tears)** **Metal Point in Horses** **Earth Point in Dogs** **Confluent Point of the Dai mai** **(Shu-Stream and Wood point in Humans)** *In horses:* Just distal to the tarsus (hock) on the dorsolateral aspect of the third metatarsal bone, between the lateral digital extensor tendon and the base of the fourth (lateral) metatarsal bone.

	In dogs: It is on the paw-dorsum, between metatarsals 4-5, one and a half inch above GB43. *In humans:* It is on the foot-dorsum, between metatarsals 4-5, one and a half inch above GB43, i.e. it lies where the tears hit the foot. *Effect:* It helps the eyes, temple; mastopathy, mammary disorders and milk disorders; the waist, flank, tarsus, metatarsus and foot. It can be substituted clinically for GB42. In horses, as a Metal Point, it is of special importance for all painful symptoms along the GB meridian or within the GB process throughout the entire body. An example of such is when noise from the surrounding world "drives you crazy." In humans, as a Wood Point of a Wood Channel, it has special importance for the muscles.
GB 42	**Diwuhui (Earth Fivefold Convergence)** **Earth Point in Horses** *In horses:* In a depression just proximal to the fetlock on the dorsolateral aspect. *In dogs:* It is directly outside the joint, above and outside the hindfetlock, between GB41 and GB43. *In humans:* It is on the foot-dorsum, between metatarsals 4-5, one inch above GB43. *Effect:* It helps severe general pain, especially acute pain, strained tendons and muscular pain in general. It also helps the axilla.
GB 43	**Xiaxi (Pinched Ravine)** **Fire Point in Horses and in Dogs** **(Ying-Spring and Water point in Humans)** *In horses:* Just distal to the fetlock on the dorsolateral aspect, in a depression dorsal to the tendon of interosseus to long digital extensor tendon. *In dogs:* It is on the paw-dorsum, in the web between toes 4 and 5. *In humans:* It is on the human foot-dorsum, in the web between toes 4 and 5 (little toe).

	Effect: In my experience, this point is of little *general* importance in horses, in which its main use is for disorders of the local fetlock joint.
GB 44	**Zuqiaoyin (Foot Portal Yin)** **Ting point in all Species** **Wood Point in Horses and in Dogs** **(Jing-Well and Metal point in Humans)** *In horses:* At the coronary band, ~55⁰ dorsolateral to the tip of the toe. *In dogs:* It is 0.1 inch from posterior edge nail-root of the 4ᵗʰ claw at the hindleg, lateral side. *In humans:* It is 0.1 inch from the posterior edge nail-root toe 4, lateral side. *Effect:* It helps pain of all muscles along GB Channel and related parts, for example near BL18-BL19 and the sacral area near the top of the groove between the semimembranosus and semitendinosus muscles. Therefore, at least in horses, it stimulates and nourishes the Wood Phase. It is especially effective for "pain that moves about," or that comes and goes quickly. Trotting horses often react to pain caused by Deficiency in GB Channel by galloping when entering or coming out of a bend. They do this because of the strain they get in their side muscles when bending. Trotters that gallop when going out of the bend usually have pain in the left side of GB Channel; lameness on entering the bend indicates pain in the right area of GB Channel. In horses that have a tendency to move the leg too far against the medial side of the leg will often hit itself on the other back leg (interfering). This point helps to convey the leg outwards. In such cases it is very helpful to combine BL64, BL65, BL67 and GB44. This is relevant if the horse brushes its other hindleg in a race. It also helps the pleura.

Table 76

The special command points in the horse are as follows:

W A T E R	*Location:* Just proximal to the tip of the lateral malleolus, on the cranial border of the M. extensor digit. Lateralis. *Effect:* Influences oedema, cold and watery conditions locally and along the course of the meridian, and generally in the body when the Gall Bladder is in excess or deficiency.

S O U R C E fetlock	*Location:* At the level of the metatarsophalangeal joint, on the dorsolateral aspect. *Effect:* Stimulates the meridian.

Table 77

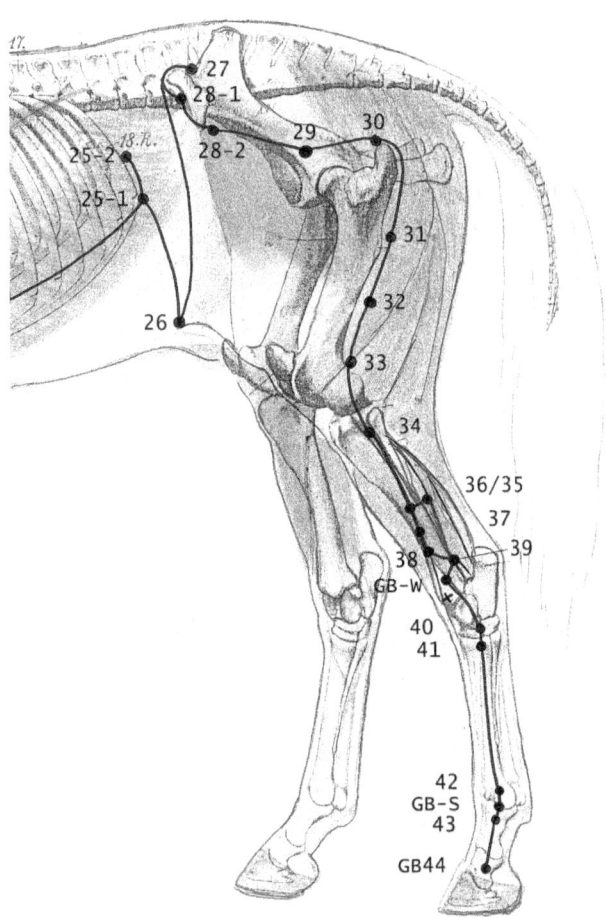

Figure 58; Illustration of several of the GB-points in the horse. Mark especially the placement of the GB Points around the Tuber Coxa.

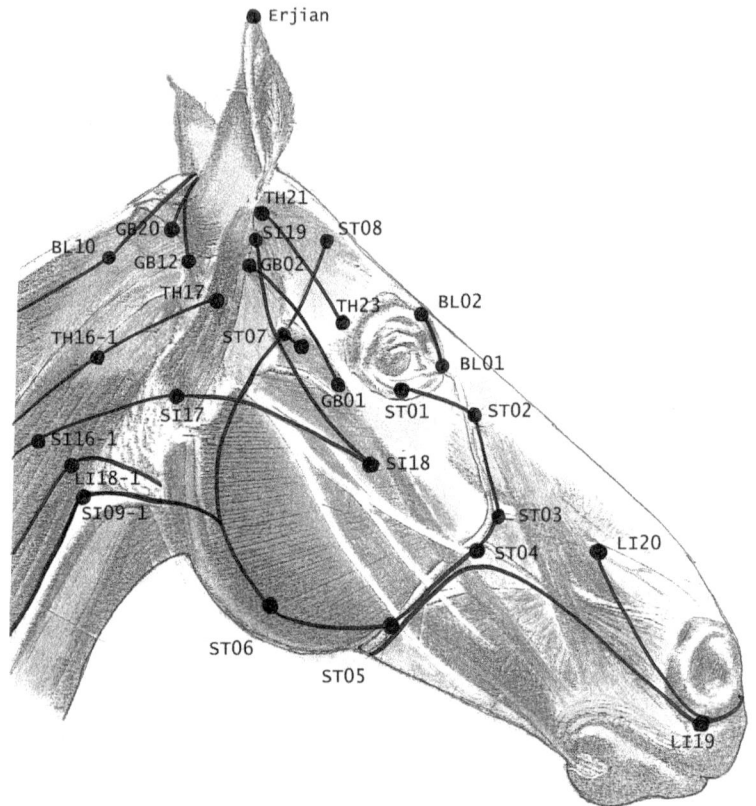

Figure 59; Illustration of some of the GB-points in the horses head. Also points on the LI/ST/SI/TH/BL meridians are shown.

LV (Liver, Foot Jueyin) Channel uses the connective tissue around *A/V. coronalis phal. III, V. digit. med., V. mtts. dors. med., V. saphena, V. saphena, A/V. femoralis, A/V. iliaca ext., A/V. femoralis prof., A/V. pudenda ext.* as the main pathways for carrying its impulses:

Anatomically it begins:

IN HORSES
The Superficial Path of the Liver Meridian:

- Begins at the coronary band of the hind foot, ~55⁰ medial to the tip of the toe; *A/V. coronalis phal. III.*

- Ascends at the dorsomedial aspect of the phalanges; *V. digit. med.*

- Continues along the groove between the medial and large metatarsal bones; *V. mtts. dors. Med.*

- Distal to the hock it turns dorsad and passes the hock on the dorsomedial aspect, dorsal to the medial malleolus.

- Continues towards proximal and crosses the medial aspect of the tibia halfway up the lower leg; *V. Saphena.*

- Intersecting the Spleen meridian at SP06.

- Ascends cranial to the Spleen meridian threequarter of the way between the medial malleolus and the medial tibial condyle, where it crosses and continues caudal to the Spleen meridian to the stifle and the medial aspect of the thigh; *V. saphena, A/V. Femoralis.*

- Continues to the pubic region via SP12 and SP13 where it encircles the genitals; *A/V. iliaca ext., A/V. femoralis prof., A/V. pudenda ext.*

- Enters the caudal part of the abdomen where it intersects the Conception vessel at CV02, CV03 and CV04.

- Continues along the lateral side of the abdomen and ribs to end in the 9th intercostal space, at LV14.

The Deep Path of the Liver Meridian;

- From LV14 it travels forward and curves around the Stomach before entering the Liver and connecting with the Gall Bladder.

- Crosses the diaphragm and spreads in the hypochondriac and costal region.

- Ascends along the neck and dorsal aspect of the throat to the nasopharynx and into the tissues surrounding the eyes.

- Passes the forehead to intersect with the Governing vessel at GV20.

The Deep Path of the Liver Meridian has 2 Important Branches:

1) One branch descends rostrally from the eyes to encircle the inner surface of the lips.

2) Another branch travels from the Liver, through the diaphragm, spreads in the Lung and meets with the Pericardium at PC01.

In dogs: It begins at LV01 at the lateral claw root of the second toe [SP01 is on the medial side of toe 2. Toe 1 (hind dewclaw) is usually absent, or is present only as a rudimentary toe]. It ascends on the dorsum of the paw to LV03 between the proximal heads of Os metatarsale 2 and 3. From here, it ascends the medial side of the tarsus and leg to LV08 (at medial side of the knee) to LV11 (on the medial thigh, 2' below ST30). From here, it ascends the ventral abdomen to LV13 (below the tip of rib 11), to end at LV14, in the 6th intercostal space.

In humans: It begins at LV01 (at the lateral nail root of the big toe - toe 1). It ascends on the dorsum of the foot to LV03 (between the proximal heads of metatarsal bones 1-2). From here, it ascends the medial side of the tarsus and leg to LV08 (at medial side of the knee) to LV11 (on the medial thigh, 2' below ST30). From here, it ascends the ventral abdomen to LV13 (below the tip of rib 11) to end at LV14, in the 6th intercostal space, directly below the nipple.

Phase	Metal		Earth		Fire		Water		Fire		Wood
Yin Channel	LU[1]		SP[4]	>>	HT[1]		KI[4]	>>	PC[1]		LV[4]
	‖		‖		‖		‖		‖		‖
Yang Channel	LI[2]	>>	ST[3]		SI[2]	>>	BL[3]		TH[2]	>>	GB[3]
Limb	Hand		Foot		Hand		Foot		Hand		Foot

(‖ and >>) mean that Qi Flow sequence is LU-LI-ST-SP, etc; ‖ = Yin-Yang Phase Mates (Partners);
[1] *Qi flow from chest to hand;* [2] *Qi flow from hand to face;* [3] *Qi flow from face to foot;* [4] *Qi flow from foot to chest*

Table 78

LV Qi comes from GB, its Yang Mate in Wood, and flows into (connects with) LU Channel. As in the case of all the other Yin Channels in animals, LV Channel is much more important than its paired Yang Channel (GB). The Wood Phase, to a great extent, relates to the nutrition of tendons and muscles. LV also has other functions in the body, such as governing metabolism, the venous blood circulation and the immune system. This makes LV Channel the most important one for animals, especially in horses. At first presentation, >60% of horses that I diagnose have a clear LV Qi Deficiency (Weak LV Process & Channel).

LV Channel has special importance for blood circulation in the longissimus dorsi muscles and the muscles in the hip (gluteal) area. Therefore, LV is responsible for equine azoturia (Monday Morning Disease), tenderness, lameness and muscle stiffness in this area. Treating LV Points effectively increases resistance to destruction of the sacral muscles (indicated by elevated transaminase blood values) and helps muscular lameness in the hip area.

LV-related digestive disorders is another important group, especially in cows. Since cows live for and from their digestion and since LV is a most important organ in the digestion process, it is very important to treat LV in times of great strain. Ketosis and inappetance are important clues.

Also, high-yielding dairy cows often have acidosis and laminitis associated with feeding on high levels of rapidly fermentable carbohydrates and high protein levels, which cause Imbalance in the digestive (ST-SP) and liver (LV) Processes. Note that laminitis is mainly a problem in the hindlimbs and that the main Channels involved (ST-SP and LV) are all hindlimb Channels. Low ruminal pH (values <6.0) and high blood levels of liver enzymes, such as GLDH, confirm that the digestive and LV Processes are under strain in those cows.

LV is very important for optimal development of the muscles around the hip in humans, horses and dogs. In dogs, it is especially important in the larger breeds such as Retrievers, Labradors, Newfoundlanders etc. The muscles play a vital role in keeping the hip joint stable; they ensure a normal development of the hip joint. Therefore, LV Points are very important to treat hip disorders, especially hip dysplasia (HD). Stimulating a single point on LV Channel easily and effectively treats HD. Also, in some cases, a single treatment can heal some HD patients permanently. I have used gold wire implant in LV03 in hundreds of dogs since 1988, and in 4 human patients (the first one I implanted in 1995, and he is still without any serious symptoms). The results of these implants are that I successfully treat more than 85% of all cases of HD. This is done by just implanting a piece of gold in LV03, either unilaterally or bilaterally.

LV is the organ of greatest significance for the development of HD. Although the Lesion-Symptom Complex manifests in the joint, ***HD is not primarily a joint disorder; it is a muscle or tendon disorder***, as in humans. HD most likely begins with a weakness or laxity in the tendons and muscles around the hip joint. This in turn leads to an improper development of the hip joint. In Germany and the USA it is known that HD can both be prevented and treated by the aid of a LV stimulating diet (see also page 490). This indicates that the development of HD depends on the liver-organ itself. The Channels only are a means to activate or regulate (further stimulate) the Processes, they are not the real cause of the various symptoms. Instead, Channels are media to re-establish the Qi balance of the Processes and the Organs. They are also indicators of where symptoms may develop. Thus, the well being of the LV is very important to the development or prevention of HD.

LV also is very significant for the immune system. Most allergies react to treatment of LV Points. In recent years, especially with the increased use of commercially prefabricated and dry food, dogs have shown a clear increase in food allergies. This food (especially dry food) can induce many allergies by placing a strain on LV functions. Abnormal quantities and qualities of protein and fat, and the presence of many detrimental products produced when a "dead" food ages in the presence of synthetic antioxidants, for example ethoxyquin, all put increased metabolic strain on LV function. The same thing occurs in children who can develop many allergies when they are fed, or allowed to eat, unsuitable diets. In such cases it is important to change the diet, reduce the protein content, improve the fat quality and stimulate the immune system and LV. A few treatments of LV Channel, in addition to previously mentioned dietary changes, can eliminate many allergies entirely (see also page 485). In accordance with the Chinese Qi Clock, around 0200h is the best time of day to treat LV Channel.

The energy in the LV meridian (Qi) may, as for the LV-process itself, be in:

- *Excess*

- *Deficiency*

Particular for the meridian the energy may also be in:

- *Destructivity*

- *Blocked*

Excess show itself rather seldom as pain, as this is a Yin meridian, and Yin meridians seldom show excesses as pain (contrary to Yang-meridians, which often show excesses as painful points or areas). An excess in the LV-meridian, although very seldom, may be the result of a deficiency in the Lung-process. An excess in the LV meridian usually passes without observation or unpleasant symptoms.

Deficiency is a much more common and serious pathological finding than excess. Such a deficiency shows itself in the same way as described under the LV-process on page 90. In addition we may find skin-changes in the form of excema along the LV-meridian.

A deficiency in the LV meridian is often the cause of an excess in the Stomach-meridian, and pain and cancer (breast/ mamma) along this meridian may be the result.

This pain is often the symptom we are confronted with in our daily practise.

Destructivity show itself as in all animals as particular viscious symptoms of the skin, erosions and wounds (see more about destructive energy on page XXXIV).

Blockage of the LV-meridian is caused by a trauma on the structures of connective tissue that lead the impulses travelling through this meridian. Such a trauma will not hurt or destroy the energy of the process itself, but hinders the Qi-flow in the meridian. This is why the pulse in such a case shows absolutely good health for the process, but the acupuncture points may show disbalance. This disbalance shows excess above the trauma and deficienct below the trauma.

LV 01	**Dadun (Great Pile)**
	Ting, Wood and Horary Point of LV
	In horses: At the coronary band of the hind foot, ~55° medial to the tip of the toe.
	In dogs: It is at the lateral aspect of the nail of hindtoe 2 (axial).
	In humans: it is 0.1" from the posterior edge of the nail-root of the 1th toe (big toe), lateral side.
	Effect: LV01 is the most important point in horses. As the Wood Point of a Wood Channel, it is the main controller of the muscles and tendons. In horses, treatment of LV01 stimulates blood circulation within the entire superficial and surface muscle mass of the hip area, the "main motor" of horses. These muscles often are strained after undergoing hard training, hard running or other strenuous activity. Many horses have chronically strained muscles in the croup. In such cases blood tests often show raised levels of muscle transaminases in blood. This Syndrome is common today in hard trained horses, especially trotters. I have treated thousands of trotters with this disorder and nearly all of them had a clear reaction to LV01 (the Wood Point). Before treatment they walked stiffly, went easily into gallop stride (undesirable) and had histories of lameness. Other colleagues usually have seen these cases and have diagnosed and treated them as arthralgia. In my experience, those colleagues have been treating symptomatically only. This is inferior treatment because the primary cause of the joint pain usually lies above the stifle and not in or below that joint, as they thought. The reason is usually strain or trauma (tenderness, spasm) of the croup muscles and compensatory changes that cause excessive strain on other joints,

	especially the stifle. Treatment of the stifle, by injecting into the joint, usually improves the horse's disorder for a while. This is because treatment can ease some or all of the most intense pain. However, the disorder soon recurs because it is the result of an imbalance in the muscular system, which has not been treated. In contrast, many of these horses improve noticeably, or are totally healed, after just a few treatments of LV Channel. A few years ago I conducted a study of the effect of LV01 on the muscles of the croup, amongst other things. In acute cases the healing period was significantly shortened. In chronically affected horses a total of 65% showed clear improvement after just one treatment and after three treatments it went up to 85%. This study involved 1700 horses and was published in an international journal (The Norwegian Veterinary Journal refused to print the article). Therefore, Norwegian colleagues were hindered in attaining this information. Ten years later, my Norwegian colleages asked to be allowed to reprint the article, which they did. LV01 is also very helpful in rectal and uterine prolapse. It helps the upper abdomen, cervix, epigastrium, male genitalia, groin, hypochondrium, inguinal area, male and female external genitalia, penis, perineum, postpartum disorders, pubis, uterus and vagina.
LV 02	**Xingjian (Moving Between)** **Ying-Spring and Fire Point of LV** *In horses:* Just distal to the fetlock, in a depression at the dorsal border of the interosseus tendon to long digital extensor tendon. *In dogs:* It is in the web between toes 2 and 3. *In humans:* It is on the foot-dorsum, in the web between toes 1 and 2. *Effect:* It increases blood circulation within the muscles and "flushes" the croup area after pain or lameness of the area. It also helps the male and female external genitalia, penis, pubis, waist, flank, tibia, fibula and sweating disorders.

LV 03	Taichong (Supreme Surge)
	Earth point in horses and dogs **(and Yuan-Source point in humans)** **Analgesic Point; Allergy Point** *In horses:* Just proximal to the fetlock, in a depression on the dorsomedial aspect of the third metatarsal bone. *In dogs:* It is between Os metatarsale 2 & 3, at its widest distance (usually between the distal 1/3 and the proximal 2/3). *In humans:* It is on the foot-dorsum, in a hole below the proximal heads of the metatarsals 1-2. *Effect:* It is not a very good Local Point for the fetlock. It helps chronic tendon disorders, cramp, spasm and calcification in the neck. Also general circulatory disorders in the muscles and in retention of urine (muscular spasm in the bladder sphincter). LV03 is of extraordinary importance in dogs. It is the most important point to treat hip joint dysplasia (HD). LV03 can be treated with needles, injections or gold implants. I have treated HD in more than 150 dogs over a period of 13 years (the first dog I implanted in 1988) by stimulation of LV03, and the results have been excellent (85-92% depending on the method). I have also implanted gold here in four humans, suffering from advanced leg Perthe, coxarthrosis and hip-dysplacia, and the effect has been very good in all patients. They have stayed well in several years (the first human I implanted was in 1994). In dogs I have noted an interesting phenomenon related to LV03; the distance between the second and the third metatarsale in the area where LV03 is situated decreases as the HD aggravates. I have especially observed that in dogs with just one hip affected; the distance between the 1 and 2 mid foot bones is noticeably smaller on the side of the more pathological hip joint. It appears as if calcium deposits occur, in this case to the same degree as the hip joint degenerates. This observation has, as far as I know, never been published before. I hope that in time this observation can become a theme for scientific research.

	Because LV has a central role in allergies, migraine, uricaemia and gouty arthralgia, digestive upsets, detoxification and eye diseases, it is a very helpful point in these disorders. It also has analgesic effects; LV03 + LI04 is a powerful combination to treat generalised pain, or pain that moves from place to place. LV03 also helps in first aid, convulsions, epilepsy, tetanus, addictions, temporomandibular joint, salivary glands, salivation; blood vessels, blood circulation, blood pressure, arteriosclerosis, ischaemia; liver, spleen, gallbladder and bileduct. Also female genitalia and reproduction. Also lowback and lumbar area.
LV 04	**Zhongfeng (Central Mound)** **Water point in horses** **(Jing-River and Metal point in dogs and in humans)** *In horses:* At the level of the medial malleolus, at the dorsal aspect of the tarsus (hock), medial to the M. tibialis cranialis tendon. *In dogs:* It is one inch anterior to the medial malleolus, between the tendon of the extensor hallucis longus and tibialis anterior muscles. *In humans:* It is one inch anterior to the medial malleolus, between the tendon of the extensor hallucis longus and tibialis anterior muscles. *Effect:* The Water Phase is often related to LV, so I often use LV04. As the Water Phase relates to oedema in general, it may be used in swollen muscles and myositis. It helps the male genitalia, male and female external genitalia, inguinal area, pubis and groin as these structures usually relate to the water element.
LV 05	**LV05 Ligou (Woodworm Canal)** **Luo Point of LV** *In horses:* On the caudomedial aspect of the tibia, just proximal to SP06, at the same level of KI09 and cranial to V. saphena. *In dogs:* On the caudomedial aspect of the tibia, just proximal to SP06, at the same level of KI09 and cranial to V. saphena. *In humans:* It is at the medial edge of the tibia, five inches above the medial malleolus. *Effect:* It connects LV Channel with its Phase Mate, GB Channel.

LV 06	**Zhongdu (Central Metropolis)** **Xi Point of LV** *In horses:* 1.5 cun proximal to LV05, 2 cun proximal to SP06, cranial to V. saphena. *In dogs:* 1.5 cun proximal to LV05, 2 cun proximal to SP06, cranial to V. saphena. *In humans:* It is at the medial edge of the tibia, seven inches above the medial malleolus, two inches above LV05. *Effect:* It helps the inguinal area, groin and testicular pain, and is useful in all acute conditions.
LV 08	**Ququan (Bend Spring)** **Local point in horses** **Water point in dogs** **(He-Sea and Water point in Humans)** *In horses:* Just dorsal to the medial end of the popliteal fossa, cranial to V. saphena, at the same level of KI10 (at the level of the femorotibial joint). *In dogs:* It is at the medial end of the popliteal crease, anterior to the semimembranosus muscle, behind the inferior end of the femur. *In humans:* It is at the medial end of the popliteal crease, anterior to the semimembranosus muscle, behind the inferior end of the femur. *Effect:* Since LV is often the cause of swellings (oedema), the accumulation of fluid, LV08 is important for all swellings in the hindleg such as tarsal swellings and swollen tendons. It helps the libido, male and female external genitalia, erectile dysfunction, penis; uterus, cervix, vagina, postpartum disorders; urethra; pubis, hip, thigh, femur, knee (animal stifle), patella and popliteal area.

LV 13	**Zhangmen (Camphorwood Gate)**
	Front-Mu point of the Spleen **Hui-Influential point of the zang** **Meeting point of the LV and GB meridians**
	In horses: Directly caudal and ventral to the ventral end of the 17th rib. *In dogs:* It is on the mid-axillary line, just below the tip of the second last rib (in dogs it is the 12th rib). *In humans:* It is on the mid-axillary line, just below the tip of the second last rib [in humans the 11th (2nd last, floating)].
	Effect: It helps the thorax, chest, ribs, sternum, upper abdomen, epigastrium, hypochondrium, liver (inflammation, jaundice, acetonaemia etc), spleen, waist and flank. Marvin Cain **combines BL20, BL18, LV13** with the **Herpes Triangle** (three points in a triangle dorsal to the external angle of the ilium) and the **Immune Point** near the jugular groove between ST10 and ST11 to treat **immunocompromised horses**, especially those with the **Equine Herpes Syndrome**. He often injects these points with Vitamin B12 +/- Echinacea or with autogenous blood from the jugular vein. He claims excellent results within 24-72 hours with this treatment. **The Mu Points of SP and LV** (13 + 14) are used especially in inappetance, anaemia, all types of organic degeneration of LV and SP and in cases of low immune resistance.
LV 14	**Qimen (Qi-Cycle Gate)**
	Mu Point of LV **Meeting point of the LV and SP meridians with the Yin Wei mai**
	In horses: In the 9th intercostal space, on a line between the point of the shoulder and the stifle joint. *In dogs:* It is distal to the intercostal space 7, on the mammillary line. *In humans:* It is in the 6th intercostal space, directly below the nipple (ST17, 4th intercostal space).
	Effect: It helps the chest, thorax, ribs, sternum and diaphragm, menopausal disorders, sweats, flushes and vasomotor disorders. **The Mu Points of SP and LV** (13 + 14) are used especially in inappetance, anaemia, all types of organic degeneration of LV and SP and in cases of low immune resistance.

Table 79

The special commandpoints in the horse are as follows:

M E T A L	***Location:*** Just distal to the tarsus (hock), on the dorsomedial aspect of the third metatarsal bone, directly dorsal to the V. saphena. ***Effect:*** Influences painful conditions locally and along the course of the meridian, and generally in the body when the Liver is in excess or deficiency.
S O U R C E tarsus	***Location:*** 0.5 cun distal to LV04, at the dorsal aspect of the tarsus (hock), medial to the M. tibialis cranialis tendon. ***Effect:*** Stimulates the meridian.

Table 80

DIAGRAM OVER DE MEST VIKTIGE PUNKTENE
PA BAKLABBEN HOS HUNDEN OG KATTEN

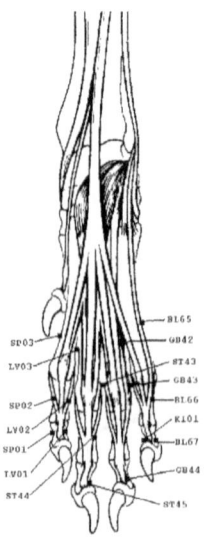

Figure 60

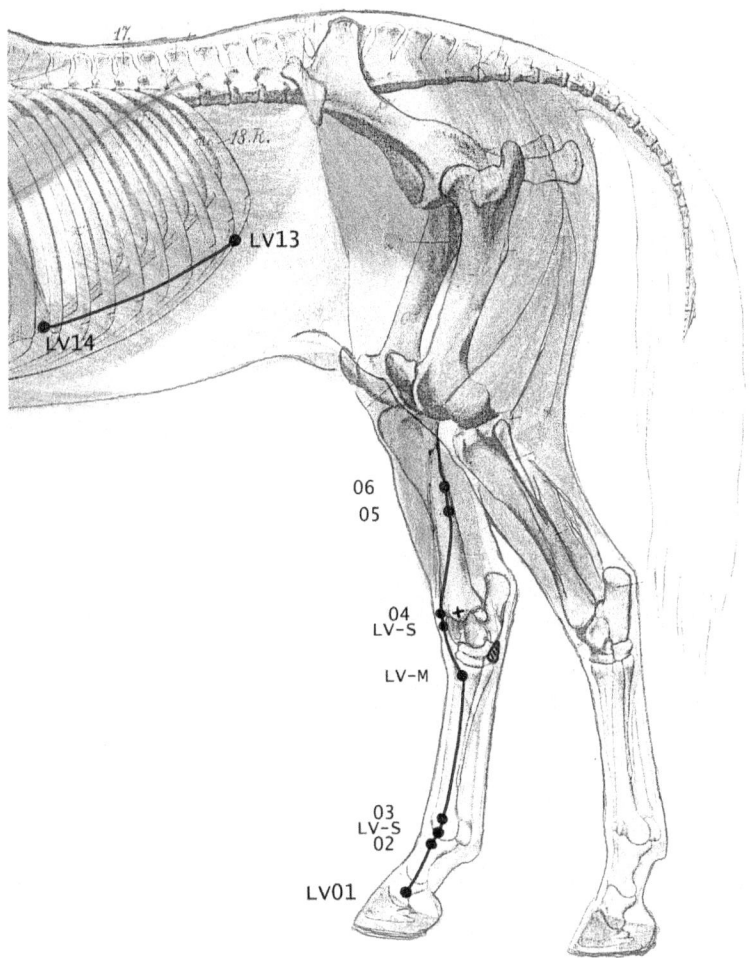

Figure 61; Picture of the points of the liver meridian in the horse.

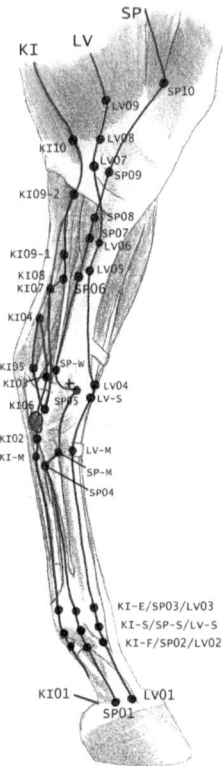

Figure62; the most importand points on the back leg on the KI/SP/LV meridians.

The Eight Mai (Extraordinary Vessels)

As well as the 12 Jing (Main Channels) and the 15 Luo (Connecting Vessels) there are Internal Channels (connecting to the related organs), Minor Channels, Tendinomuscular Channels and the 8 Mai (Extraordinary Vessels). The JingLuoMai function together to connect and keep Qi flowing in the 12 Jing, their related Zangfu (internal organs) and special parts and functions of the body. They connect the upper parts with the lower parts, the inner with the outer, the anterior with the posterior and the left side with the right side.

The 8 Mai (the so-called Extraordinary Vessels) are most important, but just 2 of them have their own points. The other 6 Mai borrow points from the Main Channels.

Dumai (Governing Vessel, GV) and *Renmai* (Conception Vessel, CV) are the two Mai that have their own points. It is important to familiarise oneself with these Vessels. They travel along the midline of the body in humans, horses and dogs.

oOo

GV Governing Vessel (Dumai) begins in the perineum at GV01, between the anus and the coccyx in humans. It ascends over the spine, in the dorsal midline, to GV03 (L4-L5 space), to GV04 (L2-L3 space), to GV09 (T7-T8 space), to GV14 (C7-T1 space). It ascends the neck and occiput to the highest point of the head (GV20) and then runs anteriorly to the nasal philtrum (GV26). It ends under the lip at GV28 (in the frenulum, opposite GV26). Ancient tradition in India taught that Dumai ends in the palate and that Renmai begins on the tip of the tongue. This was very important in the Indian system of meditation. To link these two Channels, adepts placed the tip of the tongue up to the palate when they meditated.

The superficial path:

- Begins in the lower abdomen.

- Emerges in the perineum above the anus, at GV01.

- Travels along the dorsal midline of the sacrum and the vertebral column to the atlanto-occipital area, at GV16.

- Enters the brain.

- Continues rostrally along the midline of the head to the philtrum; on a line between the lower border of the nostrils, at GV26.

- Terminates at the junction of the upper lip and the gum, at GV28.

The Governing vessel has 3 deep branches:

1) First branch;

- Begins in the lower abdomen.

- Travels to the genitals and perineum.

- Curves around the anus.

- Follows the interior of the vertebral column.

- Enters the Kidneys.

2) Second branch

- Begins in the lower abdomen.

- Curves around the external genitalia.

- Travels cranially along the ventral midline.

- Passes through the Heart.

- Continues to the throat.

- Circles the mouth.

- Terminates below the eye.

3) Third branch

- Begins at BL01, at the medial canthus of the eye.

- Follows the Bladder meridian bilaterally to GV20, converges and enters the brain.

- Emerges at GV16.

- Divides again and travels caudally via BL12 on either side of the spine to the Kidneys.

In animals, GV begins at GV01, between the anus and the tail, (as in humans). It then runs on the ventral midline of the tail to the tail-tip, and then runs cranial in the dorsal midline of the tail to GV02, as in humans. However, animals have many extra but undocumented points on the tail. Two GV tail points of great importance in animals are the Tail-Tip Point (GVTT) in all species, and the Violic Gland Zone (GVVG) in canidae. Otherwise, GV pathway in animals is similar to that in humans, but needs adjustments for GV point location because the number of vertebrae differs between animal species and differs from that in humans.

Lambrechts and Rogers (1999) discussed in detail the connection of GV01 and CV01 with the nose, sexual pheromones and genito-reproductive function in humans. The perineum connects to the vomero-nasal organ of the nose via the Chongmai and GV. The vomero-nasal organ senses ("smells") sexual pheromones in all mammals. The GVVG Point (see below) also shows the importance of the pheromones and the coccygeal / perineal area in sexual and reproductive function.

GV01	Changqiang (Long Strong)
	Luo-Connecting point **Meeting point of the GV with the CV and the GB and KI meridians**
	Location: In all species it is on GV Line, at the tip of the coccyx, between coccyx and anus.
	Effect: It helps the perineum, anus, vagina, vulva, clitoris, prolapse, tenesmus and haemorrhoids. In dogs it helps anal sac infections and rectal or anal pruritus. In horses it helps rectal windsucking and rectal or anal pruritus. It also helps diarrhoea, constipation and infertility in horses and dogs and is a very good place to vaccinate animals with enteric vaccines. Small doses of vaccine here give titres as good as larger doses elsewhere.
GVTT	**GV Tail Tip (Dumai Extra Point in all animals with tails)**
	Emergency Point in animals
	Location: It is on the distal end of the tail, the Tail Tip (TT).

	Effect: It helps to relax all the muscles of the tail and nearby areas (perineum?) and eases spasm or pain related to lifting of the tail. Combination of **TT + GV26 + sacral points** helps in apnoea, shock and emergencies, and in treating "downer animals." Like sex itself, GVTT should not be used too often as it drains Qi from the organism.
GVVG	**GV Violic Gland Zone (Dumai Extra Point in canidae)** **Prostate and Perineal Master Point in Canidae** *Location:* The Violic Gland Zone is a line of points in the dorsal midline of the tail of dogs and other canidae. The points lie over coccygeal vertebrae 5-7. *Effect:* This gland has pheromone activity and is used to attract a mate when dogs are in oestrus. Oswald Kothbauer has reported (and Phil Rogers has confirmed) that GVVG has powerful effects on the prostate and perineal area, and on the pelvic organs (rectum, bladder, vagina, clitoris and vulva). To treat this Zone, run a 2-3" needle subcutaneously over vertebrae Co5-Co7.
GVE-1	**Extrapoint in horses** *Location:* **On the dorsal midline, 2 cun caudal to WEIGEN.**
GVE-2	**Weigen** *Location:* In a small depression between the first and second coccygeal vertebrae.
GV02	**Yaoshu (Lower Back Shu)** *Location:* On the dorsal midline, in the sacro-coccygeal space; between the sacrum and the first coccygeal vertebra in all species, on GV Line. *Effect:* It helps the uterus, cervix, vagina and perineum. In animals it has effects similar to GVTT except that it doesn't have its draining effect. It also helps infertility in animals.
GV E-3	**Extrapoint in horses** *Location;* On the dorsal midline, at the level of the third sacral foramina.

GV **E-4**	**Extrapoint in horses** *Location:* On the dorsal midline, at the level of the first sacral foramina.
Bai **Hui**	**Bai Hui (Hundred Meetings)** *(Human Bai Hui is the GV20, at the top of the head)* *Location:* In the lumbosacral space. [*In humans this is the location of an Extra point;* **Shiqizhuixia** *(Below the Seventeenth Vertebra)*]. *Effect:* Increases the flow of Qi in the entire hip area. Infertility, dystocia, retained placenta, prolapse of uterus and rectum. In humans; chronic lumbar pain in both excess and deficiency patterns.
GV **03**	**Yaoyangguan (Lumbar Yang Pass)** *Location:* On the dorsal midline between the 4th and 5th lumbar vertebrae, at the level of BL25. *Effect:* Dual disorders of the lumbar region and pelvic limbs.
GV **E-5**	**Extrapoint in horses** *Location:* On the dorsal midline, between the 4th and 5th lumbar vertebrae.
GV **E-6**	**Extrapoint in horses** *Location:* On the dorsal midline, between the third and 4th lumbar vertebrae.
GV04	**Mingmen (Life Gate)** *Location:* On the dorsal midline between the second and third lumbar vertebrae, at the level of BL23. *Effect:* It helps female and male reproduction, andropathy, impotence, male infertility, spermatopathy, spermatorrhoea, prostate; female genitalia, leucorrhoea; spinal cord, lowback, lumbar, lumbosacral and sacroiliac areas, sacrum and pelvis. Jen-Hsou Lin found that it had no effect in infertility in sows.

GV09	Zhiyang (Extremity of Yang) *Location:* On the dorsal midline between the 11th and 12th thoracic vertebrae, at the level of BL17. *Effect:* It helps the diaphragm, respiration, haemorrhage, thoracic spine and back, liver (inflammation, jaundice, acetonaemia etc); bileduct, gallbladder (inflammation, calculi, obstruction etc). In horses and dogs, it is medial to BL17, or 2' and 1', respectively, cranial to BL18.
GV11-GV13	These are **immunostimulant Points**. They help in **allergies** and **immunomediated disorders**, and in **respiratory** and **cardiovascular** disorders and **cough**.
GV14	**Dazhui (Great Hammer, Vertebra T1)** **Allergy Point, Immunostimulant Point and Fever Point** *Location:* In all species it is on the GV Line, in C7-T1 space (T2 spine is the first high spineal process in horses, and T3 is the first most easily palpated in dogs). *Effect:* It helps the brain, meninges, spinal cord and their functions and parts, convulsions, epilepsy, CVA, polio, tetanus, memory; neck, cervical spine, thyroid, parathyroid, thoracic spine, back, dorsolumbar area, thorax, respiratory system, nose, nasal, sinuses, olfaction, trachea, bronchi, lung, asthma, cough, pneumonia, blood vessels, arteriosclerosis, ischaemia, skin, sweating disorders, immunity, allergy, vasomotor allergy, Blood, haemorrhage, thymus, infections (cholera, herpes, malaria, rubella, TB, typhoid, typhus, varicella etc), fever and chills.
GV15	**Yamen (Mute's Gate)** *Location:* In all species it is on the GV Line, below the occipital protuberance, 0.5' above the occipital hairline, 0.5' below GV16. *Effect:* It helps the brain, spinal cord and meninges, occiput, speech, and tongue.

GV16	Fengfu (Wind Mansion)
	Meeting point of the GV and the Yang Wei mai **Point of the Window of the Sky** **Point of the Sea of Qi**
	Location: In all species it is on the GV Line, in a hole just below the occipital protuberance, 1' above the occipital hairline, 0.5' above GV15.
	Effect: It helps chills and Wind / Wood diseases.
GV20	**Baihui (Hundred Meetings)** Human Bai Hui
	Meeting point of the GV with the LV, BL, TH and GB meridians **Point of the Sea of Marrow** **Master Point of all the Psychic Energies and Emergency Point:**
	Location: In humans it is on the GV Line, 7' above the occipital hairline, on top of the head, 5' behind the frontal hairline. In animals it is just at the top of the head, slightly caudal.
	Effect: It helps in emergencies and first aid, allergic shock, head, spinal cord, ischaemia, postpartum disorders, haemorrhoids, tenesmus and prolapse. GV20 is also called the "**Aggression Point**" because it helps horses (or other animals including man) that do not want to run or fight in races (or do the work that is expected from the individual in question). However, I prefer to call it the "**Mouse Point**," for reasons based on the following story. I had treated some horses in a stable and was talking with the owner while I was waiting for payment. Just then, a girl brought a cat that had not been known to catch a mouse for at least 2-3 years. (The cat had been bought to catch mice!). I stimulated GV20 and the cat walked off. Within minutes, just as I was leaving after the owner paid me for my work with the horses, the cat came back with its first mouse. **Note:** *In TCVM, "Animal Baihui" is in the lumbosacral space, and is coded GV03-1 or GV03 (see above).*

Yin Tang	**Yintang** (Upper Star)
	Location: On the dorsal midline of the head, at level of BL02, at the medial end of the eyebrow.
	Effect: Nasal congestion, rhinitis, nasal discharge, nosebleed, sinusitis.
GV23	**Shangxing (Upper Star)**
	In horses and dogs: On the dorsal midline of the head, at the level of the medial canthus of the eye, and BL01.
	In humans: On the GV Line, 1' above the frontal hairline.
	Effect: It helps allergic shock, allergy, vasomotor allergy; forehead, nose, olfaction, frontal and nasal sinuses.
GV24	**Shenting (Spirit Court)** **Meetingpoint of the GV with the ST and BL meridians**
	In horses and dogs: On the dorsal midline of the head, midway between GV23 and GV25.
	In humans: It is on the GV Line, on the frontal hairline. It helps the forehead and frontal sinuses.
GVE-7	**Extrapoint in horses and dogs**
	Location: On the dorsal midline of the head, midway between GV24 and GV25.
GV25	**Suliao White Bone-Orifice**
	In horses and dogs: On the dorsal midline of the head, at the level of the upper border of the nostrils.
	In humans: It is on the GV Line, on a hollow on the tip of the nose.
	Effect: Copious nasal discharge, nasal sores, nosebleed, dyspnoea. In humans this point has shown to be more effective than GV 26 in restoring loss of consciousness.

GV26	Shuigou (Water Trough), also called **Renzhong (Man Middle)** **Meetingpoint of the GV with the ST and LI meridians** **Analgesic Point and the most important Emergency Point** *In horses and dogs:* On the dorsal midline of the head, just between and at level of the lower border of the nostrils. *In humans:* It is on the GV Line, just above the center of the nasal philtrum. *Effect:* It is the most important point for use in apnoea, shock and emergencies in humans and animals. GV26 + KI01 often are combined in emergencies, with PC06 in circulatory shock or cardiac arrest. Combination of GV26 + Ear Tip Point are very effective in colic. It has a general analgesic effect and relieves spasm. Analgesic effect has been used since ancient times aided by "the twitch" (Here we also stimulate GV27 and GV28 under the upper lip on the inside of the mouth). "The twitch" is a short baton with a rope noose on the one end. Tightening this noose around the horse's upper lip induces an endorphin release and gives a degree of anaesthesia sufficient to allow slightly and moderately painful interventions to be done without too much retaliation from the horse.
GV27	**Duiduan (Mouth Extremity)** *Location:* It is on the GV Line, at the inferior angle of the philtrum. *Effect:* This helps the mouth and chin.
GV28	**Yinjiao (Gum Intersection)** **Meetingpoint of the GV with the CV and the ST meridian** *Location:* It is on the GV Line, on the frenulum between the gum and upper lip, opposite GV26.

Table 81

oOo

Renmai (CV, Conception Vessel) begins in the perineum at CV01 (between the anus and vulva/scrotum in all species). It ascends the ventral midline, through the navel (CV08), tip of the xiphoid (CV14), sternal notch (CV22), to the root of the tongue (CV23). It ends at CV24 in the hollow between the chin and the lower lip. *See the connection of CV01, GV01, the perineum, sexual pheromones and sexual function, discussed in the introduction to GV, above.*

The superficial path:

- Arises in the uterus in females and in the lower abdomen in males and emerges in the perineum, ventral to the anus, at CV01.

- Travels forward along the ventral midline of the abdomen, chest, throat and jaw, terminating cranial to the chin, at CV24.

- The interior part of the meridian curves around the lips, connects with the Governing vessel at GV28 and terminates rostral to the eye, at ST01.

The deep path has 1 branch which:

1) Arises in the pelvic cavity and travels forward along and inside the vertebral column.

NOTE!! The area between the umbilicus and the cranial border of the pubic bone is, to a great extent, occupied by the udder in mares and by the penis in stallions/geldings. The points to be found on the abdomen of humans do surely exist in horses, but they are difficult to reach/find.

Considering that points are developed to be stimulated/ treated, the points in such a difficult accessable area are probably of less importance than in humans.

We have found 3 points between the umbilicus and the udder/penis which we believe may summarise the functions of all the points found in humans in this area. These points we will call CV-E, Equine points on the Conceptional Vessel. In sharp we suggest which human points we consider to be "included" in the points found.

CV 01	**Huiyin (Meeting of Yin)** **Meeting point of the CV, GV and Chong mai** *Location:* In all species, it is on the CV Line, between the anus and scrotum-vulva. *Effect:* CV01 helps, together with GV01, in rectal air sucking, anal sac inflammation, proctitis and other rectal disorders. Constantly infected and filled anal sacs have a very clear effect on dogs. Improvement after AP at **CV01 + GV01** usually lasts for about one year. CV01 also helps the abdomen; male and female external genitalia; cervix, vagina, vulva, clitoris, andropathy, prostate, pubis and urethra.
CV E-1	**CV-E-1 [CV02 QUGU (Curved Bone) and CV03 ZHONGJI** (Central Pol)] **Front-Mu point of theBL** **Meetingpoint of the CV with the SP, LV and KI meridians** *Location:* On the ventral midline, 4 cun caudal to the umbilicus. *Effect:* A variety of urinary disorders; benefits the Bladder, regulates Qi, transforms and drains damp-heat; itching, swelling, pain of the genitals, vaginal discharge. Strong influence on the lower abdomen, especially excess patterns; stagnation of cold or heat.
CV E-2	**CV-E-2 [CV04 GUANYUAN (Origin Pass) and CV05 SHIMEN** (Stone Gate)] **Front-Mu point of both the SI andTH meridians; original Qi** **Meetingpoint of the CV with the SP, LV and KI meridians** *Location:* On the ventral midline, 3 cun caudal to the umbilicus. *Effect:* Kidney deficiency; stimulates and protects original Qi, benefits the Essence, strengthens Kidney yang and nourishes Kidney yin. Regulates the water passages; difficult urination, oedema and diarrhoea. Regulates the uterus.

CV E-3	**CV-E-3 [CV06 QIHAI** (Sea of Qi) **och CV07 YINJIAO** (Yin Intersection)] **Meeting point between the CV, the Chong mai and the KI meridian** *Location:* On the ventral midline, 2 cun caudal to the umbilicus. *Effect:* Qi deficiency; nourishes original Qi, stimulates the Kidneys and strengthens the yang. All forms of chronic diseases involving depletion of Qi. Diarrhoea. Prolapse of the rectum and uterus.
CV 08	**Shenque (Spirit Gate) or Qizhong (Navel Centre)** **Influences KI and middle abdomen; Forbidden to needle** *Location:* In all species it is on CV Line, mid-navel. *Effect:* It helps the abdomen; female infertility, functional sterility, anovulation, leucorrhoea, constipation, diarrhoea, dysentery, oedema and ascites. Moxibustion at CV08 helps many chronic and Cold Syndromes in the abdominal organs.
CV 09	**Shuifen (Water Divide)** *In horses:* On the ventral midline, 2.5 cun cranial to the umbilicus. *In humans:* on the CV Line, 1' above CV08. *Effect:* It is cranial to the navel and is used especially to treat intestinal disorders, colic, diarrhoea, constipation, oedema and ascites.
CV 10	**Xiawan (Lower Venter/Cavity)** **Meeting point of the CV and SP meridian** *Location:* On the ventral midline, 5 cun cranial to the umbilicus. *Effect:* Undigested food in the stools; dispels food stagnation.

CV 12	Zhongwan (Central Belly)
	Mu Point of ST, Master Point of the Yang (Fu) Organs, and Master Point of Upper Abdomen (ST, SP, SI, GB, LV), Digestion and Extraction
	Meeting point of the CV with the SI, TH and ST meridians
	In horses and dogs: On the ventral midline, midway between the umbilicus and the sterno-xiphoid junction.
	In humans: on CV Line, 4' above CV08, or midway from CV08 to the sternoxiphoid junction.
	Effect: It helps the mind, psyche, addictions, blood circulation, blood pressure, diaphragm, back, abdomen and its organs and functions, pain and spasm in the abdomen or its organs, epigastrium, hypochondrium, gastrointestinal tract, diarrhoea, nausea, vomiting.
CV 13	**Shangwan (Upper Belly)**
	Meeting point of the CV with the ST and SI meridians
	In horses and dogs: On the ventral midline, 8 cun caudal to the sterno-xiphoid junction.
	In humans: on the CV Line, 5' above CV08, 1' above CV12-Zhongwan (Central Belly).
	Effect: It helps the stomach and duodenum.
CV 14	**Juque (Great Tower Gate)**
	Front-Mu point of the Heart
	In horses: On the ventral midline, 5 cun caudal to the sterno-xiphoid junction.
	In humans: on the CV Line, 6' above CV08, 2' below the sternoxiphoid junction.
	Effect: It helps heart disorders. Regulates the Heart and alleviates pain; stagnation or deficiency. Descends Lung Qi and unbinds the chest; cough, shortness of breath. Transforms phlegm and calms the spirit, epilepsy, mania-disorder etc.

CV 15	**Jiuwei (Turtledove Tail)** **Luo-Connecting point** *In horses:* On the ventral midline, 2 cun caudal to the sterno-xiphoid junction. *In humans:* On the CV Line, at the tip of the xiphoid process. *Effect:* It helps the diaphragm.
CV 17	**Tanzhong (Chest Centre)** **Mu Point of PC** **Master Point of Thorax (LU, HT and PC)** **Hui-Influential point of the Qi** **Point of Sea of Qi** **Meeting point of the CV with the KI, SP, TH and SI meridians** *In horses:* On the ventral midline, in a depression at the level of the elbow joint and 7th intercostal space. *In dogs:* On the CV Line, level with the 4th intercostal space, 2/3 the way from the manubrium to the processus xiphoideus. *In humans:* On the CV Line, midway between nipples, level with the 4th intercostal space. *Effect:* It helps the thorax, chest, ribs, sternum, respiratory system, trachea, bronchi, lung, cough, asthma, pneumonia, heart, pericardium, oesophagus, diaphragm, obstetrical disorders, mammary disorders, mastopathy, milk disorders, gynaecopathy and disorders of pregnancy.
CV 22 (-1 in hors-es)	**Tiantu (Heavenly Chimney)** **Meetingpoint of the CV and the Yin Wei mai** **Point of the Window of the Sky** *In horses:* On the ventral midline, 0.5 cun cranial to the manubrium cartilage. *In humans:* On the CV Line, in a hollow 0.5' above the supra-sternal notch. *Effect:* Descends rebellious Qi; coughing, asthma, dyspnoea, phlegm and Lung abscesses. Pharyngitis. It helps the chin, throat, pharynx, larynx, tonsil, thyroid, parathyroid, oesophagus, trachea, respiratory system, diaphragm, bronchi, lung, voice, cough, asthma and pneumonia.

CV 22-2	**Extrapoint in horses** *Location:* On the ventral midline of the neck, 4 cun cranial to CV22-1.
CV 22-3	**Extrapoint in horses** **Location:** *On the ventral midline of the neck, 9 cun cranial to CV22.*
CV 23-2	**Extrapoint in horses** **Location:** *On the ventral midline of the neck, at the level of C4; the 4th cervical vertebrae, midway between CV22-1 and CV 23-1.*
CV 23-3	**Extrapoint in horses** *Location:* On the ventral midline of the neck, 3 cun caudal to CV23, just caudal to the larynx.
CV 23-1	**Lianquan (Ridge Spring)** **Meetingpoint between the CV and the Yin Wei mai** *Location:* On the ventral midline of the neck, in a depression just cranial to the larynx. *Effect:* Snoring and dorsal displacement of the soft palate. This point can be injected with 1-2 ml 15 % camphoratum in sesamy oil, at a depth of 3 - 5 cm.
CV 24-2	**Extrapoint in horses** *Location:* On the ventral midline of the head, just caudal to the chin. *Effect:* Similar to CV24-1.
CV 24-1	**Chengjiang (Sauce Receptacle)** **Meeting point of the CV with GV and LI and ST meridians** *Location:* In a depression in the centre of the mentolabial groove (midway between the lower lip and the chin). *Effect:* Facial disorders; facial paralysis. Too much or too little production of saliva, wasting and thirsting disorder.

Table 82

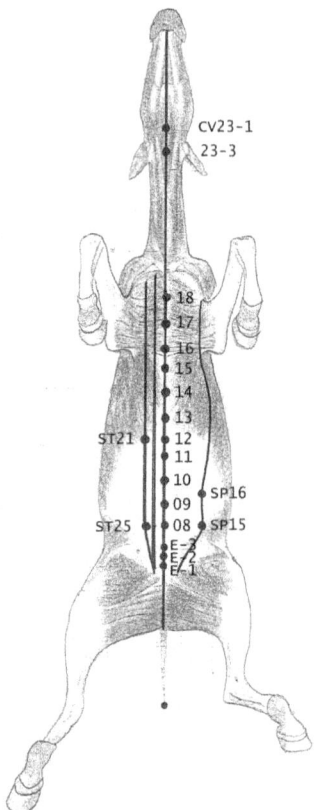

Figure 63; Diagram of the most important points on the Ren mo Channel in horses.

The Mu-points

A disorder in an organ can induce reactivity (sensitivity to palpation or other stimuli) at the related Back Shu Point and Front Mu Point. The difference between reactivity at these Diagnostic Points is:

- *Mu Point reactivity indicates a disorder in its related organ,* whereas

- *Back Shu Point reactivity indicates a disorder in the related* Channel or Organ System.

Table of Renmai (CV) and other Mu Points related to the organs. Points with a star (*) are NOT classical Mu Front Alarm Points.

CV03 BL	CV04* SI	CV05 TH	CV06* (TH)	CV07* Navel
CV08* Navel, KI	CV12 ST and Yang (Fu) organs	CV14 HT	CV17 PC and respiration	GB24 GB
GB25 KI, Ovary, Testicle	LU01 LU	LV13 SP	LV14 LV	ST25 LI

Table 83

Clinical use of the 8 extra meridians

The table below summarises and simplifies the key effects of the Mai. Two special properties characterise their effects:

1. They function as *Qi reservoirs*.

2. They *move Qi* from one part of the body to another.

Correct use of these two properties of the Mai is a very powerful therapeutic tool. Classically, correct Mai use in therapy is complicated; it must be used with caution. Excessive use empties the Qi reservoirs and induces Deficiency (weakness or emptiness) of large areas in related body parts.

Two of the Mai, Dumai GV and Renmai CV were described above. There are 6 others. The next table summarises the Activating Points of the Eight Mai and the effect of stimulation of those points. Remember to stimulate the first listed point before the second one.

Table of the 8 Mai (Extraordinary Vessels), their Activating Points and effects on Qi movement

#	Mai	Translation	Activating Points	Activation moves Qi from:
1	Dumai	Governing Vessel (GV)	SI03-BL62 (1)	Back to front
2	Renmai	Conception Vessel (CV)	LU07-KI06 (2)	Front to back
3	Yangweimai	Yang Linking Vessel	TH05-GB41 (3)	Up to down
4	Yinwei Mai	Yin Linking Vessel	PC06-SP04 (4)	Down to up
5	Chongmai	Penetrating or Thoroughfare Vessel	SP04-PC06	Internal to external
6	Daimai	Girdle or Belt Vessel	GB41-TH05	External to internal
7	Yangqiaomai	Yang Heel Vessel	BL62-SI03	Left side to right
8	Yinqiao Mai	Yin Heel Vessel	KI06-LU07	Right side to left

(1) same as Yangqiaomai but point sequence reversed

(2) same as Yinqiaomai but point sequence reversed

(3) same as Daimai but point sequence reversed

(4) same as Chongmai but point sequence reversed

Table 85

Clinical use of the Back Shu Points (BL13 to BL30)

Very important points lie on the inner line of BL Channel where it runs beside and parallel to the spine from BL10-BL30. Of these points, ***BL13-BL30 are called the Back Shu Points***. In large animals they lie about a hand-width from the midline on each side of the spine. In dogs about 1-2 finger widths from the midline. They are placed (yes, as we shall see later, they are really *placed*) between the transverse processes of the thoracic and lumbar vertebrae (BL13-BL25), lateral to the lumbosacral space (BL26), and over the 4 sacral foramina (BL27-BL30).

THERAPEUTIC PROPERTIES OF THE BACK SHU POINTS

When we have palpated the paravertebral area in our Back Shu Point Diagnosis, as described on page 107, we usually find 1-3 (sometimes up to 7 or more) reactive (sensitive or tender) Shu Points. If more than one is reactive we must determine which is the primary one to indicate the Channel with the Primary Process Imbalance for treatment. Thus we must consider each point and its Channel, as described under the diagnostic part, according to *the Five Phases and the Husband-Wife Law*. As discussed on page 113, Pain Point diagnosis (especially in horses) is not as good as detecting the Deficient point (for example the Deficient Ting Point). Painful Shu Points often indicate Excess. This Excess can disappear if therapists drain it. Initially, draining an Excess gives fast and excellent results, but the problem related to the Deficient Process still remains unaddressed. Therefore the long-term results of draining Excess are not as good as if one identifies and treats the Deficiency that usually (always) are present in pain.

THREE EXAMPLES

- If we find simultaneous tenderness, for example, at LV and SP Points, we treat LV Point first because LV is the Husband and SP is the Wife according to the Husband-Wife Law.

- If we find simultaneous tenderness at HT, SP and LU Points, we treat HT Point, as HT is the first in an unbroken Five Phase Sheng Cycle sequence.

- If we find simultaneous tenderness at HT, LU and LV Points, we treat HT Point, as HT is the first in an unbroken Five Phase Ko Cycle sequence.

Three examples

- If we find tenderness (excess) in the liver and the spleen points and additionally coldness (deficiency), we then will first treat the lung point. The lung process is placed before the liver in the Ko-cyclus, causing an excess in the liver, which in turn gives some of the excess to his wife, the spleen.

- If we find a deficiency in the heart point and tenderness in the lung point, then we must treat the heart as this is the Ko-father of the lung process.

- If we find deficiency in the heart point, deficiency also in the lung points and further excess in the liver, then we still have to treat the heart. The pathological process has just reached or evolved a step further in the Ko-cyclus.

In summary, if one chooses to treat the Shu Points directly, *we should identify and treat the primary Back Shu Point first* bearing in mind the Sheng and Ko Cycles. *After several days, we should check if the tenderness has disappeared at all points, including the primary point.* If once reactive points have lost their reactivity, we know that our treatment has been effective. If not, we must reassess the case and treat what we find at each subsequent session.

- *Indirect treatment* is much better and more skilled than direct AP at reactive Shu Points. To choose the best points for this, we must consider the Command Points (especially the Ting, and the Ting Point on the Ko (Father) Channel, Xi or Source Point of the Channel with the diagnosed Primary Process Imbalance). If indirect treatment fails to remove the reactivity within 2 weeks, then we proceed with direct treatment of the reactive point(s).

- *Direct treatment* consists of needling, fire needling or moxibustion, blistering, laser, singlet oxygen beam, or just a hard massage of the point in question (for treatment methods see page 457). As the Back Shu Points relate to the Qi system in each of the specific Processes, it is important not to treat too many points in order not to give a very confusing set of signals to the body that are difficult for it to interpret specifically.

Clinical use of the Ting (Jing Well) Points

Ting Points are *the most distal Channel points on the limbs in humans and animals.* In humans, they are just proximal to the medial or lateral angle of a nailbed of a finger or toe, except for PC09, at the tip of finger 3 (the "sex finger") and KI01, on the foot sole between the lower heads of metatarsal bones 2-3. In animals they are the most distal points on the limbs (fore and hind). They are effective points for therapy in all species. However, they have a special use in horses, in which they have great diagnostic value.

Ting Points are powerful **Command Points** *for the* **entire Channel** *on which they lie.* They influence both their own Channel and its Processes. *In horses all Ting Points command the* **Wood** *Phase Functions of both their* **Yin** *Process and* **Yang** *Processes. In humans and dogs the Ting Points of the Yang-meridians are related to the Metal Phase, while the Ting Points of the Yang Channels are related to the* **Metal** *Phase.* The **Metal/Air** Phase relates to *painful* states and the **Wood** Phase relates to *muscles and sinews.* Therefore, Ting Points are especially useful to treat *pain of all kinds,* and all *disorders in the muscles, tendons and ligaments.* Note that in contrast to humans and dogs, *the Ting points of the Yang Channels in horses relate to Wood and not to Metal.* Therefore, the Ting Points are especially well suited to horses since equine disorders most often entail painful musculotendinous disorders and sprained ligaments.

Each Ting Point also relates to its own External and Internal Channel pathways and its own related internal organ. Thus, each Ting Point is especially effective to treat disease anywhere along its own Channel.

TING POINT THERAPY

This simply involves the stimulation of the most important Ting Points. If we find only one reactive point, the case is simple. However, if several points are reactive we must use the Laws of AP to deduce the Primary Process Imbalance (the energetic origin or root of the disease) and to select the best acupoint(s) to correct the Primary Process Imbalance. The two most important Laws in this case are the Five Phase and the Chinese Clock Laws.

Two examples:

- If we find three reactive points; LU, HT and SP manifest, HT Point is most likely to be the primary point for therapy. This is because HT, SP and LU are a straight (unbroken) sequence in the Sheng Cycle. If the Process Imbalance is corrected in HT, the Process Imbalance in SP and LU often normalises quickly without further treatment.

- If we find three reactive points; LU, HT and LV manifest, HT Point is most likely to be the primary point for therapy also. This is because HT, LU and LV are in a straight (unbroken) sequence in the Ko Cycle.

When we find and treat the Ting Point of the Primary Process Imbalance in horses we see a strange phenomenon at *other reactive* (secondary) *Ting Points*. Those dry hollows (a sign of chronic problems) fill up and disappear totally within a few seconds after stimulation of the primary Ting Points. This usually happens when we diagnose and treat correctly. It shows that our treatment works throughout the whole body. Such treatment usually gives noticeable results within a few days. Some residual symptoms that have nothing to do with the primary points may persist. In such cases it may be necessary to repeat the treatment or to treat again with other methods after about 4 weeks. Allow 3-7 weeks between treatment sessions.

USE OF THE TING POINTS TO PREVENT DISORDERS

Ting Point therapy is very suitable to prevent illness. This is because the Ting Points are amongst the first points to react to stress or a Process Imbalance. By treating a reactive Ting Point as soon as we observe it we may correct the Process

Imbalance before serious symptoms arise. The Lesion-Symptom Complexes related to the Ting Points are identical to those of their related Process. They will not be described further here. I have used this method for about 18 years (since 1983). In recent years I have worked more and more with preventative treatment, usually about once a month.

SPEED OF CLINICAL IMPROVEMENT AFTER TING POINT THERAPY
Ting Points have certain characteristics which should be discussed. First, the *reaction time* (the speed of clinical improvement) depends on which is the primary reactive Ting Point or Channel with the Process Imbalance.

- When the primary imbalance shows at the Ting Points of HT and GB, the *reaction time is fastest*; symptoms usually disappear within hours.

- When the primary imbalance shows at LV Ting Point, the most important Process Imbalance in horses, the symptoms usually need 1-2 weeks to resolve.

- When the primary imbalance shows at KI Ting Point, the symptoms usually need two treatments and 3-4 weeks to resolve.

- When the primary imbalance shows at SP Ting Point, it usually needs 2-3 treatments and 8-11 weeks to resolve the symptoms. If SP Ting Point is the primary point, one should give an additional treatment to SP to get it to react quicker. In this case arsenic is most suitable. One should give a soup-spoonful/day of a 1% arsenic solution for a horse and 10 drops/day to a dog of 40 kg liveweight for 30 days.

- Another characteristic of SP Ting Point is that it acts as a secondary point when pathology has existed for about a year. If one finds a Deficient SP Ting Point that the symptoms (and Pulse Diagnosis) do not indicate as a SP Process Imbalance, one can assume that the case has existed for a year or more. This is a poor prognostic sign because if they have been present for a year or more the symptoms (and the underlying Process Imbalance) are deep seated and difficult to correct.

TING POINTS AS SYMPTOMATIC POINTS

Even when Ting Points do not show typical pathological signs on physical palpation, Ting Points may be used symptomatically in a few disorders, such as *Monday morning disease (azoturia, Tying up)* or a *bowed tendon (tendinitis)*. In these disorders the Ting Points may be used whether or not they are reactive.

- In *Monday morning disease* LV Point is used.

- In *bowed tendon (tendinitis)* in the foreleg HT, PC and LU Ting Points are used. In the hindlimb we use KI, SP and BL Ting Points.

About the Equine Mouth

WRITTEN BY DR. ANNICA NYGREN THORESEN DVM.
Tooth care, prophylaxis and what to examine (look for) at different ages.

Most horses today are not suffering from neglected dental care but rather from an excessive or wrongful one. It is important to examine the teeth regularly but that does not mean that one must float the teeth every time.

Let us start with the **young horse.** Normally there is not very much that goes wrong during the first two years of the horse's life. This, of course, provided that the horse eats and chews well and is growing normally. Racehorses or standardbreds destined to have a bit in the mouth at an early age should be examined at 1-1.5 years old. One can then determine the apposition of the teeth, maxilla and mandible, and whether brachygnathia, prognathia or normal conformation of the jaw is present.

Swedish research showed that (Thorbjørn Lundström, Swedish dentist and equine dentist) circa 45-50% of 25000 horses in the study had wolf teeth. The bit usually interferes with these teeth and >90% of horses with wolf teeth have problems with the bit. In my opinion, one should remove *all* equine wolf teeth. The wolf tooth has no function, so its removal has no adverse effects on horses.

Before 2-2.5 years of age it has not yet fused with the maxillary bone and is therefore easier to extract with the whole root intact. This is important as remnants of roots and fractured wolf teeth causes more problems to horses than the intact tooth in riding and driving but also due to a chronic pulpitis.

Horses not destined to have a bit in the mouth as yearlings and that have no problems eating, chewing or growing can be examined later, i.e. at 2-2.5 years of age. At this age the apposition of the teeth, maxilla and mandible should be similar to that of mature horses. In such horses one need not float the teeth but one should extract wolf teeth and correct hooks on 106 and 206 (the 2nd premolars in the upper jaw). This releases the lower jaw from the blockage that the hook creates; it allows the jaws to continue to grow, perhaps even to create a normal apposition between the jaws. This is good practice provided that one follows up the case every 3-6 months, as long as is necessary.

In 3-*year olds* the jaws grow markedly, both in length and width. At this time the 8th deciduous premolars (P2 and P3) are replaced rapidly. At examination one should look for deciduous caps. This can lead to food impaction, halitosis, gingivitis and disturbed normal development of teeth. ONLY loose and displaced caps should be removed. Premature removal of caps can cause hypoplasia of cement in the enamel lakes (infundibulum) of the molar teeth. At this age the mandibular growth plates can be mistaken for swellings caused by the molar teeth. Normally, 3-year olds have chewing problems because few areas are in perfect occlusion. In turn, this is due to the active replacement of the deciduous premolars. It is very important that you think twice before floating a mouth like this.

In 4-*year olds* the last deciduous premolars (109, 209, 309, 409) are replaced. It is common to get food impaction at this site. The tooth at the level of the nose band often causes ulceration in the local mucosa. It is therefore better to use a lower nose band until the horse is 5 years of age. Often 4-year olds are wrongfully diagnosed as having teeth like the waves of an ocean, but this is a question of maturity.

In 5-*year olds* the growth of the jaws is coming to an end. At this age we have the highest incidence of sharp teeth but 90% of them are physiologically normal. This means that you should be very careful if you float the teeth at this age.

A horse that gets enough roughage or grass and does not have any abnormal teeth wears his teeth very well on his own. It is very important for horses to have sharp enamel ridges to be able to crush the food. Ulcers in the oral mucosa are seldom caused by simply sharp teeth but from a disturbed mastication which is due to dental disease or pathology, high concentrate feed with small amounts of fibre or ill fitting bits, from which the horse tries to get away from opening its mouth. This results in us tightening the nose band even more. To float the teeth due to the ulcers is simply a symptomatic treatment and is only palliative.

In nature, if it is allowed to do so, a horse eats and chews for about 16 hours a day. That is why it is so important to give food as many times a day as possible and not to give concentrate. Most of the required nourishment should come from roughage. This gives horses a more physiological mastication and hence a normal wear of its teeth.

It is important to ensure that the bit suits the horse. One can measure the space between the upper and lower interdental space when the mouth is closed. Alternatively, one can measure the length of the upper and lower second premolars. Just make sure that the horse can keep its mouth shut without the bit putting pressure on the gums to signal him to open it again. Pressure from a bit that is too thick gives a reflex to open the mouth and when the horse does so, we tighten the nose band. The length of the bit, from ring to ring, is exactly the distance between the corners of the mouth. The bit should never be long enough to protrude even 0.5 cm, otherwise it may damage the mucosa badly, especially in the P2 area. The bit also works as a lever if it is hinged in two or more parts. It may then cause pressure in the upper gum so that the horse wants to open its mouth. Whether or not to use a hinged or straight bit is a matter of personal preference. It also depends on what kind of problems the horse has, i.e. what the horse's defence mechanism was to a previous bit design.

Owners should ignore current fashions and fads in bit design, unless these are based on very well designed long-term research. It would seem that many manufacturers of bits have never looked into the mouths of modern horses. Badly designed or badly fitting bits cause many problems. Let the horse decide the design that suits it best.

In the Swedish study of 25000 horses most injuries in the mouth were due to badly fitting bits. Note, however, that *oral disorders* do not necessarily originate *from (or in) the mouth*. Pain in other parts of the body can make the horse use the bit as a support; this can injure the mucosa and teeth.

In 6-**year olds** the discrepancy in occlusal contact begins to show problems. At examination it is important to evaluate the relation of the teeth in the sagittal plane and not to forget that the transversal angle of the upper teeth is very narrow.

Between 7-**10 years** the discrepancy in occlusal contact becomes progressively worse. One should examine the caudal cheek teeth for hooks and arcade balance.

Between **10-15 years** the development of the roots has come to an end. If tooth hooks are not treated properly, diastema and food impaction can occur. We can also see early signs of ageing.

Between **15-20 years** the dental changes are slowing down. One should look for fractures, caries, food impaction and normal signs of ageing.

At **20-25 years** the roots are very short. By now, many horses have worn out the enamel and the teeth are beginning to loosen. If a horse lives this long and is healthy, the quality of its teeth is the main decider of how old it can get with dignity.

The Mouth as an ECIWO System

MOUTH-ACUPUNCTURE

A very small number of acupuncturists specialise in Mouth-AP in humans. In my opinion, Jochen Gleditsch, a doctor, dentist and acupuncturist who lives in Germany, is one of the greatest exponents of this method. He mapped out the different Mouth Zones and he also showed that specific teeth relate to a specific Process. Before addressing this special subject, it is important to define clearly the teeth in question. Numbers are used to identify the human teeth.

Human Jaw	Right	Left
Upper	(incisor) 11 to 18	(incisor) 21 to 28
Lower	(incisor) 41 to 48	(incisor) 31 to 38

Table 85

Tooth numbering in horses is the same but the numbers have 3 digits.

Equine	Right	Left
Upper	(incisor) 101 to 111	(incisor) 201 to 211
Lower	(incisor) 401 to 411	(incisor) 301 to 311

Table 86

All teeth coded 01-03 are incisors, 04 is the canine, 05 is the wolf tooth, 06-08 are the premolars and 09-11 are the molars.

Now we can progress to the relationships between the Process and the different teeth starting with the human teeth (after Jochen Gleditsch).

Process	Tooth
KI-BL	11, 12, 21, 22, 31, 32, 41, 42
LV-GB	13, 23, 33, 43
LU-LI	14, 15, 24, 25, 36, 37, 46, 47
SP-ST	16, 17, 26, 27, 34, 35, 44, 45
HT-SI	18, 28, 38, 48

Table 87

The incisors relate to KI, the canines to LV, the premolars in the lower jaw and the molars in the upper jaw to SP. Finally the premolars in the upper jaw and the molars in the lower jaw relate to LU. All wisdom teeth relate to the Fire Phase, especially HT.

All this is quite different in horses. Here we must once again remember that we may not just transpose directly from humans to animals but we must investigate which Fundamental Processes reveal in the different teeth and parts. Where for example teeth fail to develop (at the beginning of the empty space (lanen)), we see SP Excess (Qi Full, a Process Imbalance with excessive SP Function); Earth Phase causes disintegration. When the teeth again start to develop, the Wood Phase is flourishing (Wood Phase gives growth). Also, as the equine nose is so much more developed than in humans, we may also expect the Metal Phase to be much more predominant than in the humans. Thus we may correlate the Processes with the teeth as follows (after Are Thoresen):

Process	Tooth
KI-BL	107 and further caudal in all jaws
LV-GB	105, 106, 205, 206
	305, 306, 405, 406
SP-ST	104, 204, 304, 404
LU-LI	101, 102, 103, 201, 202, 203
	301, 302, 303, 401, 402, 403
HT-SI	Possibly the middle part of the lane

Table 88

It is interesting that the area where the bit is placed relates to LV. This may possibly partly be, or at least aggravate, the cause that horses have so many LV disorders. It is also interesting that horses with chronic pain, especially colic, stimulate the incisors and that these teeth relate especially to the Metal Phase.

Something on the General Effect of the Commandpoints

THE PROCESSES IN RELATION TO THE ANATOMICAL STRUCTURES

It is important to bear in mind that the commandpoints relate to the *processes* and not the *organs*.

It is very easy to imagine the body consisting of organs and that the processes are connected only to them. This is not so. There are many exaples that will show the opposite, that the process has no organs, or that the process uses organs which in other species are used by another process.

In the dog water metabolism and distribution in the body is gouverned by the kidney, in the horse also by the large intestine. In humans stomach problems are often related to the spleen, in horses often to the lung.

We have to see the process at work in the body, and not connected to any organs. In trees all the processes are of course at work, as they are in single cell organisms, but here there are few or no organs to carry out the task of the process.

In humans and dogs the food is contained in the stomach but in horses by the large intestine. In cows it is contained in the oesophagus.

The command points stimulate or regulate the processes, not the organs.

The use of the command points are in this way directees to the process that show itself in the symptoms.

To make this clear, I will give you an example:

- A dog has a painful muscle on the lateral side of its back leg. The symptom is situated where the Gall Bladder meridian passes, and indicates that the Gall Bladder meridian is in excess. Then probably the Lung meridian is in deficiency (Ko-father unable to control its son). Therefore we should stimulate the Lung meridian, but what command point to use? The symptom is either dominated by wood (muscle tension) or metal (pain). If we decide that the muscle tension is the dominant symptom we will use the wood-command point and if we decide that the pain is the dominant symptom we will use the metal-command point.

Other Subjects Within Acupuncture

POINT STIMULATION.
There are many methods for point stimulation of which the more important are:

1) Needle-AP
2) Thermostimulation / moxibustion
3) Injection-AP
4) Implants
5) Blistering
6) Electrical stimulation
7) Laser stimulation
8) Magnetic stimulation
9) Light of different kinds
10) Massage

If we must rank these methods by their effectiveness, one would generally follow the numerical order shown above. There are a few exceptions in which thermostimulation is the most effective. Likewise, we find points that react best to injection-AP, blisters or laser-AP. In my experience, there are no points that react best to magnetic stimulation. In my opinion, massaging points in animals usually has the least effect.

1) Needle-AP. When using needles we should use disposable equipment avoiding all possibility of contagious infection. Disposable Seirin needles, 0.3 mm thick and 30 mm long, are excellent. The needle is placed directly into the point where it should stay for about 10-20 minutes.

2) Thermostimulation / moxibustion: Thermostimulation is very effective when we want to use heat as a superficial or internal blister to help inflammation. It is also a very effective way to convert a chronic inflammation into an acute one. Healing usually follows quickly. This method applies heat to the selected points or areas directly or indirectly. One can hold a glowing moxa stick, cigarette, incense stick or lighted match on or above the point. Alternatively, one can use modern electrical thermostimulators, infrared stimulators, or higher power lasers. In China, some therapists plunge a special red hot fire needle onto the points.

3) Injection-AP. In principle we can use many different substances for injection-AP. American colleagues often use injections. They use vitamin B6 to sedate (calm down) and vitamin B12 to tune (stimulate). Likewise a hypotonic salt solution (<0.9% NaC1) is used if the point is to be sedated and a hypertonic salt solution (>0.9% NaC1) if the point is to be stimulated. One may also inject an irritant (blister) solution, or apply a local (superficial) blister paste, in combination with manual-AP and thermostimulation. This is a method I often use if I want maximal effect.

Homeo-AP is another medical modality; it entails injecting appropriate homeopathic remedies into the corresponding acupoints. (See the relationship between AP and homeopathy go to page 546).

4) Implants. To use implants as a way to stimulate acupoints requires a veterinary license since it is regarded as a surgical intervention (operation). This method entails an operation in which we implant a foreign object into the acupoint where it is to remain as a constant stimulator. Commonly used foreign objects are stainless steel, silver and gold. I have used this method many times especially in hip dysplasia* (HD) in dogs in which I have implanted a piece of gold wire at LV03. So that the owners could spare themselves many long trips for sessions of manual-AP, I used the implants originally in dogs whose owners lived far away. However, when the result aquired through this method was just as good as in normal AP, I went more or less over to use only implants in HD. The results are very good. However, it is important to know that such operations are irreversible so the therapist must be totally sure of what s/he is doing and use the right point. Therefore, this method should only be used to treat life long chronic cases that do not change with time.

The history of gold-implants started with Dr. Grady Young (DVM) who in the early seventies started to implant gold beads as a treatment in epilepsy. He implanted the gold beads in the head and neck area. The next one to use gold implants was Dr. Terry Durkes (DVM) who in 1975 started to implant gold beads in the treatment of degenerative conditions in the musculo-sceletal system. I did the first gold implantation in 1988 in dogs in the treatment of HD and in humans in 1995 in the treatment of Leg Perthe, coxarthrosis and hip dysplacia.

Many colleges implant the gold beads at the area of the degeneration, the pain or the pathological changes (Kothbauer, Klitsgaard, Kasper). I, in contrast, have always implanted the gold bead in a commandpoint at the deficient meridian. This method is much faster, cheaper, does not require anestesia of the dog and is less invasive as the method of implanting the beads deep in the tissue around the joints or painful areas. Even the human orthopaedist Primar Helmut Liertzer (who is considered the first to implant in humans in 1998, although I did this in 1995) is critisised for the risks of putting gold in the areas that he did. This could have been solved by using my method.

5) Blistering. This method is simple. It entails dripping a drop of blister solution on the point. We can use normal 10% iodine spirit as a blistering solution here. This method has been tried in Austria to increase bovine fertility. The inseminator dropped a drop of iodine on BL22-BL23 at insemination; this method resulted in the birth of more calves (Kothbauer, personal communication). This method is useful if we desire a milder or more preventative treatment. Other blisters that may be used are; camphor oil, tiger balsam, mustard powder in oil or other substances that causes local irritation. "Blue lotion" is a usable alternative that can be purchased in stores that sell equipment for horses.

Internal blistering is an interesting method that helps to increase general blood circulation. A blister mixture which is carefully tested and composed is given as an infusion directly into the blood, lasting for 45 minutes. This mixture expands the entire blood system and transfers blood to all parts of the body. This treatment has especially been tested in the USA and I have tried it many times here at home with good results.

#
1000 ml. 0.9% (boiled*) salt solution
2000 iu Heparin
3000 mg EDTA
7500 mg Vitamin C
10 ml B complex
4000 mg MgCl
10 ml Ca borogluconate / Mg sulphate solution (strength as used in hypocalcaemic puerperal paralysis)
This mixture is infused within 45 minutes and is followed by an injection of 10 ml pyridoxine.
#

"Irritation therapy" ("reitztherapie" in German) is another form of blistering therapy. It irritates special areas or skin zones in such a way that other pathological or unwanted irritations are overcome or healed. The reasoning behind this irritation therapy may be to:

1) *Make a chronic infection acute by the help of irritating ointments locally applied.*

2) *Enhance the blood circulation to an already existing infection by the help of locally applied irritating ointments.*

3) *Stimulate specific internal organs by the help of irritating ointments applied on the reflex zones of the specific organ (for example Back Shu Points).*

4) *Stimulate specific or general physiologic Functions by the help of irritating substances that stimulate these Functions (for example, bacterial extracts that irritate the immune system).*

Ointments or remedies that may be used to stimulate specific skin areas so that the blood circulation is enhanced are **camphor, eucalyptus, turpentine, rosemary, wintergreen, menthol, mustard and pepper root. One may obtain a somewhat stronger effect by applying oil of cedar, cantharis, cayenne, capsicain and croton.**

The principle behind the different blisters used today to blister equine joints is to increase the blood flow to that particular joint and / or convert a chronic inflammation into an acute one. However, the relief obtained after this therapy usually is short-lived if we do not also eliminate the real cause of the inflammation (the Process Imbalance).

An old recipe that is quite useful (not too strong and not too mild) and which was often used in old times in Germany is:

#

Chloroform.....................5.0g
Methyl salicylate............25.0g
Mucilaginis Tylose..........50.0g
Distilled water.................ad 100.0g

#

6) Electrical stimulation (electro-AP, EAP). For this we need an electrical stimulator that generates variable voltage outputs with variable frequencies (cycles/second, or Hz). The apparatus can be connected to needles or rubber electrodes that are fastened to the skin. EAP stimulation has a stronger effect on the point than simple AP. Bipolar stimulators generate positive and negative charges on the same electrode. They are safer than monopolar stimulators, which can cause electrolytic lesions at a point if they are overused. Also, the electrodes from one socket should not cross the midline from the mid-cervical to the mid-thoracic area; stimulation across the spine in this area can cause heartblock in subjects with a cardiac disorders.

7) Lasers. Low power lasers up to Class 3b have multiple uses. They are used to treat traumatic injury, haematoma, chronic non-healing or granulating wounds or ulcers, non-bacterial infections (bowed tendon), tendinitis, bursitis, periostitis, hot splints, etc. They are used also to stimulate acupoints, especially those close to the skin, such as Earpoints and points over the distal extremities. It is important to clean the point and remove any hair. The effectiveness of the laser depends on the power and depth of penetration of the laser beam through the skin. This light resembles normal light in the respect that hair or dirt blocks it.

It is important that the point is stimulated by the right frequency. Some lasers have the possibility to change frequencies. The frequency that Nogier recommended has given good results in those cases in which I have used it.

- 2.5 Hz for disorders of cell metabolism.

- 5 Hz for digestive disorders.

- 10 Hz for injuries on the limbs

- 20 Hz for back problems.

- 40 Hz for autonomic / subconscious brain processes.

- 80 Hz for conscious brain processes.

- 160 Hz for psychic disorders.

Recently, lasers have become more and more used in AP therapy. The laser is a "light source" which emits monochromatic, polarised light (all the light waves have the same wavelength and vibrate rhythmically). Laser light can stimulate the tissue in the acupoint and can act as a substitute for needles.

Experiments have been made in order to find out how lasers can influence body temperature. The temperature of 21 people was measured before and after laser treatment. They where acclimatised in a room for 30 minutes before measurement. Before laser treatment body temperature averaged 35.4°. Laser was applied at LU05. No temperature variation was detected on the right side after laser at LU05. However, the temperature had risen on the left side. We have no theoretical explanation but undoubtedly an asymmetrical disturbance had happened because of the one-sided effect (Dr. Prof. Birger Kaada, Stavanger, Norway).

To check the changes due to laser radiation of ST36, 30 people were used, 14 of which comprised a control group; they received placebo treatment. The placebo point was chosen 1.5 cm from the correct point and Channel. The stimulation did not reach the skin properly. Urine samples were collected. The urine output and its content of steroids, minerals and phosphates were measured before and after laser treatment. In comparison to the control group, a fall in all parameters except calcium was observed. This shows that laser treatment of ST36 influences the body (Kaada).

8) Magnetic stimulation. Magnetic stimulation is performed by fastening small strong therapy magnets on to the relevant acupoint and keeping them there over a longer period of time. We can use Band Aids or super-glue to fasten them. This is a method that helps (bowed tendon); in this case, the magnets are "moulded" into the plaster when we are applying a cast.

9) Light of different kinds. I have, during the years, tried several kinds of light, but the one kind with the most effect (often even more than needles) has been "Singlet Oxygen Light."

As this kind of light is alien to most of my readers, I will explain this phenomenon in more detail:

The principle is simple and found in nature. In an activation chamber the oxygen of the air has been activated to singlet oxygen through a process called photosensitization. The ingredients for the photosensitization are:

- Light.
- Oxygen.
- A suitable photosensitiser.

This also happens when the sun shines on the leaves of plants and trees (chlorophyll is a photosensitiser) and singlet oxygen is formed on the surface of the leaves. Singlet oxygen has a distinct higher level of energy compared to oxygen in the ground state and is a very aggressive substance. Singlet oxygen (SO) acts like a free radical and can cause cell damage. Consequently, many experts considered SO to be a dangerous oxygen molecule. What many people however are not aware of is that the lifetime of singlet oxygen is extremely short. In air under normal conditions it is only a few hundred thousanths of a second, in water it is only two millionths of a second. We assume that in air with a high humidity the lifetime is close to this figure, but even in air with a normal or low humidity the lifetime is so short that no singlet oxygen can leave the equipment. A Swedish scientist, Tony van der Valk (TvdV) has been able to show that in the activation chambers used in the equipment in which singlet oxygen is really formed, but because of the short life time only very small amounts could (can) be detected.

These investigations were performed at the University of Helsinki (1993) and at the Heinrich Heine University in Düsseldorf (1995).When singlet oxygen returns to the ground state the extra energy is released. So far this energy has been impossible to measure but has powerful informative properties in respect to biological systems.One of the striking effects is that treatment of waste water contaminated with many bacteria, such as E-Coli, showed a dramatic decrease in bacterial count after only 5 minutes of treatment. After a treatment with activated light, a decrease from 3500 to 270 bacteria per 100 ml was recorded.TvdV has also noted the effect on plants, which grow faster and bigger with less need for fertilizers and pesticides. The energy can be transported with humid air but also directly as light photons, for example through a fiberoptic cable. In this case we have no transmission through other media. This minimises losses and presumably has a greater effect. There are five different singlet states, but the most important one seems to be the one which releases energy corresponding to light with a wave length of 634.3 nm. There are studies indicating that this energy can be absorbed by the vibrations of the oxygen-hydrogen bond of a water molecule. These vibrations have a peak at a wave length of 628 nm. This is probably the reason why the life time of singlet oxygen in water is so short. An investigation done in Finland with 10 high performance sportsmen (long distance runners) showed after only two weeks of treatments with activated air (totally 10 treatments of 20 minutes each) amongst others the following results:

- The blood absorbed 7% more oxygen.

- The energy production increased by 8%.

- Blood lactic acid was 8% less after performance.

The results were statistically significant to highly significant.

In another investigation done in Stockholm with 10 healthy individuals, TvdV found after only 2 weeks of inhalation (totally 6 treatments of 20 minutes each) the following results:

- Total Antioxidant Status (the capacity of blood plasma to cope with free radical production according to Randox) increased by 20%.

- Total serum cholesterol decreased by 10%

- Total serum triglycerides decreased by 25%

All results were statistically significant.

A number of investigations are currently being carried out at reputable institutions and university hospitals with very interesting results so far, especially the decrease in the production of free radicals seems to be dramatic. The effect on human beings is primarily a drastic reduction in the free radical production. Secondary effects, on top of the above mentioned, are:

- Powerful reduction of pain.

- Normalisation of processes in the body.

- Faster tissue healing.

- Healing of ulcers and open wounds with little or no scarring.

In Sweden, Dr Anders Willstedt has treated more than 600 patients with fibromyalgia with very good results. The patients experienced a powerful reduction in pain. TvdV also found that the SO activated light has a powerful effect on localised pain and can accelerate the healing process of wounds and ulcers in an unexpected way. A simple treatment with the equipment not only increases oxygen uptake and utilization (7% in healthy well trained sportsmen) but also decreases free radical production dramatically.

10) Massage. Massage is, in my experience, not of use in professional veterinary acupuncture. Massage gives to diffuse of an impulse to the points. On the other hand, I advise normal massage to relax spasm in muscles.

Acupuncture and Cancer

From a holistic viewpoint, one evaluates the Processes that control a cancerous tumour to be totally normal, even healthy. The normal biological activity is for a cell to grow and multiply. For many animals and plants this process continues throughout life. It is only in the case of highly developed animals that growth and cell division stop at a certain age. It is likewise in these species that cancer becomes a "normal" illness. If growth processes continue throughout life, cancer (uncontrolled processes) occur to a much smaller degree. The controlling Processes begin to play a more active role when growth is about to stop. They impede physical development. These controlling Processes are, to an increasing degree, present the more developed the individual is; they reach their maximum in mammals. If these controlling Processes fail in their function, growth processes regain dominance and cancerous tumours can arise.

Many reasons explain the failure of the controlling Processes. Day after day the Processes that control all cellular and bodily functions are stressed constantly. In addition to the (External)

Stressors and stimuli that adversely influence living organisms, the stressors include shock, strain on the psyche, bombardment with unwanted sounds, visual impressions, additives and electromagnetic influences (high voltage cables, geopathic stress, etc). These stressors can lead to strain on, or loss of dominance of, the Processes and especially immune function.

The aim of all cancer therapy must be to help the patient to regain this dominance and restore control of the Processes, especially of the immune system. That system is critical for good health. Time after time many methods from meditation to more or less vegetarian diets have been developed to reestablish control.

We must not underestimate the importance of the attempts of conventional medicine to find methods to hamper or kill cancer cells, even if these methods usually attack the symptoms more than the cause.

In holistic medicine it is most important to stimulate the body's controlling Processes. The idea is to "bring control" to the growth processes, otherwise they become uncontrolled, which is the basic problem with cancerous cells. If we stimulate the wrong Processes we may aggravate the disorder by stimulating tumour growth. In my opinion, working via the Ko Cycle (Controlling) is the best way to stimulate the controlling Processes of the body (See also page 28).

Treatment of Patients Suffering from Cancer

First, we must make a Channel Diagnosis, either via Pulse Diagnosis, or by a simple observation of where the tumour has arisen. *When the patient suffer from cancer it is very important to decide where the location of the lesion is. This will indicate the Channel that has lost its control.* Let us take mammary cancer as an example. It manifests on ST Channel. We must particularly avoid stimulating ST Channel, but we should stimulate LV, the Ko Controlling Channel of ST (the father of ST). For this, we could use the Ting (Wood) Point (LV01), or Earth Point (LV03). Better is to find and stimulate the ECIWO-point that is to be found along one of the metacarpal- or metatarsal bones, alomg the pathway of the meridian in question.

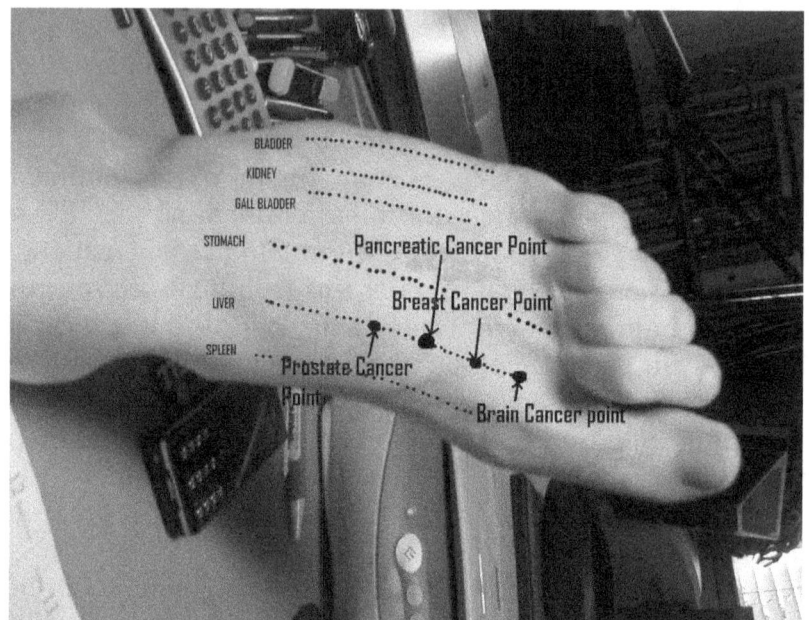

Figure 64; illustration of one og the ECIWO-systems that may be used in the attempt to stimulate the body to fight against the cancer disease.

We should stimulate *only the Ko (Controlling) Father Channel*, not for example the Ko (Controlling) Point of ST itself. During the period of treatment, we should stimulate no other Channel or Process. However, we may combine other therapies that stimulate LV.

I have tried this method over several years. Following my instructions, several colleagues in the US of A and Australia have tried it. The results have been very encouraging. Between 0-90% (depending on the organ or tissue of origin) of confirmed cancer cases have improved noticeably. The improvements included increased quality of life, better sleep, increased appetite and a glossier coat. Overall 0-90% (depending on the organ or tissue of origin) have been totally cured of the illness. Tumour(s) have, in such cases, vanished within a few weeks. Two examples:

- The first patient in which I tried this method was a Dachshund. It had mammary cancer (ST, Earth) and probably lung metastases. I treated the mammary

ECIWO-point on the LV-meridian. Within a few weeks the tumours were almost gone. Guess who was more amazed, the dog, the owner or I?!

- In liver tumours we must stimulate only LU Channel (*Metal Controls Wood*). This activates the body's adaptive / homeostatic / immune control system, so that the body itself can bring the cancerous tumours under control. If we succeed in this, the active tumour tissue shrivels within a few days and disappears within a few months. If there is considerable fibrosis of the area, the fibrous tissue remains permanently, as is true for scars elsewhere.

Sour (acidic, vinegar-like) food boost our attempted treatment of all cancers, regardless of which Channel we wish to stimulate. It seems that a more acidic diet boosts the Ko (controlling) Process in general (acid = Yang = control). Foods such as sour milk and sauerkraut* (a German form of sour cabbage) often are included in the diet of cancer patients. In this regard, it is interesting to discuss a method developed by Dr. Malchaire from Liege. He used a system of amino acids to control the Channels:

Sauerkraut is cabbage fermented by lactic acid bacteria. This is different from the Norwegian version, made by pickling cabbage in vinegar and sugar.

Summary of the amino acids to strengthen the control of the various Channels

LV	glycine, isoleucine, threonine and methionine
KI	cysteine, tyrosine*, aspartic acid and leucine
HT	arginine, tryptophan, histidine and glutamine
LU	lysine, phenylalanine, valine and proline
SP	asparagine, alanine, glutamic acid and serine

responsible for aggressiveness in Pit Bull terriers.
Table 89

The amino acids listed above have a directly controlling effect. When it is indicated that glycine, isoleucine, threonine and methionine control LV, they are used as a dietary supplement in cases of liver tumour.

The dosage is 1 g/day; it can be bought at any pharmacy.

We can use homeopathic medicine in addition to stimulating an individual Channel with needles. For each Channel there is a main homeopathic preparation that can be given simultaneously during stimulation of the specific Channel.

Table of the homeopathic remedies used in organ or Channel-related tumours or cancer;

Affected Channel	Effective homeopathic remedy
LU-LI (Metal)	Aur.met D12
LV GB (Wood)	Carbo.veg D12
SP-ST (Earth)	Stann.met D6
KI BL (Water)	Thuja CM or Ars.Alb D30
HT,SI,PC,TH (Fire)	Phos D12

Table 90

It is difficult and controversial to write about cancer, a disease that causes so much pain, anxiety and that has many taboos. However, it would be negligent not to touch on this subject when I see how a cancerous tumour, malignant or benign, can totally disappear within weeks after use of the correct treatment. Also, even in cases in which holistic methods fail to help the body to halt or cure the physical cancer, they can help many patients to attain a better psychological and spiritual status and to have a better quality of life in their remaining months or years.

SUMMARY OF MY TREATMENT OF PATIENTS SUFFERING FROM CANCER

1. Remember that you do not treat the cancer, only the deficient process that has allowed the cancer to develop.

2. It is always the father process that has failed his son. The father is always for;

   a. Heart, Pericardium, Small Intestine and Trippel Heather the KIDNEY

   b. Spleen and Stomach the LIVER

   c. Lung and Large Intestine the HEART or PERICARDIUM

   d. Kidney and Bladder the SPLEEN or the HEART or PERICARDIUM

   e. Liver and Gall Bladder the LUNG

3. Treat the father meridian, which at the time of the onset of the cancer/tumor was the deficient one.

4. The point to be chosen is the actual ECIWO-point, as described under ECIWO-biology (see page 10)

5. Treat the point every month, until the tumor has stopped growing or is completely disappeared.

Interim Clinical Results on Acupuncture in Cancer-Treatment, notes from my Casebook

On the request of Dr. Med. Ottestad, Chief Medical Officer of the mammary cancer department at the Radium Hospital of Norway, I carefully noted and measured all human patients during a certain time span; *April 22ⁿᵈ 2003 and January 26ᵗʰ 2004; they were not "cherry-picked" to show the best outcomes.* These notes are the foundation of table 90 and 91. The human patients were diagnosed by their doctor and I have just accepted the diagnosis. All patients have been followed up until 31.12.2009 (or until they died).

Important is to note that in this investigation I had still not found the ECIWO system, so only the acupuncture ponts were used (except in breast/mammary cancer, where I unknowingly already had found the ECIWO-point for the breast/mamma.

Summary of my treatment protocols and their interim outcomes in humans

#	Cancer type / description of tumour / malignancy and indication of malignant (M) or benign (B)	Patient, year of birth)	Acupoint(s) used / date of first treatment / description of progression or development and indication of positive effect (P), uncertain (?) or negative (N)
1.	Aggressive mammary carcinoma / malignant (M)	Woman, born 1962	LV-breast ECIWO / 19/11-02 / the cancer was operated and treated with medication, but the hospital gave up and sent her home to die. After treatments every month she lived for 4 years, and then died during a few weeks. (P)
2.	Prostate cancer: with multiple skeletal metastases / malignant (M)	Man, born 1942	HT09 + TH02 / September –02 / after starting the acupuncture treatment the cancer has gone "dormant." The situation is stable. PSA = 0.35. No other treatment has been performed (P)
3.	Leukaemia / benign (B)	Man, born 1944	SI18 & LU01 / 18/6-03 / the blood-values have been stable since the treatment started (P)
4.	Mammary carcinoma / 6 mm. tumour on left side / malignant (M)	Woman, born 1945	LV-breast ECIWO / 18/6-03 / she was not operated or given any other form of treatment by the hospital. The tumour went almost totally away and can now not be detected (P)
5.	Uterine cervical cancer Stage IIIB: / malignant (M)	Woman, born 1958	TH02 / 30/7-03 / diagnosed in spring 2002. After treatment with acupuncture the cancer has disappeared completely (P)

6.	Renal carcinoma / started in the right kidney with metastases in the liver where 6 metastases can be seen / malignant (**M**)	Man, born 1922	HT09 / 17/9-03 / after two treatments the man did not come, and I later learned that he had died. (**N**)
7.	Melanosarcoma / lateral side of the arm, / malignant (**M**)	Woman, born 1932	HT09 (as the cancer was situated on the LI-meridian) / 1/10-03 / the patient seem to get better and better and then suddenly died 14. January 2004. (**N**)
8.	Mammary carcinoma / 20 mm. tumour in left breast. Operated 10/2-99. Then metastases to liver and the skeleton. Also now multiple cancers in the right breast / malignant (**M**)	Woman, born 1957	LV-breast ECIWO / 28/10-03 / she was not operated or given any other form of treatment by the hospital after the discovery of the metastases and the recurrence of the breast cancer. All tumours started to shrink, then halted, and are now static. (**P**)
9.	Mammary carcinoma / 18 mm. tumour on left side / malignant (**M**)	Woman, born 1964	LV-breast ECIWO / 24/11-03 / she was operated and given additional treatment to stop metastases. Treatment to prevent metastases. (**?**)
10.	Dysplasia of the glossal epithelium / cell-changes on the tongue / benign (**B**)	Woman, born 1950	KI03 / 7/10-03 / the patient has received no other treatment, and the cell-changes are stable (**P**)
11.	Colon carcinoma / operated / malignant (**M**)	Man, born 1930	HT09 / 22/10-03 / treatment to prevent the cancer from metastasing or reappearing (**?**)
12.	Mammary carcinoma of the left breast / the carcinoma was ca. 1, cm in diameter / malignant (**M**)	Woman, born 1950	LV-breast ECIWO / 8/12-03 / the woman had undergone surgery and the cancer + 14 lymph-nodes were excised. The treatment was performed for prevention. No other treatment after the surgery is performed (**?**)

13.	Chronic myelo-monocytic leukaemia / benign (**B**)	Woman, born 1947	LV03 / 19/11-03 / no obvious change in the blood-values after start of acupuncture treatment (**?**)
14.	Chronic diarrhoea after former radiation of cancer / this is not a cancer treatment, but only damage after radiation	Woman, born 1948	PC05 + KI0+3 / 19/11-03 / the diarrhoea disappeared after 4 weeks and 2 treatments. Has stayed Ok since then (**P**)
15.	Brain cancer / inoperable / half of it benign, half malignant (**B + M**)	Woman, born 1964	TH05 + PC08 / 22/12-03 / since treatment started the patient has be stable (**P**)
16.	Mammary carcinoma, aggressive type, right side with multiple metastases / malignant (**M**)	Woman, born 1960	LV-breast ECIWO / 18/6-03 / she was not operated or given any other form of treatment by the hospital, as the doctors considered the case incurable. Since the treatment started there has been no growth of the cancer or the metastases (**P**)
17.	Carcinoma of the prostate / malignant (**M**)	Man, born 1954	BL40 / 15/1-04 / operated additionally with cryo-technique, difficult to evaluate (**?**)
18	Mammary carcinoma, aggressive. Operated, but after operation metastases to the liver and the skeleton malignant (**M**)	Woman, born 1945	LV-breast ECIWO / 26/1-03 / after the treatment started there was a stop in the growth of the cancer (**P**)

Table 91

Summary of my treatment protocols and their interim outcomes in animals

#	Cancer type / description of tumour / malignancy and indication of malignant (M) or benign (B)	Patient, year of birth	Acupoint (s) used / date of first treatment / description ofprogression or development and indication of positive effect (P), uncertain (?) or negative (N)
1	Mammary carcinoma / 10 & 8 mm tumours in both sides / malignant (M)	Female dog, Chihuahua, born 1999	LV-mammary ECIWO / 22/4-03 / the tumours went almost totally away, then reappeared, and are now stabile. No other treatment (P)
2	Perianal tumour / 12 cm. Diameter / benign (B)	Female dog, Chihuahua, born 1999	CV23 / spring –02 / the tumour was stable for 1 year, started then to grow autumn –03, and the dog was put down in November –03. No other treatment (N)
3	Osteosarcoma left front leg / 11 cm² / malignant (M)	Dog, mixed breed, born 1994	HT09 / November –02 / in April –03 the cancer was totally gone. No other treatment (P)
4	Carcinoma of the endothelium of the abdomen, with metastases to several organs / malignant (M)	Male dog, Riesenschnauser, born 1989	SP06 / 1. April –03 / the first 3 months everything seem to go better, but then the dog suddenly died in august. No other treatment (N)
5	Mammary tumour: diameter 1.1 cm / benign (B)	Bitch, English setter, born 1996	LV-mammary ECIWO / 17/7-03 / After one year the tumor was totally gone. No other treatment has been performed (P)

6	Mammary tumours (2): diameter 1.4 cm, 1,1 cm / benign (**B**)	Bitch, English setter, born 1998	LV-mammary ECIWO / 17/7-03 / After one year the tumors are 0,3 and 0,2 mm. No other treatment has been performed (**P**)
7	Carcinoma of the epithelium / 4 cm. right front paw / malignant (**M**)	Male dog, Riesenschnauser, born 1994	KI01 / 15/7-03 / the carcinoma was operated before I saw the dog, but had spread to right back leg and right axilla / after treatment the cancer was reduced with 60%. No other treatment has been performed (**P**)
8	Seminoma / Left testis 7.5 cm diameter / benign (**B**)	Male dog, Golden retriever, born 1988	LU11 / 17/6-03 / the tumour stopped growing, and has stayed stable since. No other treatment has been performed (**P**)
9	Chondrosarcoma / left side of abdomen, 12 x 12 cm / malignant (**M**)	Male dog, Mixed breed, born 1995	LU11 & LU01 / 22/7-03 / after each treatment the cancer shrunk with 20% during 1 week, but then started to grow again. This pattern has repeated itself after every treatment. Now the cancer is 17 x 20 cm. (**? P**)
10	Lymphosarcoma / have been treated for a long time with cortisone / malignant (**M**)	Male dog, Norwegian hare-hound, born 1996	LV03 / 10/9-03 / 2 days after the first treatment the dog was acutely worse, and was put down by the owner (**N**)
11	Mammary carcinoma / multiple tumours in both sides, size varying between 5 mm to 20 mm. / malignant (**M**)	Icelandic sheep-dog bitch, born 2001	LV-mammary ECIWO / 30/9-03 / she was not operated or given any other form of treatment. The tumours went almost totally away, and can now not be detected (**P**)

12	Malignant mesenchymal tumour at the inside of the knee / 10 cm. diameter / malignant (**M**)	Male dog, mixed breed, born 1999	LU11 / 10/10-03 / after the first treatment the cancer has stopped to grow and seem to be stable. (**P**)
13	Epithelial carcinoma over the ischium / 5 x 4 cm / malignant (**M**)	Bitch, big poodle, born 1992	SP01 + HT09 / 28/10-03 / after treatment started the cancer has shrunk to 1.9 x 1.9 cm. No other medication or treatments have been performed (**P**)
14	Mastocytoma / malignant (**M**)	Male dog, English setter, born 1997	HT09 / 20/12-03 / after start of treatment the cancer is reduced by approximately 70% (**P**)
15	Mammary carcinoma on left side; operated but had metastases; new cancer is developing on the right side / malignant (**M**)	Bitch, Tibetan temple dog, born 1991	LV-mammary ECIWO bilateral / 20/1-03 / since the treatment started the tumour is somewhat reduced (**P**)

Table 92

Results

Summary of my treatment protocols and their interim outcomes in 34 patients (***all*** patients during one year)

Clinical outcome [interim]	Number of Cases
Humans	18
Dogs	15
Horses	1
Total Benign tumors	8
Total Malign tumors	26
Reduced growth in benign tumors	2

Reduced growth in malign tumors	12
Total disappearance of visible benign tumors	2
Total disappearance of visible malign tumors	4
Overall positive development in number of benign tumors	4
Overall negative development in number of benign tumors	1
Overall positive development in number of malign cancer	18
Overall negative development in number of malign cancer	5
Number of patients impossible to say is positive or negative due to massive treatment in the hospital, or total removal of the cancer surgically.	6
Number of patients that died during the treatment	5

Table 93

Changes in the blood after the described treatment. Identification and isolation of pharmacopotential bioactive peptides from the human body and their preliminary application against breast cancer.

With the help of Sergio Manzetti, I have shown and detected 12 bioactive peptides with strong anti-cancer activity. The peptides were isolated from the blood of a human patient with breast cancer treated by acupuncture, re-synthesized and tested against several breast cancer cell types, 1 colon cancer cell type, a prostate cancer cell type and a healthy-cell line model. The effect of the peptides resulted to 100% cell death on the most common breast cancer cell type, MCF7, after 96 hours. The speed of cell-death was shown to be equivalent to other drugs as Tamoxifen and Doxorubicin, however differing from Doxorubicin and Tamoxifen which are highly toxic and extinguished 87% percent of the healthy cell line model, the peptides seemed to stimulate slightly the growth of the healthy cell lines and induce, not harm them. The peptides were recently tested on the common MCF7 cell line in nude mice models, and showed to induce a linear cell-death signal. The relationship between the cell tests and the mice tests suggests that the peptides have a full cell-death effect on MCF7 cells which however needs to be protected against the immune system of a multicellular organism. The protective method of PEG-modulation is under testing on mice, and will, as expected from other studies performed with PEG, prolong the half-life of the peptides in circulation, and thereby induce stronger cell-death signal to function as a complete pharmacoactive agent.

Results

SAMPLE RESULTS AND PEPTIDES FOUND IN THE PATIENT

The acupuncture stimulus of the patient yielded a pair of samples, where samples A from before acupuncture had half the amount of peptides than sample B from after acupuncture. This instigated not only the rapid effect of generation of changes in the blood after only 60 seconds of acupuncture stimulus, but also a myriad of potential peptides responsible for the internal response to the acupuncture. The key to the isolation process was a sequential choosing of crucial factors that where not only statistically probable of being in the sample of the diseased woman, but also to be related to some known factors, such as Tumour Necrosis Growth factor as an example. Out of the 70-110 peptides resulting from two different identification method, 12 were chosen based on their statistical probability of being present in the blood. The probability ranged from 95%-90% for 11 of these, and 72% for one particular. The common theme of all the peptides found was that they were fragments of proteins, suggesting a mechanism of generation of potential "medical" peptides from existing proteins in circulation.

Many of the peptides found turned out to be related to cell-cycle regulation proteins. The proteins involved in cell-cycle up and down-regulate cell-growth and play key roles in daily maintenance and control of the organisms' adaptation to internal and external changes. Table 94 illustrates the origin of the 12 peptides.

List of parent proteins of the 12 peptides originating from subject treated by acupuncture.

Protein	Statistical Probability	Function
Chain C, Hemoglobin Thionville Alpha Chain Mutant [*H. Sapiens*]	95%	Oxygen-carrier
Chain A Deoxy hemoglobin [*H. Sapiens*]	93%	Oxygen-carrier
Glutamyl Prolyl tRna synthetase [*R. Norvegicus*]	95%	Aminoacid synthesis
Zinc finger, SWIM domain containing [*H. Sapiens*]	95%	Forming nucleoprotein complex in apoptosis possibly involved with proteasome-Ub pathway
Golgin 45 (JEM-1) leucine zipper nuclear factor [*H. Sapiens*]	93%	DNA-binding protein first found in leukaemia cases, role in cell maturation
unnamed protein product [*H. Sapiens*]	77%	Liver-secreted protease inhibitor, antichymotrypsin-like
KIAA0476 protein [*H. Sapiens*]	95%	Unknown factor, detected first in brain tissue.
Winged helix domain-containing isoform B [*H. Sapiens*]	95%	Possibly involved in chromatin-interactions
unnamed protein product [*H. Sapiens*]	82%	mRNA from NT2 neuronal precursor cells treated 2-weeks mitotic inhibitor after 5-weeks retinoic acid (RA) induction (unpublished)
Regulatory Protein [*R. Norvegicus*]	95%	novel mitogenic regulatory gene which is transcriptionally suppressed in cells.
Laminin gamma 1 [*M. Musculus*]	94%	a novel transmembrane protein with a strong and developmentally regulated expression in the nervous system.
Chain A, Nmr Structure Of The Nalp1 P Apoptosis related [*H. Sapiens*]	93%	Apoptosis inducer - new member of death domain superfamily since 2003

Table 94

Cytostatic effects on cancer cells

The 12 peptides were tested at Molecular Imaging Laboratories, Ann Arbor, MI, USA. The peptides effect was focused on the most common breast cancer cell type, MCF7. The MCF7 cell line originates from a patient that had breast cancer with spreading to the lungs and bones and is a common cell type to test both commercial and experimental drugs on. The peptides were synthesized at the Biomedical Genomic Centre at the University of Minnesota and shipped to MIR for testing. At MIR laboratories the peptides were mixed in an equal dose into a complete mixture, to simulate the acupuncture stimulus, and prepared for application on the cell-plates.

The cell-death effect of the peptides has been observed already within the first 24 hours (as seen from results from earlier tests at the University of Massachusetts) to be even faster than the common drug Tamoxifen. After 96 hours of daily doses the breast cancer cells are 100% extinguished. The effect of the peptide mixture I denoted to have an IC50 of 70. This number delineates its potency. The effect was observed as a hyperbolic curve, where the highest concentrations give the fastest effect of cancer-cell death.

The effect of the 12 peptides shows also another positive aspect, it spares healthy cell lines, *in vitro.* The peptides were tested at the University of Nottingham on a healthy cell line, and shown not to harm its growth. So simultaneously as the peptide mixture kills 100% of breast cancer cells MCF7, its saves the healthy cell from its killing effect. The potential drug is therefore appearing as selective, and may be related to its origin from the body, resulting from a stimulus of acupuncture.

Cytostatic Effects on Mice Models

The twelve peptides were pilot-tested against an implanted MCF7 tumour in mice at Molecular Imaging Laboratories in September 08. The peptides' chemical structure was in this experiment in unprotected and natural state, which is a regular form to test for efficiency first. Once the results of the peptides in a natural state are interpreted, their effect can be eventually increased by adding a chemical protection.

The mice were injected with three doses of peptides, 20mg/kg, 40mg/kg and 80mg/kg peptide. The injection was given daily for a period of 21 days and the effect was visible; the highest dose gave the strongest cancer-growth retardation, the middle dose gave a lower cancer growth-retardation and the lowest dose gave the weakest anti-cancer effect. The results show that the peptides have a preserved effect in mice which follows a dose-dependent scheme. Additionally, the results show that the peptides act strongest through the blood and not when injected directly in the tumour. However, the potency of the effect must be strengthened and the central option is to prolong their endurance in circulation. The method for doing this is through a so-called PEG-ligation technology. Our contractor, Cresalus Inc, Kentucky USA, has, in early February, completed the synthesis of 240 mg of PEG-protected peptides. Molecular Imaging Laboratories are initiating the testing of PEG peptides on mice in the middle of February and results are awaited by the beginning of March 09.

Discussion

As known in western medicine and science, a cancerous condition is an uncontrolled state where the cell cycle has lost control and shows continuous progression forming an independent unit, or a tumor. Specifically, causes for this are lack of control at the genetic level, proteomic or cellular level. Each of these levels finds examples in the literature; at the genetic level mutations in the p53 promoter yield deficient expression of the p53 product thereby leading to uncontrolled transition between the G and S - phases. At the proteomic level, mutations in the p53 gene yield a deficient protein which inefficiently binds to the suppressor and cannot manage to "silence" the S - phase of the cell. Recent evidence suggests also that cancer is inducible at the cellular level, through oncovirii, as the Human T-cell Leukaemia/Lymphotropic virus type 1.

Properly used by people trained in the basic principles of traditional Chinese medicine (TCM), this protocol has few, if any, adverse effects. It is based on the following principles:

(a) The normal biological activity of bodily cells is to grow and multiply in an orderly, controlled way. For many animals and plants this process continues throughout life. It is only in the case of highly developed animals that growth and cell division stop at a certain age. It is likewise in these species that cancer becomes a "normal" illness.

(b) Holistic clinicians evaluate the Controlling Processes (CPs) - those that control, or limit, the growth and lifespan of cancerous cells - to be totally normal and essential for health. If growth processes continue throughout life in a controlled way, cancer (uncontrolled processes) occurs to a much smaller degree. The CPs begin to play a more active role when growth is about to stop. They impede further physical development. The higher up the evolutionary tree a species is, the more important normal functioning of these CPs becomes; their importance is maximal in mammals. If the function of the CPs fails, growth processes regain dominance; the cells survive past their normal time to die and cancerous tumours arise.

(c) Many reasons explain functional failure of the CPs. Constant wear-and-tear and attempts to adapt to day-to-day changes in external and internal environment stress the CPs of all cellular and bodily functions constantly. In addition to the (external) stressors and stimuli that adversely influence living organisms, the stressors include shock, strain on the psyche, bombardment with unwanted sounds, visual impressions, additives and electromagnetic influences (high voltage cables, geopathic stress, etc). These stressors can lead to strain on, or loss of dominance of, the CPs, and especially normal functioning of the immune system.

(d) The aim of effective cancer therapy and prevention must be to help the patient to maintain the dominance of, or restore the lost function of, the CPs, especially of the immune system. By preventing or limiting immuno-mediated diseases, including autoimmune diseases and cancer, the immune system is critical for good health. Many methods, from meditation to more or less veg-etarian diets, have been developed to re-establish the essential functions of the CPs. But in my experience, the most effective of all is to use the Ko-Cycle, the body's own processes to restore control.

Thus, the primary aim, the most important function, of holistic medi-cine is to stimulate the body's own control mechanisms.

- *The idea is to "bring control" to cellular growth- and lifespan-processes, otherwise they become uncontrolled, which is the basic problem with cancerous cells.*

- *If we stimulate the wrong processes, in this case the nourishing process, we may aggravate the disorder by stimulating tumour growth.*

From the summary of the results, it is impossible to make any solid claims, as the number of patients are too few and the ad-ditional factors are too unpredictable and uncontrolled.

Some of the individual results are, however, so astonishing and unexpected that they must not go unobserved by the med-ical community. The overall results indicate that it might be worth trying the described method, and that it needs further investigation.

One thing is especially interesting. I have treated, during the time span mentioned, 5 dogs with mamma-tumors of dif-ferent malignity, and 2 women with a special type of aggressive mammacarsinoma. All these patients did not receive any other treatment but acupuncture. In all 7 cases the development of the tumor/cancer was positive, and the cancer disappeared.

Acupuncture and the Immune System.

Conventional medicine is very aware of the importance of the immune system. Some medical scholars claim that most disease originates more or less in an imbalanced immune system and tens of millions of dollars are now being spent on research into new forms of immunotherapy in conventional medicine. From this we see that a well functioning immune system is of the utmost importance for health and wellbeing and that it is of great relevance for most illnesses. It is especially true today that the immune system is vulnerable to great strain in animals, humans and plants.

The relationship between AP and the immune system is very interesting and important. Many studies show that AP activates the immune system. It influences the nonspecific cellular (cell mediated immunity) and the humoral immunity. The latter is blood-related, i.e. it depends on various substances within the blood. Stimulation of certain points activate the white blood cells making them generate quicker and making them more active in their process of killing microbes and viruses. . In conventional treatment of cancer, cytotoxic chemotherapy and radiotherapy especially weaken the immune system and can cause many adverse side-effects, including leucopenia, anaemia, weakness, nausea, vomiting and inappetance. In such cases, many experiments show that AP quickly normalises most functions of the immune system and can alleviate many of the other side effects. For example, AP can accelerate the restoration of normal red- and white- cell counts, and haemoglobin. Some experiments have measured the speed with which the white blood cells travel towards bacteria and viruses. At a lecture in Tampere, Finland, Professor Pekka Pöntinen told that half an hour after AP treatment the white blood cells travel twice as fast towards bacteria than before AP treatment. It is accepted widely now that AP can stimulate the immune system.

The immune system is very important for all forms of allergies. Allergies arise when the immune system overreacts to foreign proteins and other allergens that enter the body.

Examples include allergens in pollen, house mites, food, bee-stings in sensitized people, etc. If one uses AP to stabilise and normalise the immune system, these allergic reactions become superficial or less violent and disappear eventually because the body no longer needs them.

That also applies in chronic infections, which usually are a sign of immunosuppression, i.e. that the immune system is not active enough to eliminate the infections. AP stimulation of the immune system can help it to recognise and repel the infection again. From this way of thinking one may also explain the ini-tial aggravation that often occurs in cases of immunostimulant therapy. We are exposed to infections and allergenes all the time, but when the immune system is strengthened it resumes the fight against chronic infections with rejuvenated strength. Then they flare up as acute infections with an increase in pus production and inflammatory reactions before they all recede and heal. This concept applies to most cases, eczema, throat disorders, ear disorders and many illnesses in which the im-mune system plays a large or small role. When the immune sys-tem is stimulated, all chronic illnesses related to the immune system flare up initially.

Animals usually regain their desire to eat, become more lively and are easier to satisfy, their coat becomes glossier and they gain weight after receiving immune stimulation therapy. The immune system relates strongly to LV and SP; by stimula-tion of these organs we increase the desire to eat and to live. We also observe that the immune stimulating points are on LV and SP Channels as well as on ST and LI Channels. These Channels relate to a large degree with digestion and to metabolism. All types of tumours and cancerous diseases are closely related to the immune system. When the body allows a growth or can-cer to develop it is usually due to the fact that the immune system is not strong enough to exterminate it. Therefore, an intact and functional immune system is important to prevent and treat cancer. AP has a preventative and therapeutic effect against this dreaded disease.

Acupuncture, Athletic Performance and Stamina

The fact that AP can increase human performance and stamina has been observed for a long time. Dr. Birger Kaada documented this scientifically. He used two points only in his experiments, LI04 and PC06. These points are very important for general stamina. Kaada proved this in an experiment with 21 volunteer athletes in which he assessed the effect of TENS (Transcutaneous Electrical Nerve Stimulation) on physical performance. Rather than needle or laser, he used low frequency TENS (2 Hz) for 30-45 minutes to apply electrical stimulation to the skin over the points. He tested the athletes' performance in swimming, running, biking or pure muscular endurance before and after TENS. Although individual variations were large, overall performance increased.

Low frequency (2Hz) TENS causes a widespread and prolonged increase in skin temperature both in patients who have circulatory disorders and in normal subjects. This increase also occurs in muscle tissue. This has been proven in animal experiments (Birger Kaada).

The duration of the effect of TENS stimulation was tested in swimmers. Each person had to swim 100 m 10 times with a break of only 20 seconds between each attempt. Swimmers who had TENS stimulation throughout the whole 15- or 30-minute experiments performed better (Birger Kaada). It is worth remembering that AP and TENS release neurotransmitters and hormones. These can improve physical performance through increased motivation, increased pain tolerance, increased oxygen transport to muscle and increased oxygen uptake by muscle.

I know of no experiments to assess the effects of AP or TENS on performance and stamina in animals but it is probable that results in animals would resemble those in humans. Many colleagues claim that AP effectively increases the stamina of racehorses and working dogs. Also, as it is regarded as a form of Doping, AP is banned from use within 4 days before competitive events.

Some experiments with the so-called beetroot juice mixture have shown that it can increase the intake of oxygen in competition animals as much as 20%. The test has been performed on rodents and horses and my experiments have proven that these statements are valid. For increased stamina in competitions, this mixture should be given a few hours before the event. The mixture is as follows:

- 1 liter red beetroot juice fermented with lactic acid

- 1 tablespoon ascorbic acid

- 1 dessertspoon iron sulphate

Acupuncture and Equine Joint Problems.

Acupuncture and the relationship between Meridian disturbances (deficiencies), the devellopment of joint problems and the relation to diagnostic (joint) pain-points in the horse.

This is a very complicated and much discussed item within vererinary equine acupuncture. Dr. William McCormic (DVM) has shown that the usual known joint-related diagnostic pain-points disappear after injecting a local anestetic into the joint. Although these points are situated on different meridians, this shows that they are not tender because of a possible meridian deficiency (or rather excess), but are merely reflections from a painful joint. Therefore treatment of these points cannot be considered as a causal treatment of the joint problem, as other "things" must have come before the joint problem.

This is also what I have found. The painful points are just reflectory, excessive points, and they show nothing about the primary cause of the joint problem, nothing about the underlying deficiency.

In my vieuv, there are several patterns that proceed a joint problem:

1. A trauma that hurt the joint directly with no deeper cause.

2. A Meridian deficiency which makes a certain area of the hoof grow less (se page 125) which leads to an unbalanced hoof and following joint problems.

3. A Meridian deficiency that makes the horse put more pressure on a certain area of the hoof to rebalance the Channel System (see page 125).

4. A Meridian deficiency which makes a certain muscle become sore, with a following disbalance of the movements, and thereby joint problems.

In point 2 – 4 (and usually combinations of point 2 – 4) treatment of only the joint and/or the painful diagnostic points will not take away the real underlying cause of the problem. Only finding and treating the deficient meridian will enable us to give the horse a real and causal treatment.

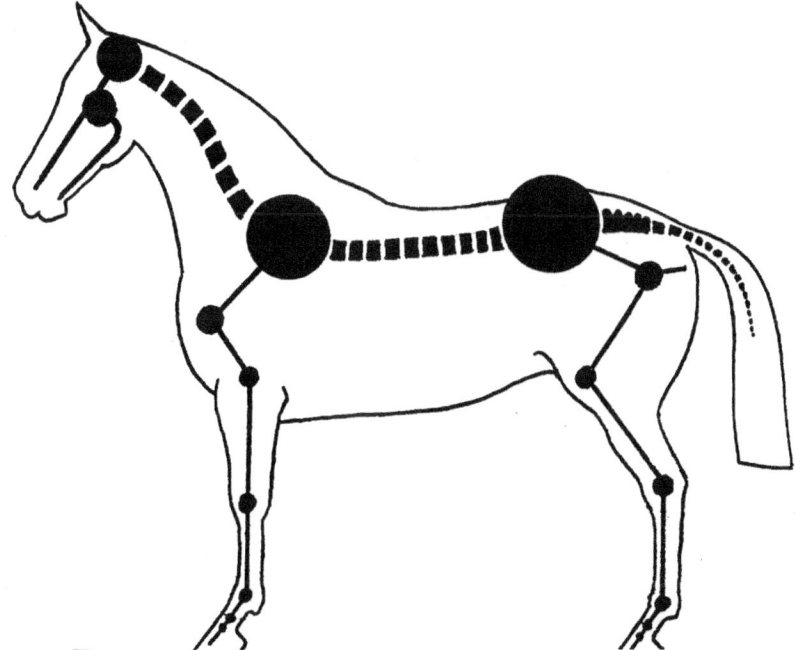

Figure 65; Illustration where I find the most common primary causes of joint pain in horses.

Acupuncture and Hip Dysplasia in Dogs

DEVELOPMENT, PREVENTION AND TREATMENT OF HD WITH ACUPUNCTURE USING NEEDLES OR GOLD IMPLANTATES

Hip dysplasia (HD) is a serious, feared and widespread disease in dogs. Out of 32163 German Sheppard's diagnosed in Germany in 2006, 21,9% of these dogs had developed HD. The numbers for Labrador-retriever was not so alarming; still 14,6% of 44009 investigated dogs showed a development of HD.

HD in its early beginning can be detected by the help of X-rays already between the 14th and the 20th week of life. Already then small irregularities in the calcification of the hip joint and the development of the interarticular tendon (Lig. accessorius) may be shown, and in dogs with such irregularities the chance of developing HD is 90%.

I have tried, by the help of needle- and gold (implant) acupuncture, to stop the development already at this stage, but that has been negative concerning X-ray changes. Concerning the symptomatic development, such an early treatment will be of great value. This is because the pain itself, deriving from the pathological changes in the joint, will lead to far more complications and problems than the changes in the hip joint itself. If we thus can stop the pain from the degenerating hip joint, many problems will be avoided.

How can the development of hip dysplasia be described?

The first step in this fatal development is, as far as I know, that;

1. Acetabulum (the hip joint) is getting more shallow. This leads to that

2. The hip joint head is forced outward. This will, in turn, lead to that the knee as well as the hock also will be turned outwards. In this position, the pressure on the lateral side of the knee become harder.

3. The lateral part of the joint capsule and menisk will receive a greater strain.

4. This will lead to a greater pain related to movements. The dog will minimise this pain by putting more tension to the muscles, especially Musculus multifidii. This will further lead to

5. A lockage of the ilio sacral joint.

6. Such a lockage or blockage in the ilio sacral joint, especially the right one because most dogs are right handed or dominant, will lead to a varying strain on all the discs along the spine. This will lead to a degeneration of these discs, which is shown by the help of MRI, and also a greater chance of prolaps of the disc.

7. The muscles of the back will react to this increasing pain with an increased contraction, and this all will end in a progressive calcification of the whole spine (akylosing or spondylosing).

8. At the end this will lead to that more and more weight will be put on the front legs, and a degeneration of the elbow will be the result.

We see by this that the HD eventually will lead to elbow degeneration. By the help of acupuncture or gold implants we can stop this development. The treatment will not cure the degenerative changes in the hip joint, but the development will be halted, and the described pathological development due to pain will be stopped.

Clinical use of Ear-Acupuncture

We have referred briefly to Earpoints in the section on diagnosis on page 137 & 146. As mentioned, Ear-AP has two forms:

- Topographic Ear-AP.

- Auriculomedicine.

The main difference between these two forms is that the topographic method is a "Cookbook Metho" that uses Ear charts to find the points, whereas auriculomedicine uses signals emitted from the body itself to find the points. Auriculomedicine is more causal [i.e. relates more specifically to the subject´s energy imbalance (deficiency)] than Topographic Ear-AP.

TOPOGRAPHIC EAR-ACUPUNCTURE

This method is the simplest form of Earpoint therapy. It uses a more or less detailed map or chart of the different reflex points on the ear. To decide which earpoint to treat one may use the diagnosis or just select points for spesific joints or organs. Then one simply stimulates the relevant Earpoints. For example, for joint disorders, we simply stimulate the Earpoints, especially reactive one(s) that relate to the affected joint(s); this is very effective. My success in treating disorders of the joints of animals was not satisfactory until I started to combine Ear-AP with other methods, such as AP and homeopathy. As I said earlier, Earpoints are used with other treatments in order to make them more effective.

AURICULO MEDICINE

Simple forms of Ear-AP were known for several thousand years. From India and China, Ear-AP spread to Egypt and North Africa. In the early 1900s, there were many French people, including soldiers in the Foreign Legion, in the French colonies in North Africa. Some of these people asked the local healers to treat their common disorders, such as backpain.

The French doctor, Paul Nogier, began to develop Earpoint therapy in 1952. He had noticed that some soldiers who had served in North Africa had burn marks in certain areas or their ears. On inquiry, he was told that the local medicine men had applied heat to these points to treat lumbago, sciatica and other back disorders. Nogier began to investigate whether there were reflex points for the whole body in the ear. He stimulated distant areas of the body in volunteers by using clips or forceps and he observed the skin of the ears for any visible changes. When he noticed a reflex change in the ear, he marked the exact reactive point or zone. In this way, he meticulously mapped the main reflex zones on the ear for the main body parts and organs. He developed this later into Earpoint therapy and auriculomedicine.

THE EAR AS AN INVERTED EMBRYO

After a long period of study, Nogier got a revolutionary idea that would solve many questions and develop the Earpoint therapy further. He imagined the ear as an image of an embryo turned upside down. This opened up to the complete picture of the body's reflex points in the ear. China, the homeland of AP, welcomed this discovery with enthusiasm. Auriculomedicine, however, was not developed until many years later when Nogier discovered ACR (Auriculo-Cardiac Reflex), or more correctly VAS (Vascular Auricular Signal). He discovered also how different colours and frequencies influence the skin and manifest in the VAS.

Earpoint therapy, the name for Nogier' method before he discovered the VAS and the sensitivity of the skin to different colours, is a reflex therapy where one applies different stimuli to the Earpoints to induce predictable organic effects. The stimulus can be needling, pressure, laser, cold or heat, etc. This form of therapy is simple and symptomatic. However, we must know that one can remove or suppress symptoms that can have a serious cause and deserve thorough examination before symptomatic therapy.

Modern auriculomedicine differs radically from Ear-AP. Auriculomedicine is based mainly on the principles of conventional medicine, while Ear-AP is based on the teaching of reflexes, something like Foot Zone Therapy.

After his discovery of the VAS, auriculomedicine was Nogier's next developmental step. Auriculomedicine is a form of therapy that is more complicated, more comprehensive and much more informative as to the energetic causes. It is based on the principles of conventional medicine but we often see that the discoveries correspond to the Laws of AP and that the

TCM pulses normalise after successful treatment. One may combine this form of therapy easily with homeopathy, herbs, AP and Zone Therapy. The equipment needed for a complete Auriculomedicine examination and treatment is:

- A pair of hands which should be as sensitive as possible.
- Colour filters.
- A thin ray of light (penlight, lamp, or laser).
- A diagnostic hammer with a black and white head.
- Needles.

ACR / VAS

The pulse reaction, called the ACR or VAS by Nogier, is an essential part of a thorough examination in auriculomedicine and in other forms of controlled AP. This pulse response is a reflex from the skin to the heart or arterial blood circulation. Stimulation of the skin over a reactive area or a point or Weak Structure activates an autonomic reaction or recognition that induces a special VAS Pulse reaction.

The place to observe the VAS pulse reaction is on the radial artery, right under the radial styloid process between the second and third classical Chinese Pulse-Positions (for GB-LV and BL-KI, respectively), as described under Pulse Diagnoses, page 152. *In the correct VAS position, one can not feel the Chinese SI HT Pulse*, that is circa 1.5 fingerwidths distal to the correct VAS position. Before starting the examination one should practice to recognise a normal pulse in several healthy subjects before one tries to use it diagnostically to assess subjects with clinical or subclinical disorders. VAS manifests in an altered quality in the pulse. VAS Pulse-changes can not be proven objectively since pulse quality is a subjective parameter.

It usually takes some time before the VAS occurs. The number of pulse beats before it occurs, is called the "*VAS latency time*," usually 1-20 beats. The duration of the VAS (i.e. the time until the Pulse normalises again is called the "*VAS reaction time*" (range 1-10 beats). *These times have diagnostic value.* Young and strong (Qi Excess) individuals have a short latency time (2-4 beats) and a long reaction time (8-10 beats). Old and weak individuals (Qi Deficiency) have a long latency time (8-12 beats) and a short reaction time. If the reaction time is long (especially with a short latency time) the prognosis is good.

Stimulation of effective acupoints usually gives a reaction in VAS.

The 12 Chinese Pulses mirror the Qi Status of their related Process. Thereby they also indicate the presence and nature of a Process Imbalance (Deficiency or Excess) in one or more Channels. In contrast, the VAS reflects the location of the injury anatomically.

Chinese- or VAS- Pulse quality is a subjective phenomenon. It has not been possible to prove objective changes in these Pulses, nor to correlate such changes with objective pathology. Therefore, diagnosis based on these Pulses may be regarded as a form of diagnostic dowsing or divining for Energetic Imbalances. See page 179.

THE COLOUR FILTERS

Colour filters are used to locate reactive Earpoints more easily. A colour filter gives a message to the body to release certain information, or select information. It reinforces the response from the ear so that we can better find the points. A filter placed on the head reduces the sensitivity. Sensitivity increases when a filter is placed on the body.

- Filter A: 2,28 Hz, nervous system, Kodak Wratten 22, yellow

- Filter B: 4.56 Hz, metabolism, Kodak Wratten 25, red

- Filter C: 9,125 Hz, movements, Kodak Wratten 4, yellow

- Filter D: 18,25 Hz, internal organs, Kodak Wratten 23A, dark pink

- Filter E: 36,50 Hz, spine, Kodak Wratten 44, petrol blue

- Filter F: 73 Hz, emotions, Kodak Wratten 98, dark blue

- Filter G: 146 Hz, personality, Kodak Wratten 30, margent pink

The filters correspond to and reinforce the response from the 7 body zones. The filter numbers relate to Kodak wratten colour filters. The 7 main colour filters can be purchased in any photo store. Each filter is then cut to size, so that it fits into a slide frame. This frame is placed wherever one wishes on the patient's body. We only need to ensure that light shines through the filter onto the body. Bill Wagner, an American vet who works with these colours, places the slide in a projector and exposes the whole animal to the projected colour. In this way, he does not need to worry whether the slide is in place or has fallen down. When these colour slides are used, the skin of the ear becomes more reactive to the VAS Pulse method. Usually we must stimulate the skin quite strongly (with a needle) to get a VAS reaction. But, in using the colour filters, it is sufficient to expose the skin to the light in order to elicit a VAS reaction. All we need is a strong concentrated source of light. The beam of light should be as thin and concentrated as possible. A Haine lamp is very convenient.

TREATMENT PROCEDURE

1. *Physical examination of the ear:* "Pull" or "roll" the ear and check for irregularities. It is a sign of good health if no dots or spots appear when you wring the ear.

   - Acute disorders usually signify Qi Excess; they often cause red dots or spots on the ear. Such imbalances need Qi to be subdued (reduced, calmed, or sedated).

- Chronic disorders usually signify Qi Deficiency; they often cause white areas or spots on the ear. Such imbalances need Qi to be boosted, stimulated or tonified.

2. Feel the structure of the ear, whether it is healthy firm and if it is even.

3. Find the right position for the VAS on your own pulse and make sure you have skin contact with the animal all the time. Place all the filters on the animal's forehead. Apply the light on the 7 colours one after the other. (Start with the A filter (orange) while you take the VAS on your own pulse. A reaction on the VAS indicates which colour filter that shall be used later on in the diagnostic procedure). Do not apply the light too long on each colour (max. 10 pulse beats in the beginning) and reduce the time as you become more experienced with the method. VAS can be completely absent in the case of exhaustion. The more sensitive you become, the clearer the VAS becomes.

4. Place the selected filter (take away all the other filters) on the body and search with the light all over the ear methodically without a break. Mark the points you find on an ear chart, or directly on the ear with a suitable pen. Be aware that even a light pressure on earpoints manifests in the Qi and the VAS response, so that marking on an ear chart is preferable. Apply needles in the points in question.

5. *Treatment time* usually is 15-30 minutes; old animals should be treated for 30 minutes.

6. *Treatment frequency* usually is 3-4 weeks between sessions (the 28-day cycle, the moon phases). The body needs 3-4 weeks for auto-cure (optimum self-adaptive Process). Thus, if the treatment is too frequent, the body can not work as much on itself.

DISORDERS THAT CAN BE TREATED SUCCESSFULLY WITH EAR ACUPUNCTURE

- *Rupture of the cruciate ligament in humans and dogs:* In this case, you should simply use the stifle point. Often all that is needed is one treatment. Dominique Giniaux, a French vet, heals 80% of these patients without operation with auriculomedicine.

- *Back problems:* Backpain often responds well to auriculomedicine.

- *Joint problems:* Joints should be treated with Earpoints in addition to other treatment. Generally it can be said that Earpoints work better than plain body-AP on physical disorders, while body-AP works better on functional disorders.

PROGNOSIS

Auriculomedicine is one of the fastest forms of therapy we have. If it does not induce a definite change after 3 treatments (improvement or aggravation), the method should be ceased and other forms of therapy suggested.

Cookbook Acupuncture: Acupoints Suggested for Common Disorders (*from the works of Dr. Phil Rogers, Dublin*)

Although expert classical AP gives better results than Cookbook-AP in complex cases, the Cookbook is very useful for more simple cases and first aid use. From a database of >55 textbooks and several dozen AP journals, Dr. Phil Rogers (1999) compiled an extensive list of Acupoint Prescriptions suggested for different diseases and organic disorders in humans. **Entries with a star*** are new data from a recent review. Earpoints are not included. The location of each point is on the internet (*http://homepage.tinet.ie/~progers/ptc.htm*)

Area, disorder or condition	1	2	3	4	5	6	7	8	9	10
Abdomen and back, its organs and functions	ST36	SP06	CV12	CV04	BL23	PC06	GB34	CV03	CV06	ST25
Abdomen lower	ST36	L_13	SP06	ST25	CV04	LI 11	ST37	CV03	SP13	CV06
Abdomen middle, periumbilical area	SP14	ST36	ST25	CV06	CV08	CV07	BL23	BL25	GB34	CV04
Abdomen upper, epigastric, hypochondriac area	ST36	PC06	CV12	BL21	BL51	GB34	BL23	LV13	LV01	BL18
Abdominal disorders*	PC06	ST36	CV01	CV08	ST37	SP09	CV06	CV12	SP06	ST25
Achilles area, heel	BL60	KI 03	BL57	BL61	KI 04	SP06	OT01	ST36	ST41	BL40
Addictions	ST36	SP06	LI 04	BL13	PC06	CV12	BL21	CV06	LV03	GB08
Allergy and allergic shock - all sources [see above; add from here in nose, head and gut disorders]	GV26	LI 20	GV20	ST25	PC09	Z_09	Z_03	CV12	GV23	SP06
Allergy [lungs, skin, gut, vasomotor etc - all sources]	LI 04	LI 11	ST36	PC06	KI 01	SP10	GB20	BL40	GV14	LV03
Amenorrhoea, oligomenorrhoea and delayed menarche in women*	CV03	CV04	SP06	BL23	Y_18	BL20	BL32	CV06	ST36	Y_11
Analgesia, pain control (general)	LI 04	ST36	LI 11	TH05	OT05	SP06	LV03	GB34	A_22	GB38
Andropathies (all headings)*	BL23	BL32	CV04	SP06	CV01	CV03	GV04	ST36	CV02	BL31
Ankle, tarsus	BL60	ST41	KI 03	GB39	GB40	SP06	BL57	OT01	ST36	SP05
Anovulation*	CV03	CV04	SP06	Y_17	Y_18	BL23	CV08	GB26	BL18	TH05
Anus, tenesmus, prolapse, haemorrhoids	GV01	BL57	GV20	BL32	SP06	BL25	BL31	BL33	BL30	BL34
Arm, humerus	LI 11	LI 15	LI 04	SI 09	SI 11	TH06	LI 10	TH08	LI 14	PC03
Arteries, veins, arteriosclerosis, ischaemia	ST36	GB20	BL10	CV06	SP06	GV20	GB21	LV03	GV14	OT05
Axilla	HT01	GB40	GB42	GB22	SI 09	PC01	GB38	PC05	LI 15	TH12
Bladder, lower ureter	SP06	CV03	BL23	BL28	BL32	CV04	SP09	CV06	BL30	CV02
Blood, body defences, haemorrhage, thymus etc	BL17	ST36	BL20	LI 04	LI 11	CV04	GV14	SP06	CV06	SP10
Bones, joints (general)	OT05	OT06	ST36	LI 04	OT01	GB34	LI 11	TH05	BL11	BL23

Brain, its functions and parts, meninges, polio, convulsions, memory, tetanus, CVA etc	LI 04	LI 11	ST36	GB34	ST06	LI 15	GB20	GB30	ST04	GV14
Brain, meninges	LI 04	GV15	GB20	ST36	GV12	LI 11	GB34	BL64	KI 01	GV14
Bronchi, lung, pneumonia, asthma	BL13	CV22	CV17	GV14	LU05	BL12	PC06	LI 04	LU07	ST36
Buttock	GB30	BL36	OT01	ST36	BL23	BL54	BL37	OT05	BL40	BL60
Cervix, vagina	SP06	BL33	KI 12	CV03	CV04	LV08	ST29	GV02	SP09	CV01
Chills	GV14	ST36	LI 04	GV16	BL40	HT06	GB25	LI 11	TH04	BL12
Chin	CV24	ST04	ST05	CV22	GV27	SI 10	SI 07	GB05	GB21	GV22
Circulation, blood pressure	LI 11	ST36	LV03	GB20	ST09	PC06	SP06	KI 01	CV12	HT07
Clitoris, vagina and vulva*	SP06	CV01	CV03	GV01	SP10	BL32	LV03	SP09	ST30	BL23
Coccygeal area	BL34	BL40	SI 06	BL30	OT01	BL37	X_35	OT05	OT06	BL35
Convulsions, epilepsy, tetanus	GV14	ST36	LI 04	GV26	KI 01	GV20	LV03	LI 11	GB20	PC06
Cough general	BL13	LU05	LU07	ST40	CV22	LU10	GV12	BL12	CV17	GV14
CVA, polio, paralysis, hemiplegia	LI 04	LI 11	ST36	GB34	ST06	GB30	ST04	LI 15	TH05	GB39
Diaphragm	BL17	PC06	CV12	ST36	CV15	CV17	LV14	GB24	ST13	CV22
Diarrhoea, dysentery, constipation	ST25	ST36	CV04	CV12	SP06	TH06	CV06	BL25	CV08	SP09
Dorsolumbar spine and area	BL40	BL23	X_35	BL60	OT01	BL37	GB30	GV14	OT05	OT06
Dysmenorrhoea and menorrhalgia*	CV04	SP06	ST29	ST36	BL23	PC06	SP10	BL20	CV03	CV06
Ear, hearing, Meniere's disease, Eustachian tube, mastoid etc	TH17	GB02	SI 19	TH21	TH05	GB20	LI 04	TH03	ST36	GV20
Ejaculation*	BL23	BL32	CV03	BL33	CV04	SP06	SP09	BL27	CV02	ST36
Elbow	LI 11	TH05	LI 04	HT03	LU05	LI 10	OT01	LI 12	TH10	SI 07
Emergencies	GV26	KI 01	ST36	PC06	A_01	LI 04	PC09	GV20	LU11	LI 11
Eye, eyelid, sight etc	BL01	LI 04	GB20	ST01	Z_09	BL02	ST02	GB14	TH23	BL18
Face, cheek	LI 04	ST06	ST04	ST07	ST02	LI 20	BL02	GB14	TH17	ST03

Fallopian tube	ST29	SP06	SP09	CV03	CV04	CV06	ST30	BL30	BL31	BL32
Female infertility, functional sterility*	SP06	CV03	BL23	CV08	BL23	BL26	BL32	Y_18	ST36	BL18
Fevers	GV14	LI 11	LI 04	PC05	BL40	GV13	A_01	PC09	LI 01	LU10
Finger	LI 04	A_22	SI 03	LI 03	TH05	SI 04	SI 07	PC07	PC06	TH04
First aid	GV20	ST36	PC06	GB20	LV03	GV26	Z_03	LI 04	Z_09	LU11
Forearm, radius, ulna	LI 11	HT03	LI 10	LI 04	PC06	HT07	PC03	TH05	SI 08	TH09
Forehead, frontal sinuses	LI 04	Z_03	GB14	BL02	GV23	Z_09	GB20	LU07	ST44	GV24
Gallbladder, bile ducts (inflammation, calculi, obstruction etc)	BL19	ST36	GB34	L_23	PC06	GV09	GB24	LV03	BL18	GB40
Gangrene, ischaemia of extremities	OT02	OT05	A_22	L_08	LI 11	HT03	GB34	SP09	SP06	BL43
Gastrointestinal tract	ST36	ST25	PC06	CV12	CV06	SP06	CV04	BL21	TH06	BL20
Genitalia female and reproduction	SP06	CV04	GV04	CV06	SP10	CV03	GB26	BL32	LV03	ST36
Genitalia male	SP06	CV03	CV04	ST29	BL32	BL33	BL34	LV01	BL31	LV04
Gynaecology, obstetrics, mammology (all data)*	SP06	ST36	CV03	CV04	CV06	LI 04	BL23	BL32	CV17	LV03
Hair, skin: alopecia; baldness; hair loss; oppilation	BL16	BL40	GB20	OT05	LI 04	BL10	CV12	ST36	BL43	CV04
Hand, palm	LI 04	LI 11	A_22	SI 03	PC07	LI 03	PC08	SI 04	TH03	PC06
Head, forehead, vertex, occiput, temple, headaches, sinusitis etc	LI 04	GB20	Z_09	GV20	LU07	Z_03	BL10	LI 20	BL02	BL60
Heart, pericardium	PC06	HT07	BL15	HT05	PC05	ST36	BL14	PC07	PC04	CV17
Hip	GB30	GB34	GB29	GB31	BL40	BL60	OT01	GB39	ST36	LV08
Immunity	ST36	LI 04	GV14	SP06	LI 11	CV04	BL18	BL19	BL23	CV06
Indigestion, inappetance, nausea, vomiting	ST36	PC06	CV12	ST25	SP06	CV06	BL21	BL20	SP04	LI 04
Infections: malaria, TB, cholera, typhoid, typhus, herpes, rubella, varicella etc	GV14	ST36	PC05	LI 04	SI 03	LI 11	GV13	PC06	SP06	CV12
Inguinal area, groin	LV01	SP11	SP12	SP13	ST30	KI 11	LV03	LV04	LV06	SP06
Kidney, upper ureter	BL23	BL52	KI 03	SP06	SP09	ST36	BL28	GB25	CV03	CV04
Knee (stifle), popliteal	GB34	BL40	L_16	ST35	SP09	ST36	ST34	LV08	OT01	GB31

Leg, calf	BL57	GB34	ST36	SP06	BL40	GB30	BL60	GB39	ST32	LV03
Leucorrhoea, leucorrhagia, gonorrhoea*	SP06	BL23	BL32	CV02	CV03	CV04	CV08	GB26	GV04	ST36
Lips, oral muscles	ST04	ST03	LI 04	ST06	CV24	GV26	ST07	ST44	LI 20	LI 03
Liver (inflammation, calculi, jaundice, acetonaemia etc)	BL18	LV03	BL19	GV09	BL20	ST36	LV13	GB34	BL48	SP06
Lowback (lumbosacral, renal, sacroiliac), lumbar, sacral spine	BL23	BL40	GB30	BL60	GB34	BL25	BL37	GV04	BL57	BL31
Lowback, lumbar, sacral and pelvic area disorders*	BL23	BL40	CV04	GB34	GV04	ST36	OT01	X_35	BL24	LV03
Lymphadenopathy	ST36	HT03	BL60	SP06	GB39	OT02	ST31	PC01	LI 01	LI 13
Male and female external genitalia and pubic area	CV04	CV03	SP06	LV08	CV07	LV04	LV12	CV01	LV02	LV01
Male infertility, spermatopathy, abnormalities of sperm count or quality*	BL23	BL32	CV04	SP06	BL33	CV03	GV04	KI 03	CV06	ST36
Mammary female	CV17	SI 01	ST18	GB41	ST36	ST16	SP18	LI 04	LV03	GB21
Mandible	ST06	ST07	LI 04	CV24	ST05	ST04	ST36	LV03	TH17	ST44
Mastopathy, mammary disorders, milk disorders*	CV17	OT02	GB21	ST18	ST36	LI 04	GB41	SI 11	LV03	TH05
Maxilla	LI 04	ST02	ST07	ST03	ST06	LI 20	ST04	SI 18	GV26	ST44
Maxilla, mandible	ST06	ST07	LI 04	ST02	ST04	ST03	CV24	ST05	LI 20	ST44
Memory: loss of; amnesia; forgetful	HT07	GV11	BL15	BL43	HT03	GV20	HT09	NL04	ST36	PC06
Menopausal disorders*	SP06	CV04	PC06	ST36	BL18	BL23	SP10	LI 04	GV26	CV02
Menopause: general points for flushes and menopausal disorders	ST36	SP06	CV04	LI 04	PC06	GB21	CV03	SP10	LV14	CV05
Menstrual cycle, contraception	SP06	CV04	CV03	CV06	SP10	ST36	BL23	LV03	BL32	BL33
Menstruation*	SP06	CV04	CV03	CV06	BL23	BL32	BL33	LV03	SP10	ST36
Metatarsal, foot	BL60	KI 03	LV03	SP06	BL57	ST41	GB39	OT01	ST42	GB41
Mouth	LI 04	LI 11	ST04	ST06	PC08	GV12	GV27	LI 07	Z_20	ST44

Muscle, tendon, soft tissues (general)	OT05	OT01	GB34	ST36	OT06	LI 04	LV03	LI 11	SP06	OT03
Neck and cervical spine	GB20	GV14	LI 04	BL10	SI 03	LI 11	OT01	GB21	GB39	SI 15
Nose, nostril, nasal sinuses, olfaction	LI 04	LI 20	GB20	GV23	LI 11	GV14	Z_03	BL07	LI 19	ST02
Occiput	GB20	BL10	SI 03	BL60	GV15	BL65	LI04	LU07	GV20	OT05
Oedema, fluid retention, ascites	SP09	CV09	KI 07	BL23	ST36	BL20	ST25	SP06	CV05	CV08
Oesophagus	PC06	BL17	ST36	LI 04	CV17	LI 10	BL10	CV12	CV22	BL20
Ovary	SP06	ST28	ST36	ST18	ST25	ST30	ST32	BL22	BL30	BL31
Ovary and PID*	SP06	CV03	CV04	BL23	CV06	SP10	LU07	Y_18	BL26	GB25
Pain, colic, spasm in abdomen or its organs, peritonitis	ST36	CV12	SP06	PC06	CV04	ST25	CV06	BL23	BL21	CV03
Pancreas, diabetes mellitus, hypoglycaemia and hyperglycaemia	KI 02	CV12	BL23	ST36	SP06	CV04	BL20	BL18	BL17	X_12
Parturition	SP06	LI 04	BL67	BL60	BL32	LV03	BL31	ST36	SP09	BL62
Parturition or abortion, before, during and after*	LI 04	SP06	ST36	BL31	BL32	BL67	GV26	BL34	CV06	LV03
Patella	SP09	SP10	GB33	OT01	OT05	BL40	LV08	BL11	ST30	SP05
Pelvic limb, its organs and functions	GB34	ST36	GB30	SP06	BL60	BL40	BL57	GB39	GB31	KI 03
Penis	ST30	SP06	SP09	LV01	CV04	BL53	BL54	LV02	LV05	ST20
Penis, urethra, libido, male impotence, erectile dysfunction*	BL23	BL32	CV02	CV04	ST36	KI 12	SP06	CV06	LV08	KI 07
Perineum	BL32	GV01	BL31	BL30	BL33	BL34	LV01	LV10	SP06	ST36
Perineum*	SP06	ST36	BL30	CV02	CV04	GV01	GV20	LV03	ST30	BL32
Pleura	BL42	BL47	BL43	KI23	ST12	KI22	BL13	BL11	GB22	GB44
Postpartum disorders	SP06	GV20	CV04	Y_16	CV02	LV01	CV03	CV07	Y_18	CV06
Postpartum uterus, cervix, vagina	SP06	Y_16	CV04	GV20	CV02	Y_18	LV01	KI06	LV08	CV03
Disorders of pregnancy	BL67	ST36	PC06	LV03	SP04	SP06	BL18	CV17	CV12	KI 21
Pregnancy: forbidden / abortion	SP06	LI04	BL67	BL60	LV03	BL32	ST36	CV04	CV03	BL31
Prostate	SP06	CV04	CV03	BL23	BL28	SP09	ST29	GB34	CV02	SP10
Prostate*	BL23	BL32	CV01	SP06	BL30	CV03	ST29	CV04	GV04	BL54
Psyche and mental disorders	HT07	SP06	PC06	ST36	GB20	LI04	GV20	LV03	BL15	CV12

Reproduction male (impotence, spermatorrhoea etc)	SP06	CV04	BL23	CV03	CV06	BL32	GV04	BL33	BL31	ST36
Respiratory system (trachea, bronchi, lung, cough, pneumonia, asthma etc	BL13	GV14	CV22	LI04	LU05	LU07	CV17	ST40	BL12	PC06
Salivation, salivary glands etc	ST40	SP04	LV03	LI04	SI05	LI10	ST43	BL59	GB07	GB38
Shoulder, scapula, clavicle	LI15	LI11	TH14	SI11	SI09	LI04	OT01	SI10	OT05	BL11
Skin	LI11	LI04	SP10	SP06	ST36	BL40	GV14	OT05	BL13	GB20
Small intestine, appendix, caecum, colon, rectum	ST36	ST25	BL25	CV04	L_13	CV12	BL27	PC06	SP15	ST37
Spinal cord	BL11	GV14	GV04	BL60	GV15	KI07	BL10	GV20	ST36	KI08
Spleen	BL20	ST36	LV13	BL51	SP06	CV12	PC06	X_16	LV03	BL22
Stomach and duodenum	ST36	CV12	PC06	ST25	BL21	CV13	CV06	BL20	SP04	SP06
Sweating disorders	KI07	LI04	HT06	SI03	SP02	LV02	LU08	LU10	LU11	GV14
Tarsal metatarsal	GB41	OT01	ST41	OT05	BL59	KI06	GB40	BL60	SP05	KI03
Temple	Z_09	GB20	GB08	GB41	LI04	TH03	TH05	TH23	GB07	LU07
Temporomandibular joint, masseter	LI04	ST07	ST06	GB02	ST05	SI19	TH17	LV03	GV26	TH21
Testicle	KI08	LV10	SP06	SP09	BL23	BL52	CV03	CV04	ST28	ST30
Testicle pain	SP06	KI08	KI12	GB34	SP04	BL23	CV03	CV04	LV06	BL23
Testicle*	SP06	BL23	CV04	ST29	ST36	BL32	CV03	KI08	KI12	ST30
Thigh, femur	GB30	GB31	GB34	LV08	ST36	BL23	LV11	BL40	BL37	SP06
Thoracic limb, its organs and functions	LI11	LI15	TH05	LI04	SI03	TH04	HT03	PC07	LI10	OT05
Thoracic spine, back area	GV14	BL40	OT01	GV12	OT05	GV13	X_35	GV09	BL60	OT06
Thorax and back, its organs and functions	PC06	BL13	BL17	ST36	LI11	LI04	GV14	GB34	GB20	HT07
Thorax, chest, ribs, sternum	GB34	PC06	TH06	BL18	CV17	BL17	LV13	BL14	LV14	BL15
Throat, pharynx, larynx, tonsil, voice	LI04	LU11	CV22	LI11	ST44	LU10	CV23	PC06	LI18	SI17
Thyroid, parathyroid	CV22	LI11	LI04	ST09	PC06	GB20	LI18	BL10	CV23	GV14
Tibia, fibula	ST36	GB35	GB34	GB37	BL40	LV03	GB36	GB30	BL62	LV02
Toe	L_08	SP04	SP06	LV03	OT05	ST36	GB34	OT01	BL60	SP05
Tongue, speech	CV23	GV15	LI04	HT05	TH17	LI11	TH05	ST06	GB20	Z_21
Tonic effects	ST36	CV06	CV04	BL43	BL20	PC06	BL23	LI04	SP06	LI11

Teeth, gums	LI04	ST06	ST07	ST44	ST05	CV24	SI18	LI03	LI11	ST03
Teeth, lower	ST06	LI04	ST05	LI03	ST07	ST44	ST36	CV24	TH08	LI11
Teeth, upper	LI04	ST07	ST06	ST44	SI18	LI20	ST02	ST36	GV26	SI05
Trachea	CV22	ST40	LI04	BL13	LU02	GV14	BL11	LU07	CV17	PC06
Ureter	BL23	CV07	SP06	CV03	ST30	KI07	CV04	CV06	LV03	ST29
Urethra	CV04	CV03	CV07	LV08	SP06	CV01	BL23	SP09	BL32	BL28
Urinary disorders*	BL23	CV03	CV04	SP06	BL28	BL32	CV06	ST36	CV02	SP09
Urinary incontinence, retention, or urination in coitus*	CV03	CV04	SP06	BL23	BL28	BL32	CV06	ST36	SP09	CV02
Urinary tract and functions	SP06	BL23	BL28	CV03	CV04	CV06	KI03	SP09	CV02	BL32
Urogenital (general disorders)	SP06	CV04	BL23	CV03	CV06	BL28	KI03	BL32	ST36	SP09
Uterus and cervix*	CV03	CV04	SP06	CV06	ST30	Y_18	BL23	SP09	SP01	BL30
Uterus, cervix	CV04	GV02	SP06	SP10	BL23	CV03	CV06	ST30	BL30	BL31
Vagina	BL30	BL31	BL32	BL33	BL34	GV02	SP06	SP09	SP10	CV02
Vertex	GV20	GB20	LV03	KI01	LI04	BL07	GV19	BL60	GB11	SI03
Waist, flank area	GB34	GB40	BL40	GB30	GB41	ST36	BL23	GB39	LV02	LV13
Wrist, carpus	TH04	TH05	LI04	PC07	LI05	LU07	SI04	PC06	LI11	OT01

Table 95

Frequency citation scores for the points in the Cookbook database, above, are shown below. In the table, the points are listed by descending citation score.

Pt	ST36	SP06	LI04	CV04	BL23	CV03	PC06	CV06	LI11	LV03
Score	.570	.525	.418	.335	.304	.259	.241	.222	.222	.222
Pt	BL32	GB34	GV14	SP09	GB20	BL40	CV12	BL60	OT01	OT05
Score	.190	.165	.146	.146	.139	.127	.127	.120	.120	.108
Pt	GV20	SP10	CV02	BL31	ST06	ST25	TH05	BL20	CV17	ST30
Score	.101	.095	.089	.082	.082	.082	.082	.076	.076	.076
Pt	BL18	BL30	GB30	BL33	GV26	LU07	ST44	CV22	GB39	GV04
Score	.070	.070	.070	.063	.063	.063	.063	.057	.057	.057
Pt	KI03	LV08	ST04	ST07	BL10	BL13	BL28	LI20	LV01	SI03
Score	.057	.057	.057	.057	.051	.051	.051	.051	.051	.051
Pt	ST29	BL57	CV01	CV08	Y_18	BL11	BL17	BL21	BL34	CV24
Score	.051	.044	.044	.044	.044	.038	.038	.038	.038	.038
Pt	GB21	GB41	HT03	HT07	KI01	LI10	LI15	SP04	ST02	ST05
Score	.038	.038	.038	.038	.038	.038	.038	.038	.038	.038

Pt	Z_09	BL25	BL37	BL43	CV07	GB40	KI07	LI03	LV02	LV13
Score	.038	.032	.032	.032	.032	.032	.032	.032	.032	.032
Pt	OT06	PC07	ST03	TH17	Z_03	A_22	BL02	BL12	BL15	BL67
Score	.032	.032	.032	.032	.032	.025	.025	.025	.025	.025
Pt	GB31	GV01	GV12	GV15	KI08	KI12	LU05	LU10	LU11	PC05
Score	.025	.025	.025	.025	.025	.025	.025	.025	.025	.025
Pt	SP05	ST40	ST41	TH04	TH06	X_35	BL19	BL54	CV23	GB14
Score	.025	.025	.025	.025	.025	.025	.019	.019	.019	.019
Pt	GB25	GB26	GB38	GV02	GV09	GV13	GV23	LV04	LV14	OT02
Score	.019	.019	.019	.019	.019	.019	.019	.019	.019	.019
Pt	PC09	SI04	SI07	SI09	SI11	SI18	ST18	ST37	TH03	A_01
Score	.019	.019	.019	.019	.019	.019	.019	.019	.019	.013
Pt	BL07	BL14	BL22	BL26	BL27	BL51	BL52	BL59	BL62	CV05
Score	.013	.013	.013	.013	.013	.013	.013	.013	.013	.013
Pt	GB02	GB07	GB08	GB22	GB24	GV27	HT05	HT06	KI06	LI01
Score	.013	.013	.013	.013	.013	.013	.013	.013	.013	.013
Pt	LI18	LV06	LV10	L_08	L_13	PC01	PC03	PC08	SI05	SI10
Score	.013	.013	.013	.013	.013	.013	.013	.013	.013	.013
Pt	SI19	SP13	ST09	ST28	ST32	TH08	TH21	TH23	Y_16	BL01
Score	.013	.013	.013	.013	.013	.013	.013	.013	.013	.006
Pt	BL16	BL24	BL35	BL36	BL42	BL47	BL48	BL53	BL61	BL64
Score	.006	.006	.006	.006	.006	.006	.006	.006	.006	.006
Pt	BL65	CV09	CV13	CV15	GB05	GB11	GB29	GB33	GB35	GB36
Score	.006	.006	.006	.006	.006	.006	.006	.006	.006	.006
Pt	GB37	GB42	GB44	GV11	GV16	GV19	GV22	GV24	HT01	HT09
Score	.006	.006	.006	.006	.006	.006	.006	.006	.006	.006
Pt	KI02	KI04	KI11	KI21	KI22	KI23	LI05	LI07	LI12	LI13
Score	.006	.006	.006	.006	.006	.006	.006	.006	.006	.006
Pt	LI14	LI19	LU02	LU08	LV05	LV11	LV12	L_16	L_23	NL04
Score	.006	.006	.006	.006	.006	.006	.006	.006	.006	.006
Pt	OT03	PC04	SI01	SI06	SI08	SI15	SI17	SP01	SP02	SP11
Score	.006	.006	.006	.006	.006	.006	.006	.006	.006	.006
Pt	SP12	SP14	SP15	SP18	ST01	ST12	ST13	ST16	ST20	ST31
Score	.006	.006	.006	.006	.006	.006	.006	.006	.006	.006
Pt	ST34	ST35	ST42	ST43	TH09	TH10	TH12	TH14	X_12	X_16
Score	.006	.006	.006	.006	.006	.006	.006	.006	.006	.006
Pt	Y_11	Y_17	Z_20	Z_21						
Score	.006	.006	.006	.006						

Table 96

It is clear that the most used points are in the top 4 lines. The most used points are *ST36, SP06, LI04, CV04 and BL23*, followed by *CV03, PC06, CV06, LI11 and LV03*.

From the data, the most *used point on each Channel* is

LU	LI	ST	SP	HT	SI	BL	KI	PC	TH	GB	LV	GV	CV
07	04	36	06	03	03	23	03	06	05	34	03	14	04
.06	.41	.57	.52	.03	.05	.30	.05	.24	.08	.16	.22	.14	.33

Table 97

Chapter 5

HOMEOPATHY

H omeopathic concepts and theories have been the subject of discussion, study and trial in most cultures; Chinese, Indian, Persian, American and European.

Homeopathy is a very much discussed and controversial medical modality. The reason for this is the specialities of the homeopathic remedies. In herb therapy we give different plants or herbs containing pharmacologically active substances. In AP we stimulate certain points or nerves which release certain substances or endorphins. But in homeopathy, from a materialistic viewpoint, we really give nothing that can be measured chemically, except the vehicle that carries the potentised remedy (see page 540). On standard scientific analysis, the lactose pills that carry the diluted and potentised homeopathic remedies contain *no detectable compounds except lactose.* (For more detail, see the chapter on potentisation page 540).

HISTORY OF HOMEOPATHY
The fundamental principle of homeopathy is found in the sentence *"similia similibus curentur"* (*"Like things by Like things shall*

be cured", or *"Like cures like"*). In more precise terms, a homeopathic remedy cures a disease whose symptoms resemble the symptoms evoked in a healthy body, by a toxic dose of the agent itself. This principle has been known since antiquity; philosophers and healers like Hippocrates and Paracelsus also expressed the same ideas. The principle comes, of course, from an ancient holistic concept that the symptoms are manifested by the body itself, in order to help an organ or Process that is failing to perform properly.

However, **Christian Frederich Samuel Hahnemann** (1755-1843), a German physician, assembled all the ideas and theories and developed them systematically into a holistic system of therapy. Hahnemann's pioneering book, "The Organon", is still a key homeopathic reference book today. Hahnemann called this system homeopathy after the Greek words **homoios,** which means "like" or "equivalent" and **pathos**, which means suffering or malfunction (homeopathy is written in different European countries as homöopati, homøopati, homöopathie, homopati or homeopati).

Early in his medical career, Hahnemann knew that the symptoms of intoxication from a substance resembled those that the same substance could cure in very low doses. In other words, when specially prepared in minute doses, the pathogenic substance was made into a remedy. He experimented with lower and lower doses (higher and higher dilutions). During this experimentation with increasing dilutions and his testing of diluted substances, he accidentally discovered the **principle of potentisation.** This is that the tincture or substance that we want to prepare as a remedy must be diluted and succussed (potentised) serially to such a dilution that its concentration eventually approaches zero. At the higher dilutions, the laws of physics would say that there could not be a single molecule of the original material in the remedy. Paradoxically, however and in total contrast to what one might expect from principles of conventional pharmacology, this process potentises the remedy, i.e. its therapeutic effect becomes clearer, cleaner, more powerful and more exact as the dilution increases.

Two examples of clinical homeopathy

- Late on a Saturday night, a 7-year old boy grabbed a red-hot poker and threw it on the hearth to prevent his granny's carpet from being damaged. In the process, he gave himself a potential third-degree burn, 3 cm long, on his thumb and index finger. The house was many miles from the nearest pharmacy, and the boy's granny had no anti-burn or analgesic remedies of any kind. However, as it was a farmhouse, there were nettles growing within 5 metres of the kitchen door. In first-aid homeopathy, Urtica urens (common stinging nettle) is recommended for burns. For want of something better to do, the boy's father, a vet and complementary thera- pist who was visiting for the night, made a crude nettle- extract in tap water. He diluted one drop of nettle juice in a cupful of water, succussed it, and serially repeated the dilution 5 more times. He gave the boy a spoonful every 10 minutes for about an hour. The boy stopped screaming within the first 10 seconds after the first spoonful. Within 2-3 days, the lesion had disappeared without a trace. Standard university training would re- gard this as impossible - that burn should have turned septic and taken 2-3 weeks to heal. But the clinical out- come was as described - unbelievable. One wonders who would buy expensive analgesics, antihistamines or ste- roids drugs to treat burns, stings, hives, or other skin allergies if all one had to do is find a nettle-leaf in the nearest ditch and make a crude home-made dilution of Urtica urens for oral use. However, Urtica does not al- ways work as dramatically as in that case.

- Many years ago, a worried father brought his little girl to me. The girl had been struggling to live for the pre- vious two years. At age 4, she had drunk concentrated NaOH (sodium hydroxide) and her esophagus was very badly damaged; it was like dry parchment, lifeless and totally functionless. She had been through countless

infections and courses of antibiotic during the 2-3 years
that had elapsed since the accident and all her food
and drink had to be given via an indwelling nasogastric
tube. In this case the cause of the trauma or disease was
obvious; it was the corrosive action of the NaOH. I then
took some NaOH and potentised it (see page 540),
which means that I made an isopathic remedy from it.
She began to take this remedy, 5 drops twice daily. After
just a few days, vitality and function began to return to
the esophagus. After 3 weeks, the nasogastric tube was
removed. After 2 months she was able to eat normally
again and remained cured. Strictly speaking, this case
was an example of the clinical use of *isopathy*, rather
than homeopathy.

Isopathy is another modality closely allied to the *"similia similibus curentur"* paradigm of homeopathy. It can help greatly in
treating intoxication with a *known toxic agent*, detoxifying the
body of toxic heavy-metals, and in treating allergies to known
allergens. Isopathy differs from homeopathy in one main respect. *In isopathy, one gives a potentised dilution of the **ingredient(s)**
**that actually precipitated the lesion-symptom complex (iso = same,
homeo = similar or like).***

AN EXAMPLE OF CLINICAL ISOPATHY

- A lady suddenly developed severe pruritus all over her
  body in hot sunny weather. There was no eczema or
  dermatitis, although there were scratch-marks from her
  nails visible in some places. She did not know where
  to scratch most because she was so totally affected. On
  questioning, it emerged that she had changed her brand
  of suntan lotion and had applied the new lotion all over
  herself earlier that day. A crude dilution of the suspect
  lotion (1 drop of lotion in a cup of water, serially diluted
  in that way 6 times, with succussion between each subsequent dilution) was prepared. She was advised to take
  one teaspoonful every 2 minutes. The itch disappeared

within 10 minutes. She was advised to avoid that lotion in future. She bought her original brand of suntan lotion next day and used it. The pruritus did not return.

Nosode therapy is another modality closely allied to the "*similia similibus curentur*" paradigm of homeopathy. *In nosode therapy, one gives a potentised dilution of a **pathogenic microbial culture** (for example Staphylococcus aureus), a **bodily tissue, fluid, secretion, or excretion** that harbors infectious agents that are involved in the manifestation of the disease.* The succussed dilution of the material is called the **nosode.** For example, one can make a nosode from one drop of infected blood, purulent milk, secretion from the eye, nose, throat, trachea or vagina, a drop of serum from a herpes blister, or a drop of diarrheic feces, to treat infections in the udder, eye, nose, throat, respiratory tract, reproductive tract, herpes-infected tissue, or the gastrointestinal tract, respectively. Some see nosode therapy as *a primitive form of "vaccination"*. Others see it as much more - giving back the total information pattern of the body, including its pathogens. From this information pattern, the body is supposed to recognise and correct its own imbalances. However, the clinical results from nosode therapy are unreliable. Skilled practitioners, using specific nosodes for specific animals, claim some excellent results. However, when the same nosode is used in a large group of animals, regardless of their individual traits, the results can be poor. For example, in attempts to prevent mastitis in cows in Ireland and England, four independent controlled trials of nosode therapy reached the same conclusion: milk somatic cell count, milk yield, or mastitis incidence between the treated versus control groups did not differ statistically (Phil Rogers, personal communication).

Homeopathic prescribing: To be able then to prescribe the correct homeopathic remedy, one must know the *toxic symptoms* of many hundreds of different substances, in order to recognise and match these in the *total disease history and symptom picture* of the patient. Hahnemann's studies convinced him that only multifactorial causes could explain the origin of disease. He came to look at the disease as the end point of the results of three factors, the physical, psychological and inherited weaknesses of the individual. He also looked upon the disease as initiated by External Stressors like Wind, Cold etc. He also found out that the patient's symptomatic picture was the only way to find the right remedy and thus induce the healing. He thought that by studying the *Modifications* of the symptoms, we could find the correct origin of the disease, even though he did not recognise the physiological cause, merely the "remedy logical" cause. We have discussed this way of thinking under the section on diagnosis, under the Modifications (see page 151).

Hahnemann discovered that if warmth, coldness, wind, humidity or draughts, etc. caused a symptom to vary, this indicated the origin of the symptoms. These precipitating factors are remarkably similar to the External Stressors, as described in TCM (Heat, Damp, Dryness, Cold, Wind, etc.). However, Hahnemann was not so interested to understand where the cause was, anatomically or physiologically. He chose *remedies that matched the Modifications of the symptoms* and gave that remedy to treat the disease. He failed to understand the Fundamental Processes (the physiological processes) involved, at least in his teachings.

AN EXAMPLE:

- One of the first remedies that Hahnemann studied was *Cinchona bark (from the China tree)*. At the time, the bark (or an extract, quinine) was used to treat malaria. Hahnemann ingested the bark in normal doses and he began to experience symptoms of intoxication after some days; he was very sensitive. Symptoms included shivering due to cold, palpitations, strong pulse, fatigue and a recurrent fever. All these symptoms are like those of malaria itself. A patient with malaria manifested similar symptoms to a patient with toxicity symptoms induced by the China tree.

After this Hahnemann tried more and more remedies on himself, his family, his friends and his employees. He found similarities between the intoxication symptoms and the indications for use in curing disease and he became more and more convinced that *a substance that induces specific signs and symptoms of intoxication in a healthy individual cures those manifestations in a diseased patient that has similar syndrome.*

THE HOMEOPATHIC METHOD

Throughout the years that Hahnemann worked, and during the years after his death, all of the homeopathic remedies are thoroughly studied on several people regarding to which symptoms they give. These symptoms are written down in a big book called the homeopathic *Materia Medica*. If we then want to use homeopathic remedies, we must know the symptoms written down in that book. When we are introduced to a patient, we then can recognise the symptom picture and can prescribe the correct remedy.

To make this process easier, and so that we do not need to remember all the minute details, we can use another book, *The Homeopathic Repertory*. Here most of the symptoms are indexed alphabetically. Here we may look under the right column to find which remedies can evoke the symptom(s) in question. If we for example have five symptoms to work with and China is labelled under all five, then we look up in the Materia Medica to see if China fits with the general symptomatic picture. The repertory is in this way a helper to find the right remedy but we must confirm the totality of symptoms in the Materia Medica. Today, one can buy computer software that has the complete homeopathic repertory in a user-friendly format. One can enter all the lesion-symptom complexes and modifications and the software returns the "best match" to suit all the data entered.

Conventional medicine is gradually accepting the therapeutic value of AP. Unfortunately; this is not the case with homeopathy. The reasons for this are multiple but one of the main reasons is that the remedies, at the usual dilutions, do not contain one single molecule of the initial substance. Another reason is that the clinical effect of homeopathy often seems to disappear in double-blind studies. We will consider this in more detail later.

Homeopaths describe what is left in the remedy as the "information structure of the substance", some kind of "resonance" or hidden information. Of course, scientifically-minded doctors or researchers find this difficult to grasp or acknowledge. That the vehicle, be it water, alcohol solution or lactose, can carry the information of a plant or metal, without one single molecule present, is in itself incredible. That this "information" can communicate with the body and induce the body to heal its diseases, such as psoriasis, depression or rheumatoid arthritis, is totally absurd to materialistic "scientific doctors". And this intellectual riddle does not get any easier when we consider the great amount of time and energy spent on trying to explain how the diluent (aqueous or alcoholic vehicle, or the lactose base) can carry this "information pattern". It is especially difficult to understand when we consider that some manufacturing methods of homeopathic pills involve the evaporation of the liquid vehicle when the pills are made. (It is interesting, however, that many atomic physicists do not find the phenomenon impossible to believe).

Homeopaths and scientists agree that continuous serial dilution of a substance eventually reduces its physical or chemical concentration to zero. But homeopathic experts claim that succussion (vigorous shaking and striking of the container) between each dilution induces thousands of small bubbles in the vehicle and preserves the "information pattern", that induces the therapeutic effect of the remedy. They suggest that succussion induces a structural change in the water molecules in the surface tension layer between water and bubbles. In this way, the remedy-free vehicle preserves the information structure or therapeutic signal of the remedy that induces its clinical effect. According to Avogadro's Law the number of molecules in 1 g of any substance is 6×10^{23}. When we dilute any substance 24 times at 1:10 each time (i.e. D24), the concentration is 1×10^{24}. Theoretically there are no molecules left in the solution at that dilution. In practice it is not possible to detect the substance even at dilutions like D7-D8. Conventional medicine classes homeopathic remedies above D6 as having no possible toxic effect. At least it cannot reject homeopathic remedies on grounds of toxicity or lack of safety!

STUDIES OF THE BIOLOGICAL EFFECTS OF HOMEOPATHIC REMEDIES
Many studies have tried to investigate and explain the actions of the potentised substances. Such studies have focused mainly on biological systems. Many showed some effect on the growth of yeast cells, detoxification in animals and some other processes. However, it is interesting to note that when critical and scientifically minded people repeated such studies, they could not reproduce the results. It seems that investigators must have a *positive and believing mental state,* if such studies are to produce positive results. This indicates that *the investigator's mental state* is important; similar phenomena apply in research into quantum physics. *Also here the investigator seems to influence the results. The investigator's, or clinical therapist's,* **intention and focused will** *are important as regards to the outcome.* This may also explain why homeopathy seems to function more in the clinic than in critical double-blind studies.

If we carefully read Hahnemann´s (The founder of homeopathy, see page 510) last edition of his writings [the 6. edition of "Organon der Heilkunst", finished in 1842 (the year before Hahnemann died) and published in 1921], we may find strong indications that also he was aware of the importance of the therapists will and intention.

In § **288** he thus writes: *"through the strong will of a person with positive intentions, when such a person touch the patient, yes he even don't have to touch the patient, then a sort of healing power flows over from that person to the diseased one. This kind of healing is one of the most powerful there is".*

Also in § **265** we find a very interesting observation made by Dr. Samuel Hahnemann. Here he writes: *"It is very important that the sick patient gets the right remedy, and it is also equal important that the therapist gives the remedy to the patient from his own hands, and also that the therapist has made the remedy himself".* He also adds: *"to be able to follow this important and fundamental principle in my teachings, I have, since I discovered it, had to suffer or endure much persecution"*

What Hahnemann here describes, resembles very much my description of healing under "Antroposophical medicine", page 605. As Hahnemann did not conduct double-blinded trials, and as he did not let machines make or give his remedies, he surely could not observe that this described "power" was one of the most important factors in all healing (as Rudolf Steiner described in 1920, see page 605).

Also, the diagnostic part of homeopathy, i.e. how and which remedy to choose, is highly individual; it depends on finding an exact match for the precise symptom picture of the patient. (The same applies in AP; two people with a common cold do not get the same treatment because one may have clear mucus and the other may have purulent yellow mucus and these differences alter the selection of the remedy). Therefore, it is very difficult to design large clinical studies to test the therapeutic effects of homeopathy. Few studies have been published that show beyond doubt that homeopathy works.

Apart from the difficulties in their design and implementation, the scarcity of clinical homeopathic studies is due mainly to lack of research funding. The remedy-costs of homeopathic treatment are only a tiny fraction of the costs of medical and veterinary pharmaceuticals. This generates very small profits within the industry. The multibillion-dollar international pharmaceutical industry simply does not want to show that homeopathy has wide clinical benefits; that result would erode their lucrative market heavily. Therefore, the industry is most unlikely to finance expert independent homeopathic studies.

VETERINARY HOMEOPATHY

The first published reports of homeopathic treatment of animals were not from veterinarians but from physicians. Hahnemann treated animals homeopathically. Spanning a period of more than 100 years, dozens of manuscripts on veterinary homeopathy are archived in the library of the University of Leipzig. Dr. Lux (1773-1849), a German veterinarian, was official founder of veterinary homeopathy. In 1833 he published the first treatise on the subject. More veterinarians followed in his footsteps, especially in Germany.

Today, veterinary homeopathy has its greatest use in Germany and France, where it is common for veterinarians to use it routinely in their practices. Studies have shown that 25% of all treatments performed in these countries have used homeopathy as a greater or lesser part of the treatment. It is taught in several German veterinary schools and in at least two schools in France (Nantes and Paris). In other European countries and also in the USA, South America and India homeopathy is used more and more, both in humans and in animals.

In summary, homeopathy in medical and veterinary practice lacks "scientifically acceptable proof" of its efficacy. However, it is a system that, correctly used in the opinion of its practitioners, is more effective in clinical practice than most other systems. This is a paradox; like many other aspects of life, it seems to contradict itself. Can the multitude of homeopathic users be wrong? Should the proponents of EBM be allowed to ban homeopathy, or tie it up with so much legalistic red-tape that manufacturers of homeopathic remedies will cease their production, because of the heavy costs involved in registering each remedy? Only time will tell. Unfortunately, because nobody knows what is happening when homeopathic remedies are given, the proponents of EBM are winning the first battles to ban homeopathy. The European Union (EU) has decided to ban its use in food animals since 1995. (A better proof for the effect of homeopathy can not be found!). Finland banned the use of homeopathy in food animals since 1997.

THE METHOD
The classical method
Diagnostic and therapeutic methods used in *classical homeopathy* are simple. Classical homeopaths observe as carefully as possible the *signs and symptoms*, their *specialities* (unique symptoms) and *modalities* (*modifying factors*). They then choose the *simillimum*, the one (best) remedy that resembles the *total symptom picture* as closely as possible.

In noting the symptoms, one must pay great attention to the **specialities** *of the symptoms and their modalities (the factors that* *modify them)*. Head colds and backache are common symptoms but are not special symptoms (i.e. are non-specific). We will fail to find the best remedies if we consider the common symptoms as the only data to help our decision-making process. For example, because they have different *specialities* (unique symptoms) and *modalities*, the following types of head cold are different and need different specific remedies:

- (a) Rhinitis, with *green, excoriating mucus* (acting corrosively on the skin), *worse* in the *morning* and *better* in the *evening;*

- (b) Rhinitis, with *clear, non- excoriating, watery mucus,* (non irritant to the skin), *worse* in the *evening* and *better* in the *morning.*

Similarly, the following types of backache are different because they have different *specialities* and *modalities*. They also need different specific remedies:

- (a) Backache, *worse* when *bending down,* and *better* when *resting, straightening up* and when eating *spicy food;*

- (b) Backache, *worse* when *lying down,* and *better* when *standing up.*

To select the best homeopathic remedy, for each patient, we must note the *specialities* and *modalities* of the symptoms. When we become as aware as possible of the symptoms, their specialities and their modalities, we may consult the *Materia Medica* to find the remedy that most specifically resembles all these observations.

One would need a photographic memory to remember the details of the symptom patterns of so many homeopathic remedies. Few people have that great gift and most of us could not remember so many specific details. Therefore we have the *Repertory*. For example, to help a patient with a head cold, we search the Repertory under "cold" and check all the rubrics until we find a *"cold with green mucus, worse in the morning; excoriates the skin, like acid"*.

The number of remedies for consideration decreases greatly as the detail of the search (including the modalities and symptom specificity) increases. If we are very accurate and specific in our clinical observation and questioning of the patient, the rubrics help us to eliminate many possible remedies, so that we are left with only one or two remedies that fit all the known symptoms. Then we study the full symptom picture of those one or two remedies in the *Materia Medica and ask further questions* to help us pick the *one* remedy that matches *all the known* symptoms of the patient, including demeanour. A perfect homeopathic match of the patient's symptoms with the symptom picture of the remedy indicates *the* best remedy for *that* patient at *that time!*. We then prescribe that remedy, the **simillimum.**

DIAGNOSIS BASED ON THE PROCESS IMBALANCES

As discussed earlier, with respect to AP, one can rationalise the Process Imbalances down to twelve fundamental functions, the Channel Processes. It should therefore be possible also to relate the different homeopathic remedies to these twelve Primary Processes. Classical homeopathy puts great emphasis on the individual symptoms and their combinations. Just as we have done in AP, Hahnemann put the greatest weight on symptoms that related to variations in the Internal or External environment. We can recognise the different Process Imbalances when we examine the relationships between the Modalities (the Factors that change the symptoms) and TCM Theory (Channel Theory, Five Phase Correspondences, the Qi Clock, etc.). Below, we will try to recognise the Process Imbalances of TCM in the symptom picture of a case that presented for homeopathy. We will then search the Materia Medica for the homeopathic remedies that fit the different Process Imbalances.

- For example, a patient has a heavy head-cold, green mucus and blurred sight. If symptoms aggravate at 0200h and after drinking red wine, we may deduce that the head-cold has its origin in a Process Imbalance of LV.

In that case, we need not find an individual and "difficult" remedy. Instead, we can give a general LV tonic to stimulate LV function. And such remedies exist. (See relationships between the remedies and Fundamental Processes, page 469).

Classical homeopathy puts great emphasis on recognising the more individual symptoms and their fluctuations. These data are used to search the repertory or the Materia Medica to find the simillimum, the right remedy. Without access to a good digital homeopathic database, this may be tedious and take a long time. Also, this work may not bring us closer to understanding the disease. However, we may also analyse these data systematically by **consideration of the Process Imbalances involved.** From AP theory, these symptoms help us to recognise the Process Imbalances in one or more of the 12 Channels. I strongly emphasise that this way of practising homeopathy is not opposed in any way to Hahnemann's thinking. The Greek homeopath *George Vithoulkas* tried to find the exact characteristic of each remedy. He sees it as a goal to characterise this remedy with just one single sentence, or even just a single word. These characteristics may be like "cold greed", "sorrow after parting", "warm wind" etc. By analogy, we may recognise connections to the Chinese names for certain points, for example:

Translation	Acupoint	Translation	Acupoint
Abdominal Bind	Fujie-SP14	Spirit Hall	Shentang-BL44
All-Round Flourishing	Zhourong-SP20	Spirit Path	Shendao-GV11
Anemic's Inspiration	Pinxueling-X_32	Spirit Pathway	Lingdao-HT04
Bathing the Unclean	Zhouyu-X_14	Spirit Ruins	Lingxu-KI24
Blood Pressure Point	Xueyadian-NX02	Spirit Seal	Shenfeng-KI23
Bowel Abode	Fushe-SP13	Spirit Storehouse	Shencang-KI25
Brain Clearing	Naoqing-NL04	Spirit Tower	Lingtai-GV10

Brain Door	Naohu-GV17	Spirit Treasure	Lingbao-L_42
Contain Tears	Chengqi-ST01	Spleen Heat Point	Pirexue-NX10
Eye-Pupil Bright	Jingming-BL01	Spleen Shu	Pishu-BL20
Gallbladder Point	Dannangxue-L_23	Sprain Point	Niushangxue-NA08
Gallbladder Shu	Danshu-BL19	Spread Smile	Sanxiao-Z_17
Kidney Shu	Shenshu-BL23	Spring in the Foot	Quanshengzu-L_10
Knee Yang Joint	Xiyangguan-GB33	Squatting Bone-Point	Juliao-GB29
Leaking Valley	Lougu-SP07	Stand Erect	Zieli-NL27
Lift and Support Point	Tituoxue-NY04	Stiff (Neck) One Half	Luolingwu-NA03
Lift Shoulder	Taijian-NA11	Stiff Neck	Luozhen-A_23
Lower Back Shu	Yaoshu-GV02	Stiff Neck	Luojing-Z_27
Lower Back Yang Joint	Yaoyangguan-GV03	Stomach Heat Point	Weirexue-NX07
Lung Heat Point	Feirexue-X_06	Stomach's Comfort	Weishu-NX14
Malaria Door	Nuemen-NA02	Stomach's Happiness	Weile-NY02
Mute's Gate	Yamen-GV15	Support Sinews	Chengjin-BL56
Nursing the Aged	Yanglao-SI06	Support Spirit	Chengling-GB18
Phlegm and Wheezing	Tanchuan-Y_02	Support Uterus	Weibao-Y_16
Qi Abode	Qishe-ST11	Taking Flight	Feiyang-BL58
Qi Centre	Qizhong-Y_10	Thigh Joint	Biguan-ST31
Qi Door	Qihu-ST13	Tonsil	Biantao-Z_26
Qi Door	Qimen-Y_15	Toothache	Yatong-NA01
Qi Point	Qixue-KI13	Tuberculosis Point	Jiehexue-NX06
Qi Sea	Qihai-CV06	Ulcer Point	Kuiyangxue-NX13
Qi Sea Shu	Qihaishu-BL24	Ulna and Radius	Chirao-A_36

Qi Surging	Qichong-ST30	Upper Arm Convergence	Naohui-TH13
Qi Wheezing	Qichuan-X_09	Upper Arm Point	Naoshu-SI10
Quiet Sleep_1	Anmian_1-NZ27	Upper Arm Upper	Naoshang-NA14
Raise Arm	Jubi-NA10	Urgent Pulse	Jimai-LV12
Recover Flow	Fuliu-KI07	Uterus Palace Point	Zigongxue-Y_18
Reflection Abode	Yishe-BL49	Water Way	Shuidao-ST28
Rigid Heel	Luodi, Genjin-NL09	Welcome Fragrance	Yingxiang-LI20
Ring of Jumping (Hip Joint)	Huantiao-GB30	White Ring (Anus) Shu	Baihuanshu-BL30
Root of Spirit	Benshen-GB13	Will Chamber	Zhishi-BL52
Sauce Receptacle	Chengjiang-CV24	Wind Gate	Fengmen-BL12
Severe mouth	Lidui-ST45	Wind Mansion	Fengfu-GV16
Sighing and Giggling	Yixi-BL45	Wind Market	Fengshi-GB31
Sinew Contraction	Jinsuo-GV08	Wind Pass	Fengguan-A_04
Sinew Seat	Zhejin-GB23	Wind Pool	Fengchi-GB20
Skull Rest	Luxi-TH19	Wind's Cliff	Fengyan-Z_28
Spasm Vessel	Chimai-TH18	Woman's Knee	Nuxi-L_09
Spirit Court	Shenting-GV24	Woodworm Canal	Ligou-LV05
Spirit Gate	Shenmen-HT07	Yang Assistance	Yangfu-GB38
Spirit Gate, Navel Centre	Shenque, Qizhong-CV08		

Table 98

Dose and strength of homeopathic remedies

The dose of a remedy may vary from 1 drop or pill or tablet, to 10 g. The remedy may be given once only, or 1-2 times/day, once/week, or once only. It may be given in different strengths or potencies: D6, D12, D30, D200, D1000, D10000, D100000, C6, C30, C200, or 1M, etc. Sometimes the remedy must be used at a special time. For example, *within 5 minutes of the full moon,* one may give homeopathic Kali.Carb to treat parasitism in animals and humans. *[NOTE "at the exact moment" of full moon is NOT practical if one must dose 100 cattle or sheep!!]*

In homeopathic prescribing, D stands for decimal. That means that the original remedy or substance is diluted 1:10. The number indicates how many times the remedy is diluted and the letter indicates the degree of dilution. D=10, C=100, M=1000 and LM=50000. For example a D6 potency is diluted 1:10, six times (10^6) and potentised by succussion (i.e. stirring, shaking and hitting) at each step in the dilution process. A C12 potency means that the remedy is diluted 1:100, 12 times. A LM6 potency means that the remedy is serially diluted 6 times at 1:50000 each time.

To choose the **correct point(s)** *is the most important criterion* in **AP**, in **homeopathy** *it is to choose* **the similimum,** *the* **correct remedy**. The dose usually is less important; it is not nearly as important as the choice of the similimum. In this respect, the homeopathic dose is like the thickness of an AP needle, which is of much less importance than the correct choice of acupoint.

To choose the **correct point(s)** *is the most important criterion* in **AP**, in **homeopathy** *it is to choose* **the simillimum,** *the* **correct remedy**. The dose is usually less important; it is not nearly as important as the choice of the simillimum. In this respect, the homeopathic dose is like the thickness of an AP needle, which is of much less importance than the correct choice of acupoint.

In chronic cases however, the remedy should be given several times, usually in low potencies (D6-D12) once/day, or once/ week in higher potencies (D30-D200), or just once at very high potencies (above D1000).

FREQUENCY OF DOSING

Homeopaths argue endlessly about how often to give the remedy and in what potency. My procedure is as follows: For:

- *physical* symptoms: use D6, 1-2 times/day;

- *psychological / mental* symptoms: use D12 once/week

- *spiritual* symptoms: use D30 or 200 once/month

- Potencies above D30 address the higher spiritual levels of the patient. If we use these, we should know what we do (which we usually do not), and how to counter any unexpected reactions.

- C potencies are used like the D potencies; (LM potencies are special; consult special literature before using these).

HOMEOPATHIC REMEDIES
Below, the most important remedies used most often in veterinary medicine are classified according to consideration of:

- **Process Imbalances:** *the imbalanced* **Channel Processes** *that they help*

- **TCM theory:** *which* **organs** *they help*

- **Classical homeopathic theory:** *which* **symptoms** *they help*

Note: Classical descriptions of a specific homeopathic remedy usually show only the symptoms that it helps; they do not show the organs or Channel Processes that it helps, because most homeopathic authors do not know AP or TCM in depth. In this respect, this book differs from others on the topic, in that we view the remedies in relation to the earlier description of Channel Functions and Process Imbalances. The description of the remedies is more complete than might seem at first glance. The following table lists the most commonly used homeopathic remedies, the Processes that they help, and the typical indication of the remedies:

Homeopathic remedy and the Process that it helps	Typical indications
Acid.phos and KI	Acidum phosphoricum is produced from phosphoric acid and shows a strong relation to KI Process. The symptoms resemble those of KI Deficiency, manifested by Qi exhaustion, tiredness, rapid (excessive) growth, menopausal disorders and old age. The animal has painless diarrhoea, poor digestion, decreased bone strength (fragile bones) with decalcification later; the patient seems exhausted and tired of life.
Acon and GB	Aconite is from monkshood, Aconitum napellus, a plant of the Ranunculaceae family. It grows well in higher areas of mountains. The plant contains aconitine, a very toxic alkaloid. This gives a strong burning sensation and a sharp taste in the mouth, followed by a heavy desire to spit, recurrent hot sweats, fast pulse and hypersensitivity. Later, high blood pressure, breathing disorders, fast pulse and diarrhea may occur. Later, the heart rate slows and blood pressure falls. A lethal dose causes paralysis, fainting, coma and death. Acon. symptoms essentially occur rapidly, especially when high fever becomes acute, followed by body tremors and a beating pulse. These symptoms often appear after rapid cooling of the body (Cold), or after exposure to severe draughts (Wind). The mucosal membranes are red and Dry and the skin is Hot and Dry. The symptoms aggravate in the evening, and in conditions of Heat or sudden Cold. They improve in fresh air and with cold water. Severe fear usually follows Acon. Although homeopathic texts do not relate it to any specific organ, Acon. sedates GB Process.
Apis and LV (and BL KI)	Apis is from the honeybee, Apis mellifica. Symptoms that Apis helps are easy to deduce; they resemble those evoked by bee stings. These are burning pain, swellings that are Hot and red and that improve with Cold compresses. They include "Hot and Cold" (fever and cold shivering) without thirst. Headache, sleepiness and a pink skin with swellings often follow these symptoms. There may be sensations of choking, dyspnea and suffocation. Although homeopathic texts do not relate Apis to any specific organ, it stimulates LV Process and helps the Water Phase (BL, KI).

Arg.met, KI	Argentum metallicum is produced from pure silver. Arg.met. especially helps KI and especially helps to fight infections. A German homeopathic firm, Wala, uses Argentum as a main ingredient in a specially formulated mastitis complex, called «Lachesis Argentum compositum». I have used this to treat mastitis for 15 years. In my opinion and that of several Norwegian colleagues, the complex is excellent to treat acute and chronic mastitis. It rarely fails to help cows with longstanding serious infection.
Arg.nit, LV	Argentum nitricum is a remedy that helps blood circulation and the mucous membranes above all else. It helps especially the throat, stomach and intestines. It helps sore throat and green coloured diarrhea, with burning sensations. The symptoms aggravate on eating sweet things and immediately after feeding. Muscle cramps usually follow. The symptoms usually improve after Hot, not sweet, drinks. Therefore it relates with metabolism and especially LV Process.
Arn and LU	Arnica is from the plant leopard's bane, Arnica montana, which usually grows in places where water and wind flow freely. This is the next best remedy (the best remedy is Symphytum) to treat all kinds of trauma, injury, crushing, bruises and falls (also psychic injury and bereavement!). Arnica is given after traumas where the bodily fluids have not left the body (closed wounds). In open wounds where blood or other body fluids leave the body, that is flow freely, we use Symphytum. Arnica does not thrive with stagnant liquid (edema) and therefore heals where liquid; hemorrhage and edema have "fallen out" of the system. The symptoms improve by resting and when the animal lays the head low; movement and touch aggravate them. Arnica may be used before and after operations to prevent bruising and hemorrhage. It helps internally or externally. Arnica helps especially the area along LU Channel, i.e. on the inside of the forelimbs and it helps LU Processes.

Ars.alb and SP	Arsenicum album (white arsenic) is produced from the notorious poison, arsenic. Symptoms of arsenic poisoning manifest mainly in the digestive tract, especially ST and SP. Severe ST pain, diarrhea and vomiting are prominent symptoms that improve when the animal flexes the spine. Pain in ST, SI and LI usually feel as if it is burning. It gets worse after a meal and is accompanied by shivering. Usually the patient partially loses appetite. The diarrhea is mostly dark and has a foul smell. Ars.Alb. also relates closely to all SP Processes; it is the most general remedy available to stimulate SP in SP Deficiency. [In TCM, SP relates to digestion, to immunity via its effects on Blood and to the deep muscles of the hip, especially musculus iliopsoas. Pain in this muscle is better if we bend down, and exactly this detail is also predominant in the symptoms of Ars. Alb.]. In horses it helps especially the deep muscles (psoas major and minor) in the hip. When the equine inner hip muscles are loaded because the strain on SP, the horse has problems towards the end of the race and the pelvis comes under the body. Ars.alb. also helps immunomediated eczema, whether itching and weeping, or dry. Emaciation and fear usually follow the symptoms.
Bell, fever and Yang Processes	Belladonna comes from deadly nightshade, Atropa belladonna. It contains the strong poison atropine, which dilates the pupils. Women used to use nightshade extract to make the eyes appear more striking, hence the name beautiful woman (bella donna). Together with Acon. and Ferr.phos, Bell. is the prime first aid remedy in fever. But compared to Acon., which is accompanied by dry fever, the Bell. fever is hot and sweaty. The patient's face becomes red, especially on one side. Since it is difficult to observe sweating in animals (and some animals do not sweat), the best way to distinguish Acon. and Bell. patients is that the Acon. patient has excessive thirst, while the Bell. patient has not. Bell. centres on the head and Acon. on the chest. Bell. stimulates mainly all the general Yang Processes.

Bry and KI	Bryonia is from wild hops, Bryonia alba. Its symptoms are characterised by dryness, or lack of water. Everything (the mucosal membranes, skin, hair and stools) seems to be dried out and the patient constantly wants to consume large amounts of water. The mucus or phlegm in the throat is dry, sticky and difficult to cough up. The patient avoids all touch and movement. The sexual cycle may be absent because of dehydration. Because of its relation to Water, this is a remedy that helps KI. By acting on KI, it also has a special effect on the joints generally and especially on the stifles.
Calc.carb and LU	Calcium carbonate is from oyster shell. The remedy helps mainly LU Process. It has a great influence on calcium metabolism and may be used in multiple calcifications and exostoses. It may also be used when there is deficient calcification. The patient also behaves like an oyster; American readers can remember this picture, "like a clam", or "clammed up". The patient is uncommunicative, quiet, introverted and withdrawn. Another way of expressing this is that Calc.carb. helps childish, big and quiet young animals, who show slow development. This type of behaviour usually relates to a decreased metabolism, as in hypothyroidism. This is why the symptoms usually improve in Heat and aggravate in Cold.
Calc.fluor and LU	Like most calcium compounds, calcium fluoride acts through LU Process (gaseous exchange). The most important symptoms relate to different infections in the pharynx, larynx, epiglottis and trachea. The infection is characterised by venous stasis. This shows in the fact that the mucus membranes are somewhat bluish or purple and a thick, viscous exudate is excreted. Sensitivity to Cold is marked and the symptoms are followed by exhaustion and cachexia.
Calc.phos and LU	Calcium phosphate helps the LU Process. It helps especially in poor or deficient development of the teeth and the bones. Teeth and bones break easily, the patient looks pale, lost and retarded and completely exhausted (as in severe Qi Deficiency). Calc.phos. is a prime remedy for underdeveloped and young animals that seem to have lost their vitality (Qi Deficiency).

Canth and KI	Cantharis is from the Spanish Fly. In large doses, it was used as an aphrodisiac, because it irritates the urinary tract and external genitals. Canth. helps KI. Drinking and Heat (warmth) aggravate the symptoms, which include infections with a great degree of burning pain, hypersensitivity and cramps, especially in the urogenital tract. Also the throat, esophagus and entire digestive system are prone to pain and bleed easily. Canth. is given especially in burning infections in the ureter, sexual area (especially priapism, cystitis, vaginitis) and throat.
Caust and KI	Causticum (Caustic soda) helps KI Process. The symptoms resemble those described under Canth., with burning pain and infections in the throat, urogenital tract and sexual organs. Like Canth., Heat (warmth) improves the symptoms but only cold air (not drinking) aggravates the symptoms. This means that the Metal Phase is involved and not the Water Phase. As the Metal Phase is involved, we might find a tendency to depression, a state of mind usually related to Metal.
Chel and LV	Chelidonium is from celandine, Chelidonium majus, a little yellow plant. It relates especially to LV Process; its symptom picture is typical of many LV diseases. Symptoms aggravate at 0300-0400h and at 1500-1600h, as in the biorhythm of LV in the Chinese Qi Clock (see page 31). The throat, pharynx, stools and urine are yellow to greenish. Green also agrees with a Process Imbalance in LV. LV area in the right side of the abdomen often shows marked tenderness and LV Shu and Mu Points (BL18, LV14) may be tender to palpation. Diagnostic symptoms include rheumatism in tendons and muscles and infections in the throat, LU and digestive organs. Chel helps Imbalance in LV, while women often suffer from disorders related to a Process Imbalance in KI. I have used Chel (together with needling at LV03) to treat 16 people, 15 men and 1 woman, with a diagnosis of "Cluster headache"; 14/16 recovered well or became completely free of symptoms; the first patient has remained well for 15 years.
Cinc and SP	"Cluster headache", also-called "Horton's disease", or suicidal headache. This is a special form of headache, mostly occurring in men. As we know from before, men often suffer from disorders related to a Process

	Cinchona (and its extract, quinine) is from the bark of the china tree. Hahnemann made his first experiments with Cinc It is a very important remedy to stimulate SP in SP Deficiency. As discussed at the beginning of this chapter, the symptoms are fevers that come and go regularly, like the tide. These are typical of malaria. They also include severe diarrhea, skin disorders and hemorrhage. The most typical of all SP/Cinc symptoms is the rhythmical aspect; symptoms come and go rhythmically. Cinch. is also very useful in patients convalescing from chronic diseases and for animals that do not recover properly after other treatments. We know that when a disease has lasted for more than a year, SP is Deficiency. SP Deficiency hinders recovery, as SP has very important roles in digestion, immunity and blood quality.
Con, LV and ST	Conium is from poison hemlock, Conium maculatum. Its main use is against cancer in animals, especially mammary tumours in dogs. Conium regulates ST Channel but has its main effect via LV, as in the Ko Cycle (Wood controls Earth; see AP and cancer, page 466)
Digitalis and HT	Digitalis is produced from the plant Digitalis purpurea. This remedy has a special reference to the heart and the activity of the heart. In Heart deficiency we may observe symptoms like irregular beating, heat sensations, fatigue, a feeling of weakness in the chest region, pale skin, bluish skin and edema in the legs. As we understand, all Heart symptoms. In animals, as described under the Heart process, all kinds of symptoms may occur, all over the body, wherever a structural weakness may be present.
Dros and LU	Drosera is from the plant sundew. It helps LU Process to reduce exudation, phlegm/mucus development and growth processes (tumors). It may be used against strong cough that aggravates in Heat and at night, especially after midnight. It has been used successfully against tuberculosis.

Ferr.met and GB	Metallic iron is a very important remedy. It helps GB Process, especially its "Fire" Process, i.e. the active, expansive, outward directed functions. Ferr.met may be used in anemia, biliary disorders, gallstones and GB Deficiency. It represses aggression (stops outward directed activity). Metallic iron is associated with the active and outward directed aggression. Swords were made from iron, swords that act like the will-powered hand that strikes all arguments to the ground. In this connection it is interesting to note that the famous Vikings, fearsome and gruesome, had a genetic damage in their DNA, causing an elevated ferrum-content in their blood. The hordes that terrorised Europe, around 1000 AD, had the craving of the iron in their blood and iron in the heart of their prey.
Gels and BL KI	Gelsemium is from wild jasmine. It helps BL and KI Channels. Therefore the symptom picture resembles influenza, or is like the common cold. The patient is exhausted, tongue-tied and sleepy, or may be terrified or have panic attacks. Gels. aggravates in Heat and improves in Cold fresh air. It is often called "the actor's remedy" because it helps to prevent stage fright, or panic attacks before examinations or interviews.
Graph and TH	Graphite is from black lead, or plumbago. It helps the blood circulation of the skin and epithelium, especially of the pharynx and mucosa of the throat. It helps TH. A typical symptom picture in a Graph. case presents as "thick, stupid and lazy". We may also see a certain stupidity of the patient and symptoms like eczema, pharyngitis and stagnation in the digestive system. All the infections are characterised by sluggishness, apathy or laziness. The exudation is usually yellowish and sluggish; it may arise from the skin, the throat or digestive tract. Similar exudate may also be seen from wounds.

Ham and LV	Hamamelis is from witch hazel, Hamamelis virginica. It works in many ways like Gels. but as a Gels. patient has a sluggish arterial blood circulation; the typical Ham patient has a sluggish venous blood circulation, especially in the skin. Since the cause of these symptoms lies in the venous circulation, Ham. mainly helps LV. It is therefore often used in hemorrhoids, in diffuse hemorrhage from a wound, in slow nosebleeds and in hemorrhage from the sexual organs in women. The hemorrhage lasts for days and is a slow oozing, i.e. just a drop now and then. The blood is often unclotted.
Hepar.sulph and LV	Hepar sulphuris calcareum (Hahnemann's calcium sulphide) is the main remedy against eczema, unclean skin, pimples (acne, pustules) and exudation from wounds, nose, throat and eyes. It helps LV Process and is indicated especially to treat purulent exudates and in purulent mastitis. In eczema it may help to give the animal a bath in a physical (not homeopathic) solution of Hepar.sulph, made by dissolving 10 g/l of water.
Ignatia	Ignatia (St. Ignatius' bean; ignatia = ignition) helps hyposensitive patients that have little or no reaction or ignition to most common stimuli. The patient is quiet, full of sorrow, withdrawn and often suffers great homesickness. This remedy also helps nervous, tense, hypersensitive individuals with hysterical tendency, nervous disorders, cramps and a tendency to bite. As discussed earlier, a remedy may work on both extremes of the scale. This applies to Ign. also. Ign. patients usually improve with activity and aggravate with quietness, Cold and strong external stimuli from sounds and light.
Ipec, LU, LI and SP	Ipecacuanha is a Native American medical plant root. It has been used for centuries to cure cough but it has many other therapeutic applications, especially when symptoms are spasmodic. It helps when the symptoms are "tossing something out" of the body, a quality that is seen in its Norwegian name; "vomit root". The air is expelled from LU and the feces expelled from LI (rectum / anus). This may look like a SP-related disease, with the rhythmical tendency and the remedy helps SP Channel.

Kali.carb and BL	Kalium carbonicum (potassium carbonate) is one of the main remedies to stimulate BL Channel. It may be used for all kinds of backache, muscular cramps in the legs, back or the neck. BL Channel-related headache is also a good indication. Parasitism is a special indication. I have used Kali.carb many times successfully to rid an animal of parasites, even heartworm. But, to have a good effect, it must be given at the exact time (+/- 2 minutes) of the full moon. The D200 potency is advised. The effect appears after 14 days, when all the dead worms leave the animal (dog). Is it as good as modern anthelmintics.
Lyc and LV	Lycopodium (Wolf's claw) is made from club moss. Lyc. especially helps symptoms on the right side of the body; this also shows its affinity to LV. The symptoms aggravate around 0400 and 1600h (related to LV also). Lyc. helps many symptoms like rheumatism (especially with urinary involvement), muscular pain, pain in the right side of the abdomen, right sided KI or GB colic and weak digestion.
Merc.met and SI	Mercurius metallicum is made from mercury. It helps SI Process and its symptoms mainly reflect those of a Process Imbalance in SI. It may be used to help alleviate the adverse effects of mercury poisoning. It also helps disorders in the mucosal membranes, mouth, teeth and in the digestive tract.
Nat.mur and KI SP	Natrium muriaticum is a remedy made from common salt. It helps mainly via KI but its symptoms seem to have their origin in SP and Nat.mur has a very clear influence on SP. As SP has a controlling action on KI (Earth controls Water in the Ko Cycle), Nat.mur. seems to stimulate the SP Process of controlling KI. This remedy may be used when the control of KI has been lost. Other symptoms are cracked tongue, like a map, dry skin and dehydration.
Nux.vom and ST	Nux vomica is from the vomiting nut or poison nut, used in the past to poison foxes and vermin. It contains strychnine. This poison mainly influences ST. Homeopathic Nux.vom helps ST Channel. It sedates

	ST activity in Excess states, for example in vomiting, gastric ulcers and stomach pain. It also stimulates ST in hypofunction (Deficiency), as in ruminal atony in cows. It helps generalised muscular cramps in the anterior muscles of the hindlimbs (quadriceps muscles).
Phos and KI	Phosphorus is the main KI stimulating remedy. It may be used in all KI-related symptoms: headache, excess, weak sexual cycle, abortion, infections and fear. Phos. also has some effects on LV but these come mainly through KI, from the nourishing action of KI on LV. KI also partly dominates digestion, especially the last part of the colon (rectum) and Phos may be given in disorders of defecation, diarrhea and obstipation. This remedy helps animals that are "fast, fearful and florid".
Phyto and ST	Phytolacca decandra is poke root. It helps especially the mammary gland. It is one of the main remedies in mastitis, acute and chronic. The glands are hard, tender and Hot and the milk often contains blood and / or pus. The remedy probably helps ST Channel.
Psor and excretion	Psorinum is from the scabies vesicle. It accelerates excretion over the mucosal membranes. It may be used when mucus production is decreased, or if we want the excretion Process (intestinal/urinary) to accelerate. We can use it in a chronic cold or bronchitis, which we want to make acute. It is in this way possible to say that the remedy acts on "cold Sulph. patients". Relationships to Channel Processes are uncertain.
Puls and LV	Pulsatilla is from the windflower, Pulsatilla nigricans. It is especially a female remedy. The patient is observant and friendly but retracts as soon as something frightens or threatens it. The feminine features predominate and the temperament is as variable as the symptoms. The patient easily becomes depressed and the symptoms usually are seen as mucosal infections, edemas, venous congestion, otitis

	media, fever and gastrointestinal disorders. It helps mainly LV Process of stimulating Blood; Blood is the Fire Phase of LV. Here we see the relation to the sexual cycle and disorders near parturition (dystocia).
Rhus.tox and GB	Rhus toxicodendron is from poison ivy. It helps the GB Process. Thus it has a special effect on the muscles and tendons, especially the tissues at the origins and insertions of tendons. The symptoms are pain and stiffness at the start of movement (after rest) but symptoms improve after 30-40 minutes of movement. These pains are clearly connected to the tendons and may reappear after sudden movements or unusual postures.
Sabal and KI	Sabal serrulata, from the plant saw palmetto, has limited use. Sabal helps the KI Process. It is seldom used in humans and in horses but in cats it has a very certain area of usage, which is FUS, Feline Urogenital Syndrome. This is a problem for male cats that are neutered and the urinary tract may become obstructed by calculi. The cat stops drinking and urinating and is quickly diseased, dying in uraemia. The symptoms are most prevalent at night and a vet should confirm the diagnosis. It may also be used to treat prostatitis in dogs.
Sars, KI and BL	Sarsaparilla is from sarsaparilla root, the smilax plant from South America. It helps BL Damp, humidity, or when any contact with water (even washing) aggravates all symptoms. Symptoms include skin disorders along BL Channel, dysuria or bladder pain during urination and pain in the joints. BL and KI Processes (Water Phase) are of special importance for bone and joints all over the body.
Sep, KI and LV	Sepia is a very interesting remedy, from the ink of the cuttle fish. It helps KI, especially KI that has lost relationship with LV. Thus the symptoms reflect both KI and LV. As co-operation between KI and LV regulates sexual function, several of the symptoms are related to this part. Sep cases are depressed, with disturbed sexual cycle, and desire to be alone. There

	is a tendency for prolapse of the uterus (and rectum). Also aggression may arise, especially against the male and towards the same race. LV Deficiency develops and may be dire and malnutrition may arise. Shape of the different tissues may be lost. Symptoms aggravate after urination or defecation.
Sil and TH	Silicea is a very important remedy from silica, or pure flint. It works very widely and deeply. It helps the skin, connective tissue and metabolism and symptoms that also manifest in the digestive area, ears, eyes and LU. The symptoms are characterised by generalised infections. The eczema is dry, the otitis is chronic, and the mastitis has hard glands with little change in the milk. Metabolism is decreased, the animal loses weight, eating is decreased and Qi (life energy) is generally Deficient. The animal avoids Cold; it has cold extremities and cracks in the paws and hooves. Wound healing is slow and the exudate from the normal orifices is thin and acidic (excoriating). Sil. is indicated in all kinds of otitis and in pain from old scars, chronic Processes, foreign bodies and the like. Sil. helps TH Process. Silica also has the effect of incarnating, which means making the patient more present, more participating in daily life, more awake and aware, both in mind and body.
Sulph and LV SP	Yellow sulphur is a most important remedy. Sulph. stimulates all metabolisms. Where Sil. helps chronic and longstanding infections or disorders, Sulph. helps recent and acute disorders. Thus, Sulph. is known as "the acute Silicea". Sulph. stimulates mainly LV Processes but also has a strong effect on SP. The symptoms arise mostly from the gastrointestinal tract, LV and metabolism. Symptoms are characterised by yellowish green exudate and an unpleasant smell, as from sulphur. Sulphur type eczema is itchy and burning and tends to have a purulent exudate; wounds and scratches turn septic, with green or yellow exudate. Sulph. may also be used to induce a chronic disorder to become acute. For example, it is very useful if we can safely convert a chronic infection into an acute one. Many different therapies can treat acute disorders or infections more easily

	and effectively than chronic disorders. However, it can be dangerous to deliberately cause an acute flare up in a chronic Process Imbalance. If the flare up is very acute, it can be lethal. One example of this is traumatic indigestion in cows, where abscesses have developed within the body, close to the heart or large arteries. If we give Sulph., one of the abscesses may burst into the blood and the animal may die instantly. A Sulph. patient longs for fresh air, is Hot and feels thirsty but refuses to drink Cold water.
Symph and KI	Symphytum is from comfrey, Symphytum officinale, also-called "Bone Set" in English, or "lus na gnambh briste" (the herb of the broken bones) in Gaelic. In European tradition, this plant was used to accelerate healing in bone fractures and wounds. In medieval times it was a great insult to give a woman flowers together with Symph. This meant that the giver thought that the woman should "grow up", or get herself together, i.e. that she was a broken woman, "sleeping around". Symph. is a common remedy to help trauma cases; it greatly helps the healing of fractures and wounds. It may be used together with Arn. and Hyp, which also enhance wound healing. The effect of Symph. is extraordinary. The most astonishing example I can remember was a young man that had a non-union fracture of the leg for 3 years after a motorcycle accident. When he met me, his doctors had decided to amputate the leg in 6 weeks if it had not healed by then. I injected 1 ml of Symph. D12 over the fracture. After a few days, the whole leg began to itch. The fracture was healed when he reported to the hospital 6 weeks later. Amputation of the leg was unnecessary.
Thuja and SP	Thuja is from the tree of life (Arbor vitae), Thuja occidentalis. It helps SP Processes and may be used in all kinds of SP Deficiency. Thuja may be used with great success after post-vaccination disorders. The immune system is stressed to a great degree after vaccination of animals or humans. If the immune system is weak beforehand, allergies and other

	immune-related disorders, including leukaemia and Hodgkin's disease may arise. The immune system depends especially on SP and LV. Thuja stimulates SP in such a way that the post-vaccination disorders disappear. SP Process also relates to cancer and tumours. This is especially for those Processes that have left the domain of the body for the domain of gravity, the Earth Phase. Thuja is a specific remedy in cancer, tumours, warts, polyps and ordinary tumours of the connective tissue.
Urt and LV	Urtica is from the common stinging nettle, Urtica urens. The symptoms for which it is useful are very similar to the ones you experience when you burn the skin on nettles, this special plant. Itchy, Hot and red rash which is improved by Damp and Cold wrappings. Urt. helps LV.

Table 99

POTENTISATION IN PRACTICE

At the moment, it is not essential for beginners to know how to make and potentise the remedies at home. This is because homeopathic pharmacies can supply all the different remedies and potencies. The remedies come ready for use in any desired potency, usually in small bottles of about 10 g. Common potencies are the D6 or C6, D12 or C12 and D30 or C30. However, it is easy (and in my opinion, better) to make remedies at home. Although it may take some time, it allows great flexibility in making whatever remedy and potency one needs. It can save a lot of money on homeopathic pharmacy bills. *In the future, however, it may become very important for practitioners to be able to make their own remedies and to potentise them at home. This is because the detractorss of homeopathy want to ban the commercial manufacture and sale of these valuable remedies, because they threaten the sales of the multibillion-dollar drug industry. Under the guise of demanding "proof of clinical efficacy", the EU (European Union) Medicines Boards and the US-FDA (Food & Drugs Administration) may legislate for this. Also, it may become difficult and expensive to purchase the raw ingredients if "commercial" homeopathy is banned.*

For example, one may treat diarrhea in calves by making remedies from the shell of the poppy, mixed with carbon from the birch. The results have been excellent. Most of the plants needed and almost all minerals and other substances, are usually easily obtained from a commercial company, or from nature, especially organic gardens and forests. Therefore the method to make your own remedies is summarised below.

To make a remedy from a plant, one must start with the plant, or the correct part of the plant. Some remedies are from the root, the stem, bark, leaves, fruits, or the whole plant. One should check which part(s) are needed.

To make the Mother Tincture, take 10 g from the most appropriate part of the plant and add 90 g of a 30% solution of alcohol. Store the mixture in a clearly-labelled clean brown glass bottle. After 1 week, the Mother Tincture is ready.

To make the D1 potency (1/10) of the remedy, dilute 10 g of the Mother Tincture with 90 g of water; stir, shake and succuss very thoroughly for 3 minutes. Hahnemann used to hit the little bottle against a leather bound Bible. This process, regarded as essential by Hahnemann, was called succussion; it creates millions of tiny bubbles in the solution. Then let the bottle stand for another 3 minutes.

To make the C1 potency (1/100) of the remedy, dilute 1 g of the Mother Tincture with 99 g of water and proceed as above. To make higher potencies, make serial dilutions from the D1 or C1, as needed, repeating the procedure (diluting, shaking and succussing) as many times as necessary. For example, to make the D2 potency (1/10 of 1/10) of the remedy, take 10 g from the D1, add 90 g of water and proceed as before. To make the D3 (1/10 of 1/10 of 1/10), take 10 g from the D2, add 90 g of water and proceed as before.

Remember to preserve the final potencies with alcohol to prevent spoiling by bacterial growth. In this way you may ascend the potentisation ladder. If you have the patience, you can reach D200 after a few weeks.

- Potency D6 may be used in physical disorders and in chronic cases

- Potency D12 may be used, for example in psychic disorders (disorders of HT and LU).

- Potency D30 helps acute cases and in behavioural disorders.

SINGLE HOMEOPATHIC REMEDIES VERSUS COMPLEXES

The pioneers of homeopathy believed that it was best to give *only one remedy at a time* and wait until they could evaluate its effect before they gave another. In the earlier described thinking process regarding Channel-Organ System Functions, if only one Process Imbalance (one Excess or Deficient Function) exists, it may be correct just to give one remedy. This is the usual situation today; it allows us to assess what helped the case or not. As we shall see later, it is permissible to give more than one remedy, provided that the remedies are selected after consideration of the Process Imbalances involved and not from the viewpoint of the symptomatology. Unfortunately many, less-experienced homeopaths use the latter method.

EXAMPLE OF BEST PRACTICE:

A common coryza (sore, runny eyes and rhinitis) with green exudate, that Wind or draught aggravates, indicates a Process Imbalance in LV (LV - Wood - typically is green, controls the eyes, and is susceptible to Wind). To heal this disorder, we may try to stimulate LV in many ways. For example, we may use several acupoints, several different diets, different herbs and *several homeopathic remedies.* These remedies may have different symptomatic pictures but they all are used to stimulate LV. We may combine remedies like Ars.alb, Echin. or Ham. On the contrary, we should NOT combine remedies that help a cold in general. One remedy may help a cold with *green exudate*, another *acidic exudate*, another *watery exudate*, another *thick exudate*. All these types of cold indicate different causes of this cold. If we would combine all these remedies as a blunderbuss attempt to treat the cold, we would stimulate different Process and achieve little or nothing. Even if the different remedies work against a cold, this combination is too non-specific to be of use. It is better to select *one specific remedy for one specific symptom picture.*

In the past few decades, especially in German-speaking countries, homeopathic complexes have become commonplace. The complexes may contain 2-50 specific remedies in combination. Each of these remedies gives a specific message to the body. Therefore, in my opinion, the clinical results may be haphazard and disappointing if the complexes are not formulated according to Channel Functional thinking, as discussed in the chapters on AP.

Of course, the same applies to all medical disciplines, including conventional medicine. If a doctor prescribed 50 remedies to cure a certain disease, then all would think that the doctor was insane or incompetent. The same applies to an acupuncturist who uses 50 needles. In conclusion, it requires great knowledge to formulate a complex of several remedies; one must know the Process Imbalance or Primary Process that they stimulate. Therefore, I recommend that novices use just one or two remedies at a time.

THE RELATIONSHIP BETWEEN ACUPUNCTURE AND HOMEOPATHY
(Beginners may find this to be very difficult. Please read it slowly and carefully several times.)

During the last hundred years, several practitioners have tried to correlate homeopathic remedies and the functions, or clinical indications, of individual acupoints. If we, with great care and accuracy, consider the effects of the acupoints and correlate them with the effect of the different homeopathic remedies, then we are struck with a remarkable resemblance. Sometimes the indications for an acupoint and a homeopathic remedy are almost identical. When we think that completely different people from different cultures and different times wrote these descriptions, we might conclude that the remedies and the points help the same Qi Processes and work within the same system of cause and effect. We might then presume the following: *The effect of homeopathic remedies follows the same patterns and Laws as are described in AP. These patterns and Laws were documented several thousand years ago in the old book of wisdom*

I Jing (Book of Changes) and the medical *"bible", the Nei Jing (Yellow Emperor's Canon of Internal Medicine).*

After many years of clinical observations and practice, I have found that the most important Laws are the following:

- *Ko Cycle* in The Five Phases (Elements),

- *Qi (Energy) Cycle* in the Chinese Clock and

- *Yin-Yang Cyclical Change.*

When we combine these three rules, we arrive at the following (complicated) rule of action. When we ingest a homeopathic remedy, the succession of the healing effect in the body follows in three distinct ways:

(a) **Every second organ** in the *Qi-Cycle sequence.* For example, if we start in **GB**, the first step is **LU** and the next is **ST** (**GB-LV-LU-LI-ST**), etc. In this, we see that the organ progression is always to opposite polarities

(b) The remedy influences these organs *following the sequence of the Ko-Cycle.* For example, if GB (in the previous example) is influenced in a **"Fire"** way, then **LU** is influenced in a **"Metal"** way and **ST** in a **"Wood"** way.

(c) Alternating *sequential change* from *stimulation* to *sedation.* For example, if GB is stimulated, then LU is sedated, and ST is stimulated.

From these relationships, one can tabulate the remedies to see all the effects of each remedy, and even *predict those still not described.* One can also understand the different species-to-species effects of these remedies (see page 5).

*NOTE: As AP texts describe where to put the needles, in the table below each remedy first influences the organ in its own left hand column as indicated by the font face. **Lower case** means **sedation** and **upper case** means **stimulation.***

If this seems incredibly complicated and impossible to understand, please re-read the previous few paragraphs. It really is quite simple! However, I will show two examples; follow them in the table. The table is constructed with the Five Phases in the horizontal row and the Chinese Qi Clock in the vertical column. We can easily find the next (or following) effect of any homeopathic remedy by going to the second next row (i.e. two organs down in the QI Cycle and two columns to the right (the next Phase in the Ko Cycle).

A *THEORETICAL EXAMPLE:*

If we give APIS, this *stimulates* LV in a *Watery* way, we can expect this effect to show up in LI (two rows down), but here it *sedates.* And its effect will be "Fire"-like. We may say that if we give APIS, then the remedy acts first to stimulate LV Water and then to sedate LI Fire. The effect will cycle according to the Qi Clock, changing from Yin organ to Yang organ, changing from stimulation to sedation and influencing in a way that follows the Phases in the Ko Cycle. For strong remedies, or for the strong acupoints or herbs, this effect continues for several steps; for weaker remedies, the effect continues for only one or two steps.

A *PRACTICAL EXAMPLE:*

(remedies in *lower case letters sedate,* those in *UPPER CASE LETTERS STIMULATE*)
Acon sedates GB Fire Process. (See the table page 546). The next step (two organs down and two Phases to the right) shows that Acon stimulates LU-Metal Process. The next step (two more down and two to the right) shows that Acon then sedates ST Wood Process, etc.

Each remedy is summarised where I think it starts its initial effect, and it travels from there through the body organs, as described above. In order to keep the table brief and more understandable, I have omitted many less important remedies.

Table of the correlation between the most common homeopathic remedies and the Five Phases and the Channels.

	Fire	Earth	Metal	Water	Wood
GB	Aconitum, Ferr.iod, FERR.MET, Crotalus, STRONTIUM, Ptelea tri, Stellaria	SABAL, SANGUIN, FERR.ARS, Vipera, FERR.BROM, Chionanthus, HAEMATOX.	COLOCYNTHIS, Taraxacum, FERR.ACET, Spigelia, Ecbal elat, Eupionum, Paris, MYGALE	CHELID, Rhus.Tox, FERR.MUR, Mandragora, FERR.PHOS, BENZIN, CHENOP.A, EUONYMUS, FERR.PICR, PULEX, Strychnin	FERR.SULPH, SPONGIA, ACONITUM
LV	ARS.ALB, HEP.SULPH, Ipecac, PSORINUM, PULS, Sulphur, Aesculus, ANT.SULPH.A, CHINA, Aethusa, Cinnamon, CLEM.VIT, CYCLAMEN, Cytisus lab, Ginkgo,	Solidago, ZINCUM, ANT.ARS, Agaricus, Hedera, YUCCA, ASARUM.E, Chloroform, Filix, GOSSYPIUM, Merc.Dulc, ONOSMOD, RADIUM, THL.BURS.P	ECHINACEA, EUPHRASIA, Kal.chlor, Anagallis, ANT.TART, Gambogia, Rheum, ARS.SULPH.R, BADIAGA, CALAD.SEG, CLEMATIS, Cornus c, FRAGARIA, Jalapa	APIS, STANNUM, ALOE, PODOPHY, SULPH.IOD, Dulcamara, ARS.IOD, ANT.CRUD, HYDRASTIS, KAL.SULPH, MAG.SULPH, Carduus b, AGAR MUSC, CAULOPHY,	HAMAMELIS, Alumen, NUX.VOM, Kal.ars, Myrica, Juglans, Betonica, DOLICHOS PUR, DUBOISA, GEUM URB
	HELONIAS, Hyoscyamus, INDIUM, CARD.MARI, LAC.DEFL, VISC.ALB			Copaiva, CROCUS SAT, FRAXINUS, GARDENAL, GENISTA, Lactuca, LEPTANDRA, RHODODEN. SSECALE, USTILAGO	

LU	ARNICA, CALC.IOD, CALC.SIL, COCCUS C, CISTUS CAN, INULA HEL.	MERC.SOL, SENEGA, CALC.MUR	CALC.FLUO, CALC.BROM	CALC.PHOS, CARB.ANIM, OPIUM, RUMEX, Ammon.carb, CALC.ARS, ELAPS.COR, ERIODICT, Eugenia j	CALC.CARB, Drosera, CARB.VEG, AMMOM.BE, AMMOM.BR, Ammom.mur, CALC.SULPH, Myrtus, RANUNCULUS
LI	CALENDULA	MANCINELL.	MERC.COR, CICUTA, BERYLL.ME.	EUCALYPT, Lemna min	Cajeput, MICA
ST	CADM.SULPH, Baptisia, Emetinum m.	CONIUM, Lappa, Menyanthes	BROM, Crot.t, BISMUT, ILLICIUM	PHYTOLAC, NAJA, ASPARAGUS,? ASTERIAS	CHRYSAROB, CALTHA PAL, COMOCLAD, Trombidium
SP	CAPSICUM, GENTIANA, IRIS VERS, LITH.CARB, Ricinus, ACID.LACT, CHININ ARS, Cimex lect, Fagopyr, Helianthus, NATR.NITR, SANICULA	CHINA, PLUMBUM, PYROGEN, GNAPHAL, NATR.LACT,	THUJA, NATR.CHLOR, Indigo, ASCLEPIAS	NATR.MUR, ANACARD, CIMICIFUGA, Petroselin, Bellis per, Castoreum, CEANOTHUS, NATR.SALIC, NICCOLUM	Urtica, COLCHICUM, Natr.phos
HT	AURUM MET, DIGITALIS, IBERIS AMA, LAUROCER	AURUM MUR, VERAT.ALB, TRILLIUM	CACTUS, Crataegus, STROPHAN, SCILLA MAR	IGNATIA, AURUM IOD, CONVALL.M, VERAT.VIR, CEREUS B	HYPERICUM, KALMIA, MAGNOLIA, AUR.MUR.N
SI	Euphorbia, Hura bras	DIOSCOREA	Lycopus vir, Cenchris	ARUM TRIP, Caesium met.	CAINCA
BL	ACID.PICR, Borax, Cubeba	GELSEMIUM, SARSAPAR, VERBASCU, CHIMAP.UM, Doryph.dec	Lycopodium, SABADILLA, CANN.SAT, BRUCEA	BERBERIS, Nepenthes, CORTISON, ARISTOLOC, COCA	PRUN.SPIN, Kal.carb, CANN.IND

KI	BRYONIA, Sepia, Rauwolf, MAG.MUR, Coffea, COLCHICUM, BAR.IOD, COBALT, KRESOL, Cyprip.pub, GRATIOLA, Guaiacum, KAL.BROM, Lachnant, LILIUM TIGR, MAG.PHOS, Raphanus, Sabina	PHOSPHOR, Cuprum, MERCURIUS, CUPR.ACET, CUPR.ARS, TABACUM, Bar.carb, CALC.BROM, COCHLEARIA ERYNG.YU ??, EUPATOR.V, EUPATOR.P, EUPATO.PU, PETROLEUM, RATHANHIA	SYMPHYTU, FORMICA, LACHESIS, SAMBUCUS, ASA.FOET, NUX.MOSC, Aquilegia, Bufo rana, Cupr.sulph, DAPHNE IND, Hydrophob, MAG.CARB, MEZEREUM	SELENIUM, ARG.MET, Chamomilla, MEDORRHIN, BAR.MUR, IODOFORM	Cantharis, CAUSTICUM, ACID.PHOS, EQUISETUM, Valeriana, ALL.SATIV, Calc.ars, COCCULUS, HELLEBOR, Jugl.reg, KREOSOTUM, LEDUM, Platinum, SCUTELLARIA, SCENECIO, TEREBINTH
PC	Hedeoma	MUREX, Stramonium, TARENTULA, VIBURNUM	GRINDELIA, SUMBUCUS, Heloderma		STAPHISAG, Moschus, Millefol, MELILOTUS, Carb.sulph
TH	SILICEA, ANT.CRUD, FLOR.DE PI, KAL.MUR, Kal.bichrom, Glonoinium, Merc.Iod flav		Iod, SAMBUCUS, Corall, OLEANDER, GYMNO.CAN, Naphthalin	BELLADON, CINNABAR??, ALUMINA, All.cepa, Asimina t, ERIGERON, HYDROCYT, LUESINUM, LAP.ALBA, Tarent.hisp	Arg.nitr, Graphit, HECLA, MANAGANUM, CHLORAL HY, COLLINS CAN, Euphor.res, TELLURIUM

Table 100

HOMEOPATHY AND (INFECTIOUS) MASTITIS

I started my veterinary career by treating bovine mastitis. My treatment methods had marked effect and the cows that received homeopathic treatment improved more than those that did not. At that time I injected the remedies at a point over the sacrum (near BL28-29). I learned later from Oswald Kothbauer that this area helps mastitis. I did not know that at that time, at least not consciously. Later I also learned from Prof. Pishinger that any injury in the connective tissue activates the immune system. I also learned at a Swiss congress for homeopathic vets that just 5 minutes of attention to the cow lowered the milk cell count by 25% (Jörg Spranger's lectures). The results from their studies were that:

- 12% of all mastitis is cured by antibiotics
- 8% of all mastitis is cured by homeopathy
- caressing the cows for 5 minutes reduced milk cell count by 25%

The conclusion of all this was that:

1. Homeopathy does not kill bacteria.
2. Homeopathy may prevent mastitis when given to healthy cows
3. Homeopathy does not cure acute mastitis

A LIST OF REMEDIES FOR DIFFERENT DISEASES
Symptomatic treatment
Here is a list of the most used remedies and the symptoms that indicate their use. The table on page 546 summarises a very good way of finding symptomatic and causal remedies for any disorder but its use requires knowledge of AP and Five Phase Theory. However, novices will find the following list of symptomatic homeopathic remedies of value:

Organ or part	Symptomatic homeopathic remedy (for novices only)
Abdominal oedema	Apis, Carduus, Kali.carb, Convallaria, Stannum
Achilles tendon	Kali.carb
Arm, Forelimb	Ammon.carb, Silicea, Aluminium,
Arteriosclerosis	Calc.carb.
Axilla	Arnica
Back	Phos, Calc.carb, Kali.carb, Merc.viv
Claws of the cow	Sil, Lach
Bladder	Kali.carb, Berberis
Blood pressure	Kali.carb., Hyssop
Blood sugar	Flor de piedra, Stannum, Lycopodium, Chelidonium
Blood vessels	Hyp, Aurum, Silicea
Bones and joints	Phos, Calc.carb., Berberis, Symphytum, Ruta
Brain	Phos
Bronchi	Ammon.carb., Ant. tart., Aconitum, Bryonia, Ipecacuanha
Circulation	Hyp
Colic	Colocynthis, Phos, Opium, Nux.vom., Chamomilla, Plumbum.acet, Belladonna, Podophyllum
Cough	Ipecac, Cupr.acet, Phos, Drosera, Bryonia
Cramps	Cinch, Sulph, Rhus.tox, Bry, Cuprum
Diarrhoea	Ars.alb, Calc.carb, Nux.vom, Veratrum alb
Ear, hearing	Phos, Causticum
Eye, eyelid, sight	Stannum
Face	Nux.vom., Sil, Phos
Fever	Lach, Pyrogenium, Sil, Belladonna, Echinacea, Acon, Ferr.phos, Bry
First aid	Acon, Arn
Forehead	Sil, Phos
Gallbladder	Ferr.met
Heart	Aurum, Digitalis, Crataegus
Help in the birth process	Puls, Hyp, Stannum, Arnica, Hamamelis, Caulophyllum
Hindlimb	Phos, Stannum, Ars.alb., Nux.vom
Hips	Stannum, Lycopodium, Chelidonium, Colocynthis
Tarsus (Hock)	Ferr, Ferr.ars, Acon

Intestines	Merc, Phos
Jaws	Ferr
Ketosis	Stannum, Chelidonium, Flor de piedra,
Kidney	Phos, Merc
Stifle	Calc.carb, Phos
Leg	Kal.carb, Arn, Hyp
Lips	Arn
Liver	Stannum, Chelidonium
Liver disorders	Lycopodium, Phos, Carduus.mar.
Loss of hair	Phos, Arg
Lumbago	Dulcamara, Bry, Rhus.tox.
Lumbar area	Phos, Kali.carb
Mammary gland	Puls, Arg, Sep, Phytolacca
Masseter muscle	Stannum, Ferr
Mastitis	Lachesis, Arg, Puls, Hepar, Acon, Bry, Chamomilla, Belladonna, Phytolacca, Urtica
Meninges	Phos
Mouth	Aurum, Arn, Plumb
Neck	Plumbum, Stannum
Obstipation (constipation)	Nux.vom., Opium, Chelidonium
Pain in the groin	Stannum
Pain killer	Opium, Rhus.tox.,
Pancreas	Acid.phos
Patella	Nux.vom
Paws	Sil, Echinacea, Hepar
Pleura	Belladonna, Bry
Rectal prolapse	Stannum, Phos, Ruta
Reproduction female	Aurum, Graphites, Bufo, Sepia, Puls
Reproduction male	Aurum, Hyp, Staphisagria, Murex
Sexual organs female	Arg, Sepia, Puls, Lilium tig
Sexual organs male	Aurum, Staphisagria, Puls
Shoulder	Arn
Sinuses	Sil, Aurum, Phos
Skin	Sil, Aluminium, Phos, Ammon.carb, Graphites, Sulphur
Spleen	Ars.alb, Plumbum
Stomach	Ars.alb., Nux.vom
Stomach, lower part	Ferr.met, Phos, Arg.nit
Stomach, middle part	Nux.vom, Ars.alb., Bry
Stomach, upper part	Sil, Carbo.veg.,

Tendons	Stannum
Throat	Sil, Hepar, Cinnabar (or Zinnober)
Tongue	Aurum
Trachea	Arn, Ammon.carb
Under arm	Tarentula, Alumina, Sil
Upper jaw	Nux.vom
Ureter	Berberis, Arg, Hyp
Vomiting	Ipecac
Weakness after parturition	Stannum, Phos, Kali phos
Wound infection	Hepar, Sil
Wounds with hemorrhage	Arn, Hyp, Millefolium

Table 101

At the end of this chapter, I will label some very interesting information which **Dr. Chris. Day DVM** has kindly and generously given me to use as an appendix to this chapter.

For the heart:
Lachesis, Belladonna, Hyoscyamus, Coffea, Crocus, Causticum, Cannabis indica, Cocaine, Stramonium, Veratrum album, Strophanthus.

For the liver:
Nux vomica, Lycopodium, Chelidonium, Phosphorus, Antimonium crudum, Anacardium, Carduus, Berberis.

For the lungs:
Tabacum, Calc. carb., Arsenicum, Nat. mur., Pulsatilla, Ipecac, Lobelia.

For the kidneys:
Aconitum, Arsenicum, Pulsatilla, Stramonium, Phos., Lil. tig., Argent. nit., Lycopodium, Causticum, Gelsemium.

For the spleen:
Carbo veg., Æsculus, Pæonia, Hamamelis, Ginkgo, Crotalus, Hamamelis, Muriatic acid, Natrum mur.

For External Pernicious Influences:

<u>Wind:</u> *Aconite, Lycopodium, Tub. bov., Rhododendron, Euphrasia, Hepar sulph., Nux mosch., Badiaga, Sepia.*

<u>Cold:</u> *Aconite, Badiaga, Tub. bov., Camphora, Causticum, Nux vom., Kali carb., Psorinum.*

<u>Dampness:</u> *Rhus tox., Dulcamara, Nat. sulph., Aranea, Gelsemium, Calc. phos., Colchicum, Phytolacca, Elateria, Guaiacum, Asterias, Baptisia, Thuja.*

<u>Heat/Fire:</u> *Glonoinium, Belladonna, Sulphur, Graphites, Bryonia, Ledum, Antimonium crudum., Pulsatilla, Drosera.*

<u>Dryness/Summer Heat:</u> (less easy to define) *Glonoinium, Belladonna, Nat. carb., Gelsemium, Podophyllum, Nat. mur., Bryonia, Aconitum, Lachesis.*

For the Meridians:

<u>Triple Heater:</u>   <u>Chest</u>: *Aconite, Phellandrium, Aspidosperma*
    <u>Abdomen</u>: *Lycopodium, Carbo veg.*
    <u>Pelvis</u>: *Sepia, Pulsatilla, Helonias*

<u>Heart</u>: *Digitalis, Strophanthus, Convallaria, <u>Cactus</u>, Glonoinium, Lil. tig., Spigelia*

<u>Lung</u>: *Phellandrium* .

<u>Liver</u>: *Chelidonium, Berberis.*

<u>Gallbladder</u>: *Berberis, Rhus tox., Gnaphallium, Phytolacca, Kali bich.* (tearing pains in tibia too), *Kali. carb.* (pain in knee too, recorded as pain in side of knee!), *Colocynth.*

FOR THE DIFFERENT KINDS OF PAIN:

Quality of pain	TCM interpretation	Homœopathic medicine
Ameliorated by heat	Cold	*Arsenicum, Causticum, Rhus tox.*
Ameliorated by cold	Heat	*Apis, Bryonia, Iodum, Pulsatilla., Sulphur*
Ameliorated by touch or pressure	Deficiency	*Bryonia, Colocynth, Pulsatilla, Thuja*
Aggravated by touch or pressure	Excess	*Apis, Bell., Hep. sulph., Lach., Lyc., Merc*
Ameliorated after eating	Deficiency	*Iodum, Phosphorus, Sepia*

Aggravated after eating	Excess	*Aloe, Lycopodium, Nux vom., Sulphur*
Ameliorated in humid weather	Dryness	*Causticum, Kali carb., Nux vom.*
Aggravated in humid weather	Dampness	*Aranea, Calc. phos., Nat. sulph., Rhus, Thuja*
With bloating or sense of fullness	Stagnant Qi	*Carbo veg., Lycopodium, Sepia, Sulphur*
Sharp and usually fixed location	Congested blood	*Aconitum, Bryonia, Hepar sulph., Nitric acid*
Sensation of heaviness	Dampness	*Gelsemium, Nat. mur., Petroleum, Sepia*
Moves from place to place	Wind or stagnant Qi	*Cauloph, Lac caninum, Pulsatilla*
Slight, with fatigue	Deficient Qi or dampness	*Conium, Gelsemium, Sepia, Silica*

Table 102

For the single acupuncture points:

Aconitum	PC6, HT7, GV26 (pain in left fore SI3)
Æsculus	BL26, BL14 (laminitis e.g.)
Apis (Nat. Mur.)	ST6, LI19, BL2, GV25
Aristolochia	CV1, BL23, BL31, SP6
Belladonna (laminitis)	SI3, TH5, LI11, BL2,
Belladonna (meningitis)	BL2, BL8, BL10, SI3 (spastic)
Bellis	GB30, GB26, GB34
Berberis	BL11
Berberis (liver & kidney	BL18, BL23
Bryonia	BL11, GB34, TH5, BL40
Chelidonium	BL18
Coffea/ Chamomilla	GV26, BL60 (& +ve Shu points)
Colchicum (autumnal arthritis)	GB34, BL11, BL60
Colchicum (frothy bloat)	TH15, Shu points
Colocynth (crampy colic)	SI3, LIV13
Colocynth (hip pain)	GB30
Digitalis & Cratægus	CV14, HT5, HT7, BL14, PC06, BL23/28
Equisetum	BL28, BL23, BL22

Flor de piedra	KI8, SP6, BL26
Formic Acid	BL26, BL40, BL60, GB30, BL11
Ginkgo biloba (laminitis)	KI8/SP6, SI2, TH5, LI11, BL18
Glonoinium (heat stroke)	GV26, BL40, PC6, GV14
Gnaphallium (sciatic pain)	BL40, GB32, BL60, GB30, BL31-35
Graphites (skin/wounds)	BL40, LI4, LI11, ST36
Graphites (limb pain)	BL26-31
Graphites (laminitis)	BL18
Gunpowder (osteomyelitis)	BL11, LI11
Harpagophytum	BL11
Hepar sulph.	LI11, GV14
Kali carb. (weakness)	BL26, BL31
Kali carb. (lumbar pain)	BL24-25
Kali chlor. (chronic kidney)	BL23
Ledum (arthritis)	BL11, GB34, TH5, BL60
Mag. phos. (pain/colic)	SP6, KI8, BL40, LI14
Merc. corr. (acute kidney)	BL23
Nat. phos. / Nux vom. (Setfast	GB34, BL40, KI6, LI4, BL13, SI3
Nux vom.	BL18, LI4
Passiflora/Scutellaria/Valeriana	GV26, GV20, GV25
Phellandrium	BL13, LU1
Rhus tox.	TH15, BL11, TH5, GB34
Ruta grav.	BL11, GV14, BL60, + Shu points
Sarsaparilla (laminitis)	TH5, LI11, BL18
Sarsaparilla (kidney)	BL23, BL28
Solidago	BL23, BL28
Symphytum	BL11
Thuja (vaccine/sarcoids)	LI11, GV26, GV14
Thuja (tonsils)	LI14
Thuja (headshakers)	LI11, LI19, BL2, GB34, ST6
Thuja (skin)	BL40, LI4, LI11, ST36
Thuja (glands)	LI4, LI11, TH5, TH17, ST6

Chapter 6

HERBAL THERAPY

Herbal therapy is one of the oldest forms of therapy; it has been used for millennia. Many of the traditions and the knowledge that we had in Europe were lost during the dark age of the Inquisition. Today we are rediscovering and applying the knowledge clinically to a great degree, especially in Germany and in France. It is most important to regain this knowledge, as foreign (especially Chinese) herbs are being used more and more.

By herbal therapy we mean the administration of effective medicinal herbs. They are given according to the same thinking process – the same philosophy – as any other holistic therapy. Their purpose is to influence, stimulate or subdue specific Processes in the body. They are not given as a part of the diet in the usual sense.

Administration of specific plant-derived extracts or medicinal substances, for example digoxin, is not herbal therapy; it is conventional medicine. The given substance acts alone, not in the same way as the whole plant. In contrast, when we give the whole plant, the effect is different than if we gave the single substance, even if this substance is the main active ingredient. The effect of a plant is holistic and the action is *regulatory* in the organism. Like AP or homeopathy, it stimulates holistically the autoregulation mechanisms of the body. Then the effect is greater, more complete and lasts longer. This effect seems to be somewhat like AP, for example stimulating or sedating the specific organ systems.

Herbs with potent effects have toxic potential if overused, or used wrongly. They often taste foul or strong, or have other special traits. Therapeutic herbs usually contain volatile (aromatic) oils. These herbs can be given as a complete plant or in extract. I have experimented with extracts from the volatile (aromatic) oils from different herbs; the oils function well. I usually administer drops of the volatile (aromatic) oils on a sugar cube. Most animals, especially large animals, will eat this. Generally, a dose for a horse or a cow is one small handful of crude herb daily. The dose for small animals (for example, dogs and cats) is 1-2 pinches of the herb. The dose of extract (tincture) or volatile oil is 1-5 drops for small animals and 20-50 drops for cows and horses. [In homeopathic and herbal dosage, 1 ml = 20 drops].

Eastern herbs

Herbal medicine has been an essential part of Asian medicine for several millennia. It has very highly developed documentation, which spans more than 3000 years. It was, and still is, thought to be more important than AP. Herbal combinations, single herbs and extracts have been used for most illnesses. A high proportion of Eastern medicinal herbs are unknown in the West. However, using the general diagnostic methods of AP, those who are interested may consult the listings given below that I have tried to compose. Most of the information listed here was given by **Dr. Cheryl Schwartz DVM** at a seminar she held for Scandinavian veterinairians in Oslo in 1998. She has been using these herbs in small animal practise for several years, and her knowledge is considerable.

Myself, I have been using mostly European herbs, and I will list those afterwards, in the next section of this chapter.

Usually Chinese herbs are listed after a diagnosis based on the "Eight Principles", a diagnostic method which I do not use or like at all. I will therefore try to list the herbs after a "Process Diagnosis", which we are used to in this book. The Chinese herbs may need to support any AP treatment. These herbs must be ordered from the East or from wholesale businesses in the West.

HERBS FOR THE SPLEEN

- Ginseng

- Atractylodes

- Hoelen

- Licorice

- Tang Kuei

- Cimicifuga

- Citrus (Chen Pi)

- Bupleurum

- Oak Bark

- Dioscorea Combination

These herbs can be used for gastrointestinal weakness, including poor appetite, weight loss, slow recovery after illness, borborygmous, fatigue, weakness of the limbs and tendency for prolapses.

Ginseng - warms and circulates the Qi, stimulating appetite.

Atractylodes and Hoelen - strengthen the transforming process of the Spleen.

Licorice - acts as a harmonizer between the Liver and the Spleen.

Tang Kuei - nourish blood of Spleen and Liver

Cimicifuga - lift the Qi, relieve prolapses

Citrus (Chen Pi) - regulate, circulate Qi

Bupleurum - smoothes Liver Qi and harmonizes with Spleen, upward and outward moving.

Oak Bark - is an astringent herb aiding the Spleen Yang. It restores integrity to intestinal cells, as well as the cells of the capillary beds and veins. The active ingredients are tannin and quercin.

Dioscorea Combination - a traditional Chinese folk remedy that strengthens Spleen Qi and Yang, drains Dampness. (It contains: Dioscorea, Eurale, Coix, Lotus Seed, Hoelen to drain dampness, and to astringe mucous membranes. These herbs are neutral, sweet or bland.)

HERBS FOR THE STOMACH

- Healthy Peaceful Pills

- Chamomilla

Healthy Peaceful Pills (Also available as McZand tincture "Curing Formula" (It contains: Gastrodia Elata and Angelica for wind dispelling, headache, Chrysanthemum, Mentha, Pueraria and Tricosanthes to reduce fever or feverish feeling, Atractylodes, Coix, Hoelen to drain dampness

Saussarea, magnolia, red tangerine peel (pericarpium citri erythrocarpae) and agastanche to regulate Qi and remove stagnation, Oryza sativa to disperse food accumulation

Chamomilla is the "baby remedy", the remedy for babies of any age." Peevish, whining, complaining, demanding attention, low pain tolerance, wanting to be carried, but not wanting to be picked up. Camomile calms nervousness (calms shen). It harmonizes between the liver and the stomach by releasing liver tension and allowing the Qi to run smoothly. This removes the "attack of the liver on the stomach" and any pain that might be associated with vomiting, stomach aches or ulcers. Camomile cools the stomach and decreases acidity.

Herbs for the Lung

- Asclepius asperula (Immortal)

- Milkweed

- Er Chen Wan

- Limpid Sea

- Longevity formula + Lavender

- Ma Huang & Morus

- Ma Huang & Ginkgo

- Platycodon & Fritillaria combination (Qing Fei Tang)

- Elecampane + Mullein + Coltsfoot

Immortal is used as a Lung Qi tonic and to dry Phlegm dampness. It specifically acts as a bronchodilator in cases of bronchitis or bronchial asthma. It helps to expel Phlegm from the lungs. Since it has both warming and cooling potential, the Phlegm can be sticky and clear or milky white or yellow.

It is also helpful with Liver Qi Constraint and Stagnation, where there is pain around the rib cage and anxiety around breathing.

N.B. Contraindicated during pregnancy, as it is a uterine stimulant.

Milkweed This is a bitter, neutral herb that has both warming and cooling potential. It serves the Lung, Heart, Kidney Yang and Conception Vessel meridians.

It has a huge root, with milky juicy pith. The roots resemble lymphatics or fine capillaries. Immortal is good in increasing circulation, especially of the smaller vessels. It is also an excellent lymph drainer.

Er Chen Wan "Two Aged Decoction". Available as a patent herb, extract granules (called Citrus & Pinellia) or liquid (McZand). This is the classic formula for Stomach and/or Lung Phlegm Damp Cold. (Contains: Pinellia (Ban Xia) – Citrus (Chen Pi) – Hoelen (Fu Ling) – Licorice and Ginger).

Limpid Sea (Three Treasures, Maciocia line). This is a variation of Er Chen Wan with the addition of Bamboo to reduce coughing and Mume to avoid dryness of the Lung during long-term use.

Longevity Formula + Lavender, "Eight Immortals Long Life Pill" for deficiency of Lung Yin and Kidney Yin. Lavender is a Qi regulator and help the herbs circulate. [Contains: Rehmannia – Ophiopogon (Mai Men Dong) – Schizandra (Wu Wei Zi) (Astringent) - Cornus (Shan Zhu Yu) (Astringent, Tonify Kidney) - Dioscorea (Shan Yao) – Hoelen (Fu Ling), Alisma (Ze Xie) – Moutan (Mu Dan Pi)].

Ma Huang & Morus   Utilizes Ma Huang which contains ephedrine, pseudo-ephedrine and related alkaloids and is a mild CNS stimulant. Ma-Huang is effective where wheezing is prominent, especially when breathing is worse on exhalation. (Some cats appear to be sensitive to Ma-Huang, showing signs of extreme lethargy, anxiety or increased heart rate. This might be similar to reactions some cats have to valium or aminophylline. Part of the reaction to Ma Huang might be due to an underlying Kidney Yin Deficiency, as Ma Huang has a drying effect, and it might be possible to add a small amount of Yin or Blood Tonic to counter these effects. I suggest that any administration of Ma Huang be first tested on the animal by giving small doses of the formula on a trial basis.) [Contains: Ma Huang – Hoelen – Apricot Seed - Perilla Fruit - Morus Bark (antitussive) - Licorice – Citrus (Chen Pi)].

Ma Huang & Ginkgo: This formula is used when the animal shows more heat signs, such as having a very large thirst. [Contains: Ma Huang - Apricot Seed - Perilla fruit – Tussilago - Morus bark (anti-tussive) - Licorice – Scute – Gingko].

Platycodon & Fritillaria combination (Qing Fei Tang) is especially suited for lung inflammation [Contains: Bamboo – Fritillara – Platycodon – Scute – Gardenia – Morus - Apricot Seed – Citrus - Hoelen – Schizandra – (astringent for Lung) – Ophiopogon - Asparagus - Tang Kuei – Ginger - Jujube and Licorice].

Elecampane + Mullein + Coltsfoot are also in this combination especially suited for treating Lung inflammation.

HERBS FOR THE KIDNEYS

- Rehmannia Six a.k.a. Six Flavor Tea (Liu Wei Di Huang Wan)

- Borage (Borago officinale)

- Alfalfa (Medicago sativa)

- Rehmannia Eight Combination

- Lycium Formula – Huan Shao Dan

- Gravel Root (Queen of the Meadow, Joe Pye Weed)

- Eupatorium Purpureum.

- Cleavers (Galium aparine)

- Polyporus Combination

- Rehmannia & Akebia

Rehmannia Six a.k.a Six Flavor Tea -- Liu Wei Di Huang Wan [Contains:
Rehmannia (cooked – Di Huang) (decreases blood pressure and Cholesterol, high in potassium - Cornus (Shan Zhu Yu) (astringent, decreases blood pressure, high potassium) - Dioscorea (Shan Yao) (tonifies Spleen) - Moutan (Mu Dan Pi) - Hoelen (Fu Ling) – Alisma (Ze Xie)].

Borage (Borago officinale) The leaf is used. It is cold, moist, and salty and strengthens Lung and Kidney.

Alfalfa (Medicago sativa) The whole plant is used. It is neutral, moist and contains eight digestive enzymes.

Rehmannia Eight Combination, a/k/a Sexoton Pills or Golden Book Tea. This is the Rehmannia Six formula with the addition of warming herbs of processed Aconite and Cinnamon (note: Aconite and Cinnamon may cause vomiting in cats).

Lycium Formula – Huan Shao Dan – Elixer for Returning the Lost:[Contains: Rehmannia – Cornus - Lycium (Gou Qi Zi) – Eucommia – Morinda – Cistanche - Achyranthes (Niu Xi) – Fennel – Dioscorea - Jujube - Schizandra – Hoelen – Polygala).

Gravel Root (Queen of the Meadow, Joe Pye Weed)

Eupatorium Purpureum. Eupatorium Purpureum adjusts the balance of waters and solids in the urinary tract. Gravel Root can bring minerals out of solution or bring them back in. This makes it good for sand and gravel formation in the tract. Its purple flower and stem are the signature for septic states, and tissue breakdown. Gravel Root helps with lumbar pain and painful micturition. It is also helpful with prostate problems. Gravel Root acts to keep the solids and fluids in balance. "The folk doctors held that Gravel Root dissolved calculi, while the professional doctors claimed that it merely helped remove them." Gravel Root promotes urination and soothes irritation, "especially in cases of reddish and reddish brown urine where there is a deposit of reddish sand."

Cleavers (Galium aparine). It softens stones and activates the lymphatics, especially of the lower body, clearing toxins and promoting their outward flow through lymph and urine. It is also helpful in prostate irritation. (Contains chlorophyll, saponins, tannins and trace minerals).

Polyporus Combination - A Chinese herb combination for dysuria or stranguria with painful urination, urethritis, cystitis, hematuria, painful distended lower abdomen. (Contains: Polyporus (Zhu Ling) - Alisma (Ze Xie) - Talc (Hua Shi) - Gelatin – Hoelen).

Rehmannia & Akebia. Freeze dried granules that address the imbalance between the Kidney Yin and Heart. Clears heat in Small Intestine and heart. (Contains: Rehmannia – Lophatherum – Bland Bamboo leaves - Akebia – Licorice).

Herbs for the muscles

- Du Hu Ji Sheng Wan
- Brocade Sinews
- Nourish the Root and Clear Wind

- Dipsacus sylvestris

- Kang Gu Zheng Sheng Pian (Combat Bone Hyperplasia Pill)

Du Hu Ji Sheng Wan – helpful in arthritis that is worse in damp and cold with stiffness, sciatica and weakness of the hind legs. The condition usually improves with pressure and massage. (Contains: Eucommia – Rehmannia – loranthus - tang kuei – Codonopsis – ginger - cinnamon bark - licorice - Du Huo - Loranthus and Hoelen).

Brocade Sinews - a Macioca formula. (Contains: Codonopsis - Tang Kuei – Coix – Peony – Lycium – Loranthus – Atractylodes – Hoelen – Acanthpanacis – Chaenomelis - Morus bark – Clematis).

Nourish the Root and Clear Wind - a Macioca formula. (Contains Clematis & Stephania Combination).

Dipsacus sylvestris (Teasel) - a member of the thistle family, this herb has an affinity for the bones. It is used for joint injury. Its Chinese cousin, Dipsacus japonica is called "Restore what is Broken" and is used for trauma to the joint and tendons. Teasel promotes circulation and unblocks stagnation, relieving pain and stiffness. It is especially suited for excess individuals who injure themselves with great force behind it. Large muscle groups are affected: shoulders, low back.

Kang Gu Zheng Sheng Pian (Combat Bone Hyperplasia Pill). This formula is good for spinal inflammation and intervertebral disc syndrome, both acute and chronic and as a preventative for recurrence in adjoining areas. (Contains: Rehmannia – Dioscorea – Erodium - Pyrola – Hedera – Liquid amber – Tokoro – Cistanches - Tiger bone (I believe it is cow bone) to strengthen Bones and Yang.

HERBS FOR THE SKIN

- Ho Shou Wu, Shou Wu Pian

- Tang Kuei & Tribulus

- Tang Kuei & Gardenia

Ho Shou Wu, Shou Wu Pian polygonum multiflori, is from the rose family, a cooling Liver Blood Tonic. They help with luster-less coats, small dry eruptions, some forms of miliary dermatitis in cats.

Tang Kuei & Tribulus - a granular herb combination. (Contains: Tang Kuei – Peony - Ho Shu Wu – Siler - Tribulus – Astragalus).

Tang Kuei & Gardenia. (Contains: Tang Kuei – Cnidium – Peony – Rehmannia – Coptis – Scute – Phellodendron – Gardenia).

HERBS FOR THE IMMUNE SYSTEM

- Radix Isatidis
- Enhance
- Red Clover
- Astragalus membranaceus
- Astragalus 10
- Mellitia nitida

Radix Isatidis. One of the major ingredients used for treating HIV, EBV and chronic colitis (Krohn's disease). In veterinary medicine we can use it in formulas to treat acute upper respiratory infections, acute and chronic ulcerative colitis, infections during and after chemotherapy and for active infections with FIV and FeLV cats, especially those with fevers.

Enhance (Health Concerns). This is a combination product to stimulate immunity and guard against infection. Contains Yang tonics to invigorate the Blood with Heat clearing herbs to fight infection. It is useful in Lymphoma in dogs and FIV, FeLV cats.

Red Clover – Trifolium Pratense, the flowers of this plant are used. Red clover is good for single encysted lymph node enlargements, especially of the neck, axilla and mammary gland. *Astragalus membranaceus* (Huang Qi). This is a herb that modulates the immune system. It is a member of the leguminosae family and has a long fibrous root that is cooked and sliced diagonally. Astragalus is sweet, slightly warm and slightly moist and serves the Spleen and Lung. It is a Qi tonic, to strengthen after illness, by increasing stamina, stabilizing the exterior by strengthening the Wei Qi, increasing digestive absorption, decreasing thirst, enhancing urination, enhancing blood production and circulation, decreasing platelet aggregation and dilated blood vessels.

Astragalus contains flavones, which are most likely responsible for increasing circulation. Astragalus also contains polysaccarides and in human trials, it appears to increase survival rates in cancer patients after chemo or radiation therapy by increasing IgA and IgG.

Astragalus 10 (ITM/Seven Forests, Health Concerns) ASTRA 8 (Contains: Astraglus – Ganoderma - Eleutrhero Ginseng – Atractylodes – Codonopsis – Licorice - Ligustrum - Schizandra - Ginseng (red) - Ophiopogon -and Morus fruit).

Mellitia nitida is a member of the Leguminosa family and contains miletol aclohol. This herb is good in combination with other Blood tonics and Astragalus to increase platelet counts and in cases of leukopenia.

Western herbs

Westerners usually are more familiar with, and interested in, Western herbs, because we can pick many ourselves, or buy what we need in a herbal pharmacy. Herbs bought commercially include dried herbs, alcoholic extracts (10% tincture) or oil extracts. As we discussed in the description of the homeopathic remedies, in herbal presentations we ought to see the herbs in a broader energetic perspective also. Medicinal herbs influence bodily Processes and should be understood in relationship to these. Therefore, the descriptions of the different bodily Processes are included in the description of some of the herbs, so that readers can see the Processes that they influence.

For example, if we see below that dandelion stimulates LV, this means that it influences all the previously described Processes concerning the TCM and western Functions and pathological expressions of the liver.

Herb	Action
Achillea millefolium L	Yarrow stimulates LV in a similar way to dandelion. It also can be used for immunomediated disorders, such as colds, chronic bronchitis and diarrhoea.
Arctostaphylos alpina L	Bearberry has a special disinfecting effect on the Water Processes (KI and BL Channel). It helps infections of the lower urinary tract (lower ureteritis, cystitis and urethritis). It cannot be used for renal infection (nephritis). The dose is from one teaspoon for small animals, up to a handful for big animals three times a day for 14 days. In addition to mulberry, you can successfully use Equisetum arvense and Chamomilla. These plants influence BL.
Arnica montana	Arnica is one of the best healing plants, and the tincture may be used in all kinds of trauma where the skin is not broken. That is, where the body fluids do not flow out of the body.
Berberis vulgaris L	Barberry stimulates GB and biliary secretion and helps those who suffer from LV disorders, gallstones and hepatitis.
Betula verrucosa	Birch leaf extract strongly stimulates KI and increases urinary excretion. Considering that KI also relates to dry eczema, extracts from the bark help chronic dry eczema.
Calendula officinale L	Marigold helps non-healing wounds. Mostly it is used as a 10% tincture or as an ointment but it can also be used as a fresh or dried herb directly on the wound. Flowers from this herb are used directly in salads and other food.
Cetraria Islandica	Icelandic moss contains large amounts of starch and loosens up the mucus and is a laxative. It helps coughs and colds and has its effect via LI Channel. This plant is also used as food and animal feed.

Echinacea	(Echinacea purpurea L.) Has been mentioned several times in this book. It is one of the plants, which has the most potent immune stimulating effect. For allergies, eczema and chronic infections related to immunity, one can give a handful of the dried root daily for a horse, or a couple of pinches for a dog for one to two months. It stimulates the immune system. Together with other therapy, it is possible to heal chronic infections and allergies.
Equisetum arvense L	Horsetail has a very high content of silica and has a similar effect as silicea (homeopathic medicament). It has a stimulating effect on KI and BL function. It also has a stimulating effect on the metabolism, similar to TH Point (Channel). The herb must be boiled for 10 minutes to allow the silica to be released. There are very few herbs that must be boiled in order to work – Equisetum Arvense is one of these. It is used over a long period of time without any significant damage.
Gentiana purpurea L	Gentian stimulates the appetite. It helps all sorts of ST disorders as a powder, extract or tincture. It influences LV and ST.
Humulus lupulus L	Hops are vines that grow year after year. Extract from the fresh shoots (buds) is being used as a sedative for anxiety and nervousness. This herb had its main effect on KI.
Hypericum perforatum L	St. John`s Wort has a good effect on blood circulation. It relieves the pain and contracts wounds. Rubbing it into scars increases blood circulation, counteracts blockages and reduces the formation of keloids. It mainly influences HT Channel.
Juniperus, Picea and Pinus	Juniper, spruce and pine contain strong volatile (aromatic) oils. They can be boiled in hot water and the steam can be inhaled for colds, bronchitis and throat infections. The oil is used in rubs to help rheumatic and sore muscles.
Matricaria chamomilla L	Chamomilla contains volatile (aromatic) oil, which can be bought and used separately. The plant sedates KI but should not be used for more than 14 days, as it has a relatively strong effect on KI.

Menyanthes trifoliata L	Buckbean has a similar effect to red beetroot. It increases the appetite and stimulates LV and GB. It is particularly effective for belching, borborygmus, flatus and other gastrointestinal disorders.
Petasites ovatus H (hybridus L)	Coltsfoot is an old medicine plant that sedates coughs and dissolves mucus. It helps throat infections, asthma and bronchitis. The effect works via LU and SI Process.
Plantago major L	Plantain is a plant that has been used since ancient times as a bandage for chronic non-healing wounds. It is used as whole leaves under a bandage, or as an ointment, or crushed.
Prunus padus L	Buckthorn is an excellent laxative. Its bark is used for tea. The laxative does not irritate the mucous membrane of ST. One teaspoon of bark is added to a cup of cold water and brought to boil. It should be drunk in the evening and used for not >14 days.
Pulmonaria officinale L	I have used Lungwort especially for horses with many lung disorders. Chronic lung disorders, lung bleeders, retention of mucus, cough and fatigue often respond. A small handful is given daily for 1 month.
Quercus robur L	Oak contains tannic acid in its bark, so finely ground oak-bark is very good for diarrhea. Powdered oak-bark has an astringent effect and can thus be used for intestinal hemorrhage.
Symphytum officinale L	Comfrey is a most important plant to stimulate LV. It stimulates the healing process of broken bones and all kinds of wounds. In Norwegian it is called the plant of the battle ground, as it is said to heal all wounds from the battle ground. This plant is used frequently in Africa and is said to halve the healing time of bone fractures. This plant is, in my opinion, the most important healing plant there is. The tincture, put on wounds or fractures, reduces the healing time by 50%. As the plant has a strong effect on the liver process, overuse of this remedy may induce cancer, and the plant is thus said to be cancerous. It must then only be used externally, and internally only in Liver Deficiency and over no more than 14 days.

Taraxacum officinale	Dandelion is a most important plant to stimulate LV. The fresh leaves can be given as animal feed in the springtime. During the summer and fall one can make tea from the leaves.
Tussilago farfara L	This plant may be used especially in long-standing coughs.
Urtica dioeca L	Most people know Urtica urens, the common stinging nettle plant. It has a high iron level. Urtica dioeca is a relative. Nettles are great stimulants for LV and Blood. It can be taken as a tea, or as a green vegetable, chopped into mashed potato or stews.
Vaccinium myrtillus L and Vaccinium vitis idaea L	Blueberry and cranberry leaves help diarrhea, infections in the urinary tracts, gout and rheumatism. It mainly stimulates LV-GB.
Valeriana officinale L	Valerian is a sedative except for cats, which, contrary to all other animals, are stimulated by this plant. For restlessness at night, one should give valerian extract, or as a tea at night. It has a sedative effect on KI.

Table 103

FIVE SAMPLES HERB RECIPES.

The equine dose is the whole amount, given over 1 week. In all, 4 times the amount are given over 4 weeks and a cure usually takes 4 weeks. The human dose is the whole amount, but given over 6 weeks, which is the length of the cure in humans. The canine dose is in proportion to human bodyweight, and the length of cure is 6 weeks also.

The first recipe stimulates blood circulation, the second SP-ST, the third and fourth LU-LI, the fifth KI and the last LV.

To stimulate Fire (HT-PC) and blood circulation	Hypericum perf.	200g
	Capsella bursa pastoris	100g
	Betula verr.	100g
	Crataegus mon.	100g
	Cytisus scop.	50g
	Liquorice root	30g
	Ginger root	15g
	Convallaria herba	15g
	Digitalis purpurea	15g
To stimulate Earth (SP-ST)	Echinacea	100g
	Calendula	100g
	Viscum album	100g
	Agrimonia eup.	80g
	Rhamus Frangulae	80g
	Gentiana lutea	30g
	Liquorice root	30g
	Chelidonium maj.	30g
	Cortex Quercus	20g
To stimulate Metal (LU-LI): little recipe	Pulmonaria officinalis	100g
	Achillea mill.	90g
	Tussilago farfara	80g
	Arnica montana	80g
	Hedera helix	50g
	Ipecacuanha	50g
	Liquorice root	40g
To stimulate Metal (LU-LI): extended recipe	Cetraria islandica	200g
	Pulmonaria officinalis	100g
	Hypericum perf.	100g
	Achillea mill.	90g
	Thyme	90g
	Tussilago farfara	80g
	Arnica montana	80g
	Hedera helix	50g
	Ipecacuanha	50g
	Liquorice root	40g
	Aniseed	20g
	Fennicel-seed	20g
	Caraway seed	15g

To stimulate Water (KI-BL)	Betula verr.	100g
	Alchemilla vulg.	100g
	A. Uva Ursi	100g
	Rhamus frangulae	100g
	Veronica off.	80g
	Hummulus lup.	50g
	Valeriana off.	50g
	Chamomilla	50g
	Juniper com. fruit	40g
	Liquorice root	30g
To stimulate Wood (LV-GB)	Lycopodium ann.	100g
	Taraxacum off.	100g
	Pulmonaria off.	100g
	Polypodium vulg.	80g
	Hyssop	80g
	Plantago	80g
	Urtica dioica	50g
	Berberis vulg.	40g
	Chelidonium maj.	30g
	Liquorice root	30g
	Ginger root	20g

Table 104

The herbal compositions of Gerhard Rodal

Gerhard Rodal was a famous therapist using herbs. He lived in Sandefjord, Norway. He used the following compositions, and they had a very good effect in patients.

In traumas;
Fol. Rosmarin + Herb. Arnica + Fol. Urtica urens + Cort. Frangulae

In circulatory problems;
Viscum album + Frukt. Crataegus

In stomach problems;
Cort. China succ. + Fruct. Auranti imm. + Gummi Myrrhae + Pulv. Aloe succ. + Rad. Gentiana lut.

In geriatrics;
Fruct. Crataegus fol. + Avena sat. + Herb. Cactus gr.

In lung problems;
Herb. Drosera rot. + Herb. Hedera helix + Herb. Ipecac.

In coughing;
Herba capsella Bursa pastoris + Herba Cochlearia

In psyological problems;
Fol. Melissa off. + Rad. Valeriana off.

In kidney problems;
Herb. Solidago virg. + Fol. Potentilla ans. + Fol. Betula + Herb Poligonium ans. + Rad. Ononis sp. + Herb. Viola tric. + herb. Equisetum arv. + Fruct. Juniper com.

In pain;
Herb. Mentha pip. + Flos Lavendula spica + Herb. Hypericum perf.

HERBAL OINTMENTS

Most of the herbs that have been mentioned here can also be bought as ointments. The most frequently used ointments are:

- Arnica ointment and Hypericum ointment helps bruises and injuries.

- Majorana / Melissa ointment for KI-related eczema

- Graphites ointment helps SP-related eczema

- Calendula ointment helps wounds heal

- Honey, beeswax and propolis ointments help wounds and eczema

If the cause of the disorder is External (wounds or injuries, non-healing wounds, or reactions to External causes), I find it completely legitimate to use these ointments. But if the cause of the disorder is Internal, use of these ointments would be just symptom suppressive. We can certainly do this as well, provided that we also treat the cause itself. The cause can also be treated with ointments.

- If the eczema is due to LV imbalance, applying Stannum, Chelidonium or Taraxacum ointment over LV can treat it.

- If KI is the cause, we can apply Cuprum or Argentum ointment over the renal area. Infants having colic due to KI Deficiency, often respond well to a 0.4% copper ointment over the renal area.

VOLATILE (AROMATIC) OILS

In addition to the herbs, which we have mentioned here, there are several extracts of foreign plants rich in volatile (aromatic) oils. These oils can be bought in the pharmacy. For dogs and smaller animals, the dose for these are one drop daily, for cow and horse it is 5-6 drops daily. One may use these oils in ointments for application over the organ to be influenced. I have been using these oils with success for many years and I have systematised them according to which points (Channels) they influence.

Volatile (aromatic) oil	Has an affinity for, influences, stimulates or helps the Processes of
Myrrh	LU
Basilicum and Bergamot	LI
Cardamom, pepper and gentian	ST
Majorana and cypress	SP
Hypericum, rose	HT, PC
Salvia (sage)	SI
??	BL
Jasmine and melisse	KI
Neroli	TH
Pennyroyal	GB
Juniper, finical, cypress, chamfer and lavender and several other plants	LV
Hyssop	Very effective for high blood pressure related to LV and SP

Table 105

One may combine these oils successfully with AP in order to give further stimulation to the Weak Process.

Chapter 7

OSTEOPATHY, CHIROPRACTICS AND CRANIO-SACRAL THERAPY

These methods arose from older forms of "bone setting". Dr. Andrew Taylor Still (1828-1917), who was inspired by the great homeopath Dr. James T. Kent, was the main pioneer of osteopathy. He also learned a lot from his father (who treated many American Indians) and from Indian Medicine Men (shamans). Dr. Still had many students. The most famous were J.M. Littlejohn, who brought osteopathy to Europe, and Jim Atkinson, who wrote the principles of Chiropractic, and D.D. Palmer (1845-1913), who is considered to be the father of chiropractic. Osteopathy and chiropractic consist of manipulating the different joints or bones to reach a diagnosis as well a therapeutic effect.

Osteopaths, especially W.G. Sutherland (1872-1950) and John Upledger, developed craniosacral therapy. In 1983, Upledger introduced the craniosacral concept for the entire body.

Osteopathy

Osteology is the science of the bones and joints. *Osteopathy* is the science of how subluxation, stiffness, or decreased range of movement in jointsaffects the body, which of course often is due to tensions of the muscles, and the therapy should thus more often be called *"muscleopathy"* rather that *"osteopathy"*, can be caused by, or cause, illness. It is also the name of a method, which uses the joints or bones or muscles as its tool and uses the relationship of the bones, which meet in the joints, to each other as basis for diagnosis and therapy. Osteopaths use this muscle/bone/joint system as their microcosm. Concerned mainly with the ability of bones/joints to move freely, they examine the ability of the vertebrae and the large and small bones of the limbs (including the small bones of the digits) to move. Then, they analyse the total movement to reach a diagnosis. Having examined the subject and diagnosed the affected joints, osteopathic therapy consists of relaxing spasms of the muscles and restoring the functional integrity, by bringing the bones and joints into a normal position and range of movement. Without knowing the theory in detail, it is possible to make an osteopathic diagnosis and to perform an osteopathic therapy. Where one finds that joints or movements are locked or blocked, one must work to relax, release or unblock them. In most cases, manipulating the movements/joints does this. [Contraindications include severe osteoarthritis, spondylosis and spinal infections, such as tubercular spinal pathology]. In suitable cases, one first tries to relax the spasm by moving the joint carefully, both in its small movements and in its big movements. You can try this yourself with a finger joint. After some time one can feel that finger joint movement improves considerably.

Osteopathy originated in the United States with Andrew Taylor Still, who suddenly "saw" the osteopathic method on the 22nd June 1874, at 10 o`clock in the morning. It is a system of healing that places emphasis on the structural integrity of the body as being vital to the well-being of the organism. The principals of osteopathy are that the body, through a complex balance system, aims at auto-regulation and self-recovery and that the body is an entity in which structure and function are mutually and reciprocally interdependent. Chiropractic treatment evolved from osteopathy but is directed principally at restoring joint mobility, with manipulation directed to the local site of dysfunction. The osteopathic diagnostic approach is based on identifying patterns of dysfunction, with minimal reliance on appositional factors and emphasis on the interactions of the entire body. Treatment is aimed not only at restoring local function, but also at identifying and removing factors that predispose to acute relapse. The central nervous system is continuously provided with information from the environment gathered by receptors of the α-afferent system, e.g. touch receptors or the β-afferent system, pain receptors or nociceptors. When an injury is present the β-afferent system is encountered. A painful stimulus is conveyed to the spinal cord and passes on to the brain to register pain, and stimulates motor neurons in the ventral horn, resulting in paravertebral and peripheral muscle spasm. It also stimulates sympathetic activity in the lateral horn causing reduced blood flow to the skin. To avoid constant discomfort, a control mechanism exists at the level of the spinal cord that is mediated by the α-afferent input of touch and proprioception and by descending inhibitory activity, creating a gate for painful stimuli. The balance between α-afferent stimulation and β-afferent input determines the activity of the interneurons and the sensory, motor, and autonomic responses. The α-afferent activity from joint receptors is reduced if the movement is restricted. Thus inhibitory effects on the interneurons are reduced and β-afferent activity may even increase and register pain, without direct stimulation of pain receptors. If the β-activity is intense or prolonged, it will cause changes in the chemistry and structure of the interneu-rons. These changes reduce the threshold for interneurons fir-ing in a process called facilitation. The interneurons become supersensitive to afferent input and to internal network activ-ity within the spinal cord. Facilitation underlies hyperesthesia, production of pro-inflammatory neuropeptides and increases central stimulation thus creating a spinal cord response out of proportion to the peripheral stimulation. This may explain horses with recurrent joint and soft tissue swellings and also some of the non-specific lameness and back pain where no pathological condition of tissue can be demonstrated by radi-ography, scintigraphy or nerve blocking.

Osteopathy offers techniques to manually test and nor-malise all joints of the body. To be able to make an osteopathic diagnosis the osteopath has to be familiar with the equine anat-omy, physiology and biomechanics. The clinical investigation begins with palpation of the muscles, tendons and joints. With the information gathered the osteopath then continues with biomechanical tests of suspected joints. Ascertening what is the site of primary injury and what are secondary changes may be difficult, but in horses, the engine, the muscles of the hip joint, seems to be of outmost importance for the whole body. The major cause of injuries is the demanding work performance horses have to do, rather than the result of direct trauma, in combination with how the horse uses its body.

The biomechanical tests reveal which movements in the joint are restricted and give directions to how the joint is to be manipulated. The Sacro-iliac and hip joints are tested holding the leg up and slightly bent. Ilium carries out a slight rotation around a transverse axis through the dorsocranial pole of the joint surface of the sacrum. The movement is a combination of rotation and gliding in a transverse plane ~30 degrees to the horizontal. Ilium is tested in four different directions; dorsal, as in flexion, ventral as in extension, lateral, as in moving the leg in adduction and medial, as in moving the leg in abduction, with one hand around the fetlock, moving the leg in different directions, and the other hand on the sacral tuber, feeling the movements of the ilium. The movements of the sacrum are very complex and are tested, with the tail as a lever, over three different axes. These are flexion and extension around a transverse axis through the center of the SI-joint, rotation and lateral flexion around oblique axes, left and right, and from the coxal tuber on one side to the great trochanter on the other side. The fingertips of one hand feel the movement of the sacral base. Mobility of the hip joint is tested by moving femur in six different directions; flexion-extension, abduction-adduction, lateral and medial rotation. The cervical-, thoracic- and lumbar vertebrae are tested by passive lateral flexions of the vertebral column, in either neutral position or flexion, while deciding if the tested vertebra is rotating in the physiological direction.

Osteopathic treatment aims to reverse changes in the areas of somatic dysfunction by restoring normal joint motion in all directions/planes, restoring normal pain sensibility by removing pain, inhibition, and restoring normal sensitivity, facilitation, and improving altered tissue function for muscle, connective and vascular tissues.

There are different kinds of techniques to treat one and the same joint. The technique of choice is decided by which direction the mobility is restricted, the state of the tissue of the area, the temperament and size of the horse. There are soft tissue techniques, articulatory techniques, and mobilization and functional techniques. These techniques result in increased α-afferent input from the muscles and joints, inhibiting the interneuron pool and blocking incoming pain signals from the β-afferent system. Usually 2 – 3 treatments 2 – 3 weeks apart are necessary. Often the outcome of the first treatment is good, but to maintain the result it is necessary to do follow ups. In my experience most of the trotters, and other high performance horses, need checkups routinely every 3rd to 4th week to avoid relapses and secondary lameness due to overload from an altered gait pattern.

Veterinary osteopathic manipulation is especially common in France, where colleagues Francois Lizon and Dominique Giniaux pioneered its use in small animals and horses, respectively. Impressed by the results of their French colleagues, vets in many other countries, including Australia, Canada, Europe, UK and USA, now use osteopathy routinely in their practices.

The Ilio-sacral joint

In horses, as well as other species including humans, sacroiliac dysfunction (SID) is an important cause of diseases and problems concerning movements, and of poor performance in horses. In the horse the most consistent clinical symptom of poor performance is a lack of impulsion from one or both hind limbs. Changes in performance also include back stiffness, resisting jumps, and subtle gait asymmetries at slow speeds during groundwork or dressage movements and in harness horses at racing speeds.

In traditional veterinary medicine the hip joint is rarely a source of pain causing lameness in the horse. A more common problem described in the thigh area is the "gluteal syndrome". Pain can be demonstrated with digital pressure along a line between the wing of ilium and the greater trochanter of the femur. The accessory head of *M. gluteus medius* was identified as the deep structure that best corresponds anatomically to the characteristic pattern of pain.

To study the mobility, or kinematics, of the back, the horse has to be filmed on a treadmill with special markers glued or pinned on the studied vertebrae. The result is calculated in a special computer program. This procedure is not possible to do in every horse with back pain in an ordinary clinic situation. Instead the veterinarian may want to take x-rays or do scintigraphy and hopefully detect changes in the skeleton, and maybe perform diagnostic analgesia.

In recent years several experienced scientists have done research of the sacroiliac joint, SIJ. The major obstacle to the successful diagnosis of dysfunction of this joint, SID, is that it is inaccessible for veterinary methods. The SIJ cannot be reached for intra-articular analgesia or radiology. Scintigraphy of the SI-joint is a diagnostic test of low sensitivity and low specificity, which means that the results are difficult to interpret. The obtained information from sacroiliac ultrasonography must be interpreted in light of thorough physical and lameness examinations, sacroiliac stress tests, periarticular SIJ analgesia, and nuclear scintigraphy. This means that in a clinic situation the veterinarian must rule out any other cause to problems of the horse, before he can diagnose pain or dysfunction of the SIJ.

Because the vertebral column and the SIJ are so inaccessible for veterinary methods, for diagnosis as well as treatment, and problems of the hip joint is mainly related to the muscles, osteopathy is a better way of diagnosing and treat injuries in these areas. The concept of somatic dysfunction is fundamental to osteopathy; somewhere in the course of entering information from the environment and body, processing the information in the central nervous system, and then generating a motor response, something has gone wrong. This manifests itself in a horse with clinical symptoms such as stiffness, poor performance, gait asymmetry, where no pathological process can be identified. Osteopathic treatment is directed at changing the signals to the neural network to modify the way sensory information is processed and thus to correct the motor response generated in the central nervous system. Equine osteopathy offers biomechanical techniques for testing and manipulation of the ilium and sacrum as well as for the vertebrae and hip joint (femur). Restriction of mobility, in the SIJ, hip joints and/or vertebrae is an important cause to overload of the joints, ligaments and tendons of the fore- and hindlimbs.

BIOMECHANICS OF THE HORSE

When the horse is moving, the pelvis is the centre of power, or the engine. The energy is coming from the hip joint. The muscles of the pelvic area have two main functions; with force move the body forward, and to stabilize the pelvis during stance. The movement is largest in the hip joint. The most important function of the stifle joint is to stabilize the hindlimb during stance. During stance the stifle joint is flexing and the large extensor muscles of the knee might act to resist gravity as opposed to power locomotion. The tarsal joint also has an important role during stance. Tendons and ligaments of the area behave elastically to store and return energy to be used in propulsion. The power from the proximal hindlimbs is transferred via the sacroiliac joints to the thoracolumbar vertebral column. The forelimbs act as a pivot that move the body forward until the hindlimbs can take over again.

The forelimbs are only connected to the body with strong muscles and ligaments. The shoulder joint does not have any collateral ligaments but are surrounded by strong muscles and tendons. During stance the shoulder- and elbow joints are flexing and the extensor muscles as well as the adductor muscles might act to resist gravity and abduction. The shoulder- and elbow joints behave like a stiff spring that allows forces to be transmitted through them to the proximal shoulder- and torso musculature. These muscles absorb and/or return energy, thereby functioning as a shock absorber. The main action of the muscles and tendons along the forelimb is stabilization during stance. The carpal-, metacarpophalangeal- (fetlock) and distal interphalangeal joints behave collectively as elastic systems storing and returning energy with the ability to recover up to 40% of energy during stride. The elasticity is driven primarily by the metacarpohalangeal joints in the fore- and hindlimbs thanks to the superficial and deep flexor tendons and accessory ligaments, and the third interosseous muscle (suspensory ligament). Stabilization of the carpus during stance is done by the *M. ulnaris lateralis* and *flexor carpi ulnaris*, both relatively stiff muscle-tendon units. The head and neck help to keep the horse's balance.

As long as the shock-absorbing musculature of the scapula and torso function normally, there should not be any overload of the distal joints and tendons. What interferes with this function? Is the main problem the condition of the track or training surface, bad shoeing, poor conformation, inherited or congenital bad composition and stamina etc.? These all play a part in the problem, but primarily, in most cases, I believe it is a combination of workload and motor laterality.

Chiropractic

Chiropractic is more understandable and clearly arranged than osteopathy. Like osteopathy, it has both diagnostic and therapeutic aspects. While osteopathy uses all the joints of the body in its system, chiropractic mainly uses the vertebrae. It is relatively well known in Norway and is accepted fairly well by the public health sector.

THE DIAGNOSTIC METHOD

Diagnosis of spinal disorders begins with examination of the vertebrae, from the atlas to the sacrum and hip. One must identify which vertebrae are misaligned, incorrectly positioned, or in any way restricted or blocked in their movement.

We recognise three degrees of spinal injury or restriction:

- Stage 1 is *blockage*, or reduced ability to move.

- Stage 2 is *subluxation* (almost dislocated joint), or misalignment (vertical, horizontal or in the long axis of the body); in Stage 2, the vertebra is slightly luxated or misaligned.

- Stage 3 is *total luxation*, i.e. complete dislocation of the vertebra.

All 3 Stages involve a "blockage" at one or more of the vertebrae. This means that the affected vertebrae have reduced mobility or range of movement that causes pain, "guarding", stiffness and other signs of abnormal function and behaviour. There may be accompanying reflex disorders in the skin, muscles and internal organs that share a common spinal innervation with the affected vertebrae. When physical examination identifies the affected vertebrae, one proceeds to "release the blockage". This involves manipulation of the spine and its muscles so that the affected vertebrae return to their correct alignment and normal range of movement.

Oseopathic and chiropractic methods are as effective in animals as they are in humans. However, it is important to differentiate between horses and other animals. Dogs can have any of the three stages: reduced vertebral mobility, subluxation and luxation; the vertebrae must be checked for all three possibilities. If necessary, the affected vertebra must be manipulated back to normal position. In horses, however, Stage 1 (blockage, or reduced vertebral mobility) is the most common finding; Stage 3 (full luxation) in the development of the spinal disorder is almost impossible in horses. The examination of horses consists of checking each vertebra, feeling whether it has normal mobility, or if its mobility is restricted even slightly.

CERVICAL VERTEBRAL TRAUMA AND PAIN

Disorders of the cervical vertebrae, nerves and spinal cord are common in humans and animals. Cervical trauma in humans often occurs in car accidents (whiplash injury). Cervical trauma in dogs and horses usually has a different cause.

- *In dogs* it usually is due to improper use of the leash, especially if the owner applies too much traction on the leash to control the dog. It may also occur if susceptible dogs jump down from a height.

- *In horses* it usually is due to serious falls, or improper use of the halter or lunge rope. It may also arise in show- or dressage- horses whose freedom to move the neck naturally is prevented by the use of tight straps from the chin ring to the girth strap.

Neck injuries can manifest many different symptoms. These include neck and thoracic limb pain, paraesthesia, paresis or circulation disorders; ataxia or hindlimb paresis or paralysis (Wobbler Syndrome); digestive disorders (LI, SI, ST,

GB Channels); reproductive disorders (TH Channel) and headache, tinnitus, facial disorders and fatigue.

In horses and dogs the most common symptom is neck pain, tenderness, or guarding / spasticity. As a result, the animal does not walk in a straight line, or walks awkwardly at an angle, like a crab. Dogs may have difficulty turning around, jumping off a chair, or walking downstairs. Horses tend to both pull away from the painful side and turn in a circle more easily **towards** the pain side. This is because they want to get away from the pain, and avoid extension of the affected side, which often increases the pain.

In all cases of suspected cervical disorders the atlas (vertebra C1) deserves special attention; because of its anatomy, C1 is especially vulnerable to trauma. Treatment of an injury to C1 is difficult; it requires the care of a trained vet or chiropractor.

TREATMENT OF EQUINE BACKPAIN

Although non-veterinary "spinologists" often diagnose "slipped disc " in horses, this diagnosis usually is incorrect. Intervertebral disc pathology is common in humans and animals but so-called a "slipped disc" is very rare, especially in horses. Discs usually can NOT slip out of place! Because of the anatomy of the equine spine and its powerful ligaments and muscles, disc misalignment, or disc herniation (rupture of the annular ligament with escape of the nuclear pulp) is almost impossible in horses. Also, disc-calcification, which is common in older humans, horses and dogs, and which can restrict spinal agility somewhat, seldom causes pain or other serious clinical problems *per se.*

A horse with backpain or vertebral blockage seldom is seen to "shake through" the entire vertebral column from the atlas to the tail, or to fully roll with its back to the ground. It protects its back and does not want to stretch it. It may have difficulty grazing short grass, because this extends the neck and the whole spine, via the attachment of the nuchal ligament at the withers. As mentioned earlier, experiments with anaesthetised horses showed that it is very difficult, if not impossible, to dislocate equine spinal discs (Giniaux). The spinal processes automatically return to the correct position in anaesthetised animals.

Primary anatomical causes of equine backpain include:

- poor saddle fit;

- sprain or strain of muscles, ligaments or vertebral joints, due to:

    ° poor riding skill,

    ° excessive stretching or contraction of the paravertebral muscles, as in a bad fall, or struggling when fallen in a box or stall, sudden fright or backing up in a restricted area, causing a lumbar (KI area) or sacral wrench;

    ° strain on the spine or facet joints, which have a very sensitive innervation;

    ° Backpain in the rider, which causes the horse to move unevenly.

- sacroiliac subluxation;

- spondylosis (calcification across the intervertebral space):

- "Kissing" dorsal spinal processes, etc [any other primary causes].

- Pain due to poor teeth-management

All of these can cause the osteopathic Syndrome of **vertebral blockage**. This is due to a slight misalignment of the spinal processes.

Secondary equine backpain is very common, probably more common than primary backpain. It can arise in:

- *Compensatory "guarding"* to protect a weak joint, tendon, or other structure in the limbs, especially in the forelimb (carpus or fetlock), or hindlimb (stifle, tarsus, fetlock);

- *Referred pain from a Process Imbalance in a Channel* (disorders in the gastrointestinal tract, HT, SP, LU, KI, ovary, testicle, uterus, LV, etc);

- *Metabolic disorders,* especially azoturia (a Process Imbalance in LV) and thyroid disorders, etc.;

- *Nutritional imbalances,* especially excessive protein, excessive carbohydrate, Ca/P imbalance, trace element deficiency (especially Cu, Se, I), vitamin deficiency (especially Vitamin A, D3 and E), etc.;

- *Infections: viral* (equine herpes, influenza, etc.); *protozoal* (EPM (equine protozoal myositis)); *bacterial, fungal and parasitic diseases;*

- *Immunosuppression from stress:* This is very common in horses. In such cases, the horse may show sensitivity at BL20 (SP), BL18-BL19 (LV-GB), and at SP06.

Whether it is primary and secondary, all equine backpain has a **strong muscular component** that involves "guarding". Spastic muscles can contract easily but extension or stretching of the muscle increases the pain. In this way, the horse "protects" its back against further pain by "locking" the affected area, i.e. by a reflex spasm of the local paravertebral muscles. This means that the horse hinders its back movement by using its own muscles. Many French chiropractors and osteopaths have realised this fact.

We may use two main ways to treat equine backpain:

1. muscular therapy, especially by AP and

2. vertebral adjustment therapy

1. *Muscular therapy, especially by AP* is very effective. Because of the marked involvement of the paraspinal muscles in backpain, several colleagues began to use AP in order to correct the reduced range of movement in the equine spinal

processes. If one can release muscular spasm and induce correct muscular tone, the vertebrae resume their normal function and movement spontaneously. This indicates that equine chiropractic/osteopathic therapy is a combination of vertebral therapy and muscular therapy and that reduced spinal function and movement is due to reflex muscle spasm. To treat such cases, we use AP at Local Points (Back Shu Points), or other common acupoints, even the Ting Points. Simple AP often corrects cases of spinally-related pathology. This indicates that Process Imbalances (deeper causes of disease) reflect in pathological blockage or misalignment of the equine vertebrae. Correction of the Process Imbalances restores function to the spine.

2. *Vertebral adjustment therapy, chiropractic / osteopathy* uses several approaches:

   (a) *The chiropractic hammer and block:* A special weighted hammer and wooden or polythene block is used to apply a short sharp power strike to realign the spinal processes, or rather to restore its range of movement by releasing the blockage. Untrained people (including vets) should not use the hammer. *Trained people seldom use a hammer; they use their hands instead. In the thoracic and lumbar area the hammer is used ONLY to adjust a rotational subluxation.*

   (b) *Atlantic adjustment:* The atlas, vertebra C1, influences all of the other spinal vertebrae. Adjustment of the atlas (using the hammer, or using a more gentle method to apply corrective stretch and rotation to the joint) can release the blockage in the neck. This can help to release a blockage in a distant vertebra, but additional readjustment mey be needed at the other vertebra also.

   (c) *The bending method:* Method (c) is probably the most applicable for owners and handlers untrained in methods (a) and (b). The idea is to *get the horse to move the blocked vertebra,* so that it comes back into its normal line with those before and behind it. One simply "bends the horse" by using gentle force, or by coaxing the horse (carrot, sugar, or hay) to bend his body in such a way that the misalignment becomes a normal part of the curve. Keep that position for 30-60 seconds before allowing the horse to resume its normal resting position. The blockage often resolves itself at that stage.

- *The abdominal pinching method*: If one vertebra protrudes above the others, i.e. if the affected vertebral spine stands slightly higher on the back than its neighbours, one should NOT try to press it down. Instead, one should pinch the horse under the abdomen. This induces the horse to arch (raise) its back and raise the other vertebrae, so that they come into line with the subluxated vertebra. This eases the pain and muscular spasm and allows the muscles to return to their original relaxed state and to function normally. When the horse then bends its back to its original position, it "brings along" the affected vertebra, which resumes its correct alignment, thus restoring normality.

All methods of therapy have indicators of a successful outcome, which are obvious to even casual observers:

- *The horse realises* that the pain is gone, or is much less. The horse often gives an almost comical "sigh of relief". Its attitude improves clearly, sometimes within minutes of successful treatment. It manifests its relief in its ears, eyes, social interest, general relaxation and improved movement.

- *The reactive acupoints disappear (i.e. lose their hypersensitivity)* over a period of a few days;

- Immediately after successful therapy, *the horse may spontaneously "shake through" the entire vertebral column, from the occiput to the tail.* If the horse does not do this spontaneously, one can often induce it to "shake through" by gently tweaking or elevating a few hairs in the lower part of the mane, as Marvin Cain teaches.

The next table summarises the relationship between the equine vertebrae, BL Points (mainly the Back Shu Points) and their related Process and other functions (Processes) as taught by the TCM, and Drs. Lizon and Giniaux of France:

Equine verte bra	BL Point	Back Shu Point and related Channel and Process () = not a Back Shu Point	Other related functions, not necessarily the same as those of the Back Shu Points
C1	BL10	(Wind)	LV and senses
C2			GB and oesophagus
C3			KI
C4			TH, sex and balance
C5			SI or LI, intestine
C6			SP
C7			ST, circulation, blood pressure (HT, PC)
T1	BL11	(joints, bones)	SI and circulation, (HT, PC)
T2			KI and circulation (HT, PC)
T3	BL12	(Wind)	LU
T4			PC
T5	BL13	LU	HT
T6			LI
T7	BL14	PC	TH
T8			LV
T9	BL15	HT	GB
T10	BL16	GV, spine, spinal cord	ST, LU
T11			BL, LU
T12	BL17	Diaphragm, respiration, haemorrhage	Diaphragm, LU, SP
T13			KI, ST
T14	BL18	LV	GB, LV
T15			LU, sweat
T16	BL19	GB (horse has no physical GB)	LV, LI and colic
T17			LV, LI and colic
T18	BL20	SP	HT and colic
L1	BL21	ST	LV and uterus
L2	BL22	TH, metabolism	KI

L3	BL23	KI	SP
L4	BL24	Qihaishu-Qi Sea	LU (LI, uterus)
L5	BL25	LI	HT and colic
L6	BL26	Guanyuanshu-Gate Origin	uterus, BL, colic
S1	BL27	SI	
S2	BL28	BL / KI	
S3	BL29	Zhonglushu-Midback	lowback pain
S4	BL30	Baihuanshu-White Circle (anus)	rectum, perineum, anus, vulva

Table 105

TREATMENT OF CANINE BACKPAIN

Treatment principles in dogs are similar to those used in horses.

Vertebral misalignment in dogs: Dogs often have vertebral misalignment. As in horses, *the vertebrae may be displaced vertically or rotationally.* When one locates the affected vertebra, one can apply manual force (leverage) to realign it. One can also bend the body, as described in horses, above, so that the neighbouring (normal) vertebrae "catch" the affected one and bring it back into line when the body is straightened out into the normal position. Chiropractic hammers are not needed in dogs, as manual manipulation, or the bending method, can usually restore alignment. However, some dogs have seriously luxated vertebrae. Those dogs need more extensive treatment over a longer time to restore complete vertebral alignment.

The best treatment in severe vertebral misalignment is to combine vertebral adjustment, AP, rest and good nursing care. Simple AP alone gives mediocre results. Simultaneous administration of *homeopathic Arn, Hyp and Rhus.tox* helps also.

Disc disease in dogs: In contrast to horses, dogs often develop clinical signs due to of disc disease in the neck, thorax or lumbar area. Contrary to popular belief, because of the strong ligaments that hold them in position, affected discs are very seldom "slipped". *They do NOT need to be "put back" because they are NOT seriously out of position.* Common disc lesions in dogs include degeneration, diminution of the disc space, calcification, or occasional rupture of the annulus and extrusion of the disc pulp into the spinal canal. A combination of AP, rest and good nursing is the best treatment for these cases. Simultaneous administration of *homeopathic Arn, Hyp and Rhus.tox* helps the effect of AP.

Cranio-Sacral Therapy

This special therapy was develloped by **Dr. William Sutherland**, who was an osteopath. Therefore this form of therapy is taught by and considered a part of osteopathy. Osteopaths consider this therapy as a part of their curriculum. The term Craniosacral Therapy was originally coined in the 1970s by American Osteopathic physician Dr John Upledger. When Sutherland introduced his concepts to the Osteopathic community it was ignored by all but a handful of his colleagues. It was not Osteopathy as they knew it, at this time largely a therapy based on gross manipulation of the body. How could such subtle work achieve such profound effects? Clients can also be sceptical – until they notice the results!

I will refere some of the arguments used at that time, and the answers;
Comment; In my opinion Cranio-Sacral therapy has little to do with osteopathy, more with healing, really, although the theories in Cranio-Sacral therapy is developed from osteopathy, and then C-S seems to be related to osteopathy.

Statement; Life expresses itself as motion. Deep in our physiology all healthy tissues "breathe" with the motion of life - a phenomenon that produces rhythmic impulses which can be palpated by sensitive hands. The presence of these subtle rhythms in the body was discovered by osteopath Dr William Sutherland after examining the specialized articulations of cranial bones.

Comment; As we know, all physical is the expression or secondary revelation of the primary source; the ethereal body, the energy of life. The enrgy moved in rhythms, and lemniscates, which feels as physical movements.

Statement; Dr Sutherland realized that cranial sutures were designed to express small degrees of motion. He demonstrated the existence of this motion and eventually concluded it is essentially produced by the body's inherent life force, which he referred to as the "Breath of Life." Furthermore, Dr Sutherland discovered that the motion of cranial bones he first discovered is closely connected to subtle movements that involve a network of interrelated tissues and fluids including cerebrospinal fluid, the central nervous system, the membranes that surround the central nervous system and the sacrum.

Comment; Agree

Statement; The Breath of Life produces a series of subtle rhythms that may be palpated in the body and which make up an integrated physiological system. At least three subtle rhythms have been identified in this "primary respiratory system", each having a different rate and producing rhythms within rhythms. These three "tides" are referred to as the cranial rhythmic impulse, the mid-tide and the long tide.

Comment; Agree

Statement; The emphasis in Cranio Sacral Therapy is to help resolve the trapped forces that underlie and govern patterns of disease and fragmentation in both body and mind. This involves the practitioner "listening through the hands" to the body's subtle rhythms and any patterns of inertia or congestion. Through the development of subtle palpatory skills the practitioner can read the story of the body, identify places where issues are held and then follow the natural priorities for healing as directed by the patient's own physiology. The treatment is to enhance the body's own self-healing and self-regulating capabilities. Furthermore, the practitioner's deep and clear quality of presence can become a reflective mirror for the patient and an invaluable cue for their potential for change.

Comment; Agree, this can be explained through "Mirror neurons"

Statement; This underlying vitality is expressed throughout the body as rhythmic motion - Cranio-Sacral motion.

Comment; This ethereal rhythm is not limited to the sacrum and the cranium, although the rhythm was first discovered there. It was explained to be as the result of the movement between Os parietale and Os spenoidale

Statement; Any disturbance to health and wellbeing - physical or psycho-emotional - influences this movement, creating asymmetries or restrictions to Cranio-Sacral motion.

Comment; In my opinion this is just the opposite; a change in the rhythm is the primary sourse of disease. First come the change in rhythm, then the illness.

Statement; The Cranio-Sacral Therapist can therefore diagnose and identify the nature and source of the condition through the corresponding patterns expressed through the Cranio-Sacral system. By responding appropriately to these patterns - following the subtle internal pulls and twists manifested by the Cranio-Sacral System until points of resistance are encountered and dissolved - the Cranio-Sacral Therapist can facilitate the release of restrictions, thereby restoring the free flow of the Breath of Life and consequently restoring a healthy, balanced state.

Comment; Again, in my opinion this is just the opposite; the therapist first restores the free flow of the Breath of Life which leads to dissolution of resistance and then health is restored.

Statement; All Cranial Osteopaths and Craniosacral therapists are individuals and the emphasis of their work will vary as will their skills. The foundation of the work remains the same whatever the title, and most cranial workers are in agreement as to its effects. They all agree that the PRI can be felt anywhere on the body, that its integrity is vital to health, and it seems to be transmitted via the Cerebrospinal Fluid (CSF) and a system of membranes that surround the brain and spinal cord.

Comment; Agree partly, but again this emphasis on the CSF in which I do not agree.

Statement; Sutherland referred to the physiological system that carried the PRI as the Primary Respiratory Mechanism (Nowadays generally called the Craniosacral Mechanism or System). This consists chiefly of the CSF, the Dura Mater (a tough membrane surrounding the brain and spinal cord), and those structures intimately related to the Dura, notably the intercranial membranes (*Falx cerebri, Falx cerebelli* and the *Tentorium* – continuations of the Dura within the cranium), the cranial bones and the sacrum (hence the name, Craniosacral therapy).

Comment; I do not agree, as I think that the ethereal energy is everywhere.

Statement; Sutherland observed a rhythmic movement of the cranial bones and sacrum, a movement reflected through the whole body. It is a movement of expansion and contraction which was driven by some kind of inherent fluctuation within the CSF. At the end of the expansion phase the tension built up in the dural membrane system (called the Reciprocal Tension Membrane by Sutherland) causes a reflex contraction back to the beginning of the cycle. The brain and spinal cord moves along with this tidal flow of the CSF. Modern computerised tomography shows that Sutherland was right about the movement of the brain – it does change shape along with the movements of the craniosacral system. Ultimately Sutherland believed the driving force to be the "Breath of Life", a subtle organising energy that seems to echo similar concepts of life energy that have emerged under various names through the centuries. Sutherland was not alone in believing that the CSF was one of the body's prime self-healing and self-correcting mechanisms. Andrew Still, the founder of Osteopathy called it "the highest known element" in the body and Randolph Stone, the creator of Polarity therapy said the CSF "...acts as ...the liquid medium for life energy radiation, expansion and contraction."

Comment; I do not agree, as I think that the ethereal energy is everywhere.

Statement; Whatever the driving force, the effects are real enough to make this a very effective therapy in many conditions. Because the dural membrane is intimately linked into the connective tissue or fascia of the body it is possible by gently restoring correct function to the craniosacral system to effect changes in the fascia and vice versa. Fascia is continuous throughout the body and connects every part to every other part. It connects and supports the bones, the muscles, the organs, the viscera, the endocrine system, the nervous system, everything. It gives solid physical evidence for the holistic concept in health. Thus the scar from an operation, a localised infection, toxicity or irritation, for example, may have a disturbing effect far from the site of the problem. Craniosacral therapists have refined their sense of touch to the extent that they can sense and correct such dysfunctions and imbalances by "tuning in" or "listening" with their hands resting lightly on a part of the body remote from this site. This is often done by monitoring the state of the craniosacral system and making subtle adjustments. An experienced cranial worker is able to shift attention between the bones, the membranes and the fluids of the craniosacral system. They can access "body memory" of past emotional or physical injury and help the body-mind towards resolution of the injury.

Comment; Agree. This description shows the wholeness of the ethereal energy. It also shows that the real healer in all forms of therapy is our *intention.*

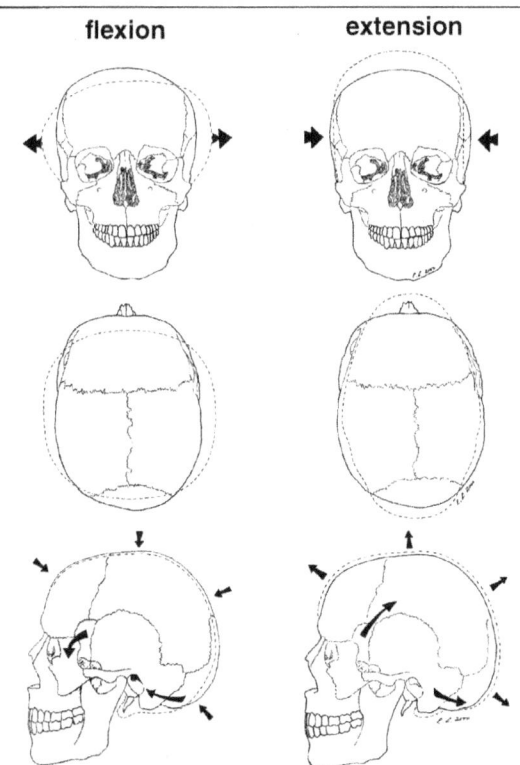

Figure 66; Illustration on how the Cranio-sacral rhythm is thought to work or function.

Neural therapy

In Germany, Neural therapy is considered part of conventional medicine. In spite of this, there are very few people in Norway who are familiar with this form of therapy. Neural therapy (NT) is a basic medical diagnosis and method of therapy. In British publications it is referred to as Sekunden Phanomen (*Instantaneous Phenomenon*) therapy. The reason for this name is that the results of a successful treatment often manifest within seconds.

Dr. Ferdinand Huneke, the medical doctor who discovered and publicised the method in 1928, researched it until his death in 1968. His work was based on two basic observations:

- *He gave his sister an intravenous injection of an analgesic agent for a migraine attack; this was more effective than expected. He discovered later that he had made a mistake; he had given her procaine instead. This effect, caused by procaine, was not known at the time.*

- *He had a female patient with bilateral frozen shoulders and chronic pain. Her disorder seemed to be incurable because of its long duration. She also had a tubercular wound on her right leg. This wound had to be cleansed surgically and a local anaesthetic was given to facilitate this. Her right shoulder became free of pain only seconds after the injection of procaine was given. This effect lasted for a long time and after repeated local anaesthetic on the same spot on her leg, the left shoulder was completely cured.*

Having discovered a phenomenon completely unknown to him at the time, Huneke started working with his observations. Even though Dr. Leriche, the great French surgeon, and Professor Esnaurrizar at the University of Mexico City, had noted similar phenomena before him, Huneke's greatest strength was that he realised the importance of his discoveries. He organised and documented his notes into a very complete system that was based solely on his clinical experience. He did not try to explain anything; he did not even try to develop a theory. This was probably the reason why he did not experience the big breakthrough that he wanted so much.

Although some German medical experts knew that his observations were correct as well as important, in his lifetime Huneke did not receive the medical recognition that he deserved. However, value of his work was recognised posthumously when scientists at the University of Vienna confirmed his results. They proved that the effect was purely physical and they managed to explain the physiological mechanisms that cause the effect. Professors Fleischacher (Internal Medicine), Pishinger and Kellner led that medical research. Their observations silenced Huneke's critics and cleared the way for increasing international acceptance of NT.

The important aspects of NT are as follows: Throughout life, Disturbance Fields in local injuries and scars in any part of the body can disturb the total harmony of bodily functions and these disturbances can last a very long time. Huneke used the German term "Störfeld" to designate these Disturbance Fields. The word means "an area which disturbs". A Störfeld can work like a time-set bomb: it can be latent for a long time and then suddenly "explode" to cause an acute disorder.

In NT theory, it is most important to find the actual Störfeld. In practice, this can be very difficult. Huneke usually analysed the whole medical history of the patient and systematically administered "durchspritzen", i.e. he injected all scars or damaged areas that the patient could remember. Often this would mean many small injections and the result depended on the patients' ability to remember their scars. This ability is rather poor, even if the person has medical education and a good memory. Such people normally remember <50% of their medical history.

Dr. Doch was probably Huneke's best student. One of Doch's patients, a veterinarian, came to him in a wheelchair; polyarthritis had left him an invalid, unable to walk. Doch gave him several injections in all possible scars, even in the upper part of the tonsils but without result. Finally Doch went to a hospital in Leipzig where his patient had been shortly before the onset of his polyarthritis. The hospital could not help. The veterinarian then remembered that he had treated a cow and had pricked his own finger with a dirty needle before his problems arose.

The sore had developed into an infected boil that had burst and healed soon afterwards. He discharged himself from hospital, went home and injected Impletol (2% procaine plus 1% caffeine) at the old site of the boil on his finger. Immediately he experienced a Sekunden Phanomen (Instantaneous Effect). The polyarthralgia disappeared and, five minutes later, he could walk again.

Forty-nine years is the longest time on record (Dr. Doch) between the formation of a Störfeld and the onset of symptoms that could be traced back to it with certainty. The patient was a taxi-driver who had sciatica that had failed to respond to any form of treatment. Measurements of the temperature of the skin signified a possible scar on the inside of the left heel, on the same side as the sciatica. The man could not remember any injury on this spot until he suddenly remembered that he had hurt himself with an axe when he was 7 years old (49 years earlier). Using a magnifying glass, Doch found the scar and injected it with Impletol. That treatment cured the patient's sciatica.

Pain or other symptoms induced by a Störfeld can appear anywhere in the body, and in any organ. The problem may occur on the same or the opposite side of the Störfeld. Until now, the only way to confirm whether a certain Störfeld is the cause of a specific ailment, is to inject a local anaesthetic into the scar and wait for the classic sign that shows whether there is a relationship or not. If the "Sekunden Phanomen" (Instantaneous Phenomenon) occurs, it proves the relationship. For example, pains or other clear signs of illness, such as skin discoloration, often disappear within seconds. The anaesthetic must be free of additives, adrenaline, or other vasoconstrictors.

Huneke recommended using Impletol, which contained 2% procaine and 1.42% caffeine. I use 0.5% xylocaine (lidocaine) without additives. Instantaneous phenomena ought to come immediately and should last at least for 20 hours. Huneke was quite definite about this. However, those of his students whom I know thought that the reaction needs not occur immediately and needs not last for 20 hours.

Finding the relevant scar, and then finding the Störfeld within it is the most important part of NT. But how can we find it? Sometimes we simply get the information from the owner of the animal. Typical significant information from the owner is:

- "The cat has been ill since it was castrated", or

- "The horse has been lame since the operation on its throat", or

- "The cow has been seen in heat since her ear tag was pulled out", or

- "The dog has been aggressive since the tail was docked".

I have seen all of those examples and many more in my practice. Such causes are not as rare as we would tend to think. However, animal owners often forget that the disorder started after an injury.

Although a Störfeld often arises after trauma or a wound, it can arise in other circumstances also. For example, a Störfeld can arise after a sore throat, an abscess, an infected tooth socket, or an apparently insignificant scar. An invisible and old trauma, or a calcified abscess site, can also be the cause.

NEURAL THERAPY IN PRACTICE

In German studies, 10% of operations create a Störfeld (personal communication, Georg Bentze). Thus, it is important to check post-operative scars, for example in spayed or castrated animals. I have treated many functionally impaired horses after castration. They showed sensitivity in the TH area of the neck, or the TH or KI areas of the lumbar, sacral or hindlimb muscles, unpredictability or poor racing performance. Before the horses could function properly, they needed treatment of a Störfeld in the operation wound. One should include an internal examination of the cervix, vagina and rectum, especially in females that have given birth. Vaccination scars should be noted also. Several times I have seen that the vaccine itself has not caused the problem but rather local scarring after infection of the needle track.

A Störfeld on the tiniest scar can be as important as one on a big scar. It requires a very thorough whole-body examination to locate scars that may contain a Störfeld. When scars are present, one should try to confirm when the trauma occurred in relation to the onset of the illness. It is important to note that trauma influences the body at the time that it occurs but a disorder like a gallstone may have an effect for a long time before the symptoms manifest.

Neural therapy is the most effective way to treat disorders that originate in a Störfeld. Treatment of the blockage - the reactive parts of the scar or the place of injury - usually improves the disorder within seconds. It is as if one resets a tripped electronic fuse; suddenly the power is restored to the circuit again. We should examine for a temporal relationship between onset of the disease and prior injuries or operations that induced *Störfelds* in scars. Here is an example:

- After his tail was docked, a Doberman became irritable and began to bite his hindquarter. He had obvious pain in the tail area. Later, he developed a KI disorder and heavy proteinuria (+++). The symptoms disappeared within a few days after injection of local anaesthetic into the scarred area of the tail stump. Treatment about six times per year kept this dog healthy for several years.

Surgery (tail docking, castration, spaying, etc.), injuries and ear tagging can induce a blockage (Störfeld). I have seen on several occasions that eartags can inhibit the expression of oestrus in cows; the tag usually is inserted in the reflex Earzone that relates to the endocrine system. Also, I have seen that rings in the ear can induce serious symptoms of humans.

Where possible, *avoid making transverse abdominal incisions and avoid incising directly over the ventral midline (the Renmai, CV).* Where possible, surgeons should *incise **between** Channels, or **slightly off the ventral midline**.* Transverse abdominal scars (from surgery) can obstruct the free flow of Qi in many Channels, especially KI, ST and SP. Incisions in the midline may obstruct CV. The CV has 6 Mu Points (CV03, CV04 and CV05 for BL, SI and TH; CV12, CV14 and CV17 for ST, HT and PC). Reactive (hypersensitive, tender) points in scars at these locations can obstruct Qi flow and induce symptoms in the related Processes. Treatment of reactive points on scars can relieve many symptoms that relate to the obstructed Process. *However, one really can not avoid cutting some Channels, or other "side branches", as the body has many, many energy pathways apart from the Main Channels. Disturbance Fields on scars anywhere can cause problems. Therefore, the best solution is to treat all scars routinely about 5-6 weeks after surgery. If the scar is treated just a few days after surgery, the neuraltherapeutic treatment does not seem to work.*

Anthroposophical Veterinary Medicine

Diagnosis and therapy of animals via the human energetic system versus via their own energetic system.

MYTHICAL BEGINNINGS

Rudolf Steiner created the theory behind and the myths related to the evolution of Anthroposophical medicine. I suspect that Steiner was wrong in some of his theories, but I share without doubt the effect of the relationship between humans and animals and the importance of the human will and intent in these interactions.

According to Steiner, treatment of disease dates far back into prehistoric times. According to myth, Atlantis, a prehistoric continent, had sunk into the sea and humans had to work with the more condensed materialistic world. (Although Plato mentioned it, there is no historical evidence of this mythical continent). At that time strange life forms, mixtures of human and animal, were said to be present. These forms had evolved as a result of a great misuse of life forces by black magic, which finally caused the destruction of Atlantis. Today, we have a pale memory of these forms in the concept of the Centaur.

According to clairvoyants of this century, for example Edgar Cayce (American psychic and a man who claimed to be able to see both back and forward in time), initiates at the beginning of historic time felt responsible for these creatures, created by the former misuse of black magic. This was especially so in ancient Egypt. Using powerful etheric forces, which the initiates were able to use, they divided the animal-human hybrids into the animal-like and the human-like. Thus, human souls, in human form, could work themselves back to human consciousness.

However, as a consequence of and in contrast to this, the domestic animals of today arose. These were formed as two groups: those with hooves and those with cloven hooves. This division was widely known in folk medicine up to 1800, which can be seen in the fact that up to this time health advice was separate for horses, humans and cows. Thus, in esoteric theory (especially Steiner's theory), our domestic animals have a dual origin from the human entity.

For the first type of animal origin, all the animal kingdom has emerged from the human development as described by Dr. Hermann Poppelbaum (a student of Rudolf Steiner). In his book "Animal and Man", he says: "When you look at the tree of human evolution, it shows how human development is the trunk from which all the other forms spring. The lower, higher and highest forms of animals have sprouted as branches, always at higher places from the upwards striving human trunk".

The second type of animal origin was from the deformed human-animal hybrids previously described. In the splitting of the human-like and the animal-like, they sacrificed themselves **(or humans sacrificed them)** for human misdeeds. In the service of humanity, this sacrifice continues today.

We shall see later how the evolution that took place especially in ancient Egypt repeats itself in a similar way today. From the solutions of the Egyptian initiates, we can find new ways of treating our animals. However, in our hands, we have the power to destroy as well as to heal. We can misuse our powers; such misuse of power is said to have caused Atlantis to sink into the sea. The destructive force was the misuse of etheric forces for the sake of egotistic purposes. This was especially in manipulating life forms, which were put into human service against their will. This is seen clearly today in genetic manipulation of plants and animals.

MAGICAL HEALING RITES

Advice on how to treat animals by magical rites and spells was common.

- For example, to cure a cow with mastitis, the farmer was asked to draw a little milk from every other cow and put the milk in the middle of a circle made by hot glowing coals. From here, the milk would trickle into a mixture of sulphur and carbon from burnt wood (ashes) (advice from Martin Luther, 1483-1546).

- We also find advice to cure hemorrhage in verses as: "Blood be standing in the vessel, as Christ was carried on the cross. Blood be in the wound, as Christ was nailed on the cross".

- For eye disorders in horses: "if a horse has pain in the eye take then a little honey mixed with some butter and stir with some free white copper smoke (sulphur + zinc oxide) and rub in the eye (advice from Ole Hodtvet 1796).

The "Sixth Sense" is just another sense; is most important for survival in harsh, unpredictable and dangerous environments, such as in jungles, mountains or open plains. During evolution from prehistoric to modern times, "civilised man" has lost many instincts and innate survival skills; urban dwellers and hunter-gatherers need and have different emphasis on these innate abilities. The instincts and survival skills of so-called indigenous peoples (jungle people in Borneo, North- and South American Indians, Esquimos, Australian aborigines, etc), who must live in very close harmony with nature, contrast sharply with those of urban dwellers.

Human magical rites have lost much of their power in "civilised" society. We have lost most of the esoteric knowledge of the difference between the evolution of human and animal types, karma and etheric structure. Few people in modern society have, or even know of, the skills and powers to work directly with human and animal etheric structure. The rediscovery of homeopathy by Dr. Samuel Hahnemann (1755-1843) was a very important first step to regain the ability to work with the etheric structure of humans, animals and plants. However, even Hahnemann did not appreciate the esoteric knowledge of human-animal differences, or the power of human magical rites. This knowledge still remains alive in shamanistic traditions and practices.

Dawn of scientific materialism

The more rational folk medicine expelled magical advice from its repertoire. As folk medicine evolved, botany, pharmacy and medicine slowly emerged as a unity out of the magical and mythical forms. However, as the Age of Enlightenment proceeded, medicines for similar disorders in humans and animals became more and more alike, until they became identical. Similar symptoms in all species are supposed to have the same causes and, today, usually are treated with the same medicines and therapies.

The Age of Enlightenment continues as modern medicine, agriculture and animal breeding develop. But what is happening as we go down the road of this scientific, profit oriented, intensive animal and agriculture system? Our animals are being drained of their etheric forces. Their original forms are being destroyed. The old harmonic proportions, which our animals had and which stood in direct communication with the macrocosmic world, are being lost. Powerful drugs, such as growth promoters, beta agonists, synthetic hormones, antibiotics and steroids allow greedy producers to force unnatural levels of production and further drain the animals' Qi. Also, intensive methods of animal production, and unnatural feeding practices (such as urea, fat and high levels of concentrate feed, etc) have greatly increased stress-related, digestive and metabolic diseases. The latest effects of unnatural feeding methods are bovine spongiform encephalopathy (BSE) and its human form - new variant Creutzfeldt-Jakob Disease (nvCJD) - due to the feeding of recycled animal waste as infected meat and bone-meal. That disease threatens to destroy the multi-billion dollar beef trade in Europe.

RETURN TO COMPASSIONATE WAYS

Now more than ever before, we need a total reform of animal husbandry, management, breeding and veterinary therapy. Here, as in also other areas, Anthroposophy may point to an answer. Already in the name of Anthroposophical veterinary medicine we are beginning to feel the possibilities of renewal. We are working toward a humane veterinary medicine, where humans become conscious of their responsibility for these un-happy forms (the animals) and offer their own human ethe-ric forces or structure as a sacrifice. We also can carry on our shoulders responsibility for ourselves and the development of the earth to its fulfilment (karma). In particular, we need to in-fluence our Governments to rethink their attitudes towards the free movement of animals and animal products across nation-al borders from countries in which highly contagious diseases like Foot and Mouth disease and Swine Fever are endemic.

Like so-called "primitive peoples", we can work to return to more natural ways of living, in which we show essential respect for our natural environment and embrace all of creation in a universal love. We, who work closely with domestic animals, can work into the etheric structures of the animals in the same way as the old Egyptian initiates, who worked formally, directly and helpfully into the etheric animal forms. By sacrificing our own structure, our own etheric process, to the healing process of the animals, we can make atonement for human misuse of animals in the past and say "thank you" to them for their pa-tient and faithful service to humanity.

Many healers do this subconsciously all of the time. It is possible because animals have the memory of a human etheric structure within themselves from the common development of all mammals. Thus, in the domestic animals (and of course in the wild ones also), one can find the corresponding Channels and the working of the corresponding human homeopathic remedies.

TWO (AT LEAST) ENERGY SYSTEMS IN ANIMALS

The human etheric system occurs in animals in addition to their own etheric structure. This is the energetic system that we usually have used, probably because of our attempts to transpose the theory and principles of human AP / TCM, including Five Phase Theory, the Channel pathways and their acupoints to animals. Thus, two different medical systems can be applied to domestic animals.

We can see this most easily in equine energetics. Transposition of the human Channel system is used widely in horses. Apart from having no physical gallbladder, horses have a GB Channel, similar in many ways to that in humans. But we may also consider the equine energetic system as unique in its own right. It is at one with itself, a completely balanced system: the substantial (material) horse is an expression of the etheric (immaterial) horse. As Goethe said, "the material is the secret revelation of the invisible". In that idea, we find an up to now unknown system of etheric energy. By looking at horses in this way, especially the distal limbs, we find that **human etheric analogues do not apply directly to horses**. This is easily seen in regards to the locations of the Command Points. The reality of these differences has been shown previously by the author, for example in his work on the equine Ting Points.

Although both systems work, by treating horses according to the theory of Goethe, I find AP points that are more effective than points transposed directly from human AP concepts. This shows that animals have more than one energy system. This theory also applies to humans, both in Tibetan medicine and in European esoteric traditions concerning the presence of a "doppelganger" (the personal double). This is a double in the human body that calls on the nervous system to function as its working instrument. Thus, the nervous system, the blood system and the etheric system are not identical.

When treating animals directly, we may use both etheric systems (human and animal), although the animal system is the more effective. But by treating via the human etheric system we must use the human-animal system. Into this last system we can sacrifice our own etheric forces. How is this possible? We have seen that human etheric forces are in continuous and direct contact with human surroundings and other etheric forces. This communication is not random or by chance. As a key fits a lock, it is possible to work therapeutically **only with similar etheric forces**, ones with a structural congruence or empathy, a similar feeling, or those in direct communication.

We often see that etheric weaknesses in the owner manifest in the animal attached to him or her. This is easy to see in regards to temperament shared by the dog owner and the dog. But this communication applies to all animals - cows, horses, sheep, pigs and their keepers. A nervous, irritable owner often has nervous, irritable animals.

Use of etheric concepts in diagnosis and therapy of animals

Now we are at the kernel of this article: techniques of using the human etheric system to treat animals. We can regard animal and human disease as an etheric or energetic imbalance. This Qi Process Imbalance can manifest in physical symptoms. The cause of the Qi Imbalance can vary from time to time and from case to case. It can have nutritional, parasitic, toxic, allergic or immune-mediated causes. Other causes include atmospheric, climatic, geographic, constitutional and managemental (human-induced) causes, as mentioned already. In practice one finds many causes from all of these groups operating together.

To prevent further disease it is important to recognise and remove (or alleviate) these causes. However, a more direct therapy is necessary as a first aid veterinary treatment. This may involve direct etheric intervention but, first, we need an etheric diagnosis on the animal.

ETHERIC DIAGNOSIS

On the basis of etheric intercommunication, special diagnostic methods are used. Etheric diagnosis is discussed in separate articles. There are many different methods. One method relates closely with diagnostic crystalline precipitation patterns or metal blots formed by the combination of silver nitrate and copper chloride salts with specimens of body fluid (blood, saliva, urine, etc.), as used in Anthroposophical medicine. (See also the sections on Pulse Diagnosis, radiaesthesia, medical divination, etc, discussed elsewhere in this book).

ETHERIC TREATMENT

With one exception, any healthy human can give etheric treatment. The exception is *the person who is the cause of the disease, if we have found this to be the case.* The therapeutic approach is to *strengthen the same Processes in the treating human that are Weak in the animal,* i.e. if the animal has a Weakest Process in SP, tonify SP Process in the therapist. When this is done the therapist spends a few *minutes in contact with the animal, with a conscious, loving intention to heal.* Then the necessary etheric forces can flow over from the human to the animal, or organise the etheric forces in the animal so that they balance themselves. During this therapy the therapist may feel certain exhaustion but this feeling soon vanishes when the therapy is over.

SUPPORT THERAPY

Anything that works energetically can be used as support therapy: homeopathy, AP, Anthroposophical medicine, reflex therapy, herbs and others.

CLINICAL RESULTS

I have tried etheric methods on several cases since 1985 with very good results. (See case reports at the end of this article). In my experience, the effect of this therapy far exceeds that of conventional therapy given impersonally (without compassion or a feeling of love) to the animal. I have found this to be true even in disorders such as arthritis, heart failure, traumatic indigestion, hormonal and other difficult disorders. In addition to its efficacy, I believe this method to be ethically correct. This type of diagnosis and therapy is possible not only between humans and animals but also between adults and children, humans and plants and between a human as microcosms and the whole macrocosm. Humans have a clear responsibility to Nature and Creation. We can and should use our powers in the healing processes in our companion creations, the animals.

CASE 1: A 4-year old female cat had a 5 cm wound on the left foreleg. The wound had not healed for at least 6 months. It had been treated unsuccessfully with various ointments. Its owner, a 20 year old female, was told to place "Heilsalbe" (a complementary healing ointment from Weleda) on her own left arm in the area analogous with that of her cat. She applied the ointment, as directed, in the evening while the cat was in her lap. The cat became anxious and ran out into the night. The wound had closed when it returned in the morning.

CASE 2: A 55 year old farmer presented a 5-year old cow with reticulitis, reticular pain, anorexia, ketonemia and icterus. An acupoint in the farmer's ear showed reactivity when the farmer was placed in contact with the cow. A permanent needle was placed into this point *in the farmer's ear.* Very soon the farmer reported heavy pain in his stomach. Within a day or so the cow began eating. The icterus and ketonemia gradually disappeared. After three weeks, the farmer slaughtered the cow for human consumption. After slaughtering the cow, the farmer's stomach pains subsided.

CASE 3: A 6-year old horse was presented with lameness of the left forelimb for three years. On Pulse Diagnosis, the horse had BL Deficiency (Weak Process in BL Channel). The owner, a physiotherapist, did not believe in AP at the time. However, when requested to remove his left shoe and place his hand on the horse's back he agreed in disbelief. Placing a needle for 20 minutes in his BL67 treated the owner. He reported that he was drained of energy at the end of treatment. After this treatment the horse became sound. The owner has since become a certified acupuncturist.

*One can not overemphasise the power of love and willed, directed intention in healing. It is very important that we activate and project our intention to heal our patients, i.e. we really want to make the treatment work and we visualise that this is happening. I have mentioned this above several times and will do so again. Late in life, Rudolf Steiner had a revelation after he had met the well known German naturopath, Marie Ritter. He realised that healing did not depend on the remedies themselves but on the awareness or intention of the therapist at the time of prescribing or administration of the remedies. Rudolf Steiner wrote: "In reality it does not depend on the **remedy** given but on the intention of the one **making** the remedy" (may be the therapist then often made the remedies themselves?) (R.Steiner,1920). Even without remedies, without needles or direct treatment of any kind, **focused intention can heal**. Sometimes it can work even better than a treatment given directly.*

Summary of the relationships between Anthroposophy and acupuncture for these initiated in the thinking process of both of those disciplines:

Zodiac sign	Channel	Human faculty	Sense of	Musical Note
Aquarius	SI	Sleep	Movement	B
Pisces	BL	Dream	Sight	F
Aries	LV	Sleep	Balance	C
Taurus	TH	Inspiration	Hearing	G
Gemini	LI	Dream	Taste	D
Cancer	ST	Sleep	Life	A
Leo	HT	Imagination	Warmth	E
Virgo	KI	Sleep	Feeling	H
Libra	LU	Intuition	Thinking	Giss
Scorpio	PC	Awake	Words	Ciss
Sagittarius	GB	Intuition	I (the self)	Fiss
Capricorn	SP	Dream	Smell	Diss

Table 106

On the relation between the ethereal and the physical
Do we need modern scientific parameters to confirm the clinical suc-
cess of our energetic treatment? For example, does clinical cure depend
on normalisation of biochemical anomalies (such as blood parameters,
mineral composition of tissue fluids, etc.), or normalisation of physi-
cal scans (such as ECG, myelography, ultrasonography, radiography,
scintigraphy etc.)? Conversely, does absence of change in "scientific"
lab tests or scans mean that our treatment has failed to induce clinical
cure?

These are very important questions. To both, the answer
is NO! Astonishing clinical results often occur in spite of no
change in the lab tests or scans. The following two examples
show this so well that little more need be said:

- *Example 1 was from my human practice: A woman had seri-*
  ous menstrual irregularity, many abortions, eczema, migraine,
  heavy uterine hemorrhage and had a very unstable psycho-
  logical life. Standard medical blood tests revealed that the hor-
  monal balance was out of control. I then treated her with AP
  and homeopathy and all her Lesion-Symptom Complexes disap-
  peared slowly. However, a blood test when she was well showed
  that the hormonal balance was as abnormal as before.

- *Example 2 was a dog with serious hip dysplasia (HD) and*
  severe intervertebral calcification in the back (spondylosis).
  When I put my hands on his back while he was walking, it felt
  as if stones were grinding and cracking in his spine. After 3
  treatments with AP at LV03, the dog could walk without pain
  and acted like a puppy again. A new radiograph showed that
  the hip and spinal lesions were unchanged. When I palpated
  his back as he walked, I felt the same sensation of grinding and
  cracking in the spine as before. In spite of those lesions, the dog
  continued to remain clinically sound and he did not need an
  additional treatment for another year.

How is this possible? I emphasise that I do not doubt the clinical val-
ue of the methods used, but it is hard to understand how the ener-
getic therapy had such good clinical effect on physical health without
a corresponding improvement in the scientific parameters used in the

*pretreatment assessments. A probable answer to the examples above is that the **ethereal or energetic body has little influence on the physical body**. **Energetic / ethereal therapies influence Life Processes and Life Expressions, more than they influence the physical body or lesions.***

*Holistic therapy has less potential to change the physical, material body than the physiological processes. It changes white blood cell **activity**, or **how** hormones influence the body but it may have little effect on their levels or amounts. (Some research, especially with AP, has shown clear effects on blood parameters, neurotransmitters, etc. This may be explained by assuming that the body has reservoirs of all these components, and after activating these components, it seems to be elevated, while they are more detectable).*

It is possible that the physical (material) body may be changed over a long time. This is certainly true of the material body of children or young animals as long as the body is growing (because the Processes govern the changes then). It is very important to be aware of these relationships, so that we do not promise our patients more than we can fulfil. An important exception is when we diagnose etheric changes that are abnormal or incompatible with healthy etheric formations or Processes as the root cause of the material pathology. When these are the root cause of cancer or exostosis, we can expect the material manifestations to disappear soon (in many cases) if we can correct or eliminate the abnormal etheric aspects. In that way, if we can banish, correct or control the causal abnormalities in the etheric body, it is quite easy to induce exostoses or tumours to diminish or disappear.

Chapter 8

HOW TO START THE PRACTICE OF HOLISTIC MEDICINE

By now, readers must understand that holistic medical practice does not appeal to all professionals. This is partly because proof of its validity is not as strong as those committed to "Evidence based medicine" (EBM) would like, and partly because holistic medicine involves the LIKEM Principle, (Love, Intuition, Knowledge, Empathy and Mysticism, as well as imagination, inspiration and sensitivity) and emphasizes the importance of **intention**. Those committed to EBM focus almost exclusively on the K (knowledge), whereas holistic practitioners put great importance on ALL elements in LIKEM; that inevitably involves the use of psychic methods. For further discussion of these topics, see Rogers (1998c).

When novices reach the point when they want to try to practice these methods, they encounter two questions:

- How to start?

- What disorders to treat?

The answers depend on the type of practice (horses, farm animals, companion animals, mixed practice, etc) and what therapeutic goals the novice has. *It is essential to regard these methods as complementary or addition to normal veterinary practice. A holistic veterinarian should be first a good clinician and practitioner!* It is important that s/he checks the sick animal to find out if the main Lesion-Symptom Complexes threaten the life of the animal, or cause great discomfort. I have seen many unsuccessful attempts by non vets to treat bone fractures, KI disorders and dystocia. These cases have convinced me of the importance of co-operating with a skilled veterinarian. *We all make mistakes but veterinarians, especially those trained in holistic methods, make fewer mistakes in diagnosis and treatment than untrained lay people.*

Holistic veterinarians emphasise the following methods together with, or sometimes instead of, conventional veterinary treatment:

1. To avoid having an adverse effect on our patients, we should keep ourselves physically, mentally (psychically and emotionally) and spiritually in good condition and balance, as far as we can. We should not train or treat a horse if we feel aggressive or depressed. However, it can also happen that working with animals can make us forget or overcome our negative emotions. Animals often help humans in this way.

2. We should record all atypical symptoms. These are very helpful as a guide to the selection of the correct homeopathic remedy in the early stages of the pathogenesis.

3. We should try to make the correct holistic diagnosis from the data discussed in the section on diagnostic methods. The key is to determine the Process Imbalances (Qi-, Channel-, Energetic-, or Functional- Imbalances) that allow the disease to manifest. It takes years of training and experience to become proficient in making a correct functionally oriented diagnosis.

4. We should record all scars and check them for blockages (Störfeld). We should note especially whether the symptoms occurred before or after specific injuries or operations.

5. We should examine all Back Shu Points routinely and record any reactivity (tenderness). These should be evaluated – and treated if necessary. Years of training are needed in order to perform correct interpretation of Back Shu Points.

6. We should examine all Ting Points in horses at each session and treat the reactive (deficient) point(s). If a point does not go away, we must not treat it too often. Every third week is sufficient.

7. We should identify, counter, or eliminate any External Stressors (Heat, Damp, Dryness, Cold, Wind, etc) and other adverse environmental influences.

8. Finally, we must identify and map any geopathic radiation, high voltage power lines and aquifers, so that we do not confine animals in such zones of radiation.

9. Having diagnosed the Process Imbalance(s) and the causal factors involved in the onset and manifestation of the symptoms, we should start the most appropriate therapy. That may be AP, homeopathy, herbs, ointments, manipulation etc., and/or conventional treatment if necessary, following the principles described in this book.

It is important that a veterinarian should make a conventional western diagnosis first. After that diagnosis, we can assess whether we should use conventional medicine only, or also help with holistic medicine. Conventional veterinarians seldom exclude totally the use of holistic medicine. Conventional and holistic medicines often constitute two sides of a rapid and effective healing.

We can consider practical advice for three groups of animals:

- Food-producing animals, such as pigs, cows and horses
- Sports horses
- Pets, such as dogs and cats

1. FOOD-PRODUCING ANIMALS (PIGS, COWS AND HORSES)

It is very important to cooperate with the attending veterinarian when one treats food-producing animals. For example, one should not try to use AP, or birth-promoting homeopathic remedies such as Caulophyllum, to assist an immature heifer to calve naturally; such heifers usually need immediate caesarean section. Also, all acute disorders such as milk fever, grass tetany, severe bloat, acute mastitis, fever, and acute toxicities etc., need immediate conventional treatment.

I recommend beginners to start by treating chronic mastitis, inappetance, chronic ketosis, chronic diarrhea, poor health, absence of health and various painful musculoskeletal disorders. This is because these disorders often respond poorly, or with difficulty, to conventional medicine. In those disorders, we should try holistic therapy after a poor response to conventional therapy.

In theory, it is very important to make a correct conventional diagnosis before attempting to select an effective therapy. However, we often can help cases for which there is no definitive scientific diagnosis. For example, we know that some individuals and well defined Syndromes often have the same cause from one individual to the next. For example, stimulating the immune system usually helps to treat chronic mastitis. As regards common disorders in farm animals, we can especially try to stimulate KI, LV and digestion (ST, SP, SI, LI, TH).

- *Chronic infections:* First, we should consider homeopathic medicaments (Arg., Cimicifuga., Sulph., Ars.alb. and Phos.) in addition to any Back Shu and Ting Points. Immune stimulating points, such as LI10 and SP06, should be stimulated.

- *Diarrhea (often related to SP Deficiency):* We can treat with Coffea, Carbo betula and Ars.alb. Remember points like ST16, LI04, LV03 and BL23-BL30.

- *Digestive disorders:* We should treat by stimulating LV with Stannum and SP with Ars.alb. Herbal options for consideration include Gentiana. Above all, we should not forget the dietary advice, discussed in the section about preventing illness (see page 649).

- *Disorders of fertility (anestrus, lack of sexual drive):* Consider Arg, Puls, Sep and Major / Melissa ointment applied at BL23.

- *Inappetance:* LV or SP Deficiency usually causes inappetance. We can stimulate LV and SP with herbs, medicaments or AP.

- *Ketosis and other LV-related disorders:* We can consider Stannum, Chel and Sulph. and Flor-de-Piedra, and/or use AP at LV Points

- *Mastitis:* We can stimulate acupoints BL28, ST16, ST36 and LV03, and/or consider Phytolacca, Lach, Bell and Acon.

While they are learning to use holistic methods, veterinarians may have limited success in treating the common disorders by those methods alone. *For the good of their patients, and for their own self-confidence, veterinarians should add conventional treatment in serious cases, or if improvement is slow.* However, as veterinarians become more confident in diagnosis, they can help in many other disorders.

If veterinarians learn to use Pulse Diagnosis, or are very sensitive in detecting reactive Back Shu Points, they also can treat many preclinical disorders, days, weeks or months before the symptoms would manifest otherwise. This is excellent prophylactic or preventative medical practice (see chapter 9). Even if they are not supersensitive, veterinarians who apply holistic principles often can promote animal health by preventing many different illnesses. For example, they can use holistic methods to stimulate:

- KI before the mating season;

- LV after parturition;

- LV and SP before changing the feed;

- LI, LV and SP when calves have tendency to get frequent diarrhea.

For example one may stimulate the relevant Process by leaving an AP needle in one of its relevant acupoints for 15 minutes. Alternatively, one could use homeopathic or herbal remedies to attain the same effect.

SPORTS HORSES

Sports horses respond particularly well to AP. I have treated thousands of horses that compete or race with very good results. I use mainly Ting Point diagnosis and treatment. However, I also must note the precise location of the pain, and along which Channels (points) the disorders have arisen. I must then treat this Channel, regardless of clinical findings from Pulse Diagnosis or the Back Shu- or Ting- Points. If this is difficult, for example in joint disorders, we then must rely on tenderness in the Back Shu- or Ting- Points and Pulse Diagnoses.

Some French veterinary schools (Maison Alfort) teach that 60% of joint disorders occur because the joints have been forced to carry excessive loads. Finding the cause of uneven loading of affected joints allows us to treat pain or infection in the joints. However, the presenting joint disorder often is not the primary one. Instead, it is a secondary effect, an attempt to compensate for, or to limit, pain or muscular imbalances elsewhere, i.e. in the back, neck or other joints, especially in the diagonally contra lateral limb. My experience confirms this.

First, we must examine and treat (balance) the whole horse in order to correct joint pain. Then, we should treat the joint itself via Ting Points or Earpoints related to the affected joint, plus Local Points around the joint. Better still, we should treat acupoints related to the Primary Process Imbalance (see page 84). Blisters or stimulant rubs to the affected area should be used in addition to this. Injection of synovial fluid substitutes (hyaluronic acid) into the joint or into the blood (Legend) may be appropriate in chronic joint disorders.

- *Arnica + Hypericum + Symphytum* is particularly useful in trauma, as a tincture or as homeopathic remedies. A bandage thoroughly sprinkled with a tincture of these three herbs can be applied to a wound, or to a traumatised area. Alternatively, we may give the homeopathic dilution via mouth, vagina or anus.

- It usually helps to add Distant and Local Points on the Channel(s) that pass (es) through or nearest to the injured area.

- We can also apply a bandage or plaster medicated with *Arnica + Hypericum + Symphytum* along an injured sinew or tendon. However, stimulating the Ting Point on the Channel that runs along the affected sinew is the most successful treatment for such injuries, together with a cast of 7-14 days.

- Stiffness that improves with exercise usually responds well to *Rhus.tox*. If the pain aggravates with exercise, we should use *Berberis* instead. Add acupuncture points like LV01 and Bai Hui.

- Crooked, crabby walking or trotting ("hanging on the rein", or favouring one side and avoiding the other) often is a symptom of neck, Para vertebral- and / or limb-pain on the disfavored side. For example, if a horse hangs on the right rein, or turns easily to the left but resents turning to the right, the problem is usually on the right side. When examining such horses, pay special attention to the back and neck.

- In horses more than 90% have a problem in their *right Iliosacral joint*. This must be treated in all horses with that problem.

To prevent disorders is not as easy in *sports horses* as in cows. However, we can still do it to a certain degree. Some horses have a weakness in their Gluteal muscles (in connection with problems of the iliosacral and hip joints), and we can prevent this by stimulating LV. During a change of feed, we should stimulate SP; in Cold weather, we should stimulate KI; in Hot weather, we should stimulate TH and LI. Stimulation of these different organ-Processes can also be done homeopathically according to the chart on page 546.

DOGS AND CATS

Specific disorders are different in dogs and cats than in farm- and sports- animals. Therefore it is not as simple to establish what to prevent, or to give prescriptions to treat specific illnesses. The different illnesses usually have individual causes and the animal must be examined according to the program that I have described in this book. It is still possible, however, to give some general advice and tips:

- Stimulation of LV03 greatly relieves most cases of canine hip dysplasia (HD). In dogs, the point is on the foot dorsum, between the upper heads of metatarsals 2-3. In HD, I needle LV03 to a depth of about 1 cm and retain the needle for 10 minutes. In these cases I usually treat the dog once every 4 weeks. Almost all dogs with HD-related disorders recover considerably or completely within a few weeks of receiving this therapy. They may need "booster treatments" 2-3 times/year when symptoms return.

- An interesting variation is to implant 24-karat gold wire in LV03. Since 1990, I have tested this method with good results in >100 dogs; 85% became asymptomatic after gold-wire implantation at LV03. The "total cure" rate increased to 95% when I added an additional gold wire implant at KI01. Only 5% of dogs showed no improvement to gold wire implants at LV03 + KI01. When I say, "totally cured", I mean that the dogs appeared to be free of pain and had an increased range of movement. However, the radiographic lesions showed little or no positive or negative change. This indicates that the symptoms are not due to the physical lesions per se; they arise due to **the process** of the illness, and its effects on the musculature in the hip area. This explains why certain rheumatic illnesses can self-cure ("burn out"). The pains in Bechtrew's disease disappear when the Process Imbalance stops, even if the physical changes remain.

- LV03 is also an interesting area when it comes to diagnosing hip dysplasia. I have noted that the "LV03 gap" (between the middle and the distal third of metatarsal bones 2-3) reduces as hip joint degeneration increases; in cases with severe and long lasting HD, it can be almost impossible to find space even for something as small as an AP needle there. As mentioned earlier, this observation has not been published before; it can be verified by independent researchers.

- AP at LV03, between metatarsal bones 2-3, helps mammary cancer. LV03 is needled to about 1 cm deep; the needle is retained for 10 minutes. After one session, in 75% of cases show a diminution of the mammary tumor. 95% show improved general condition, and 75% show a reduction of metastases.

- Epilepsy often has its cause in a Process Imbalance in KI or HT. These should be treated homoeopathically (phosphorus or aurum) and via acupoints or Ear points.

- Pseudo pregnancy often has its cause in a Process Imbalance between LV and KI. Homeopathic sepia, or AP at points for the LV, KI, TH/PC (TH05/PC06) and ovary, uterus and cervix can help.

- Giving Bearberry and "Renodoron" from Weleda can treat urinary tract disorders, especially in cats. Dosage of the Bearberry is 1 teaspoon X 4 times/day for 14 days in the food. Don't forget to put needles in KI and / or BL Points. Lyc. and Sabal serratus also seem to have a positive effect on urinary disorders in cats.

- In dogs and cats, holistic methods can help to treat infections (see "food-production animals"), and wounds and injuries (see sports animals).

- Back disorders in dogs respond well to Nux Vomica and chiropractic. Also, local Back Shu Points should be treated; use of BL60, LI03, KI03 and LV03 can prevent disorders from recurring later.

Adverse or unwanted side effects

Iatrogenic disease is very common in allopathic medicine and surgery. Such diseases result directly or indirectly from adverse or unwanted side effects of therapy - the medicines, therapy, or surgery used cause these effects. The medical professions have known of the high incidence of iatrogenic diseases for several hundred years. The old adage, "kill or cure", came from the early days of medicine, when heavy blood letting and highly toxic compounds, such as salts of arsenic, antimony and mercury were widely used as "medicines".

Today, most countries have formal mechanisms whereby practitioners (including veterinarians) must register any suspect cases of adverse drug reactions. These data are fed back in summary form to the practitioners each year. In the USA, the Food and Drug Administration (FDA) monitors all reports of adverse drug reactions and take steps to ban medications for which there is an unacceptably high risk, provided that safer alternatives are available. However, the FDA still allows licensed experts and practitioners to use highly toxic compounds in cases where no suitable alternative is available.

The list of iatrogenic diseases runs to several hundred. A few examples are:

- *Unintended effects of active ingredients, poisons or infective agents in medicaments,* such as:

    ° Onset of serious, often fatal, disease (including Hodgkin's disease) within months after vaccination; inadvertent contamination of vaccines and sera with other infectious agents.

    ° Allergic and anaphylactic reactions to antibiotics and other drugs.

    ° Nausea and vomiting from cytotoxic chemotherapy.

    ° Cushing's disease from chronic steroid use.

    ° Gastric hemorrhage from excessive use of aspirin, N.S.A.I.D.s or steroids.

    ° Multiple drug resistant bacterial infection and candidiasis from misuse or overuse of antibiotics, etc.

    ° Creutzfeldt-Jakob Disease (CJD) from infected pituitary extracts, used as sources of gonadotropin releasing hormones (GnRH) or growth hormone (MSH).

    ° Hepatitis, AIDS and possibly CJD from injection or transfusion of infected blood products.

    ° Congenital malformation after use of drugs, such as thalidomide

    ° Drug dependency / addiction from overuse of sedatives or sleeping tablets.

- *Unintended effects of surgery or cytotoxic irradiation,* such as:

    ° Intravascular clots, causing cardiac, pulmonary or brain embolism or infarct.

    ° Sudden death in the days or weeks after coronary angioplasty.

- ° Paralysis of a muscle or function after accidental sectioning of a motor nerve.

- ° Ileus, urinary retention, or urinary incontinence after lower abdominal surgery.

- ° "Dry eye" and other eye diseases after corneal "cosmetic" laser surgery.

- ° MRSA (methicillin- resistant Staphylococcus aureus) infections of incision sites in hospitals.

- ° Creutzfeldt-Jakob Disease (CJD) from infected tissue transplants, surgical or dental instruments.

- ° Hepatitis and AIDS from infected needles or instruments.

- ° Immunosuppression or leukemia from repeated use of radiography, radiation burns and tissue inflammation from onco-radiotherapy.

- *Inevitable results of radical surgery,* such as

  - ° Male impotence, sterility and KI Deficiency after radical surgery +/- surgical or chemical castration for prostatic cancer.

  - ° "Zombie" mentality after primitive use of lobotomy.

- *Unintended effects from inexpert spinal manipulation,* such as

- Spinal fracture or paralysis after unwarranted manipulation of a spondylotic, osteoporotic or tubercular spine.

- *Unintended effects from unwarranted or inexpert use of electroconvulsive therapy (ECT), TENS (transcutaneous electrical nerve stimulation) or electro-AP,* such as

  - ° "Zombie" mentality after primitive use of ECT

- ° Heart block if TENS or electro-AP electrodes are stimulates across the midline from the midcervical to the midthoracic area

- ° Aggravation of pain in some patients

Especially since the growth of Internet usage, the general public is also becoming aware of the extent of iatrogenic disease. Anyone can use the Internet to publicise anything that is legal within their national legislation. Those who suspect that they have an iatrogenic disease can search the Internet to see if others have had the same experience. In this way, special interest groups, including email discussion groups, can form to exchange data. In some cases this has led to Class Action cases, whereby a group of sufferers can sue a hospital or pharmaceutical company for damages in court. Such Class Actions are likely to increase in the future.

Proponents of holistic medicine, like acupuncture, herbal medicine, homeopathy, healing, etc., often claim that these are without serious side effects. Some claim that they are totally free of risk, a sort of "one way medicine". This is untrue. In particular, some herbal medicines contain potent active principles; they also can contain contaminants, such as heavy metals, bacteria and prions. Serious adverse effects can arise after their misuse, or the use of herbal medicines from companies that have poor quality control. Failure to know the contraindications or interactions of herbal remedies with other therapeutic agents can kill the recipient. How to classify and define the side effects of therapy is discussed below.

To get a better insight of the complexity of the problem, one must understand how the different therapies work and how one chooses to define the side effects. In this regard, it is appropriate to classify therapeutic modalities into two main types, information pattern therapies and direct acting therapies:

- *Information pattern therapies* include homeopathy and AP; they act only via information about, or by influencing, the body's Fundamental Processes

- *Direct acting therapies* include

- Substantial therapies, such as herbal medicine or aromatherapy

- Physical and reflex therapies, such as chiropractic and physiotherapy

Also, the side effects can be defined as either:

- Unwanted effects of the given substance or stimulation therapy

- Unpredictable or indeterminable effects of these therapies

When one considers therapies classified as above, one can clearly find the answer to the complexity of the problem as regards side effects.

- When used properly, *information pattern therapies* have few side effects. If they occur, they usually are predictable and often favour the healing response. For example, AP and homeopathy sometimes trigger an aggravation, or a return of earlier (forgotten) Lesion-Symptom Complexes before a resolution of the Lesion-Symptom Complexes. However, AP can have many side effects, some of them serious or fatal; these effects are due to the abuse of AP, rather than to AP *per se* (Rogers 1998b).

- *Direct acting therapies* that work via their own specific Processes (prescribed physical remedies such as arsenic or herbs, or external physical impulses, such as chiropractic manipulation) may have clear side effects, like arsenic poisoning or paralysis. Some herbal remedies have side effects that depend on the pathophysiological status of the recipient. Badly prepared remedies have additional side effects, including heavy metal toxicity, increase in paralysis, or pain and several other effects (lead or arsenic in Tibetan herb-pills). Also, fecal bacterial contamination of raw herbal ingredients can be a problem. It is most important that practitioners who use herbal remedies purchase their supplies from reputable sources that have a high degree of quality control. Also, the data sheets that accompany the remedies must be printed in a language that the practitioner and the client understand. It is illegal in the European Union to use herbal remedies that are unregistered. This is a separate issue for the future.

Vaccination and holistic medicine

Vaccination is a most useful means to prevent infectious disease. However, before deciding whether or not to vaccinate animals (or children), we must consider and evaluate all the facts objectively in the light of recent knowledge about the pros and cons. Therefore, we must decide

- Against which diseases should we vaccinate?

- How often should we vaccinate?

- At what age should we vaccinate?

- Should we vaccinate all individuals, or only those at most risk of the disease(s)?

- Under which conditions and in which situations should we vaccinate, or not vaccinate?

ADVANTAGES OF VACCINATION

The ultimate aim and the main advantage of successful vaccination are to induce specific immunity against specific infectious disease(s). This immunity also reduces the danger of transmission by natural infection(s) to individuals and the environment. In the case of smallpox, for example, the aim of mass vaccination of populations in, or people who wish to travel to, smallpox areas is to eliminate the disease completely.

Also, most shows, races, competitions and other events that involve the assembly of animals (dogs, cattle, horses, etc) from many different sources and environments require vaccination against specific diseases.

DISADVANTAGES OF VACCINATIONS

Because vaccines are so important to modern medical science and because they generates much income, the pharmaceutical trade and professionals who use vaccines seldom publicise their negative aspects and other disadvantages.

Vaccines can trigger many serious adverse effects, especially in two main areas, the *nervous system* and the *immune system.*

1. *Adverse effects on the nervous system:* Several research projects have shown that vaccination can cause lysis of existing myelin and inhibit the growth of the new myelin. Vaccinations early in life have a massive effect on the nervous system and the damage increases as the number of vaccines given simultaneously increases. Therefore it is important to vaccinate as late in life as possible.

2. *Adverse effects on the immune system:* Research in psycho-neuro-immunology has shown recently that close relationships exist between the nervous system, the psyche and the immune system. An influence on one system can influence the others. Happiness stimulates the nervous system and thereby also the immune system. Stress and depression weaken the immune system. Therefore, the immune system suffers when vaccines adversely affect the nervous system.

   Vaccination stresses the immune system directly. In clinical practice we see a clear increase in the incidence of allergies after vaccination. Also, we see an increase in the recurrence of chronic infections. Researchers compared children who had been vaccinated against measles and unvaccinated children who had developed and overcome measles; allergies were twice as prevalent in vaccinated- than in unvaccinated- children. A Danish report showed that children who overcame measles develop considerably less cases of cancer than vaccinated children. Women vaccinated against mumps had a higher incidence of uterine cancer than unvaccinated women.

3. Vaccination as a means to total eradication of an infectious disease works best when the pathogenic agent (bacterium, virus, protozoon, etc) is specific for one species and can not survive long in the environment without recycling in its natural host species. Unfortunately, many pathogens thrive in various animal species, including humans, birds and wildlife. The outbreak of foot and mouth disease (FMD) in 2001 in animals in the UK, and its spread to other European countries is an example. Countries that use vaccination to control FMD are at high risk of having FMD become endemic. At great cost, such countries must vaccinate all susceptible stock for many years, if not indefinitely. This is because the virus survives in many species of wildlife (for example, deer, wild pigs, wild goats, etc) which can not be caught for vaccination, or otherwise vaccinated effectively. Also, countries that vaccinate against FMD may lose their export markets for animal produce to those that are free of that dreaded disease. Bovine tuberculosis is another example. As the TB bacillus also can infect humans, deer, possums, badgers etc, cattle vaccination alone can not eradicate tuberculosis. Where infection can be transmitted directly or indirectly, vaccination of the main species (say cattle) can not eradicate the disease unless all host species can also be vaccinated.

In summary, vaccination can have adverse effects on the nervous and immune systems and, unless all susceptible species can be vaccinated, it will fail to eradicate infections that can cross species lines.

Conclusion

In spite of many negative aspects, vaccination is here to stay. Therefore, we must learn to live with it and consider how to use it in the optimal way:

- What diseases should we vaccinate against?

- Which individuals should we vaccinate?

- In what condition should the individual be when we give a vaccine?

- In which situations should we or should we not give a vaccine?

- At what age should we start to vaccinate?

- How often should we repeat each vaccine?

The answers to these questions are relatively easy. We should vaccinate as little as possible and rather evaluate the epidemiological situation. How great is the risk of the animal catching the disease and what is the risk if the animal should develop the disease? We must remember that we do not get healthier by not getting sick, rather the opposite is the case. It should not be necessary to vaccinate really healthy people or animals against illnesses like colds, coughs and flu. For example, horses may develop a contagious cough once or twice a year and an epidemic only strengthens the immune system and raises the resistance level of the population.

However, in endemic areas, we must use vaccines to prevent life-threatening diseases like distemper, rabies, tetanus and blackleg, etc. but we should wait until the animal is as old as possible. In my opinion dogs should be 6 months and horses should be 12 months of age before vaccination. Animals should be in balance as much as possible and not be exposed to stress immediately before or after the vaccination. We should not vaccinate animals that are ill or animals that have a weakened immune system. The same applies to animals suffering from allergies, eczema or cancer.

At the time of vaccination, the recipient should have as good an immune system as possible. Also, we can increase immunity (the effect of the vaccination) if we stimulate SP06 (and/or LI04, LI11, ST36 (the Immune Points)) after each shot. Alternatively, one treatment with Echinacea (herb) is advisable at the time of vaccination.

If vaccines cause undesirable side effects, to counteract the adverse reaction we can give Echinacea (herb), Thuja D30 or stimulate SP06 or LI10, or BL17 + BL20.

Some experiments have shown that the immune response of pups is stronger when vaccinations are given infrequently rather than frequently, even if the antibody (the blood titre) is larger in more frequent vaccination. In other words, the dog has the greatest possibility to fight diseases of puppyhood if it is vaccinated every third year rather than every year.

Holistic or conventional medicine:

AN ACADEMIC CONCLUSION

An objective approach to reality (truth) needs calm evaluation of all aspects of a complex case. A useful starting point is to assume that all honest parties in the discussion basically are correct in their evaluation, but that different groups see it from different standpoints. In relation to complementary medicine, there are mainly two opposing views:

- *Most informed and honest conventional medical therapists know of the weaknesses and adverse effects of conventional medicine. Nevertheless, they regard their methods as being superior to holistic medicine. This is because they think that holistic medicine lacks an acceptable level of proof of its* safety, efficacy and quality-control. *These are the three main criteria by which conventional medical therapists assess any therapy, or therapeutic agent.*

- Most informed and honest holistic medical therapists know of the weaknesses and adverse effects of conventional medicine *and of* complementary medicine. Most

think that their more integrated approach usually sur-
passes the results of most conventional medicine. That
is why holistic veterinarians or MD´s have taken the
time, often many years, to study holistic methods and to
use them routinely in their practices.

Let us accept that both groups in the debate in conventional
versus holistic medicine are correct in their observations. Let
us also accept that they observe aspects of reality that are true
for them and that they present their reality truthfully to the
best of their ability. We must therefore try to understand how
these diametrically opposed conclusions can coexist in scientific truth.

First let us assess the situation from the viewpoint of conventional medicine. Typical conventional therapists see and defend the excellence of their medicines and methods. Modern
antibiotics can suppress an acute bacterial infection within
hours; they are much better than any herbs or teas in such
cases. After a viper-bite, cortisone can remove unbearable itch-
ing or swelling in an arm within minutes. Potent analgesics and
anaesthetics can remove pain almost immediately or induce
narcosis for surgery. Similarly, conventional medicine uses very
advanced technology that can give rapid information on blood
values, bone structure, fracture morphology or degree of calcification in joints, etc.

Let us now look at the situation from the viewpoint of holistic medicine. If we think of the example of the girl who had
drunk concentrated NaOH (see page 511), or other examples
from this book, we cannot but wonder in awe of the effectiveness and usefulness of holistic therapy and its relative absence
of side effects.

In order to understand the distance between the conventional and holistic viewpoints, it is important to differentiate
between

- Holistic *methods and remedies*

- Holistic *thinking and diagnosing*

If used on the basis of *conventional thinking processes*, holistic methods, must fail almost totally when compared to the conventional methods, unless the latter have serious side effects. Because conventional therapists tend to think in conventional ways, they prefer their medicines to the remedies of holistic medicine. *What they fail to consider, is that holistic methods must be used within the model of holistic concepts and thought processes.* The advantage of holistic medicine lies in its understanding of the causes, effects and development of illness, its understanding of illness in energetic terms, and of the interactions between the soma, psyche and spirit in ways unacknowledged by conventional therapists.

It is not so much that the methods used in holistic therapy are especially effective, but rather that they are applied at the correct point, and/or are used to help the Process Imbalance that allowed the Lesion-Symptom Complexes to manifest. It is the Process Imbalance that helps the body to help itself when it manifests the Lesion-Symptom Complexes of the disease. For example, the symptom of pain is the body's "call for help" from its innate resources as well as for external help. Similarly a national epidemic, such as human nvCJD in UK, or an international epidemic, such as foot and mouth disease in animals, is an "alarm cry" to examine seriously, *and to correct if possible*, all the environmental, social, managemental and political factors that triggered the epidemics.

The holistic model of thinking is difficult for conventional therapists to accept. *De facto*, if they accept it, they would be no longer be true to their beliefs if they continued to practise conventional medicine only. To follow their instincts, they would have to move into the realm of holistic medicine. Therefore, we accept that holistic medicine will remain a marginalised medical model reserved for those who can change their thinking processes to embrace a holistic view of the world. It also follows that conventional medical practitioners probably will continue to regard holistic medicine as inferior to theirs, and they may continue to try to enforce a ban on all therapies that can not meet their criteria of "Evidence based medicine". We have a parallel to this in the white man's way of looking at the Australian Aborigine's boomerang in comparison with his own rifle. Certainly, though much more costly, the rifle is a more powerful and lethal weapon than the boomerang. However, in the context of the close-to-nature conditions in which many Aborigines wish to live unhindered in the Australian bush, their skills in using the boomerang, and its minimal effect on the environment and on their society, the boomerang is much more effective and desirable than the rifle.

The importance of double-blind studies to prove the efficacy of acupuncture therapy

BACKGROUND TO PARADOXICAL THERAPEUTIC RESULTS

Most veterinary acupuncturists who use AP, or gold implants at the acupoints, find them to be most successful and effective to treat canine hip dysplasia (HD). Clinical experience from several colleagues (Drs. Terry Durkes, H. Grady Young, Pål Hanson, John Limehouse, Phil Rogers, Allen Schoen and others), with overall success rates of 80-90%, supports this opinion.

Recently, although they used slightly different methods of implantation, three independent uncontrolled retrospective clinical studies on the effectiveness of gold implants to treat canine HD in 218 dogs in Denmark (the late Jens Klitsgaard, 100 dogs), Norway (Are Thoresen, 50 dogs) and Germany (Erhard Schulze, 68 dogs) reported a clinical success rate of near 90%.

However, the clinical response to gold bead implantation AP to treat canine HD was evaluated also in two double-blind studies. One was in Finland by Anna Hielm et al (1998) and the other was in the USA by Bebchuk et al (1998).

- Anna Hielm gave me a summary of her article in Finnish. The dogs were treated in a double-blinded study; the owners did the evaluation. Both groups of dogs showed positive results but there was no difference between the two groups.

- Bebchuk's study was a communication from his university. He also treated the dogs in a double-blind study but the evaluation was objective; it used force-plates to measure the force exerted by the dogs on the treated limbs. Neither group of dogs improved, and there was no difference between the two groups. The dogs in the treatment group tended to get worse.

Both studies show the same result: gold-implantation in the hip area had no positive effect on the dogs and some dogs in Bebchuck's study got worse! Assuming that all five studies, referred to above, were true and honest, let us discuss how the clinical results could be so divergent: they show two apparently different parts of reality.

PHILOSOPHICAL BACKGROUND

After Aristotle, philosophy stated that if A is different from B, then A could not be the same as B. This philosophy has prevailed since that time. Before Aristotle, already in the time of Plato, A and B could be the same, yet different, at the same time. This can be possible because different people observe the phenomena from different viewpoints (as in the story of the three blind men examining the elephant). Honest observers that differ in individuality, purpose and intention can observe different realities when faced with the same phenomenon. This philosophy has survived and is held widely, even today in some Asian, religious and shamanistic traditions, traditions that deal with living forces, etheric powers and religion, which all depend on individuality. Modern Quantum Physics and the Uncertainty Principle have rediscovered this philosophy also, observing that the personality of the experimenter changes the results of the experiment.

The purpose of the following discussion is to investigate if the five studies, three having opposite results to the other two, may all be true on the basis of pre-Platonian philosophy and the theory of different people and intentions interrelating with the result of the experiment. We also will discuss two very important issues:

- Can the act, or fact, of "double-blinding a study" change the premise of the study in a way that alters its outcome? This is especially important as regards an energetic spiritual therapy, such as that involved in AP.

- Is it true, as in the words of Heraclitus, that: "Nature likes to hide itself".

Discussion

The practice of medicine and of the healing arts operates on many levels. One can classify these levels in many ways:

- GP medicine v specialist medicine

- allopathic v holistic

- mechanistic v energetic

- materialistic v mystical

- corporal somatic v ethereal spiritual

- personal v impersonal

In human medicine, the role of "*bedside manner*" and "*doctor patient trust*" are well known. At its best, AP is a high form of *physical-energetic-spiritual medicine*. It combines full consideration of the client's history, psyche (emotions, spirit, symptoms) and soma (lesions, signs) and the importance of balance and imbalance in and between the interior and exterior environment. AP accepts the *Law of Change*. The skilled AP therapist aims specifically to rebalance the circulation of the client's Qi and Blood, and to remove Stasis or Obstructions, in order to help the natural homeostatic mechanisms of the body and psyche spirit to adapt to his or her unique realities in the optimal way.

Most energetic spiritual therapies operate on the basis of LIKEM, a combination of love, intuition, knowledge, empathy and mysticism:

- *Love:* Compassion for the patient is of great importance for the outcome of AP therapy. This is held to be true also in Asia.

- *Intuition* is the interrelation between the energetics of the healer and the patient. It helps the healer to feel or decide the most appropriate treatment, one that may give better results than if the healer used the intellect alone.

- *Knowledge* is undoubtedly of great importance for successful treatment but knowledge alone makes for poor therapy. Some doctors, regardless of their academic knowledge, make poor therapists. Rightly or wrongly, they project negative signals (impersonality, greed, hurry, impatience, uncertainty etc) to their clients.

- *Empathy* creates a trust within the patient that enhances the healing process.

- *Mysticism:* Many holistic physicians hold that all healing comes from God. The human healer is only an extension of God's love for creation, *a Mystical Impersonation*, the actual incorporation of the Spirit in human form.

To each of the 5 components of LIKEM, skilled therapists and natural healers add one most important factor - directed intention (will). They know how important it is to direct their intent and energy to the task of healing their patients.

All of the above are crucial factors in healing. The fact that they change greatly the results of therapy (by AP or other energetic therapy), indicate that the qualities of the therapist influence the outcome of the treatment or the experiment. Modern quantum physics has precedents to suggest that the observer can change the outcome (information given during conversations at the 1998 Annual Congress in Veterinary AP, Taiwan). If this is true, it follow that *the best medicine must be based on love, respect and the willed, focused intention to heal.*

As well as in recent email discussion groups between practising acupuncturists, many serious AP books from China expressed this opinion, for example:

- *Chapter 26 of the Suwen:* "... That which differentiates craftsmen is that which is not manifested to be observed externally and that all cannot observe. Therefore observing that which is obscure means seeing that which has no form and tasting that which has no flavour. *This [capacity] seems to be divine*".

- *Scheid & Bensky:* In pre-Han China, yì (intention) was considered a pre-requisite of the knowledge and understanding required for and derived from the divination practices based on the Ijing. "*Yì is what the sages used to search profundity and study the all encompassing. As it is profound, it can penetrate throughout the purpose of the sub celestial realm. As it is all encompassing, it can penetrate throughout the affairs of the sub celestial realm. As it is divine, it is fast but never hurries; it arrives but never travels*".

- *Zhenjiu Dacheng:* "The importance of AP lies in *concentration of the mind*"

- *Guo Yuzhi:* "needling ability rests with whether [acupuncturist] can *focus his attention on the heart and hand* during the needling".

- *Xu Yinzong:* "*Medicine is intention; it is in one's thoughts and deliberations.*

Also many scientific experiments have been carried out in recent years on the effects of Qigong (the emission of Qi (directed will and intention) from the practitioner). The results showed that will and intention could kill bacteria, cancer cells, and lower blood pressure and improve the level of the immune system (investigations of the English healer, M. Manning)

Can such qualities be present in double-blind controlled trials? As discussed above, most energetic-spiritual therapies operate on the basis of a combination of LIKEM (love, intuition, knowledge, empathy and mysticism), *plus directed intention.* We argue that *the combination of those qualities cannot easily be maintained in a double-blind study.* If these qualities are as important as ancient Chinese texts and modern holistic and colleagues maintain future research studies must consider them in a very different way than has been the case up to now and especially in controlled trials.

It is difficult to imagine how the described qualities can be maintained in double-blind studies. If they are as important as we think, there are important implications for future studies on the mechanisms and clinical effects of AP.

Conclusions

- Because the clinical results are due, at least in part, to the qualities, intention and empathy of the investigator, double-blind studies do not fit well within energetic therapies such as homeopathy or AP. This is not to say that the results of AP and homeopathy depend on the belief of the patient in the therapist. If that were so, the hip-dysplastic dogs in the retrospective clinical studies would not have been better. Instead, the results depend in part on the mental capacity and quality of the therapist, which directly influence the healing powers of the body of the patient.

- Conventional scientists ridicule holistic practitioners' arguments that double-blind studies are not valid to test some of their methods. The claim, however, it *not an admission of reluctance to be assessed;* it merely states that new methods of research and new ways to assess holistic therapies need to be considered.

A probable explanation why most of the effects of AP, homeopathy, Zone Therapy, divining rods etc. disappear when submitted to critical assessment or double-blind study, is that these effects are (at least part-ly) the product of the therapist's focused intention or directed will. In other words, the instruments of the water diviner, homeopathic remedies or AP needles are nothing more than "aids to concentration", or objects to help to focus the directed intention of the operator or therapist. Once therapists realise this, they can dispense with this equipment, or simply visualise it in action as if they had the material instruments in hand.

Chapter 9

PREVENTING DISEASE

Importance of nutrition

Properly balanced diets are important for good health and well being and to prevent disease in humans and animals. Internationally, universities and scientific institutes have done extensive research to establish data on nutritional requirements, for example for fiber, protein, fat, carbohydrates, vitamins and minerals. Nutritionists must consider many factors when they attempt to formulate a perfectly balanced diet. These include the nature, physiology, productivity and stress levels of the animal(s) being fed, the composition of the raw ingredients and supplements, variation in the quality of feed ingredients, the specific times for consumption, contents of pesticide and other chemical residues in the plants, use of artificial fertilisers and the use of herbs and spices, etc. However, expert opinions on optimum balance of animal diets are being updated continually. Thus, the quality of animal diets may need further revision.

Some specific factors that I feel are very important in compromising animal health are summarised and discussed below. Factors that adversely affect animal health include the use of:

- artificial fertilisers

- synthetic pesticides and crop sprays

- grass monocultures in pasture and conserved fodder for farmed animals

- Animal feed with inadequate dietary fiber and/or chop length (threads)

- mineral licks containing a combination of salt and minerals for animals

- dried fodder for animals

- "processed food" for dogs and cats

- antioxidants (i.e. ethoxyquin) in commercially prepared animal feed

- excessive or poor quality protein for LV and KI

- poor quality fat and its importance for LV function

- excessive sugar and its importance to LV function and the immune system

Where possible, we should remove, limit or rectify these conditions immediately.

ARTIFICIAL FERTILISERS
Today production of large amounts of highly digestible fodder is a primary goal in animal production. However, rapid grass growth, especially on rotational paddock systems, involves increased forage levels of non-protein nitrogen (amino acids, amides, nitrate and nitrite). Also, increased grass growth and reduced transit time through the digestive tract reduce the net absorption of major and trace minerals from the forage.

This is an example of the conflict between quantity and quality of forage. Although it increases the amount of forage produced per hectare, intensive use of artificial fertilisers adversely affects some aspects of the quality of animal fodder. Therefore, many professionals believe that we should advise farmers to avoid feeding animals on forage from intensively fertilised areas.

INSECTICIDES AND PESTICIDES

The quality of groundwater has deteriorated in the past 20 years. This adversely affects the quality of human water supplies, but also threatens the health and survival of fish and other animals that live in our rivers, lakes and seas. Water pollution is due mainly to pollution from farming, urban and industrial practices. Pollution of the environment (including marine mammals and ground water) with pesticides, insecticides and other chemicals is an increasing problem. This is alarming because these chemicals have a negative effect on reproductive function, LV and the immune system. Therefore, in order to reduce disease incidence in humans and animals, we should avoid food and animal fodder, which contain chemical residues.

MONOCULTURE SWARDS

The immune system relates mainly to the Processes of LV and SP and that these organs "taste" and must process the food that we eat. If the digestive system receives too many monotonous impulses, this may weaken the immune system (see the importance of variation in the Weak Structure, page 40).

In German research, inclusion of >29 species of wild herbs in cattle fodder stimulated the immune system, but <20 species suppressed the immune system (Jürg Spranger). This is something to consider when produce forage for optimum animal health; we should strive towards the greatest possible richness of lively tastes and aromas.

In Norway, I have seen hay organically grown in the mountains and lowlands that were much better for the immune system than hay from cultivated areas that were fertilised, sprayed with weed killers, or otherwise "forced". Such organically grown hay usually consists of 30+ botanical species. According to Asbjörn Lavoll, farmer and agriculturist in Sandefjord, one can grow excellent organic hay in previously cultivated fields, by reseeding with 10-12 species and by avoiding chemical weed killer sprays. The seed mixture can consist of timothy (Phleum pratense), rye grass (Lolium), dog grass (Dactylis glomerata), Meadowgrass, Yorkshire fog, cocksfoot, bentgrass, etc [(Poa pratensis), (Agrostis tenuis) and (Festuca pratensis)]. The content of energy, protein and other feed components are better in grazed and conserved herbage from reseeded ryegrass monoculture. Reseeded ryegrass is usually a much better feed for cattle than grazed or conserved old permanent herbage (**Teagasc** Advisory Services, Ireland). However, in my experience, old, multi-species pasture is better for the immune system.

DIETARY FIBER AND CHOP LENGTH
The content of dietary fiber and chop length (threads, fibers) are important for all species, including humans. For optimal bovine ruminal movement and function, the chop length of herbage cut for fodder, should be >2.5 cm (Jürg Spranger). Fiber is also important for normal peristaltic function in LI. Increased fiber content in the food also reduces the incidence of colon cancer in humans (the Norwegian Journal of Medicine) and animals. Additional fiber in the food of dogs and cats reduce the incidence of KI disorders. This is because the ratio of free- and protein bound- nitrogen is shifted to a more desirable state.

SALT LICKS
Although I can not be sure for other species, I often see in my practice that horses that can choose freely between salt

and standard mineral mix consume **10 times** as much minerals as salt. Excess salt stresses KI, and when I through Pulse Diagnosis discover a KI-deficiency, this deficiency will usually vanish much faster if I take away the licking-stone of the horse. In my opinion, salt and minerals should be given in separate bowls to which the animals have free access. Salt blocks or licks should not combine salt and other minerals; that combination forces animals to consume excessive quantities of salt if they want minerals. These observations refer to Norway, a very cold country with low summer temperatures. It may be, and probably is, quite different in other climates. These observations refer only to KI Qi. Otherwise animals can ingest enormous quantities of salt safely, provided that they have access to *ad libitum* water. Also, MOST National Advisory Services recommend the combination of Ca, P, Na, Mg, Cu, Co, Mn, Se, I and vitamins A, D3 and E in balanced mineral mixtures.

PELLETED (DRY) FOOD FOR SMALL ANIMALS

For small animals (dogs, cats), pelleted (dried) food is "dead" food. Traditionally, herbivores (horses, cattle, sheep, goats) thrive well on diets that include dried forages (hay, straw) and concentrate-feeds (grains, soyabean, cottonseed, etc), especially in the winter. However, herbivores thrive better and have less digestive upsets, if they eat crushed or rolled grains (coarse-feeds) rather than finely-ground and pelleted feed. I have often seen improved health in horses after substitution of coarse feeds for pellets; coarse feeds and whole grains are more "alive" (have more Qi) than pelleted feeds.

Degeneration of food quality begins as soon as pelleted food is produced, and degeneration increases with length of storage. By-products of food degeneration may have adverse effects on the body. Such food that is stored for long periods will contain food mites. Mites or their excreta can cause allergies. We see many allergies in dogs and cats that are being fed commercially prepared dry and pelleted food. This undesirable practice is becoming very common today. Even when it is produced to the highest technical standards to match the recommended requirements of dogs and cats at different stages of their lives, commercial dried and pelleted food can be dangerous, inadequate or undesirable. This is because it usually contain antioxidants, vegetable fats (margarine), remnants of mites and other insects, bacterial contamination by birds and vermin in the manufacturing plant or storage depots, diverse breakdown products that are effected by time, fungal toxins, etc. All of these adversely affect animal health.

The health of dogs and cats is better if they eat food that is prepared fresh at home and that is of the same quality that we eat ourselves. This applies even if the quality of the food that we eat is not as good as it should be. I have seen the health of many dogs improve dramatically soon after the owners began to share their family's food with their dogs.

PRE-PROCESSED ANIMAL FEED
We must not underestimate the value of fresh food compared to old, preserved food, whether it is pelleted or canned (dried whole grains are not dead, they are absolutely alive and have no adverse effects). Most medical doctors agree that fresh food, prepared daily, is healthier than canned food for humans. Also, I and several colleagues have noted that pre-processed (canned and dried) food has negative effects in animals in comparison to "living", fresh food. For example, I have observed that dogs that are overweight, or that fail to lose weight, when fed scientifically formulated foods, immediately start to lose weight when fed fresh, home-made food, even if this food contains more calories then the pre-processed food. Also, several colleagues have observed that dogs with reduced pancreatic function have improved after a change of diet from canned to fresh food.

ANTIOXIDANTS IN PRE-PROCESSED ANIMAL FEED
Antioxidants in food are necessary to prevent the development of rancidity. Rancid fat is bad for the organism but recent experiments have proven that synthetic antioxidants, for

example ethoxyquin, weaken the immune system. Where possible, food should contain only natural antioxidants such as vitamin E and C.

DIETARY PROTEIN AND FAT

The liver must metabolise the products absorbed from the digestive tract. Feeding of high-protein, high-energy diets puts great stress on LV Function.

Many diets have grossly excessive amounts of protein for animals. In my practice, many diseases of the liver and kidney in horses and dogs have improved greatly after the owners reduced dietary protein inputs on my advice. Excessive protein intake damages especially the kidney and the liver, or at least the Qi of these organs or Processes. In recent years, expert animal nutritionists have recommended less and less dietary protein. Even for pups, dog food with >20% protein is potentially poisonous. In my experience, dietary protein for pups and adult dogs should not exceed 15% and 12%, respectively. Also, horses should not be fed a total diet in which the protein exceeds 12% dietary protein.

Notes on the energy and protein requirements of horses

All horses: *Energy and crude protein (CP) requirements differ between horse breeds (standardbred trotters - warm bloods - and Finnhorses - cold bloods) and physiological activities (pregnancy, lactation and work). Dry matter (DM) intake (DMI) of lactating mares was 2-3.5 kg/100 kg; DMI of working horses and pregnant mares was 1.6-1.8 kg/100 kg. Individual variation in energy intake among working horses is high, especially in Finnhorses (Saastamoinen 1993).*

Mares and foals: *In the first month of lactation, mares produce 2-0-3.5 kg milk/100 kg (Doreau 1994). Other references say that the capacity of the mare's udder is 1.5-2.5 l and that the foal suckles 5-7 times/d, taking 8-17 l/d. Mares secrete milk with 20-22g protein/l. They need 49 g digestible protein or 75 g CP/kg milk. A mare loses 200-300 g protein/d in 10-15 kg milk and needs 750-1100 g total dietary*

CP to compensate for that (Kosharov et al 1984). Protein requirement (as L-amino acids) for critically ill foals and adults was 200-300 and 100-150 g/100 kg/d, respectively. Fluid requirement was 10-17 and 1.5-5.0 l/100 kg/d, respectively. Parenteral feeding prevented digestive complications but was expensive and labour-intensive (Schusser 1994). Protein deficiency reduces foal development but giving protein at levels greatly above the US-NRC requirements for the average total ration (16% DM) is of no value (Hintz 1986a). Weanling foals are sensitive to the quality of dietary protein, i.e. amino acid supply. Lysine and threonine are first-limiting amino acids for growth. Dietary protein quality influences the amino acid profile of serum. The energy requirements of weanling foals depend on age, growth rate and proportion of the utilised growth potential. Requirements for growth are influenced by ambient temperature and the type of energy source fed to foals (Saastamoinen 1996). Newly weaned New Forest and Welsh ponies (fillies, about 6 months old, c. 105 and 120 kg, respectively), were given the same diet of concentrate to maintain a constant weight or to grow at a predetermined rate. Apparent digestibility of dietary CP was 0.70. CP intake to maintain constant weight in New Forest and Welsh ponies, respectively, was 113 and 125 g/d. Weight gains of 378 g/d and 301 g/d, respectively, required CP intakes of 332 and 281 g/d (Ellis & Lawrence 1980).

Young horses: *Fed to a maximum of 3% bodyweight, high forage diets (60% lucerne cubes (18% CP and 0.80% lysine) and 40% concentrate) can meet the energy and protein needs of young growing horses. The NRC (1989) protein and lysine requirements are adequate for forage-based diets (Coleman et al 1997).*

Adult and working horses: *Feed digestibility decreases as the content of crude fiber of the diet increases. Therefore crude fiber content of horse diets should not exceed 20% of total DM, with a minimum of 15% to avoid colic. Energy demands for maintenance of a 500-kg horse are circa 73 MJ/d, but depend on bodyweight, breed, temperament and performance (130.0 MJ/d for heavy work), etc (Galler 1997). Energy demands increase dramatically as work increases from walking* *to galloping. For strenuous work, horses of 500 kg need 110-151 MJ of energy or 10.5-14.4 feed units (Patterson et al 1985).*

There is no evidence that increasing dietary protein above maintenance level increases muscle mass or energy production of racehorses. By oxidation and gluconeogenesis, protein can produce energy during exercise but it is not the optimum source of energy (Miller-Graber 1991). CP requirement for maintenance and heavy work, respectively, is 350 and 480 g. It is important to avoid an oversupply of protein (Galler 1997). Dietary CP of 6% is adequate for mature horses, regardless of workload. In athletic horses, high input of dietary protein (>9% DM) has no benefit and may have adverse effects; it is certain that water requirement increases with high protein inputs. Most hays and grains satisfy the estimated protein requirement (Hintz 1986b). However, horses doing hard work may need supplementary protein to offset 38 g nitrogen (equivalent to 238 g CP) lost in sweat, and the fall in plasma amino acid concentrations that occurs in chronic sub maximal exercise. Increased protein intake may lower blood lactate concentration and improve performance (Custalow 1991).

Ireland is world-famous for its thoroughbred horses. However, it has high-N grass because its rainfall is dispersed throughout the year (thus its green countryside - the Emerald Isle) and the application of N-fertilisers and recycling of slurry for early grazing. Crude protein (CP) levels in the dry matter (DM) of Irish herbage, grass-silage and hay on cattle and sheep farms are circa 22 (range 6-39), 15 (range 6-37) and 8 (range 5-13) % DM, respectively (Rogers & Murphy 2000). Thus, on ruminant farms, the CP levels in herbage and grass silage often are too high for horses. Irish horse owners usually use hay and concentrates as the main feed for horses; they use old (usually unfertilised) pastures, or bare pasture as exercise areas to limit the protein intake of their horses.

In conclusion, *the CP requirement of horses is controversial. Lactating mares and rapidly growing foals may need 14-18% CP in the dietary DM, whereas adult horses may be satisfied with CP levels* *in the total dietary DM as low as 6-9% CP. Feeding excessive protein is bad policy.*

Fat: The type of dietary fat is very important for LV function. All kinds of **margarine** stress LV Function in monogastric species and slowly weaken the immune system and induce allergies (Dr med. Wollf, personal communication). Gastric, pancreatic and hepatic enzyme systems can not metabolise fully the new "synthetic" fats that are available in foods today (Dr. Wollf). Because imbalanced LV Function is an essential causal factor in the development of HD in dogs, exclusion of vegetable fat also can be important in preventing HD. I have had success in treating many cases of allergy and food intolerance in both humans and dogs simply by excluding pre-processed vegetable fat (such as margarine) from the diet. Also, exclusion of pre-processed vegetable fat (to make it hard, not liquid) is very important when feeding calves. Milk substitutes for pre-ruminant calves should not contain such fats (for example "hardened" coconut-fat) to which they are unaccustomed (Prof. Magne Aas Hansen, Veterinary Highschool of Oslo). In contrast, adult ruminants can handle most vegetable- and animal- fats without difficulty as long as the total inputs are not excessive.

DIETARY SUGAR

LV Function has the same role and importance in metabolising dietary sugar as it has in fat metabolism. LV has a day-night rhythm, which is maximal at 0300h and minimal at 1500h. In the anabolic phase (0300-1500h) LV synthesises glycogen from glucose; in the catabolic phase (1500-0300h) it breaks down glycogen (my teacher in Physiology at the Vet. School). It is therefore important to avoid eating sugar (sweet) during the anabolic phase of LV. Thus, sweet food should not be consumed until after 1500h (Dr. Victor Bott, France, personal communication). As with margarine, I have in my own practise, treated very many allergies successfully only by excluding sugar consumption between 0300 and 1500h.

Notes on diets for sick dogs (and cats)

Diet to help LV Function in dogs prone to HD	Diet to help LV Function in pups from parents prone to HD
Lower dietary protein content drastically (15% for pups, 12% for adult dogs)	Give 2-4 g sodium ascorbate/day to the pregnant bitch
Avoid food with synthetic antioxidants; use Vitamin C and E instead.	Give 100 mg sodium ascorbate/day to pups <3 weeks old
Avoid all margarine; use pure vegetable oils or butter	Give 500 mg sodium ascorbate/day to pups 3-4 weeks old
Avoid sweet-tasting foods	Give 2 g sodium ascorbate/day to pups 4-24 months of age
Feed a lot of vegetables, especially broccoli	
Add extra sodium ascorbate (2 g daily)	

Table 107

Diet for dogs with KI disorders	Diet for cats with KI disorders
2 eggs	¼ cup hamburger meat
½ cup of meat	¼ cup azuki beans
2 cups rice	¼ cup brown rice
2 tablespoons vegetables	2 tablespoons cottage cheese
1 teaspoon honey	1 tablespoon vegetables

Table 108

Notes on diets for healthy dogs

Referring to what has been said earlier, this section is a brief summary of how to prepare an optimal diet for healthy dogs. To prepare a complete meal, we first need a good carbohydrate source; bread, pasta, macaroni, rice, potatoes, beans or cereals are adequate. This part can be prepared for three days at a time. Into this, we mix protein as eggs, meat or fish. Finally, we add minerals, vitamins, a little oil and lastly a sardine or sprat. Here are two examples of a menu:

Menu 1	Menu 2
400g chicken	3 eggs
3 cups of potatoes	2 cups of rice
1 sardine	1 sardine
2 teaspoons of olive oil	1 teaspoon rapeseed oil
¼ teaspoon bone powder	¼ teaspoon bone powder
¼ multivitamin pill	¼ multivitamin pill
a little salt	a little salt

Table 109

NOTES ON DIETS FOR HEALTHY HORSES

Great care is needed to provide horses with *fresh water ad libitum*, preferably fed from a clean *bucket*. When horses return to the stable after heavy work, they can be very thirsty. Automatic drinkers in the stable are very convenient and save labour but they usually are too slow to fill. Thirsty horses can not get the water quick enough and may suck a lot of air in trying to do so. They also usually get too little water from such installations. For the horse to get to drink enough water, the drinking device must give at least 6 litres of water/minute. This can be a factor in causing digestive upsets and colic.

It is important that healthy horses get hay composed of many (at least 30) species of grasses, herbs, flowers and harmless weeds, lactic acid fermented silage, crushed or whole oats that are fresh or alive, a mineral supplement without salt, pure salt separately and vitamins. It is also important that the high energy feed (oats, etc.) is fed at the same time every day (preferably after 1500h). Sudden changes of feed stress LV and SP. Change of feed (including hay) should be very gradual, over a period of at least 14 days and the new feed should be given in gradually increasing amounts. Even a new load of hay from the same farmer should be considered new feed, since it may have been harvested from a different field.

NOTES ON DIETS FOR SICK HORSES

In general, sick horses need good care and good nutrition, including good water, good mould-free oats and hay from at least 30 botanical species. Before we formulate other aspects of the diet for sick horses, we must first establish the Process Imbalance (root cause of the disease). For example:

Process Imbalance (root cause of disease)	Advice
LV disorders	**Use forage and coarse feeds only.** Remove all pelleted food. Avoid all processed vegetable fats (margarine) and sweet feeds (molasses). Reduce dietary protein content to 12% or less. (See note on protein for horses, above, page 510). Give additional lactic acid (acid from fermented lactose).
Muscular disorders (LV,SP)	Give a LV diet (as above).
SP, ST, SI, LI (digestive) disorders	I advise good hay, hay and more hay (plus more oats). Also give Gentiana (gentian plant), as well as general dietary hygiene and advice as above.
KI disorders	Remove all salt. Give other minerals (ordinary mineral/vitamin mixtures). Use a woollen blanket over the lumbar area to protect the KI area at all times.

Table 110

The importance of the environment

THE IMPORTANCE OF VARIETY OF STIMULATION

Monotony is boring and has adverse effects! If we are constantly exposed to the same sounds, the same tastes the same colours etc., we get very bored and we seek change. Like humans, animals need interesting surroundings. They need variation in stimulation via all the senses - sight, hearing, touch, taste and smell.

- I have seen many cases where, after two months in the same stable, horses with the same type of training and feed, became bored; they lost their ability to perform well. However, as soon as the manager introduced variety (music, change of feed, change of paddock and change of training area), the performance and wellbeing of the horses increased dramatically.

- I have seen experiments in which milk yield increased when cows were exposed to music in the stable; yield increased even more when the music was turned off after a while.

This shows that variety (changing environmental stimuli) stimulate all living organisms.

SOUND (NOISE IN CONTRAST TO MUSIC)

Monotonous and mechanical sounds weaken the immune system (Peter Tompkins and Christopher Bird: "The Secret Life of Plants"). Continuous noise especially from ventilation in stables and animal rooms can have a negative influence. I have seen often that the temperament, appetite and the well being of animals improve greatly after reducing or changing this noise (by a simple change of the site of the fan-motor from below in the stable to top of the ventilation tube). Low, beautiful music, played for 2-4 hours/day, also has given positive effects on animal health and well being. Animal preferences for music type have been investigated: Classical Indian music was best, hard rock worst (Peter Tompkins and Christopher Bird: "The Secret Life of Plants"). Music even influenced the growth of plants. The results were similar as for animals - Indian ragas and Mozart was best and rock music was worst.

COLOURS AND SMELLS

The colour of the room, box or stable is important. Certain colours and nice furniture make wounds heal faster than if the furniture is dull coloured and ugly (Professor Pekka Pöntinen). In Finland, research on hospital environments showed that wounds healed faster if the patient had a window with a nice landscape outside, than if it was a motorway outside the window.

Animals are sentient creatures with a developed aesthetic sense; ugly environments depress them. They also have a sense of smell that is far more developed than in humans. We can imagine what stress this can cause when we confine pigs and poultry, for example, for life in small, narrow, foul smelling spaces that often are unbearable for humans.

In ancient Chinese Five Phase Theory, special colours stimulate specific Bodily Processes. The colours for the Main Processes are as follows:

Colour	Stimulates the Phase of:
Red	Fire
Yellow	Earth
White	Metal-Air
Black	Water
Azure(bluegreen)	Wood*

It is helpful to paint the inside of the stable in a blue green Mediterranean colour because LV function is most important (and Process Imbalances in LV is the most common disorder) in horses. This does also apply for dogs with HD.

Table 111

I have noted often that patients with a Deficient Channel seek the colour that stimulates the Process of that Channel. I remember an artist that painted pictures only in yellow. She was famous for these pictures. After treating and healing her SP Channel, to her disappointment she was unable to paint much in yellow anymore.

Fengshui and the importance of room orientation and placement

Fengshui *(Wind and Water)*, an element of Eastern architecture, is a subject of special interest. Its principle is simple - man-made structures should be designed in relation to natural pre-existing earth energies (ley lines, geophysical energy lines, etc). Even if it is appreciated little in western culture, Eastern culture considers it to be very important. For example, in Hong Kong, a bastion of capitalism, many of the commercial buildings are planned and oriented with that idea in mind. Several courses in this discipline are held in the West.

In Fengshui Theory, *the direction of doors, windows, walls in relation to other elements in the immediate surroundings are important.* Also the direction towards which living creatures are forced (by humans) to orient relative to the elements mentioned is important. This applies absolutely in relation to compass orientation and relatively in relation to the other elements. We will consider three aspects:

- Orientation of doors and windows

- Orientation of the head in humans and animals

- The presence of geopathic radiation, to be discussed further in the appendix (see page 667)

ORIENTATION OF DOORS AND WINDOWS

Doors and windows should not be placed facing a road, a pile of feces or other so-called "negative" energies. I suspect that roads and feces are not intrinsically negative. However noise and movement (opposites of quiet and calmness), characterise the Qi of roads and rotting and decay (opposite of growth) characterise the Qi of feces. Thus, constant exposure to these Qi forms could have adverse effects.

ORIENTATION OF THE HEAD IN HUMANS AND ANIMALS

Most humans spend 7-9 hours, circa 33% of their time, in the same bed, and in the same part of the bed. Apart from its quality (back-support and comfort), and its position (whether over geopathic fields or not, see below), the *orientation of the bed* is important; humans who sleep with the head oriented towards a nearby road may suffer adverse effects. The orientation of the head in restrained animals is important also; animals that must stand with their face towards a road may suffer adverse effects. As most animals are not restrained in individual stalls, and can choose their preferred sleeping place, this is less important in animals than in humans.

THE PRESENCE OF WATER LINES (AND THE IMPORTANCE OF THE DIRECTION)

Underground water flows in natural rock fissures called aquifers. These fissures can be from 5 to several hundred metres deep in the underground rock. An aquifer usually has negative effects on humans and animals confined directly over it, for example in a bed or a tie-up stall. The direction from which the water flows in the aquifer is important for the way in which this negative energy affects the animal or human. These directions are summarised below. If a water line "attacks" from north, it can harm KI. If it "attacks" from the east, it can harm LV. The place (bed, or stall, etc) directly over the crossing point of two aquifers, usually at two different depths underground, is especially harmful to most humans and animals.

THE IMPORTANCE OF THE DIRECTIONS
The habitual direction in which humans or tied-up animals that sleeps in the same bed or stall is important. Different energies come from the different parts of the cosmos, as indicated below. Energies:

From north stimulate (or hurt)	KI
From south stimulate (or hurt)	HT
From west stimulate (or hurt)	LU
From east stimulate (or hurt)	LV

Table 112

Note: *If the cosmic or terrestrial energy is beneficial, it helps and stimulates the organ in question. If it is noxious it can injure the organ in question. In Indian tradition, the cosmic energies are usually beneficial while the earthly energies usually are harmful.*

Many ancient cultures knew this. Today, farmers in southern Germany, Switzerland and Austria still retain traces of this knowledge. I have been told that knowledgeable farmers have their cow-stalls with the head facing north, while their tied-up horses face east. This directional orientation stimulates the Processes that farmers in the area would like to strengthen at that time - KI in the cows for reproduction, and LV in the horses for muscular work. Today, because of the present state of the liver in all species, I would advise farmers to face their cows *and* horses towards the east.

It is most beneficial if we can change the orientation of animal. This allows one to orient a diseased animal to face towards the correct direction that stimulates its Deficient Process. To do that, we must know the Weakest Process involved.

- face a cow with mastitis (ST Imbalance) towards the east

- face a cow with ketosis (or a horse with azoturia) (LV Imbalance) towards the east

- Face a pig with reproductive disorder (KI deficiency) towards the north.

APPENDIX OF INTEREST TO ANIMAL OWNERS AND HUMAN PATIENTS WITH UNEXPLAINED DISEASES

To decide what is most beneficial as regards the orientation and placement of the bed or animal stall we must know:

- *the individual weakness of the subject (Weakest Process or Structure)*

- *the possible presence of aquifers or geopathic energy lines, especially lines that cross underneath areas in which the subject spends much time each day - the bed, work area (the precise work station at which the person spends c. 8 hours in a factory or office, etc), or the favourite armchair in housebound patients, etc.*

The principle of correct orientation and placement of the bed is simple:

- *Seek the compass direction that strengthens the Weakest Process in question*

- *Sleep with the head towards the direction that stimulates the Weakest Process.*

- *Avoid spending much time daily directly over aquifers and geopathic energy lines (see page 674); they and their directions further weaken the Weakest Process in question*

Move at least 0.5 metre away from aquifers or geopathic energy lines, especially those that intersect or cross beneath the bed, the precise work station, or favourite armchair of patients that are housebound.

Biorhythms

Biorhythm AP has been used therapeutically in all species. I have tried it, mainly on cows, with very good results. The method is simple and builds on experiences from Japan, where it has been used for years with results just as good as with conventional AP (personal communication from Dr. Bentze). Also, the biorhythm method seems to be a most promising way to prevent disease.

The unique principle of biorhythm AP is that the points are chosen according to the time of the day at which treatment is given, i.e. on the principle of the Horary Points; in this system, points are not chosen according to the usual criteria (Lesion-Symptom Complex, Command Points, Mu + Shu Points, Local + Distant points, etc.). While an AP therapist who is unfamiliar with this concept usually examines the patient, asks questions and checks the pulse, one familiar with biorhythm AP only checks the time in relation to the Qi Clock. S/he notes the time and needles the point that corresponds to that time of day. As mentioned earlier, this method gives results as good as those from conventional AP.

This disturbed me for several years. However, after having seen how difficult it is for a farmer to diagnose correctly in order prevent bovine diseases, it dawned on me that the Biorhythm method of AP could be ideal for this purpose. Since then, my personal experience has confirmed that it helps in about 60% of the cases.

Before I describe how to use this method, I want to describe the mechanisms that cause the effect.

MECHANISMS OF THE BIORHYTHM EFFECT

If we view the body Processes moving rhythmically like a pendulum, any Process Imbalance may cause an irregularity (or "wobble") somewhere in the movement of the pendulum. This irregularity repeats itself every time the "pendulum" passes that point (the location of Process Imbalance). There are then two ways to correct this.

1. One can determine the Process Imbalance, and stimulate this particular Process. (This book generally explains this way of thinking).

2. One can give the "pendulum" an extra push wherever it is, at any time, so that the energy of the swing increases. Thus it gets more power, greater impulse, so that it corrects the Process Imbalances by itself, i.e. it auto-cures.

THE BIORHYTHM METHOD

The method used in biorhythm therapy is to *stimulate one or more different biorhythms when they are at their highpoint,* i.e. when they are at their maximum Qi level. Hereby the Qi generally is increased to prevent or cure illness.

We choose the intensity of treatment. Depending on how soon we wish the condition to improve, or how much we want to prevent disease, we can treat one rhythm once/week or we can treat twelve rhythms/day. If we treat one, two, three or four Processes at their highpoint every day, over periods of 3-4 weeks, with a few months interval between courses of treatment, we can create a balance in the body and treat irregularities before it is possible to discover them through Pulse Diagnoses or the Lesion-Symptom Complexes.

Channel	Qi Clock time (best time to treat)	Hour (Horary) Point*
LU	0400h	LU08
LI	0600h	LI01
ST	0800h	ST36
SP	1000h	SP03
HT	**1200h**	**HT08**
SI	1400h	SI05
BL	1600h	BL66
KI	1800h	KI10
PC	2000h	PC08
TH	2200h	TH06
GB	**2400h**	**GB41**
LV	0200h	LV01

Table 113

As long as we treat at the best time (see the table, above), it does not matter whether we stimulate the Horary Point, the Back Shu Point, the Ting Point, or the Source Point of the selected Process, or give the homeopathic remedy that corresponds to the Channel - all these methods can help. We can combine several of these therapeutic modalities by giving the homeopathic remedy at the same time as we needle the selected Point in question. In this way we can prevent illness.

Table of homeopathic remedies used to stimulate the different Processes; it is best to give that remedy at the time of maximum Qi in the Process in question

Phase	Yin Channel	Stimulant remedy	Yang Channel	Stimulant remedy
Wood	LV	Stann.met D6	GB	Colocyntis D12
Fire	HT	Aur.met D12	SI	Plumb.met. D30
Fire	PC	Staphisagria D12	TH	Silicea D30
Earth	SP	Thuja or Ars.alb. D30	ST	Nux.vom. D12
Metal	LU	Carbo.veg D12	LI	Aluminum.met D12
Water	KI	Phos D12	BL	Kali.carb. D6

Table 114

Appendix

GEOPATHIC RADIATION AND DISEASE

Ley-lines

*The following description of the history of earth radiation was written by me in the years 1982 – 1989. During this time I related to the tra-ditional description and observations of the earth radiation, although already in 1985 I had started to **see** the radiation with my own eyes, and also observed several phenomena that did not entirely correspond with the tradition.*

On the 4th *of February 2006 my observation of the all-embracing energy matrix or network in the nature made a great leap, and this changed my view of earth radiation totally during the following years.*

In part two, I will describe my altered view in detail, but first, in part one, I will describe the traditional explanation of earth radiation and its effect on life.

Part 1 – the traditional explanation, observation and view of earth radiation

I have often heard people say that they become ill from sleeping in certain places. They had slept there for 5-20 years and when I ask them why they have not moved, they were astonished. They replied "surely that can't make any difference if I sleep elsewhere?"

A farmer called me to treat a cow with mastitis. When he commented that all the cows confined to that particular stable had became ill at some time in the past, I asked him why he used that stable if that was the case. He had no answer. On closer study, we found that there were two aquifers crossing directly under the stable. The energy distortion above the aquifers* weakened all animals that were kept in the stable above them. I advised the farmer to use that stable as a tool-shed instead and to move the cows elsewhere. After that, the health of the cows improved greatly.

These examples show that some people realise that certain precise locations are not good for them or their animals, but they do not take the necessary steps to avoid the pathological influence. The examples also show that there is a lack of general knowledge about this type of influence. People often know that something affects them, but do not know what it is and therefore find it hard to believe in it. They often draw conclusions about the effect of this "power" but are uncertain about how to protect against it. It is important to talk freely about these phenomena, so that people will know how to take protective measures according to available knowledge.

It is most important to avoid confining people or animals over geopathic areas! Moving away from the area by as little as 0.5-1.0 metres can benefit health greatly.

HISTORIC BACKGROUND

Radiation from the earth and from aquifers (natural water lines in underground rock fissures), has a long tradition. The earliest reference that I could trace is in the books of Moses. The story tells of the Israelites thirsting in the desert. Moses took his stick and hit the rock, and out gushed water. The German expression "Rotenschläger" (to hit or beat something with a rod), refers to the European tradition of diviners using twigs or Y-sticks from hazel or other trees to locate water or metals underground.

There are many references in such events throughout history. It is mentioned in China that emperor Kuanggu made laws already 2400 BC about how a piece of land for building on should be examined beforehand concerning geopathic radiation. Several Indian cultures in America have the same rules. If a tent was to be put up or a camp built, one must sit down and talk with the spirits and feel the effect of the spirits to be able to find the right place. This is a tradition especially with the Hopi Indians in America. In India we find the same tradition, where it is of great importance to find the right place for a bed to be placed. Several woodcarvings from 14-16th century show diviners (branch-bearers) searching for water lines.

THE EARTH'S ELECTROMAGNETIC FIELDS (EMFs)

Referring to the summary of Dr. Becker's research on page 185, the essential conclusions are:

- Through millions of years, our biorhythms have developed in the earth's fluctuating electromagnetic fields (EMFs), and depend on these.

- Illness occurs both when the EMFs (especially manmade EMFs) and are too strong, and also when the earth's own EMF is distorted.

BIORHYTHMS

Biorhythms guide the body and the variations in our Processes are manifestations of these rhythms.

The life rhythms that we adopt (our usual patterns or set times for sleeping, eating and working, etc.) influence our bodily functions and energetics, and *vice versa.*

Environmental EMFs influence us. Electric fields, radio and TV, high frequency radiation such as alpha-, beta- and gamma-radiation, cosmic radiation and geopathic radiation, influence us. We meet this influence in our everyday life as sound, light and other electromagnetic radiation that we normally do not register with our senses.

All these types of EMFs interfere with each other and these complicated patterns influence the organs of the body, Processes and biorhythms. Therefore, the influence varies from one individual to the next and from one place to the next. That is why we cannot predict the human or animal that will develop disorders, the places that will manifest the disorders, or the specific disorders that will arise. However, despite that, it is very important that we can diagnose the cause.

As Dr. Becker concludes, it is important to disturb normal EMFs and magnetic fields as little as possible and to limit in so far as is possible man-made and artificial fields, or excessive natural fields. As far as is possible, we should therefore avoid:

- Strong artificial EMFs from mobile telephones, high voltage transformers, electric equipment and high voltage cables, etc.

- Strong geopathic radiation, especially over crossing aquifers.

We should try to develop our ability to detect these stimuli (or get help from others to do so) and we should make as many people as possible aware of these noxious effects. In clinical practice, we should check for their presence in all difficult cases.

Below are summarised some of the symptoms and effects that one may expect as a result of chronic exposure to excessive EMFs or geopathic radiation, especially from (crossing*) aquifers (underground water streams).

Effects of geopathic radiation

PLANTS

The effect of geopathic radiation on plants was recorded in the late 1800s; the first observations were from Germany. They observed that fruit trees, especially apple trees, try to grow away from geopathic radiation. They become crooked and deformed; the trunk may split in two and the branches that grow directly over the area of radiation become deformed. Cherry- and sweet cherry- trees develop stunted, malformed branches and cankers, such as we often see in birch trees. Cankers or tumours on birch trees are quite common in areas of strong radiation. Here we can see whole groups of birch trees full of so-called "crows nests" or cancerous tumours. In garden hedges we can clearly see the effects of geopathic radiation, in that the bushes have few and small leaves and do not look good.

It is proven that viruses cause these tumours on trees but this does not explain why some trees are attacked and others are not. It is the same as in humans and animals; viruses and bacteria surround us but disease can manifest only under certain conditions. *It is most important not to try to explain disease as due to the viruses or bacteria per se, but rather by stress-induced immunosuppression, i.e. by a reduction of the organism's resistance to these organisms.* Reduction of resistance occurs when we are exposed to excessive EMFs over a long period of time, i.e. geopathic radiation, electric installations, TV or heating cables in the floor, etc.

ANIMALS

In my practice, I have found it almost impossible to treat such animals or humans successfully as long as they remain exposed to a precipitating Stressor. In contrast, my clinical results improve greatly if I can show the owner or subject how to escape from, or neutralise the Stressor. Chronic stress and geopathic radiation decrease immunocompetence and weaken the immune system. Animals that are free to roam where they wish seem to avoid areas of noxious radiation. This is the case with most of the known domestic animals. However, forcing animals to stay over a long period of time in the area of adverse electromagnetic influence can cause stress. Animals that are exposed chronically to geopathic radiation are more vulnerable to infection, ketosis, infertility and poor thrive than animals that are not exposed.

ANIMALS THAT SEEK OUT RADIATION

Certain animals, such as owls, bats and cats, seek out areas of strong radiation for their dwelling places. Traditionally, these animals have been associated with darkness or evil powers. Also other animals, such as ants, bees and wasps, show affinity to the earth's radiation. Bees that swarm often settle in trees that are growing over strong areas of radiation. Ants' paths usually follow a dowsing reaction line and we can often see the areas of radiation by how the ants' paths lead out from the nest. Experiments were done to shield ants' nests from geopathic radiation. The result was that the ants left the nest in the following year. They preferred not to stay for the winter in a nest that had no radiation (Rupert Sheldrake). Another possible explanation is that a nest over a strong dowsing zone usually has underground water directly below it.

Even if other animals avoid staying over geopathic radiation lines, they often follow such lines for their paths. If we take into consideration that plant growth is smaller along these lines, it would be natural for animals to move around where it is easiest to pass. In this way we cannot say that they follow the radiation path but, rather, they choose the path of least resistance.

HUMANS

As is the case in animals, excessive or qualitatively negative EMFs (geopathic radiation or other fields) affect humans adversely. The dowsing literature in many countries has a litany of hundreds of disorders that geopathic or noxious EMFs can induce. These include insomnia, neurasthenia, depression, sudden death syndrome in babies, asthma, arthralgia and arthritis, cancer, degenerative diseases such as multiple sclerosis, etc. I have seen many examples of this in my practice:

- Children who cry and cry for months, until their beds are moved 0.5 metres away from where they were.

- Older people with chronic ulcers and infections that heal quickly after their bed is moved to another place.

There are strong indications that radiation from power lines and transformers cause illness in people who live under or close to these over a long period of time. Several observations concerning kindergartens and residential houses that are situated under high voltage lines seem to show a negative effect on health of the adults and children in those places.

PROTECTION AGAINST EXCESSIVE EMFs

The literature of national Dowsers groups in America, Europe and Australia abounds with case histories, mainly of human disorders, that were caused by these effects, and that responded within weeks to their correction or elimination. *When more usual methods of conventional and holistic medicine fail to help a patient, one should always check his/her sleeping- and work- place for noxious influences from geopathic zones, or other EMFs.*

In recent years, some people have shielded their houses against all types of EMF. *This is not good practice, because it also removes the earth's normal EMF that is necessary and health giving. Total shielding from normal EMFs can have problematic consequences for our biorhythms.*

I emphasise that we should try to avoid or shield against EMFs only in areas where they are excessive or noxious. There are three main ways to protect against EMFs (radiation):

a) Vary the influence

b) Move away from the influence

c) Shield from the influence

Vary the influence: This is probably the best way to treat the disorder. In practice we see that the disorders occur when the body is influenced in the same way or by the same type of frequency or radiation over a long period of time. We can avoid chronic exposure to the negative influence if we vary regularly the place in which the animals are confined, the work place, or the location of the bed. *Sleeping with the head turned one way in the bed for one month and the other way for the next month can do this also. If one has a double bed, one can sleep on one side of the bed one month and on the other side the next month, first with the head turned one way, then with the head turned the other way.*

Move away from the influence: If we want to move from the noxious zone, we first must confirm its exact location. Then we must find a place where the radiation is absent, or only mild.

Shield from the influence: Because of limited space or money, most people have difficulty finding new places to sleep or rest, or to vary those places regularly for themselves and the animals. In such cases, shielding can be very useful. Shielding is based on three methods:

- Diversion of the radiation
- Accumulation and discharge of the radiation
- Modification of the radiation

Diversion of the radiation: To divert geopathic radiation, we can use electric cable, usually a copper wire or coil. The coil is tightened around the box, the stable, the bed, the chair or the place to be shielded, and is earthed by soldering it to a metal water pipe, or to a copper spike buried in the earth. Other materials that seem to shield or divert electromagnetic radiation include turf (peat), swamp turf and lead plates. Älma company (Sweden) markets bed pads of swamp turf that seem to stop or modify the effects of EMFs. Also, lead plates that are thick enough may block EMFs. German experiments suggested that the plates must be several cm thick. Thin lead plates (a few mm thick) may be effective initially but they lose their blocking effect after a few months. This may be due to microperforations, which can be seen by electron-microscopy (personal communication from Älma, Sweden).

Accumulation and discharge of the radiation: A type of accumulator made from plastic layers seems to be effective; 15-20 layers of plastic are placed under the bed and this seems to function for a couple of months. I do not know how this could be done for large animals but it should be easy to do for small animals. After this one must "discharge" the plastic by putting it on damp ground, or by washing it.

Neutralising the noxious effect: Magnets may be used to neutralise noxious radiation. If we expose the radiation to a magnetic field, it seems that we can modify the EMF so that it does not cause illness. I have seen several different arrangements of strong and weak magnets that seem to have modified geopathic radiation, so that the pathological effect was dispersed. The use of turf falls into this category, since it seems that turf modifies radiation rather than shielding or diverting it.

TRACING NOXIOUS RADIATION

Three important methods are used to trace noxious radiation:

- Divining instruments

- Technical instruments to detect electromagnetic distortions

- Bioassay, using living organisms

DIVINING INSTRUMENTS

German experiments on several hundred students in the time between the two World Wars showed how some people reacted immediately when exposed to radiation. In these and other "noxious zones", some people felt unwell or dizzy and saw dots in front of their eyes (vibrating sight). Blood pressure, measured before and when sensitive people walked across areas of strong radiation, fell by up to 20-30 mm mercury.

The dowsing reaction is transmitted via the parasympathetic part of the autonomic nervous system. This autonomic system, which usually is beyond voluntary control, controls respiration, heart rate, blood pressure, blood circulation, digestion and peristalsis of the digestive organs, urinary filtration rate and other organ functions. Measuring the blood pressure and heart rate can show the changes that occur when a sensitive person is placed over a noxious area (Rupert Sheldrake). Alternatively, as done since antiquity, one can find noxious zones by dowsing, or divining. The dowser holds a divining rod (Y-stick), or other divining instrument (pendulum, rubbing pad, angle irons, etc.) in the hands. When the body's autonomic system senses a noxious influence, it increases muscle spasm. This causes the divining instrument to move or behave differently, thus indicating the location of the noxious influence.

TECHNICAL EQUIPMENT TO DETECT ELECTROMAGNETIC DISTORTIONS

If a transistor radio is tuned to "white noise" with its antenna extended, the noise may change when the searcher moves over a zone that has a distorted EMF. Other electronic measuring equipment, such as a sensitive magnetometer that can register EMFs, gives a more objective, quantitative proof. However, this equipment is expensive and hard to locate. Research with a large range of electronic devices shows that they have the added disadvantage that they do not differentiate qualitatively between EMFs that cause disease and EMFs that are harmless. Skilled dowsers, however, have this ability as an innate reaction.

TRACING NOXIOUS INFLUENCES BY BIOASSAY USING LIVING ORGANISMS

We can prove the adverse effects of noxious radiation in a bioassay with living organisms. Noxious influences stunt or alter adversely the immunity, growth or health of plants, humans and animals. The noxious influence is confirmed by noting its effects on the growth of hedges, plants or fruit trees and where the plants thrive, or fail and wither (Peter Tompkins and Christopher Bird: "The Secret Life of Plants"). This method takes a long time and is not as convenient to prevent illness as the other methods described above.

Part 2 – my view, explanation and observation of earth radiation after being able to see it by myself

FIRST A LITTLE ON MY EXPERIENCES WITH EARTH RADIATION

1. *Seeing the "water"-lines, or ley-lines*

2. *Seeing the etheric matrix of living creatures*

3. *seeing the astral matrix of living creatures*

SEEING THE "WATER"-LINES, OR LEY-LINES

In the summer 1985 I suddenly **saw** a network of thick, black and shiny snake-like bands, transversing the mountains. I was walking together with a friend of mine (Ragnar Widerheim-Paul), skilled in using the divine rod as an instrument for finding these water-lines or ley-lines. We spent the whole day checking and re-checking the positions of the ley-lines that I had seen, and we correlated the whole time. The first time I saw these lines I was on the mountains, later I saw them at the sea front, and later everywhere. I saw that they often followed paths of human activity, graves, graveyards, churches and old trails. One special incident made me question if these lines were there before the human activity, indicating that our ancestors also could see the lines and followed their paths, or if the lines were created by human activity and thoughts. A friend of mine was to construct an area where agricultural experiments were going to be performed. We found an area free influence from the earth. But then, after he had constructed small squares where to sow the seeds, definite radiation lines appeared along the borders of his squares. The radiation was created by his thinking. I have also registered these phenomena when somebody builds a house. This changes the radiation pattern completely. My next observation was of even more astonishing character. During a course on veterinary acupuncture held in Germany, the organizer of the course had hired a skilled "water-line"-detector or earth radiation finder for an excursion. She was to show where the radiation lines were,

how to detect them and tell stories about their origin and relations. I was standing a little away, watching it all. Then I, in
my thoughts, in my imagination, moved the radiation lines 20
meters away from where they were, and then, suddenly, the
experienced ley-line finder could not find them any more. She
was very frustrated, but this incident, this experience, gave me
much to think about on the reality, the origin and the effect of
such earth radiation.

This showed that water lines or earth radiation or ley-lines
are far more connected to the human (and animals?) psyche
than I had thought. My teacher and benefactor in acupuncture, Dr. Georg Bentze, told me about the following incident;
he was summoned to a local prison to see if any of the beds
used by the prisoners were under influence of earth radiation.
Where the prisoners slept he found an extreme amount of radiation. He asked the guards to move the beds and change
their location, and the prisoners immediately slept and felt better. But, the interesting thing was that, after a short time, all the
negative radiation was back. It was created by the presence of
individuals with negative or criminal thinking.

In both historical literature and more modern papers on
earth radiation and Ley-lines, both Alfred Watkins (the first
man that in a scientific and systematic way described and investigated earth radiation and ley-lines) and Paul Devereux
(present authority on earth radiation) posed that ley-lines are
created from the human mind in certain ways.

SEEING THE ETHERIC MATRIX OF LIVING CREATURES

Living Nature process the same kind of radiation or energy
described previously. In this way energetic matrix or lines may
interconnect all living creatures, trees and animals, insects and
humans, even the earth itself.

Skiing in the forest on the 4th of February 2006, at 1443
in the afternoon, I suddenly, and for the first time, saw this
network, this matrix of living energy. The appearance was similar, although the snakes were much thinner, to the ley-lines I
had observed in 1985, and all the time since. It was like black,

shining snakes that flowed or moved between all living entities, from tree to tree, from animal to animal, from human
to human. Also between species; from trees to humans, from
animals to trees. This matrix immersed the whole nature with
its presence. The matrix included all living, yes, also the farms
that I passed, especially those having animals. I saw how these
energy power lines streamed from the forest, embracing the
houses where cows were living, where pigs were living, and also
the houses where people were living. Where animals were present the matrix was stronger than where humans were living,
though.

The network was stronger between trees of the same kind
and between animals of the same kind.

This observation made me understand that the whole creation was intertangled in wholeness, and if anything in this
wholeness is changed or made to disappear, the whole will suffer. I have long thought that Indian tribes that expressed or understood the wellbeing of the total world as dependent on their
existence or special rituals that they performed were somewhat
egocentric. But after having experienced this total network
which binds everything together in a holistic community, and
all together with the human consciousness, I have begun to
understand the feeling of such Indian tribes. We and they are
inseparable entities dwelling in this network. If anybody disappears, the whole network will suffer. The childish and egocentric mind I thought to have observed in primitive people was
really an expression of the experience of this network.

On several occasions I have observed fishermen or hunters, while killing their prey. Usually fishermen or hunters are
not aware of the described matrix, they don't feel it. But, in
the moment of killing, it seems that the whole matrix opens
up for them, and they feel connected to the wholeness of creation. For a few minutes they are one with everything, and will
have an intense communication with the cosmos. This might
be one explanation that hunters and fishermen so often justify
their actions with natural experiences. While people who have

this feeling or connection all the time do not have to kill to experience the wholeness of creation.

This will explain why sacrificial offering was an important part of the old connection to God. In the blood of the lamb, the closeness of God was felt. But it is better to have this feeling all the time, and not kill.

SEEING THE ASTRAL MATRIX OF LIVING CREATURES, OF THE WHOLE NATURE

On the 12th of March 2007, at 0625 in the morning, suddenly, after having contemplated the art-sculptures of a woman who feels the forces in nature (Inger Sannes), the whole astral matrix of the nature revealed itself to me. It was like a firework of energy, white and sparkling. A deep contrast to the dark and quiet and strong manifestation of the ethereal energy.

EARTH RADIATION AS A NAVIGATION SYSTEM FOR ANIMALS, OUR INTERNAL GPS WITH SAVING POSSIBILITIES

If all actions, deeds and movements of animals, birds and fish leave a trace, a trace stronger and stronger and more and more obvious the more entities that have done the action or wandered the trail, this gives a good explanation of how animals, birds, fish and insects can navigate. This system will in addition contain all information of what has happened along the trail, what kind of dangers, what kind of honey is to be found or which enemies are to be expected. Animals who can tap into this kind of information will then chose to dwell in the zones of radiation, and are described as radiation seeking animals like cats, bees and crows.

There are certain people, who can describe what has happened previously in certain places just by being there, who get pictures or imaginations from times gone by. In some traditions this may be described as a kind of "chronicle", a sort of history book, where all that has happened is written, "the Akasha-chronicle". May be it is so?

Later on, in 2012, I came to the realisation that all these shiny snakes were in fact living enteties, called elementals, created by our own thoughts, actions and deeds. That is why they respond to our imaginations, our intentions, our thoughts and our actions. They relate to us as children relate to their parents. More of this in the Requiem, page 675.

A simple method to detect or diagnose if the patient has been or is under the influence of earth radiation

I have developed, or rather found a simple method that may detect a potential influence of earth radiation. Patients that do not react to treatment might be under such influence. With this method we also find out, in case there really is such influence, in what angle the line hits the body. Then we also know in what direction to move the horse or the bed to avoid this radiation, and we will also know what organ system is most vulnerable for this kind of radiation.

To obtain all this information, we need a plastic square, 5x5 cm. On this transparent sheet we draw, in black waterproof and permanent ink, the figure illustrated below (the thin black arrow is not to be drawn, it will be explained later).

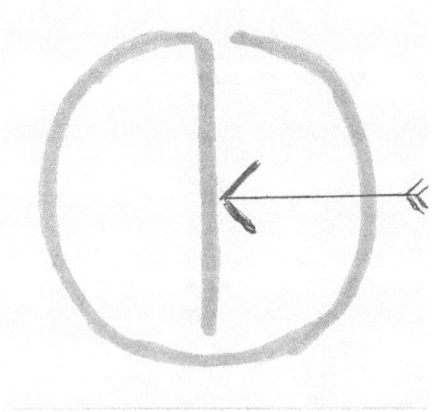

Figure 67

This sheet it then hold in front of the ear, while we carefully control the pulse of Nogier (RAC – VAS) (see page 179). We then slowly turn the plastic sheet around completely (360^0). At certain angles there will be a distinct RAC/VAS. This reaction indicates that the patient is under influence of earth radiation. The angle at which this radiation hits the body can be calculated in the following way; we have to keep in mind the following;

- The ear resembles the body itself, with the lobe as the head and the top of the ear as the butt and legs.

- This ear also carries the memory of the radiation, so that the pathological effect of the radiation is also imprinted in the ear.

- The RAC occurs when the straight line in the drawing creates an angle of 90^0 with the imprinted radiation.

- If the RAC occurs as indicated in the diagram below, it will mean that the radiation crosses or hits the body 90^0 to the longitudinal axis (to the median plane).

- If the patient then sleeps with the head to the north and the feet to the south, then the radiation line will go east-west or west-east.

- Then we know that the organ systems in danger are either the Lungs or the Liver.

- Then the patient will have to move the bed further towards the head or the feet. If he moved the bed to the side, he will not avoid the radiation.

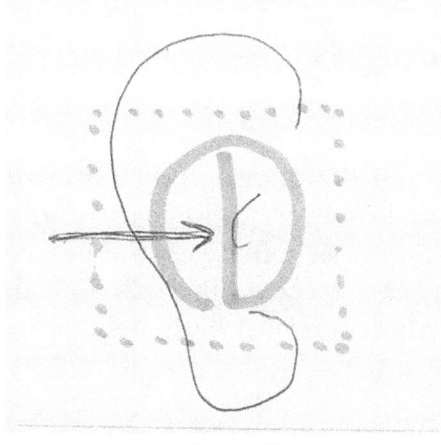

Figure 68

How to use this knowledge to treat patients?

We have to keep in mind, if we are to use this knowledge, that the direction of the radiation decides which organ system will be hurt.

From north radiation will stimulate or hurt (a little stimulates, too much will hurt)	KI BL
From south	HT, PC, SI, TH
From west	LU LI
From east	LV GB

Table 115

So, then we will know what organ system to stimulate if the patient has been or slept too long under the influence of pathological earth radiation. We may then treat the organ in question with herbs or acupuncture.

The patient should also be removed from the radiation.

The knowledge about the directions was known in ancient times by the farmers.

As I told you a little radiation will stimulate, and there is always a little radiation everywhere, earth radiation or cosmic radiation. Standing or sleeping with the head towards special directions, unless a strong earth radiation also happens to come from that direction, will be beneficial to the organ system in question.

So, if the cow is standing with the head (the head is the receiver of cosmic radiation, even the horns are like antenna) towards north, the cow will receive energy that stimulate the kidneys. And if the horse is standing with its head towards east, the energy will stimulate the liver.

Farmers in Switzerland knew this, and the old tradition there was exactly to let the cows stand with the heads towards north, and horses towards east.

Amazing!

This knowledge may also be used therapeutically. If a patient has problems with an organ system, it, she or he will then have benefit from standing or lying with the head in the direction for stimulating the organ system in question.

Epilogue

This book is based mainly on my own studies, personal experiences and practice; it has relatively few references to the works of others. The effects of AP are those that I have observed through years of working with animals and people. This applies also to the effects of herbal and homeopathic medicines.

However, I received my first training and inspiration from older and more experienced veterinarians, AP therapists, homeopaths and authors. My main inspiration in homeopathy, as well as most other subjects, came from the writings of *Rudolf Steiner*. He made me aware of the importance of intent.

My basic knowledge and insights in AP came from my teacher, the late Dr. *Georg Bentze* (who showed me the true energetics of Chinese medicine) and from the textbook "Essentials of Chinese Acupuncture" (Foreign Languages Publishing House, Beijing). The works of the ingenious French doctor Dr. *Paul Nogier MD* inspired my study of Ear-AP, but I also learned much about these topics from my colleagues Dr. *Francois Lizon DVM*, Dr. *Dominique Giniaux DVM* (who shared his ideas and Ting Point locations with me) and the great Dr. *Jaque Milin DVM*. Dr. *John Limehouse DVM*, Dr. *Marvin Cain DVM*, Dr. *Earl Sutherland DVM*, Dr. *Oswald Kothbauer DVM* and Dr. *Malchaire* **MD.** (who taught me how to take pulses in animals via my own pulse) have all contributed to my development.

Doctors in the Norwegian organisation for Anthroposophical medicine whetted my interest in Anthroposophical medicine, especially Dr. *Margit Engel MD.*

Many friends and colleagues have helped me to conceive and write this book. Dr. *Annica Nygren Thoresen DVM*, my x-wife has written the anatomical descriptions of the placement of the acupuncture points and the chapter on the teeth. Dr. *Phil Rogers DVM*, my friend and colleague stimulated and challenged my ideas, and allowed me to include some of his published and unpublished research in this new version of my book. He also corrected the language throughout the whole book. Dr. *Dominique Giniaux DVM* has kindly revised the chapter on osteopathy. Dr. *Chris Day* has kindly revised the chapter on homeopathy. Thanks to both!

Before printing Dr. *Diane Skoberg DVM (Canada)* and Dr. *Eidin Burns DVM (Ireland)* were so kind to read the whole manuscript and correct all orthographic mistakes. Thank you!

The illustrations are taken from old anatomy books and from the generous gift of several drawings from Dr. *Peggy Fleming DVM*. The artistic contributions were given by *Elisabeth Knap* and by my deceased father *Odd Thoresen*. My sincere thanks to them all!

A REQUIEM

We have come together in a journey of knowledge to the last page, the end of the "active life" of this book. By now, you should have spent several hours reading this work. If you have not done so, please go back and read it again before you proceed! One spoils the enjoyment of a thriller if one reads the last page first! I want you to read this requiem only when you have grasped the ideas in this book and you have made its thinking process an instinctive part of your thinking process.

A requiem is a formal farewell ceremony for the dead. In its briefest form, it can be a note on a grave, or tomb. It points beyond the grave, beyond death, to the afterlife. In the Christian tradition, the most common requiem is "Requiescant in Pacem - May they rest in Peace".

In a certain sense, with these last words I want to demolish all that I have said in this book, but also show the necessity of its writing. As life that dies in the leaf fall of autumn resurrects in the green shoots of spring, this requiem shows how all that has been written in this book will resurrect in a new way, in a new life of meaning and context.

Page 420 & 490 showed how easy it is to heal HD with a method as simple as a gold implant at LV03 and that this procedure does not seem to work if the practitioner's *focused will and intention* is absent. Several other results and studies within both complementary and conventional medicine indicate that the essential effects within most holistic systems depend on the interaction between the therapist and the patient, i.e. are not objective in the strict sense of "scientific assessment".

The intricate medical or healing systems that we have made and believe in, do not work in or of themselves. The most important component of healing is our own *will and intention,* which can kindle belief of the patient and auto-cure, i.e. the healing capacity of the body itself. Most people reject the idea that an animal's "belief" (if there is such a faculty) could have anything to do with clinical results. However, animal owners, and most good veterinarians (whether conventional or holistic) know that animals have highly developed instincts to distinguish "friend" from "foe". It is uncanny how often animals sense the good intentions of a holistic veterinarian. They usually respond by allowing handling or other interventions, such as multiple needling or spinal manipulations that would put many conventional veterinarians in great danger of being bitten, scratched or kicked! Holistic veterinarians know that animals see them as "friend". This intention and will and courage to cure and heal, also carries the potential to heal, or start the patients self healing abilities all by their own. As two of my teachers have said:

- "If you can really visualise the effects of a point, you need not insert a needle" (Georg Bentze)

- "If you really know the workings of a homeopathic remedy, it is enough to think that you give it to a patient" (Margit Engel).

The concepts in this book are absent from, or is hard to find in other books. However, these concepts are very important for professionals who want to improve their clinical success rates. When you have assimilated it and made it real for yourself, it becomes superfluous to your needs and you can dismiss it. When this happens, it resurrects as your own healing, intuitive powers. Then you become a true healer.

And, in becoming a true healer, the healing, health and diseases become alive for you, and you become capable of seing directly into the true reality of diseases.

There are many stories and insights from old times and old religions where disease and ailments are looked upon as separate and individualized entities, or energetically self conscious structures, described as elementals, spirits, demons or devas. Many of us have experienced that if we are too open in the moment of acupuncture treatment, the energetic pathological structure may jump over and attack us, inflict us with the disease itself. We have also seen that such pathological structures may inflict, influence or create disease in creatures connected to the patient.

We are all interwoven in an enormous web of energy, a web that connects all living entreaties in the world, may be the whole cosmos. This web is to be seen just on the other side of the threshold of the spiritual world. It is called by many names, as the Achasic record, Karma or the Matrix. This web is made of energy, but not just lifeless energy. It is made up of elementals, living etheric beings, created by our minds, our thoughts and our actions.

This web is also part of our diseases. This web is influenced when we treat energetically.

Some times, in some therapists, I have seen that their treatment pushes the disease, or may I rather say pathological-energetic-structure, to other places in the body, actually creating new diseases instead of the old one.

Sometimes the patho-structure just takes a little trip, and then returns to its original place, we say that the disease reappeared .....

Well, what I want to describe, is disease as caused by energetic, self containing structures that may influence or "attack" other beings, change or just come back. This sounds a lot like descriptions of real and living enteties.

In old times, and still we may see this phenomenon today, the doors to temples of small communities are boarded by the pictures or sculptures of ugly looking demons. This was to scare the real demons or negative spirits away, to scare diseases away.

There is a moving story about Jesus. When he in his twenties he visited one of the Esenic communities. He then realized that the sculptures around the door scared or drove the evil spirits away, but then a very important question arose in his mind; to where were the spirits driven? And then he understood that it was no solution just to drive the bad spirits away to other people, to save somebody on the cost of creating disease in others. This question and realization opened his mind to be the receiver of the Christ, the redeemer of all.

If acupuncture, at least in the way we are doing it, just pushes the ailment to another place or person or animal, then we must do the treatment in another way.

If it creates lasting health, for us all and the world, then we are on our right way.

Thank you for the company this time.
Are Simeon Thoresen
Sandefjord the 6th of June 2011

Term or acronym	Meaning
' (Cun, tsun)	The "body inch", a relative unit of distance, used to locate acupoints. In humans, there are 8' between the nipples; 1' is the distance between the creases of the phalangeal bone 2 of flexed finger 3; 3 fingers = 2'; 4 fingers = 3'; 5 fingers = 4'. In horses and dogs, 1' = the width of rib 18.
ACR Pulse	Auriculo-Cardiac Reflex Diagnostic Pulse
AP	Acupuncture
BL	Urinary Bladder Channel
Chongmai	Penetrating-, or Thoroughfare-, Extraordinary Vessel
Command Point (60 + 6 = 66)	These are the Five Phase Points (see below) on each Channel (60 points), plus the Source Points of the 6 Yang Jing (= 66 points in total). Each stimulates the whole Channel and its functions, with special effect according to the nature of the point. Wood Points command especially the Wood Processes of a Channel; Fire Points command especially the Fire Processes of a Channel.
CV	Conception Vessel, Renmai

Daimai	Girdle (Belt) Extraordinary Vessel
Dumai	GV, Governing Vessel, dorsal midline Extraordinary Vessel
EAP	Electro-AP
EBM	Evidence-Based Medicine
ECIWO	Embryo Containing Information of the Whole Organism
EMF	Electromagnetic field
External Evils	See External Stressors
External Pathogenic Factors	See External Stressors
External Stressors	(External Pathogenic Factors, External Evils): the external factors that initiate or precipitate disease by challenging the adaptive mechanisms of the body at the level of the Twelve Processes
Five Phase Points	The Five Phase Points are the Fire, Earth, Metal-Air, Water and Wood Points on each of the 12 Jing, including the Tonification (Mother) Point, Sedation (Son) Point, and Ko (Controlling-Restraining) Point. They also include the Horary Point of the 12 Jing and the Earth / Source Point of the 6 Yin Jing.
Fu	Yang (Hollow) Organs
GB	Gallbladder Channel
GuQi	Nutrient Qi, Qi derived from digestion
GV	Governing Vessel, Dumai
HD	Hip dysplasia
Horary Point	This is the "Own-Phase Point" of each of the 12 Jing (Fire Point of HT, Earth Point of SP, etc.).
HT	Heart Channel
Hun	Courage, Spiritual faculty of LV
Ijing	Book of Changes, a classical TCM text
Internal Evils	See Internal Stressors
Internal Pathogenic Factors	See Internal Stressors

Internal Stressors	(Internal Pathogenic Factors, Internal Evils): the emotional imbalances that initiate or precipitate disease by challenging the adaptive mechanisms of the body at the level of the Twelve Processes
Jiao	Heater, Burner, as in TH
Jing	The Main Channel that controls each of the 12 Main Process
JingLuoMai	Channels (Jing), Collaterals (Luo) and Extraordinary Vessels (Mai), the energetic pathways and reservoirs of Qi in the body
KI	Kidney Channel
Ko (Controlling) Father Point	Ko Point of a Channel
Ko Cycle	Restraining or Controlling Cycle of the Five Phases
LI	Large Intestine Channel
LIKEM	Love, Intuition, Knowledge, Empathy and Mysticism, the 5 fundamental requirements for healing
LU	Lung Channel
Luo	Collateral, Connecting Vessel between Channel Mates within one Phase
Luo Point	Passage (Connecting) Point of a Channel. It connects the Channel Couples within a Phase (the Phase Mates), i.e. it shunts Qi between Phase Mate Channels. For example Bu (reinforcing) manipulation of HT Luo Point shunts energy from SI to HT; Xie (dispersing) manipulation of HT Luo Point shunts energy from HT to SI??
LV	Liver Channel
Mai	Extraordinary Vessel, Qi Reservoir
Mother Point	Sheng (Tonification) Point of a Channel
Mu Point	Front Alarm Diagnostic Point of a Channel
Neijing	Canon of Internal Medicine, the most famous of the TCM Classics
PC	Pericardium, Heart Constrictor, Circulation Sex Channel

Phase Mate	Partner Channel within a Phase, for example LU-LI in Metal
PID	Pelvic inflammatory disease, usually associated with inflammation of the ovary, Fallopian tubes, uterus, or other pelvic organs.
Po	Spiritual faculty of LU
Qi	Vital Energy of Life; Channel Qi flows in the Jing Luo to reach all parts of the body
Qi Clock	Diurnal Qi Flow, whereby Qi reaches a maximum in each of the 12 Main Channels in a specific time sequence, starting in LU at 0300-0500h
Renmai	Conception Vessel, CV, ventral midline Extraordinary Vessel
Sanjiao	TH Channel, Three Burners, Triple Heater (Upper, Middle and Lower Burner)
Sekunden Phanomen	Instantaneous Phenomenon of Huneke, whereby neural therapy of a Disturbance Field (Störfeld, reactive area), especially in a scar, can give immediate release of longstanding pain or other symptoms
Shen	Spiritual faculty of HT
Sheng Cycle	Generative Cycle; Mother-Son Cycle of the Five Phases
Sheng Point	Mother Point of a Channel in the Sheng Cycle; Tonification Point of a Channel
Shu Point	Back (Association) Diagnostic Point of a Channel
SI	Small Intestine Channel
Son Point	Sedation Point of a Channel in the Sheng Cycle
SP	Spleen Pancreas Channel
ST	Stomach Channel
TCM	Traditional Chinese Medicine
TENS	Transcutaneous Electrical Nerve Stimulation
TH	Triple Heater Channel
Ting Point	Another name for the Jing (Well) Point, the most distal point on a Channel; it influences both the Channel and its Process, especially in relation to painful and / or muscular disorders.
VAS Pulse	Diagnostic Pulse, based on the Vascular Auricular Signal

Wei Qi	Defensive Qi, Interactive Qi, circulating in the skin and superficial tissues; the first line of defence against External Stressors
Xi Point	Cleft (Ravine) Point of a Channel; used in acute disease of the affected Channel
Yang	Active, male, emitting principle
Yangqiaomai	Yang Heel Extraordinary Vessel
Yangweimai	Yang Connecting Extraordinary Vessel
Yi	Reflection, Spiritual faculty of SP
Yin	Passive, female, accumulating principle
Yinqiaomai	Yin Heel Extraordinary Vessel
Yinweimai	Yin Connecting Extraordinary Vessel
Yuan	Source, Origin, Ancestor
Yuan Point	Source Point of a Channel. It commands, regulates and strengthens Yuan qi and the Yuan-Ancestral Qi Processes throughout its own Channel. LI04 (Source Point of LI) is the most powerful Source Point; it regulates and strengthens the Yuanqi (Source of Qi) of the whole body.
Yuanqi	Source Qi, Ancestral, Hereditary or Prenatal Qi; it flows in all Process but KI (and the area near GV04-Ming men) is the House or Home of Yuanqi
Zang	Yin (Solid) Organs
Zangfu	Yang (Hollow) and Yin (Solid) Organs
Zhi	Willpower, Spiritual faculty of KI

Table 116

www.ingramcontent.com/pod-product-compliance
Lightning Source LLC
Chambersburg PA
CBHW051435170526
45166CB00001B/2